Register Now for O...
to Your B...

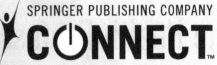

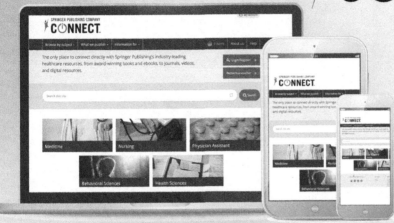

Your print purchase of *The Health Professions Educator,* **includes online access to the contents of your book**—increasing accessibility, portability, and searchability!

Access today at:

**http://connect.springerpub.com/content/book/978-0-8261-7718-6
or scan the QR code at the right with your smartphone
and enter the access code below.**

6U0WUCR0

*Scan here for
quick access.*

SPRINGER / PUBLISHING COMPANY

View all our products at springerpub.com

The Health Professions Educator

Gerald Kayingo, PhD, PA-C, is the director of the Master of Health Services, Physician Assistant Studies program, and an assistant clinical professor at the University of California (UC), Davis. Prior to his UC Davis appointment in 2014, he was a faculty member at the Yale School of Medicine Physician Associate Program and practiced at the Yale New Haven Hospital Primary Care Center in Connecticut. Dr. Kayingo has extensive experience in scholarship, education, clinical practice, and global health. He is a graduate of the Management Development Program at the Harvard Institutes for Higher Education, following a master of medical science–physician assistant degree at Yale University School of Medicine, and a PhD in microbiology from Orange Free State University in South Africa. He completed his postdoctoral education in infectious diseases at Yale, where he studied microbial pathogenesis, membrane transport, and signal transduction. He is a recent graduate of the UC Davis Interprofessional Teaching Scholars Program. Nationally, Dr. Kayingo serves as a trustee of the Physician Assistant Foundation, serves on the editorial board for the *Journal of Physician Assistant Education*, and is a member of the Commission on Health of the Public for the American Academy of Physician Assistants. He was recently inducted into the prestigious Uganda National Academy of Sciences and has been widely published in several peer-reviewed journals.

Virginia McCoy Hass, DNP, MSN, RN, FNP-C, PA-C, is associate clinical professor; former director, Master of Science Nurse Practitioner Degree Program; and former interim director, Master of Health Services Physician Assistant Studies Degree Program at the Betty Irene Moore School of Nursing, University of California (UC), Davis. Dr. McCoy Hass has more than 20 years of experience in graduate nursing and medical education and has mentored dozens of students and junior faculty. She practices as a family nurse practitioner in primary care. She is a graduate of the Rush University Doctor of Nursing Practice Program, following a master of science in nursing from California State University, Sacramento, and family nurse practitioner and physician assistant certification from UC Davis. She has extensive experience in the development and implementation of active learning strategies, simulation pedagogy, distance education using innovative technology, and instructional design strategies. She has led a variety of initiatives to create new interdisciplinary models for the delivery of primary care and student training opportunities. Dr. McCoy Hass has published in a variety of peer-reviewed journals and authored book chapters on chronic illness management. She is a sought-after presenter at regional, state, and national meetings. Dr. McCoy Hass serves on the editorial board of the *Journal of the American Academy of Physician Assistants* and the board of directors of the California Association for Nurse Practitioners, and is an expert witness for the California Board of Registered Nursing.

The Health Professions Educator

A Practical Guide for New and Established Faculty

Gerald Kayingo, PhD, PA-C

Virginia McCoy Hass, DNP, MSN, RN, FNP-C, PA-C

Editors

SPRINGER PUBLISHING COMPANY

NEW YORK

Springer Publishing Company, LLC
11 West 42nd Street
New York, NY 10036
www.springerpub.com

Acquisitions Editor: Suzanne Toppy
Production Editor: Lori Bradshaw
Compositor: Westchester Publishing Services

ISBN: 978-0-8261-7717-9
ebook ISBN: 978-0-8261-7718-6
Supplemental Faculty Material ISBN: 978-0-8261-7719-3

Supplemental faculty material is available at http://www.springerpub.com/hpe

17 18 19 20 21/ 5 4 3 2 1

The author and the publisher of this Work have made every effort to use sources believed to be reliable to provide information that is accurate and compatible with the standards generally accepted at the time of publication. Because medical science is continually advancing, our knowledge base continues to expand. Therefore, as new information becomes available, changes in procedures become necessary. We recommend that the reader always consult current research and specific institutional policies before performing any clinical procedure. The author and publisher shall not be liable for any special, consequential, or exemplary damages resulting, in whole or in part, from the readers' use of, or reliance on, the information contained in this book. The publisher has no responsibility for the persistence or accuracy of URLs for external or third-party Internet websites referred to in this publication and does not guarantee that any content on such websites is, or will remain, accurate or appropriate.

Library of Congress Cataloging-in-Publication Data

Names: Kayingo, Gerald, editor. | Hass, Virginia McCoy, editor.
Title: The health professions educator : a practical guide for new and established faculty /
    Gerald Kayingo, PhD, PA-C, Virginia McCoy Hass, DNP, MSN, RN, FNP-C, PA-C, editors.
Description: New York, NY : Springer Publishing Company, LLC, [2018] | Includes bibliographical
    references and index.
Identifiers: LCCN 2017026477 (print) | LCCN 2017027782 (ebook) | ISBN 9780826177186 (ebook) |
    ISBN 9780826177179 (hard copy : alk. paper)
Subjects: LCSH: Medical education.
Classification: LCC R735 (ebook) | LCC R735 .H44 2018 (print) | DDC 610.71—dc23
LC record available at https://lccn.loc.gov/2017026477

Contact us to receive discount rates on bulk purchases.
We can also customize our books to meet your needs.
For more information please contact: sales@springerpub.com

Printed in the United States of America by Gasch Printing.

The book is dedicated to our families, who have supported and encouraged us throughout our journey to become educators.

To Jane, Geri, Grace, and Ethan—my true heroes.

Gerald Kayingo

To David—my husband and champion; and to William F. and Lillian McCoy—my parents and first teachers.

Virginia McCoy Hass

Contents

Contributors   *xi*

Reviewers   *xix*

Foreword   Alfred M. Sadler Jr., MD, FACP; Debra Bakerjian, PhD, APRN, FAAN, FAANP; and Jonathan Bowser, MS, PA-C   *xxiii*

Preface   *xxvii*

PART I. CURRICULUM DESIGN AND IMPLEMENTATION

1. Learner-Centered Pedagogy: Teaching and Learning in the 21st Century   *3*
   Dipu Patel-Junankar

2. Curriculum Design   *13*
   Holly West, Camille Termini Loftin, and Clifford L. Snyder

3. Competencies and Milestones   *25*
   Mary L. Warner

4. Curriculum Mapping   *35*
   Carrie A. Calloway

5. Interprofessional Education: What, Why, When, and How?   *45*
   Kevin Lohenry, Désirée Lie, Ashley Halle, and Sae Byul (Sarah) Ma

PART II. ACTIVE TEACHING–LEARNING METHODOLOGIES

6. Problem-Based Learning   *57*
   Susan Hawkins, Judy Truscott, and Alyssa Abebe

7. Team-Based Learning   *67*
   Victoria Wallace and Lisa Walker

8. Flipping the Classroom Without Tears 79
   Amy A. Nichols

9. Technology in the Classroom 87
   Nina Multak

10. Using Social Media and Big Data to Facilitate Teaching and Learning in
    Health Professions 95
    Bianca Belcher and Jessica Duff

11. Distance Education Strategies 105
    Susan E. White

PART III. CLINICAL EDUCATION

12. Recruiting and Maintaining Clinical Training Sites 121
    Andrew P. Chastain

13. Simulation in Clinical Education 131
    Natalie Walkup, Carolina Wishner, and April Gardner

14. Interprofessional Education in the Clinical Setting 139
    *Angel K. Chen, Tamatha Arms, Barbara L. Jones, Jeffrey Okamoto, Noell Rowan,
    and Evaon C. Wong-Kim*

15. International Clinical Education 151
    Nicholas M. Hudak, Dennis Clements, and Michael V. Relf

16. Service Learning 167
    Hoonani Cuadrado, Sharon E. Connor, Corinne Feldman, and Mary Marfisee

17. Creating a Career Development Curriculum: Facilitating Transition
    to Professional Practice 177
    Bonnie Jo Hanson and Matt Casey

PART IV. ASSESSMENT AND EVALUATION OF LEARNING OUTCOMES

18. Diverse Learner Assessment Strategies 187
    *Marie Meckel, Nadia Cobb, Aviwe Mgobozi, Evelien E. Cellissen, Kristen Burrows,
    Theresa J. Riethle, and Htin Zaw Soe*

19. Professionalism 199
    April Gardner, Natalie Walkup, and Carolina Wishner

20. Learner Assessment and Remediation 207
    Jeanie McHugo

PART V. PROMOTING DIVERSITY, EQUITY, AND INCLUSION

21. Equity Pedagogy: Applying Multicultural Education in Health Professions
    Learning Environments 223
    *Kupiri Ackerman-Barger, David Acosta, Debra Bakerjian, Jann Murray-García,
    and Hendry Ton*

22. Minority Faculty: Recruitment, Retention, and Advancement   *237*
Karen Mulitalo, Kupiri Ackerman-Barger, Darin T. Ryujin,
and Maha B. Lund

23. Achieving Inclusive Excellence   *247*
Kenyon Railey, Jacqueline S. Barnett, and DeShana Collett

PART VI. PROMOTING LEADERSHIP AND SCHOLARSHIP

24. Effective Ways to Promote Scholarship: The Academic
Scholarship Portfolio   *263*
Douglas Brock and Susan Symington

25. Scholarship Reconsidered for Health Professions Educators   *275*
Karl Terryberry and Gerald Kayingo

26. Promoting Academic and Student Leadership   *285*
Reamer L. Bushardt, Teri L. Capshaw, and Sonia J. Crandall

27. Giving and Receiving Feedback   *297*
Craig Keenan

28. Successful Mentoring: Socialization of Faculty and Students   *305*
Ruth Ballweg

29. Creating a Faculty and Student Mentoring Program   *311*
Michael Estrada and Laura Estrada

30. Managing Up and Managing Down: Getting Along With Others   *317*
Ruth Ballweg

PART VII. PROGRAM OPERATIONS

31. Admissions Best Practices   *327*
Mariah Kindle and Douglas Brock

32. Legal Matters for the Health Professions Educator   *345*
Gerald R. Weniger and John F. Knight

33. Creating a Culture of Restorative Justice   *359*
Joao Salm, Gerald Kayingo, and Virginia McCoy Hass

34. Work–Life Balance for the Health Professions Educator   *369*
Patrick Auth and Michael Howley

35. Mindfulness for Health Professions Educators   *377*
Brenda Gustin

PART VIII. CURRENT TRENDS AND FUTURE DIRECTIONS IN HEALTH PROFESSIONS EDUCATION

36. Postgraduate Fellowships and Residency Programs   *389*
Vasco Deon Kidd, Dennis Tankersley, and Virginia McCoy Hass

37. Doctoral Education for Physician Assistants: Demand, Design, and Drawbacks   *397*
Lucy W. Kibe and James F. Cawley

38. Nurturing Social Accountability and Community Engagement   *407*
Nadia Cobb, Amy Clithero, Fortunato Cristobal, Julian Fisher, Sarah Larkins, Lyn Middleton, André-Jacques Neusy, Robyn Preston, Simone J. Ross, Roger Strasser, and Torres Woolley

Index   417

Contributors

Alyssa Abebe, MPAS, PA-C   Assistant Professor, Associate Program Director, Chatham University Physician Assistant Program, Pittsburgh, Pennsylvania

Kupiri Ackerman-Barger, PhD, RN   Assistant Clinical Professor, Codirector Interprofessional Teaching Scholars Program, Betty Irene Moore School of Nursing, University of California, Davis, Sacramento, California

David Acosta, MD, FAAFP   Chief Diversity and Inclusion Officer, Association of American Medical Colleges, Washington, District of Columbia

Tamatha Arms, DNP, PMHNP-BC, NP-C   Nurse Faculty Leadership Academy Scholar, College of Health and Human Services School of Nursing, University of North Carolina Wilmington, Wilmington, North Carolina

Patrick Auth, PhD, PA-C   Director, Physician Assistant Program, Chair, Physician Assistant Department, College of Nursing and Health Professions, Drexel University, Philadelphia, Pennsylvania

Debra Bakerjian, PhD, APRN, FAAN, FAANP   Associate Adjunct Professor, Betty Irene Moore School of Nursing, University of California, Davis, Sacramento, California

Ruth Ballweg, MPA, PA   Professor Emeritus, Department of Family Medicine, School of Medicine, University of Washington, Seattle, Washington

Jacqueline S. Barnett, DHSc, MSHS, PA-C   Associate Professor, Associate Program Director, Department of Community & Family Medicine, Duke University Physician Assistant Program, Durham, North Carolina

Bianca Belcher, MPH, PA-C   Director of Technology and Strategic Initiatives, Assistant Clinical Professor, Physician Assistant Program, Northeastern University, Boston, Massachusetts

Douglas Brock, PhD   Associate Professor, Department of Family Medicine and MEDEX Northwest, University of Washington School of Medicine, Seattle, Washington

Kristen Burrows, MSc, BHSc (PA), CCPA   Assistant Dean, Physician Assistant Education Program, Faculty Health Sciences, McMaster University, Hamilton, Ontario, Canada

Reamer L. Bushardt, PharmD, RPh, PA-C   Professor and Senior Associate Dean, School of Medicine and Health Sciences, The George Washington University, Washington, District of Columbia

Carrie A. Calloway, EdD   Director of Curriculum and Assessment, Assistant Professor of Physician Assistant Studies, College of Medical Science, School of Physician Assistant Studies, Alderson Broaddus University, Philippi, West Virginia

Teri L. Capshaw, MBA   Senior Project Manager, Department of Physician Assistant Studies, Wake Forest School of Medicine, Winston-Salem, North Carolina

Matt Casey, MBA   Professional Career Coach, Matt Casey Career Coaching, Associate Director of Career Management for Sawyer Business School, Suffolk University, Boston, Massachusetts

James F. Cawley, MPH, PA-C   Professor of Prevention and Community Health/Professor of Physician Assistant Studies, The George Washington University, Washington, District of Columbia

Evelien E. Cellissen, MSc, RM   Lecturer, Master's Physician Assistant Clinical Midwifery, Rotterdam University, Utrecht, Netherlands

Andrew P. Chastain, MSPAS, RRT-NPS, PA-C   Clinical Assistant Professor/Director of Clerkship Education, Office of Physician Assistant Education, Stanford University School of Medicine, Stanford, California

Angel K. Chen, RN, MSN, CPNP   Clinical Professor and Vice Chair, Department of Family Health Care Nursing, University of California San Francisco School of Nursing, San Francisco, California

Dennis Clements, MD, PhD, MPH   Director, Duke Global Health Institute Medical School Programs, Professor of Pediatrics and Global Health, Duke University, Durham, North Carolina

Amy Clithero, MBA   Senior Lecturer, Department of Family & Community Medicine, University of New Mexico School of Medicine, Albuquerque, New Mexico

Nadia Cobb, MS, PA-C   Director, Office for the Promotion of Global Healthcare Equity, Division of Physician Assistant Studies, University of Utah School of Medicine, Salt Lake City, Utah

DeShana Collett, PhD, PA-C   Associate Professor, Division of Physician Assistant Studies, University of Kentucky College of Health Sciences, Lexington, Kentucky

Sharon E. Connor, PharmD   Associate Professor, Director, Grace Lamsam Pharmacy Program, University of Pittsburgh School of Pharmacy, Pittsburgh, Pennsylvania

Sonia J. Crandall, PhD, MS   Professor and Director of Research and Scholarship, Department of Physician Assistant Studies, Wake Forest School of Medicine, Winston-Salem, North Carolina

Fortunato Cristobal, MD, FPPS   Dean, Ateneo de Zamboanga School of Medicine, Zamboanga City, Philippines

Hoonani Cuadrado, MSPAS, PA-C   Assistant Professor, International Rotations/Truth Home Coordinator, DeSales University Physician Assistant Program, Center Valley, Pennsylvania

Jessica Duff, MEd   Assistant Coordinator of Inclusion, National Collegiate Athletic Association, Indianapolis, Indiana

Laura Estrada, MPH, BSN, RN, PHN   College Nurse, San Bernardino Valley College, San Bernardino, California

Michael Estrada, DHSc, MS, PA-C   Founding Director and Associate Professor, Physician Assistant Program, University of La Verne, La Verne, California

Corinne Feldman, MMS, PA-C   Assistant Professor, DeSales University Physician Assistant Program, Director, DeSales Free Clinic, Center Valley, Pennsylvania

Julian Fisher, BDS, MSc, MIH   Research Associate, Peter L. Reichertz Institute for Medical Informatics, University of Braunschweig Institute of Technology, and Hannover Medical School, Hannover, Germany

April Gardner, MSBS, PA-C   Program Director, The University of Toledo Physician Assistant Program, College of Medicine and Life Sciences, Toledo, Ohio

Brenda Gustin, PhD   Owner, Union with the Heart, Sacramento, California

Ashley Halle, OTD, OTR/L   Assistant Professor of Clinical Occupational Therapy, University of Southern California, Los Angeles, California

Bonnie Jo Hanson, PA-C   Director of Clinical Education, Physician Assistant Program, Northeastern University, Boston, Massachusetts

Virginia McCoy Hass, DNP, MSN, RN, FNP-C, PA-C   Associate Clinical Professor, Betty Irene Moore School of Nursing, University of California, Davis, Sacramento, California

Susan Hawkins, MSEd, PA-C   Associate Professor/PBL Coordinator, Physician Assistant Program, Chatham University, Pittsburgh, Pennsylvania

Michael Howley, PhD, PA-C   Clinical Professor, Director, Healthcare Management MBA Concentration, LeBow College of Business, Drexel University, Philadelphia, Pennsylvania

Nicholas M. Hudak, MPA, MSEd, PA-C   Associate Professor of Community and Family Medicine and Clinical Coordinator, Duke Physician Assistant Program, Duke University School of Medicine, Durham, North Carolina

Barbara L. Jones, PhD, MSW   Associate Dean for Health Affairs, University Distinguished Teaching Professor, Co-Director, the Institute for Collaborative Health Research and Practice, School of Social Work, University of Texas at Austin, Austin, Texas

Gerald Kayingo, PhD, PA-C   Assistant Clinical Professor, Physician Assistant Program Director, University of California, Davis, Sacramento, California

Craig Keenan, MD   Internal Medicine Residency Program Director, Professor of Medicine, University of California, Davis, Sacramento, California

Lucy W. Kibe, DrPh, MS, MHS, PA-C   Director of Doctoral Education, Assistant Professor of Physician Assistant Medicine, Lynchburg College, Lynchburg, Virginia

Vasco Deon Kidd, DHSc, MPH, MS, PA-C   Orthopaedic Surgery PA Fellowship Director/ Chief Administrative PA, Assistant Clinical Professor at Loma Linda University, California State University, Los Angeles, Colton, California

Mariah Kindle, MSOL   Director of Admissions, Department of Family Medicine, MEDEX Northwest, University of Washington, Seattle, Washington

John F. Knight, JD, BA   Associate University Counsel, James Madison University, Harrisonburg, Virginia

Sarah Larkins, PhD, MBBS, BMedSci, MPH&TM, FRACGP, FARGP   Associate Dean, Research, College of Medicine and Dentistry, Codirector, Anton Breinl Research Centre for Health Systems Strengthening Australian Institute of Tropical Health and Medicine, James Cook University, Townsville, Queensland, Australia

Désirée Lie, MD, MSEd   Clinical Professor of Family Medicine, Keck School of Medicine of the University of Southern California, Alhambra, California

Camille Termini Loftin, DHEd, MPAS, PA-C   Assistant Professor/Academic Coordinator and Interim Vice-Chair for Academic Affairs, Physician Assistant Studies, The School of Health Professions, The University of Texas Medical Branch, Galveston, Texas

Kevin Lohenry, PhD, PA-C   Assistant Professor of Clinical Family Medicine and Director of Primary Care Physician Assistant Program, Keck School of Medicine of the University of Southern California, Alhambra, California

Maha B. Lund, DHSc, PA-C, DFAAPA   Director, Physician Assistant Program, Department of Family and Preventive Medicine, Emory University School of Medicine, Atlanta, Georgia

Sae Byul (Sarah) Ma, PharmD   Assistant Professor of Clinical Family Medicine, Division of Physician Assistant Studies and the USC School of Pharmacy, Keck School of Medicine of the University of Southern California, Alhambra, California

Mary Marfisee, MD, MPH   Assistant Clinical Professor, Department of Family Medicine, Program Director for Community Service Learning, David Geffen School of Medicine, University of California, Los Angeles, California

Jeanie McHugo, PhD, PA-C   Associate Professor/Chair, Department of Physician Assistant Studies, University of North Dakota, Grand Forks, North Dakota

Marie Meckel, MS, PA-C, MPH   Physician Assistant, Bay State Medical Center, Springfield, Massachusetts

Aviwe Mgobozi, BCMP   Associate Lecturer, Clinical Associate Educator, University of Witwatersrand, Johannesburg, South Africa

Lyn Middleton, PhD, RN   Program Director, Training for Health Equity Network (THEnet), School of Health Sciences, University of KwaZulu-Natal, Durban, South Africa

Karen Mulitalo, MPAS, PA-C   Program Director, Division of Physician Assistant Studies, University of Utah, Salt Lake City, Utah

Nina Multak, PhD, MPAS, PA-C, DFAAPA   Director, Primary Care Practicums, Associate Clinical Professor, Physician Assistant Department, College of Nursing and Health Professions, Drexel University, Philadelphia, Pennsylvania

Jann Murray-García, MD, MPH   Assistant Adjunct Professor, Betty Irene Moore School of Nursing, University of California, Davis, Sacramento, California

André-Jacques Neusy, MD, DTM&H   Senior Director Training, Training for Health Equity Network (THEnet), New York, New York

Amy A. Nichols, EdD, RN   Associate Clinical Professor, Betty Irene Moore School of Nursing, University of California, Davis, Sacramento, California

Jeffrey Okamoto, MD   Medical Director, Hawaii Department of Health, Developmental Disabilities Division, Assistant Professor, Department of Pediatrics, University of Hawaii Manoa School of Medicine, Honolulu, Hawaii

Dipu Patel-Junankar, MPAS, PA-C   Associate Program Director/Assistant Clinical Professor, Director of Simulation Education, Bouvé College of Health Sciences, Northeastern University, Boston, Massachusetts

Robyn Preston, PhD   Lecturer, General Practice and Rural Medicine, College of Medicine and Dentistry, Cohort Doctoral Studies Mentor, Division of Tropical Health and Medicine, James Cook University, Townsville, Australia

Kenyon Railey, MD   Assistant Professor, Department of Community and Family Medicine, Assistant Chief Diversity Officer, Duke School of Medicine Office of Diversity and Inclusion, Duke University Medical Center, Durham, North Carolina

Michael V. Relf, PhD, RN, ACNS-BC, AACRN, CNE, FAAN   Associate Professor/ Associate Dean for Global and Community Health Affairs, Duke University School of Nursing, Durham, North Carolina

Theresa J. Riethle, MS, PA-C   Associate Professor/Director, Physician Assistant Studies Program, Bay Path University, Longmeadow, Massachusetts

Simone J. Ross, MDR, BPsych   Lecturer/Project Manager for the Training for Health Equity Network, College of Medicine and Dentistry, James Cook University, Townsville, Australia

Noell Rowan, PhD, LCSW, LCAS   Professor/Associate Director, College of Health and Human Services School of Social Work, University of North Carolina Wilmington, Wilmington, North Carolina

Darin T. Ryujin, MS, MPAS, PA-C   Assistant Professor, Division of Physician Assistant Studies, University of Utah School of Medicine, Salt Lake City, Utah

Joao Salm, PhD, MPA, BL   Assistant Professor of Criminal Justice, Governors State University, University Park, Illinois

Clifford L. Snyder, MPAS, PA-C   Codirector, Sealy and Smith Laboratory for Surgical Training, Assessment, and Research, The University of Texas Medical Branch, Galveston, Texas

Htin Zaw Soe, PhD, MBBS, MMedSC (P & TM), DipMedEd   Rector, University of Community Health, Magway, Myanmar

Roger Strasser, MBBS, MClSc, FRACGP, FACRRM   Dean, Northern Ontario School of Medicine, Lakehead and Laurentian Universities, Lakehead University, Thunderbay, Ontario and Laurentian University, Sudbury, Ontario, Canada

Susan Symington, MPAS, PA-C   Associate Director/Associate Professor, Department of Family Medicine and MEDEX Northwest, University of Washington School of Medicine, Seattle, Washington

Dennis Tankersley, MS, PA-C   EMPA Fellowship Director/Lead PA, Arrowhead Regional Medical Center, Colton, California

Karl Terryberry, PhD   Associate Professor, Daemen College, Amherst, New York

Hendry Ton, MD, MS Professor, Department of Psychiatry and Behavioral Science, Associate Dean for Faculty Development and Diversity, University of California, Davis, Sacramento, California

Judy Truscott, MPAS, PA-C Assistant Professor, Program Director, Chatham University Physician Assistant Program, Pittsburgh, Pennsylvania

Lisa Walker, MPAS, PA-C Director, Department of Physician Assistant Studies, School of Health and Rehabilitation Sciences, MGH Institute of Health Professions, Boston, Massachusetts

Natalie Walkup, MPAS, PA-C Assistant Professor/Associate Program Director and Assistant Academic Coordinator, The University of Toledo Physician Assistant Program, College of Medicine and Life Sciences, Toledo, Ohio

Victoria Wallace, MEd Instructional Designer, Office of the Provost, MGH Institute of Health Professions, Boston, Massachusetts

Mary L. Warner, MSc, PA-C Founding Director/Assistant Professor of Medicine, Boston University School of Medicine PA Program, Boston, Massachusetts

Gerald R. Weniger, MEd, MPAS, ATC, PA-C Program Director/Assistant Professor, Physician Assistant Program, James Madison University, Harrisonburg, Virginia

Holly West, DHEd, MPAS, PA-C Women's Health Specialist, UT System Distinguished Teaching Professor, Senior Research Coordinator/Site Manager, Obstetric–Fetal Pharmacology Research Center, The University of Texas Medical Branch, Galveston, Texas

Susan E. White, MD Director of Didactic Education, Physician Assistant Program, Assistant Professor, Division of Graduate Medical Sciences, Boston University School of Medicine, Boston, Massachusetts

Carolina Wishner, MD, MPH Assistant Professor, Assistant Program Director, The University of Toledo Physician Assistant Program, College of Medicine and Life Sciences, Toledo, Ohio

Evaon C. Wong-Kim, PhD, MSW, MPH, LCSW Director/Professor, School of Social Work, California State University, Los Angeles, Los Angeles, California

Torres Woolley, PhD Evaluation Coordinator, James Cook University School of Medicine and Dentistry, Townsville, Australia

REVIEWERS

Craig A. Baumgartner, MBA, MPAS, PA-C, MPLC, DFAAPA   Medical Provider Legal Consultant, Baumgartner Consulting, Glenview, Illinois

Richard Bennett, PhD, PA-C   Physician Assistant, Big Horn Basin Bone and Joint, Cody, Wyoming

Oren Berkowitz, PhD, MSPH, PA-C   Director of Research & Assistant Professor of Medicine, Department of Graduate Medical Sciences, Physician Assistant Studies, Boston University School of Medicine, Boston, Massachusetts

Jeri L. Bigbee, PhD, RN, FAAN   Adjunct Professor, Betty Irene Moore School of Nursing, University of California, Davis, Sacramento, California

Jane Davis, DNP, CRNP   Practitioner of Nephrology, Nephrology Division, University of Alabama at Birmingham, Birmingham, Alabama

John Encandela, PhD   Associate Professor, Psychiatry, Associate Director for Curriculum and Educator Assessment, Teaching and Learning Center, Yale School of Medicine, New Haven, Connecticut

Deborah Fahs, DNP, MSN, FNP-C, RN   Assistant Professor of Nursing, Yale School of Nursing, West Haven, Connecticut.

Shani Fleming, MSHS, MPH, PA-C   Director of Community Outreach, Assistant Professor of Medical Education, Barry University Physician Assistant Program, St. Croix, United States Virgin Islands

Janette Rodrigues Editorial Director, American Academy of PAs, American Academy of PAs, Washington, District of Columbia

Charandip Sandhu, MD Assistant Professor, Director, Anesthesiology Resident Program, University of California Davis Medical Center, Sacramento, California

Jenna Shaw-Battista, PhD, RN, NP, CNM, FACNM Associate Clinical Professor, Director, Master's Entry Program in Nursing, University of California, Davis, Betty Irene Moore School of Nursing, Sacramento, California

Bradley Stockert, PhD, PT Professor, Department of Physical Therapy, California State University, Sacramento, Sacramento, California

Howard Straker, MPH, PA-C Assistant Professor of Physician Assistant Studies, Assistant Professor of Prevention and Community Health, The George Washington University, Washington, District of Columbia

Alan R. Titche, PhD Owner, Editorial Services, Davis, California

Laura Van Auker, DNP, RN, FNP-BC, SN-C Assistant Clinical Professor, Betty Irene Moore School of Nursing, University of California, Davis, Sacramento, California

Floris Van de Ven, PT, DPT Lecturer, California State University, Sacramento, Sacramento, California

Nancy Kim Zuber, MSPAS, PA-C Secretary, American Academy of Nephrology PAs, Oceanside, California

Foreword

This timely collection of chapters is of great practical and pedagogical value to anyone who is involved in interdisciplinary education in the health professions. The editors are very experienced educators who have served as program directors of the joint Physician Assistant and Nurse Practitioner Program at the University of California, Davis. This program is unique in the country for its ongoing collaborative learning and training of physician assistants (PAs) and nurse practitioners (NPs), which it has done since 1974, originally supported by a Robert Wood Johnson Foundation grant.

The book is filled with nuggets of "how to" information, in addition to theoretical foundations for teaching. For anyone who has grown up with the traditional lecture format, there is much to learn about new and alternate strategies from these experts. The teaching of PAs, NPs, MDs, and members of other disciplines has much in common. As educators involved in PA and NP education and policy issues for many years, we are fascinated by the excellent and varied chapters contained herein and commend the editors and authors for this work.

Thinking back to the "early days" of the 1960s and 1970s, although it was clear that PA learning would emulate medical student and residency training, the introduction of the clinical algorithm as a teaching strategy was a significant contribution to PA education and practice. Over the decades, algorithms have been widely accepted throughout medical and health education.

Competency-based testing, as developed in 1973 for the first national certification examination for assistants to the primary care physician by the National Board of Medical Examiners, was a significant departure from testing of medical students and physician specialists. The competency-based model of education and testing remains essential today and has undergone permutations and challenges resulting from the increased emphasis on obtaining advanced degrees.

The focus on "person-centered care" has also evolved; the need for the health care team to work together to achieve that common goal is receiving important emphasis in both health care and health professions education. This book addresses the need for this interprofessional approach to health professions education. For a historical perspective on person-centered care, please see Sadler, Sadler, and Bliss (1975).

Although PA education follows a similar model to that of physicians, NP education builds on the strong foundation created by registered nurses in health promotion, disease prevention, and family and child health. Advanced concepts of clinical nursing, including physical assessment, pathophysiology, and pharmacology, are integrated with primary care medicine in all NP programs. NPs traditionally follow a holistic approach to care and are prepared in a specific population-focused pathway (e.g., family, pediatrics, women's health). Yet, despite differences in backgrounds and educational approaches, PA and most NP education programs focus on primary care, and learners can benefit from interprofessional educational experiences that may also include medical students and other health professionals.

Over the past decade, a series of expert reports have brought greater emphasis on interprofessional collaboration in practice and the importance of preparing health professionals to work as an interprofessional team. The Institute of Medicine's *Report on Health Professions Education* was the first of these reports, recommending that all health professionals be educated to work on interdisciplinary teams (Institute of Medicine, Greiner, and Knebel, 2003). This was followed by "Interprofessional Education for Collaboration: Learning How to Improve Health from Interprofessional Models Across the Continuum of Education to Practice" (Cuff, 2013), a report that articulated the importance of being educated together in teams to understand each other's roles and to better communicate in ways that improve in patient outcomes.

These studies provided the impetus for six accrediting bodies from nursing, medicine, pharmacy, dentistry, and public health to cosponsor the first expert panel to develop the core competencies for interprofessional collaborative practice (Schmitt, Blue, Aschenbrener, & Viggiano, 2011). The initial set of core competencies was recently updated (Brown et al., 2016), strengthening the four competency domains: (a) mutual respect and shared values, (b) professions working together to address patient needs, (c) responsible and responsive communication, and (d) a team-based approach to care. To further promote these concepts, the National Center for Interprofessional Practice and Education, established in October 2012 at the University of Minnesota, has established a comprehensive resource center for educators and researchers. Multiple studies have shown that clinicians working in interprofessional teams improve patient outcomes, thus supporting the interprofessional focus of this text.

This book builds on fundamental team-based pedagogy and experience, integrating materials that embrace these interprofessional principles to assist the educator in designing and implementing curricula for learners from various professions. Educators will be able to use the various strategies outlined here, not only for implementing adult learning principles for the health professional, but also for adapting any type of content. Faculty who use the strategies detailed in this book, with a goal of preparing students for collaborative practice, will produce health professionals capable of stepping into a team-based care environment.

In addition to the focus on interprofessional education and collaborative practice, with the emergence of value-based models that focus on the health of populations, quality improvement, and patient safety, the past decade has seen considerable change in our approach to health care delivery. To keep pace with a quickly evolving practice environment, education for health professions is undergoing an equally transformative period. Many established health professions programs are engaged in or actively planning curricular reforms.

The shift away from an instructor-centered paradigm toward a learner-centered paradigm has catalyzed innovation in curriculum design and teaching methodologies. We now use high-fidelity simulation and other technological tools in many contexts, an array of active learning strategies instead of traditional classroom lectures, and new approaches to assess learning and competence.

We have developed a more holistic approach to promoting diversity, equity, and inclusion among educators, learners, and the patients we serve. Our appreciation for fostering and developing leadership in the health professions has matured. Educators in the health professions face the daunting task of staying current—keeping up with the latest developments in so many areas—while performing the demanding tasks intrinsic to a career in this field. In this volume, the editors have brought together a wealth of experts across all domains of health professions education to help them do just that.

Alfred M. Sadler Jr., MD, FACP
Founding Director, Yale Physician Assistant Program
Founding President, Physician Assistant Education Association
Senior Officer, Robert Wood Johnson Foundation
President, Physician Assistant History Society
Carmel, California

Debra Bakerjian, PhD, APRN, FAAN, FAANP
Associate Adjunct Professor
Former Senior Director for NP/PA Education and Practice
Betty Irene Moore School of Nursing
University of California, Davis
Sacramento, California

Jonathan Bowser, MS, PA-C
Associate Dean, Program Director
University of Colorado Child Health Associate/Physician Assistant Program
Aurora, Colorado

REFERENCES

Brown, B., Brehm, B., Dodge, H. S., Diers, T., Van Loon, R. A., Breen, P., . . . Wall, A. (2016). Evaluation of an interprofessional elective course for health professions students: Teaching core competencies for interprofessional collaborative practice. *Health and Interprofessional Practice, 3*(1), 4.

Cuff, P. A. (Ed.). (2013). *Interprofessional education for collaboration: Learning how to improve health from interprofessional models across the continuum of education to practice: Workshop summary.* Washington, DC: National Academies Press.

Institute of Medicine, Greiner, A., & Knebel, E. (2003). *Health professions education: A bridge to quality.* Washington, DC: National Academies Press.

Sadler, A. M., Jr., Sadler, B. L., & Bliss, A. A. (1975a). Issues and recommendations. In *The physician's assistant: Today and tomorrow* (2nd ed., pp. 143–151). New Haven, CT: Yale University Press. Retrieved from http://pahx.org/pdf/Sadler_Sadler_Bliss_2nd_Edition.pdf

Sadler, A. M., Jr., Sadler, B. L., & Bliss, A. A. (1975b). Organizational alternatives. In *The physician's assistant: Today and tomorrow* (2nd ed., pp. 137–141). New Haven, CT: Yale University Press. Retrieved from http://pahx.org/pdf/Sadler_Sadler_Bliss_2nd_Edition.pdf

Schmitt, M., Blue, A., Aschenbrener, C. A., & Viggiano, T. R. (2011). Core competencies for interprofessional collaborative practice: Reforming health care by transforming health professionals' education. *Academic Medicine, 86*(11), 1351.

Preface

The rapidly evolving health care landscape calls for an urgent transformation in the ways we prepare learners across the continuum of health professions education. There is a need for ongoing self-assessment of our teaching and learning approaches to address the changing demographics of learners and to improve work–life balance for educators. The current generation of students has been raised in a rapidly changing technological environment, and they view teaching and learning very differently from their professors. If educators are to adapt to this new wave of transformation, a shift in attitudes and teaching methodologies is inevitable.

One of the most limiting factors in health professions education is scarcity of experienced faculty and teaching resources. Most health professions educators are expert clinicians who do not have a formal education in pedagogy. These busy clinician educators have limited opportunities for teaching fellowships to hone their teaching effectiveness. Similar to becoming an expert clinician, the learning curve for becoming an expert educator is long. In our experience, it takes about 5 years for new educators to become fully comfortable in their teaching roles. Meanwhile, students have high expectations for quality education, and class sizes are growing.

This book provides a practical guide for new and established faculty. It is written to be the "go to" resource for health professions educators in general, with an emphasis on the needs of physician assistant (PA) and nurse practitioner (NP) faculty. It is the guide we wish we had had at the beginning of our teaching careers. In it, you will find new pedagogical approaches that are critically needed to prepare the learners and future clinicians of the 21st century. Equally important, you will find ideas to help you to maintain work–life balance and have fun while you teach.

This book is unique in a number of ways. First, it presents an interprofessional and collaborative perspective on health professions education. Health care is a team sport. Thus, it is important that future health care professionals are educated in an interprofessional environment using modern team-based approaches. The various chapter contributors were intentionally selected to represent an interprofessional perspective. Each chapter was either coauthored or peer reviewed by an interdisciplinary team of experts. Second, we have threaded a theme of learner-centered pedagogy and active learning strategies throughout the book. We believe that learner-centered pedagogy puts the student's learning at center stage and encourages learners to engage deeply with the material. We also believe that active learning stimulates critical thinking and problem-solving skills, which are vital for health professionals. The third unique feature of this book is its emphasis on technology in the classroom. We provide excellent guides to educators on how to use hybrid and online teaching formats to actively engage learners. In addition, the book provides strategies for harnessing the power of cognitive diversity and inclusion in the teaching environment. Finally, this book can be used by educators to improve their own scholarship, leadership, and work–life balance.

This book is divided into eight parts. Although the themes discussed are woven throughout, each chapter can stand alone, providing "just-in-time" information when you need it.

- In Part I, Curriculum Design and Implementation, you will find useful resources on how to conduct curriculum mapping, follow competency- and milestone-based approaches to instruction, and integrate interprofessional education in the curriculum.
- Part II, Active Teaching–Learning Methodologies, focuses on active learning strategies such as problem-based learning, team-based learning, and flipped classrooms. This section also provides resources on how to incorporate technology in the classroom and how to use social media and big data to facilitate teaching and learning.
- Part III, Clinical Education, provides state-of-the-art resources on simulation, international clinical education, interprofessional education in the clinical setting, and service learning. It also addresses a critical aspect of clinical education: How to recruit and retain clinical training sites.
- In Part IV, Assessment and Evaluation of Learning Outcomes, you will find particularly useful information on how to assess and remediate professionalism, as well as on how to assess diverse learners.

Parts V through VIII provide innovative strategies that can be used in the classroom and for faculty development.

- In Part V, Promoting Diversity, Equity, and Inclusion, you will find approaches for achieving inclusion excellence and promoting faculty and student success.
- Part VI, Promoting Scholarship and Leadership, addresses both faculty and student leadership and provides essential information on how to develop your career and navigate the academic milieu.
- Part VII, Program Operations, tackles fundamentals such as admission practices, legal matters in academia, and creation of a culture of restorative justice.
- Finally, Part VIII, Current Trends and Future Directions in Health Professions Education, explores what is new in health professions education, as well as thoughts on what is likely to be coming next.

Additional material, chosen to supplement selected chapters, accompanies this book online. It can be obtained from Springer Publishing at http://springerpub.com/hep.

Drawing on the wisdom of West African people, we represented the major themes of each book section using Adinkra symbols. These symbols have been used traditionally to communicate concepts, ideas, and wisdom across generations. The symbols and their meanings were adopted from "West African Wisdom: Adnikra Symbols & Meanings" (MacDonald, 2004).

We are deeply grateful to the contributors and peer reviewers for their timely support and attention to detail while preparing this book. We are also very grateful to our institutional and departmental colleagues for allowing us time and space to concentrate on this book.

Gerald Kayingo
Virginia McCoy Hass

REFERENCE

MacDonald, J. (2004). *West African wisdom: Adinkra symbols and meanings.* Retrieved from www.adinkra .org/htmls/adinkra_index.htm

PART I
Curriculum Design and Implementation

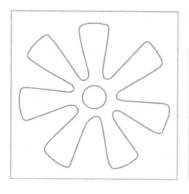

ANANSE NTONTAN
"Spider's web"

Symbol of wisdom, creativity, and the complexities of life Ananse, the spider, is a well-known character in African folktales.

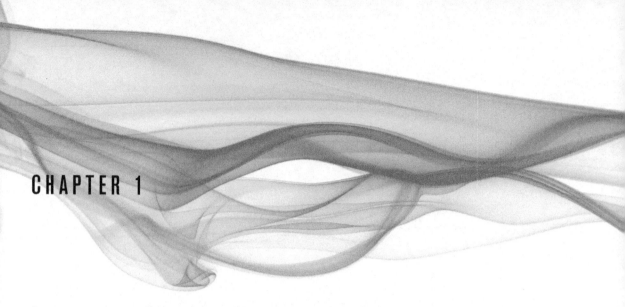

CHAPTER 1

Learner-Centered Pedagogy: Teaching and Learning in the 21st Century

Dipu Patel-Junankar

CHAPTER OBJECTIVE

- Implement strategies for engaging students in planning, implementation, and assessments that address their values and needs

---

[H]uman resources are like natural resources; they're often buried deep. You have to go looking for them, they're not just lying around on the surface. You have to create the circumstances where they show themselves.

—*Sir Ken Robinson*

Just as we educate our students that the patient is at the center of care, as educators we should know that students are at the center of our teaching philosophy. Over the past decade, a shift has occurred in the delivery of health care curricula. Health sciences schools have begun to restructure their curricula to be more inclusive of hands-on patient care, to dedicate more time to the training of academic educators, and to provide a balanced and multidisciplinary approach to health care (Parkhurst, 2015). Changes in health care economics, managed care, and an increased demand on the health care delivery system have been the catalysts for these changes. Learner-centered pedagogy, or student-centered learning, has become the focus in health sciences academia. The integration of student-centered learning and technology within the classroom has been the topic of numerous studies and continues to be the driving force for curricular changes within the existing, new, and developing health care education curricula (Keengwe, Onchwari, & Onchwari, 2009).

Learner-centered pedagogy creates an environment that speaks to the heart of learning. It encourages students to deeply engage with the material, develop a dialogue, and reflect on their progress (Weimer, 2002). It represents a shift away from the "sage-on-the-stage" mentality and puts the students' learning at center stage (King, 1993). As students gain greater access to information, it is the educator's role to guide the application and assimilation of that information into real-world problems. The foundation of learner-centered teaching is rooted in a constructivist framework of learning theory. Constructivists postulate that humans are perceivers and interpreters who construct meaning from new and prior experiences (Jonassen, 1991). Instructional design should therefore focus on providing tools and environments for helping learners interpret the multiple perspectives of the world in creating their own world (Karagiorgi & Symeou, 2005).

STUDENT-CENTERED PEDAGOGY VERSUS TEACHER-CENTERED PEDAGOGY

The anthropologist Margaret Mead said, "children must be taught how to think, not what to think" (1928, p. 246). Although health professions students are not children, the same adage applies to them. The notion of engaging students in learning and educating them to be critical thinkers requires a shift in pedagogy from the teacher being at the center of the classroom to the learner being at the center (Table 1.1). In teacher-centered pedagogy, the focus is on the

TABLE 1.1 Teacher-Centered Versus Learner-Centered Pedagogy

Teacher Centered	Learner Centered
Focus is on the instructor	Focus is on both students and the instructor
Students work individually	Students work in groups or alone, depending on the activity
The instructor observes and corrects students' responses	The instructor provides feedback and corrective action when needed
Only the instructor answers students' questions	Students may answer each other's questions and use the instructor as a resource
Only the instructor evaluates students' learning	Students evaluate their own learning, which is supported by the instructor

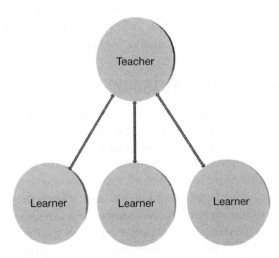

FIGURE 1.1 Focus in teacher-centered pedagogy.

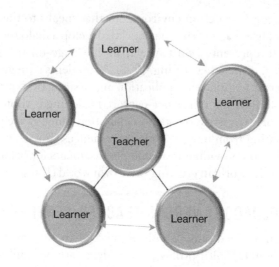

FIGURE 1.2 Focus in learner-centered pedagogy.

instructor and students work independently. The instructor controls the conversation and makes corrections to students' responses. The instructor also evaluates students' learning (Figure 1.1). In learner-centered pedagogy, the role of the teacher is more that of a coach than a person with all the answers. The focus is on both the instructor and students. Learning occurs through the process of interaction between the instructor and students and among the students (Figure 1.2). Both the instructor and students answer questions and provide feedback and corrective measures when needed. Both the instructor and students evaluate students' learning. A similar approach occurs during clinical teaching, when trainees are taught to round together and care for a patient as a team rather than individually.

Weimer (2002) discusses five characteristics of teaching that make it learner centered:

1. Learner-centered teaching engages students in the hard, messy work of learning.
2. It is teaching that motivates and empowers students by giving them some control over learning processes.
3. Learner-centered teaching encourages students to reflect on what they are learning and how they are learning it.
4. It is teaching that encourages collaboration, acknowledging the classroom (be it virtual or real) as a community where everyone shares the learning agenda.
5. Learner-centered teaching includes explicit skill instruction. It teaches students how to think, solve problems, evaluate evidence, analyze arguments, and generate hypotheses.

DOMAINS OF LEARNER-CENTERED PEDAGOGY

Student-centered learning can be implemented in several ways—as team projects, nontraditional writing assignments, role play, and service learning assignments, just to name a few. Weimer (2002) discusses five domains that need to be considered when transitioning to learner-centered teaching (Table 1.2). The role of a teacher should be to facilitate the learning process and allow shared decision making about learning with students. It is important to create the right environment for learning, and faculty must be aware of knowledge-building processes and incorporate them depending on the course and curriculum. Assessment processes should be used to promote learning and should include self-evaluation and peer-evaluation strategies. When the factors of learner-centered teaching are well balanced, learners are able to retain the knowledge and develop skills for lifelong learning.

TABLE 1.2 Five Domains of Learner-Centered Teaching

Factor	Learner-Centered Pedagogy	Example
Role of the teacher	Instructional action should focus on students' learning	Approaches that avoid the tendency to tell students what to learn: • Not "reading the syllabus" to students • Providing "how-to" study advice
Balance of power	Faculty share decision making about learning with students	Assignment choices and policy setting
Function of content	Content should be used to build a knowledge base and develop learning skills and learner self-awareness	Approaches that do not separate learning strategies from content: • End-of-class summaries • Exam-review sessions
Responsibility of learning	Cocreate learning environments that motivate students to accept responsibility for learning	Student-driven activities to create constructive classroom climates and logical consequences
Process and purposes of evaluation	Evaluation activities should also be used to promote learning and develop self- and peer-assessment skills	Self- and peer-assessment Evaluation of participation

Source: Adapted from Weimer (2002).

LEARNER-CENTERED PEDAGOGY IN THE ERA OF TECHNOLOGY AND SOCIAL MEDIA

Learner-centered pedagogy is gaining ground in the realm of online education, where the concept of a classroom without walls harnesses the power of technology. Current and future generations of students are being raised in an environment that straddles the transition from books to terabytes of information. These generations are "digital natives" (Essary, 2011, p. 50) who are hooked up, linked in, and better connected than any prior generation. Faculty need to meet this shift in order to remain current and relevant within education. In conjunction with this shift, the attitude and methodology of educators needs to adjust to ever-evolving technologies. Already the role of teachers at the K-12 education is being redefined (Johnson et al., 2014), and so should the role of health professions educators. Students enter health professions programs with a preexisting e-professional profile and "netiquette" is ingrained (Kaczmaxczyk, 2013), which, impacts their behavior as students and their journey toward professionalism. We present techniques that we have successfully used to engage the new generation of digital natives: blogging, debate, and art.

Social Media and Blogging as Tools in Learner-Centered Pedagogy

Use of social media as a communication tool has become the norm in many industries. The evolution of technological industries has led to the advent and higher acceptance rate of such tools in education (see Chapter 10 for more information). At our institution, we have used blogging as learning strategy in Professional Issues, a first-semester course in which students blog and self-reflect on a number of health care and ethical case studies.

The implementation of a student blog requires foresight and deliberative execution. The idea of the blog is twofold: to harness the student's enthusiasm early and to create a living document of the student's reflections as the student progresses. The student's advisors are also given access to the blog, providing a way to foster the mentor–mentee relationship. The creation of the student blog begins prior to the arrival of the student on campus. As soon as the student has an institutional email account, his or her blog page is created. Invitations with a message about how the blog will be used in his or her education are sent out via email. Various postings are made on the student blog throughout the Professional Issues course. Blog topics include compassion and empathy, discussions of various aspects of being a physician assistant (PA), and analysis of an ethics case. An assignment called "Gray Paper," which is the first post of the blog, provides a further example of implementation.

For the Gray Paper, students select from a variety of gray paint chips from a local hardware store and are asked to read their shade of gray and share with the class how they will embrace gray areas in health care as they navigate the upcoming year. On the paint chip they write one word that describes best how they balance the science and art of health care and then attach the paint chip next to the board in front of the classroom as a constant reminder of this reflection. This in-class activity is followed by a blog-posting assignment.

In the Gray Paper blog, students are asked to reflect on how they feel at the beginning of their journey to becoming a clinician and how they will embrace the gray areas of medicine. Students ponder how and why they chose this profession and what in their past lives led them to this point. They are further asked to reflect on what they think constitutes professional versus unprofessional behavior. Questions used to prompt reflection include (a) What experiences have you had as a consumer of health care with relation to professionalism? (b) How did those experiences impact your notion of what is considered professional versus unprofessional behavior? (c) How will that experience impact your future practice as a health care provider? Our experience with this reflective activity and with blogging in general is that students begin to see the challenges and acknowledge the difficult journey they will all navigate together.

At the end of the first academic year the paint chips are removed and, one by one, students read their words and once again reflect on their progress and their journey. They rededicate their gray message to the next year of their learning journey. They reread their initial post from the beginning of the year and make one last post to the blog about the past year, reflecting on what they have learned and experienced—physically, academically, emotionally, and mentally. As illustrated by the Gray Paper assignment, blogging is a learner-centered activity that motivates and empowers students, which encourages self-reflection and collaboration.

The Role of Debate in Learner-Centered Health Professions Education

Use of debate as an educational tool has historical roots that date back to the Greeks and Romans. Protagoras of Abdera is credited with implementing debates in the educational arena more than 2,400 years ago (Hall, 2011). However, it was not until the late 19th and early 20th centuries that debate was incorporated into American higher education.

Debate in health professions education has been used successfully to bridge the gap between didactic education and its clinical application, particularly in controversial areas such as ethical issues (Darby, 2007). Debate as a teaching–learning tool shifts the responsibility for learning to students, and requires active engagement in the process. In addition to allowing immersion in a topic, debate builds critical competencies beyond the content covered that are essential to the practice of students as clinicians. These include evidence-based practice, creation and oral presentation of logical arguments, and analysis of evidence and differing points of view (Darby, 2007). Debate requires student engagement with the health sciences literature and incentivizes the development of skills required to answer complex clinical and ethical questions in a systematic way.

Implementing Debate as a Learner-Centered Strategy

The selection of debate topics can be based on current issues involving the health care professions or system. In our case, we cross-pollinated two courses: Evidence-Based Medicine and Infectious Diseases. We use four issues that are actively evolving in the news and being debated in the media as well as in the medical literature. To keep the topics timely and relevant to current practice, they are changed every year. Debate topics used in our course have ranged from the pros and cons of Ebola quarantine to needle exchange programs.

In order to prepare for debate, students must be able to develop an answerable question and to retrieve and evaluate evidence to answer it. Predebate instructions thus include principles of evidence-based practice and how to formulate a question using the PICO (population, intervention, comparison, outcome) format (Sackett, Richardson, Rosenberg, & Haynes, 1997). To show the validity of the evidence used in their debate, students are required to turn in Critically Appraised Topic forms. An exemplar of this form may be found in the online supplement (Chapter 1 Exemplar). Using these forms, students indicate the methodology for their search and the validity of the evidence critiqued. Students are required to include at least two systematic reviews or meta-analysis papers to serve as a teaching point about interpretation of new studies concerning evolving academic, political, and socioeconomic viewpoints. Each group is assigned a "faculty coach" who guides them in formulating debate strategies, avoiding errors in reasoning and illogical connections, and using propaganda techniques.

Setting the parameters for the faculty coach role in debate preparation is crucial. The faculty coach motivates, coaches, and guides students toward a deeper understanding of the issue at hand. Rather than telling them where to look for information, guiding them to think and see the issue through several lenses helps solidify the concepts of evidence-based medicine and their application. As an example, students in a group preparing to debate mandatory flu vaccine for health care workers were struggling with how to make the argument against vaccination. They initially looked to their faculty coach to tell them the answer. The coach prompted them to think about the issue and who it impacted. While the students talked, the faculty coach wrote their ideas on a whiteboard, sorting into three categories: health care workforce, economics, and patients/communities. After just this 5-minute activity helping students visually organize their thoughts, students were able to identify new search terms and phrases, new websites to be visited, and developed deeper searches for stronger evidence. Thus, in a debate, the inquiry process alone is a learning experience. By the time students actually debate, they are more knowledgeable about the content, citing references by author and year, quoting and paraphrasing articles, and comparing studies.

The style of debate used typically depends on how much time is available and where it is integrated into the curriculum. Debate formats commonly used in health professions education include (a) online, (b) team (Karl-Popper format), (c) parliamentary, (d) legislative, and (e) public forum (International Debate Education Association, n.d.). Detailed information regarding these debate types and their uses may be found in the online supplemental material for this chapter (Chapter 1 Debate Format Types).

No matter which format is used, expectations and rules for the debate should be made explicitly clear. Parameters should address expectations around dress code, use of certain types of language, rebuttal timeline, use of visual aids, and whether there will be a "winner." If a winner is to be decided, judging criteria and who will judge must be determined. A template of a modified British Parliamentary Debate format used in our PA program may be found in the online supplement (Chapter 1 Template).

Debate is adaptable to various health professions curricula. Potential challenges to be addressed in implementing debate as a teaching–learning strategy include faculty development and preparation of educators, creating time within the curriculum, and balancing course workload for students. Overall, the benefits outweigh these potential challenges. In our experience students report that debate proficiency translates into their clinical experiences in the form of increased confidence as they address issues with patients and colleagues.

Use of the Arts as a Driver for Learner-Centered Pedagogy

The use of humanities in medical education is experiencing a revival. Observing and creating works of art allows students to engage in a nonmedical topic, and these techniques are easily transferable to learning health-related topics (Bardes, Gillers, & Herman, 2001; Dolev, 2001). Art fosters curiosity, creativity, and exploration, which are important in health professions education. Naghshineh and colleagues (2008) found that students who participated in seven or more educational sessions linking visual arts observation with physical diagnosis made 38% more observations than the control group. In addition, students who completed visual arts training provided qualitatively different evidence for their interpretations than the control group, including more supporting evidence for observations and increased awareness of pertinent negatives (Naghshineh et al., 2008).

Implementing an Arts and Medicine Curriculum

Within the curriculum of our PA program, we implemented a 2-hour medicine and the arts class in conjunction with the local museum of fine arts. Situated just prior to the beginning of the clinical phase of the program, this class consists of four exercises: visual thinking strategies, a drawing activity, a sculpture reflection activity, and a discussion about death and dying. The class was cotaught by PA program faculty and a museum docent.

Visual Thinking Activity

The visual thinking strategy is designed to make the connection between medicine and arts using three questions. While students observe a painting, they are asked to ponder, "What is going on in this picture?" "What do you see that makes you say that?" "What more can we find?" Once students are able to answer these three questions, they apply the concepts to a clinical scenario using three similar questions: "What is going on with this patient?" "What are the signs and symptoms you have found that make you say that?" "What other signs and symptoms are you looking for to confirm your findings?" Answering these three questions provides core skills for formulating a differential diagnosis and can be applied in many settings and over many skill levels.

Drawing Activity

The drawing activity is designed to foster team building and consideration of multiple perspectives. In this activity, students sit in groups of 12 around a large sculpture and, using paper and pencil, draw what they see for 30 seconds. Each student then passes his or her drawing to the left. After 12 passes, all drawings are compared side to side to see how the images come together. Typically, students comment on not knowing which one is their initial drawing and that seeing a patient from multiple perspectives would help open their minds to more creative and better care of that patient. This activity can be further extended to the clinical realm with a discussion of how views differ between a specialist and a primary care provider, discourse on the importance of precise documentation, and strategies for clear communication among the team.

Sculpture Reflection Activity

The sculpture reflection activity focuses on self-reflection. It acknowledges the hard work of providing health care and how, for students, it is often difficult to see beyond the next exam or class. In this activity, students sculpt clay into a reflection of how they feel about entering the next (clinical) phase of their education, using the process of self-reflection. This activity is coupled with a dialogue about the importance of self-care and rededication to their craft that acknowledges the difficulties of their pursuits and clarifies the big picture.

Discussion About Death and Dying

The discussion about death and dying takes place in front of an Etruscan sarcophagus. Students are given a brief history of the sarcophagus and then asked to walk around it and observe the reliefs and images sculpted on its top and sides. A discussion facilitated by PA program faculty is framed around acknowledging death and dying as a natural part of life and recognizing that it is uncomfortable to have discussions with patients about death and dying. Questions used to facilitate this discussion include "How do you think the dying process has changed over the millennia?" "What are the commonalities and differences between ancient and modern times?" "How do *you* feel about death and dying?" This activity characteristically resonates with students at a deep level. Engaging students in this discussion can be difficult, but it is important. Faculty development to assure that they are comfortable with the topic is key. In addition, appropriate placement of this activity within the curriculum is paramount. A preparatory session regarding issues around death, such as advanced directives, "do not resuscitate," and POLST (physician orders for life-sustaining treatment) orders (National POLST Paradigm, n.d.) provides the foundational language and a departure point for subsequent conversations. Similar to previous reports (Perry, Maffulli, Willson, & Dylan, 2011; Schwartz et al., 2009), the use of art in our curriculum has improved students' observation skills and accuracy in the description of physical exam findings, improved students' interpretation of patients' emotional state, and increased students' awareness of multiple perspectives. Although we conducted our sessions in conjunction with a museum docent, other data support doing similar activities without specially trained personnel or museum partnerships. Shapiro, Rucker, and Beck (2006) found that small-group training by faculty with either clinical photographs and paper cases or art plus observation of dance have the same impact and outcomes.

CONCLUSIONS

The future of learner-centered pedagogy lies in the ability of institutions to develop and foster learning communities and to harness the power of technology and innovation both within and outside of the classroom. As the delivery of health care becomes more personalized and digitized, the educational philosophies of yesteryear can no longer sustain the health care education of future generations. Innovation breeds innovation; it is imperative that we shift our focus and broaden our acceptance that students have information at their fingertips, and to innovate how students learn so that they are better prepared for the future of medicine. As reflected by creativity expert Sir Ken Robinson (2010) in his Ted Talk:

> We have to recognize that human flourishing is not a mechanical process; it's an organic process. And you cannot predict the outcome of human development. All you can do, like a farmer, is create the conditions under which they will begin to flourish.

REFERENCES

Bardes, C. L., Gillers, D., & Herman, A. E. (2001). Learning to look: Developing clinical observational skills at an art museum. *Medical Education, 35*(12), 1157–1161.

Darby, M. (2007). Debate: A teaching-learning strategy for developing competence in communication and critical thinking. *Journal of Dental Hygiene, 81*(4), 78–87.

Dolev, J. C. (2001). Use of fine art to enhance visual diagnostic skills. *Journal of the American Medical Association, 286*(9), 1020–1021.

Essary, A. C. (2011). The impact of social media and technology on professionalism in medical education. *Journal of Physician Assistant Education, 22*(4), 50–53.

Hall, D. (2011). Debate: Innovative teaching to enhance critical thinking and communication skills in healthcare professionals. *Internet Journal of Allied Health Sciences and Practice, 9*(3), 7.

International Debate Education Association. (n.d.). *idebate.* Retrieved from https://idebate.org/debate-formats

Johnson, L., Adams Becker, S., Estrada, V., & Freeman, A. (2014). *NMC Horizon Report: 2014 Higher Education Edition.* Austin, TX: The New Media Consortium.

Jonassen, D. H. (1991). Objectivism versus constructivism: Do we need a new philosophical paradigm? *Educational Technology Research and Development, 39*(3), 5–14.

Karagiorgi, Y., & Symeou, L. (2005). Translating constructivism into instructional design: Potential and limitations. *Educational Technology and Society, 8*(1), 17–27.

Keengwe, J., Onchwari, G., & Onchwari, J. (2009). Technology and student learning: Toward a learner-centered teaching model. *AACE Journal, 17*(1), 11–22.

King, A. (1993). From sage on the stage to guide on the side. *College Teaching, 41*(1), 30–35.

Mead, M. (1928). *Coming of age in Samoa.* New York, NY: William Morrow.

Naghshineh, S., Hafler, J. P., Miller, A. R., Blanco, M. A., Lipsitz, S. R., Dubroff, R. P., . . . Katz, J. T. (2008). Formal art observation training improves medical students' visual diagnostic skills. *Journal of General Internal Medicine, 23*(7), 991–997.

National POLST Paradigm. (n.d.). What is POLST? Retrieved from http://polst.org/about-the-national-polst-paradigm/what-is-polst

Parkhurst, D. C. (2015). A call for transformation in physician assistant education. *Journal of Physician Assistant Education, 26*(2), 101–105.

Perry, M., Maffulli, N., Willson, S., & Morrissey, D. (2011). The effectiveness of arts-based interventions in medical education: A literature review. *Medical Education, 45*(2), 141–148.

Robinson, K. (2010, February). *Bring on the learning revolution!* Lecture presented at TED2010. Retrieved from http://www.ted.com/talks/sir_ken_robinson_bring_on_the_revolution

Sackett, D. L., Richardson, W. S., Rosenberg, W., & Haynes, R. B. (1997). *Evidence-based medicine: How to practice and teach EBM.* New York, NY: Churchill Livingstone.

Schwartz, A. W., Abramson, J. S., Wojnowich, I., Accordino, R., Ronan, E. J., & Rifkin, M. R. (2009). Evaluating the impact of the humanities in medical education. *Mount Sinai Journal of Medicine: A Journal of Translational and Personalized Medicine, 76*(4), 372–380.

Shapiro, J., Rucker, L., & Beck, J. (2006). Training the clinical eye and mind: Using the arts to develop medical students' observational and pattern recognition skills. *Medical Education, 40*(3), 263–268.

Weimer, M. (2002). *Learner-centered teaching: Five key changes to practice.* San Francisco, CA: Jossey-Bass.

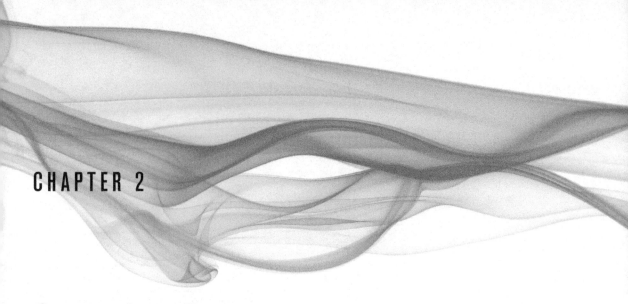

CHAPTER 2

Curriculum Design

Holly West, Camille Termini Loftin, and Clifford L. Snyder

CHAPTER OBJECTIVES

- Conceptualize, develop, and refine a curriculum, including using strategies such as longitudinal and vertical curricular integration
- Apply Bloom's taxonomy in curriculum development and in writing course and instructional objectives
- Create syllabi and develop assessment tools that clearly communicate and measure learning outcomes

---

As educators, we are only as effective as what we know. If we have no working knowledge of what students studied in previous years, how can we build on their learning? If we have no insight into the curriculum in later grades, how can we prepare learners for future classes?

—*Heidi Hayes Jacobs*

Anyone involved in the education of health professions students understands why the term *curriculum* was derived from the Latin word *currere* meaning to run/to proceed or to race a course. Providing a uniform definition of what the term *curriculum* actually means is difficult. Some refer to a curriculum as a subset of courses, others view it as an overall concept of what is being taught or learned, and many view it simply as a period of time or number of credit hours. To complicate matters further, curricula are often described with additional terms such as *hidden*, *horizontal versus vertical*, or *integrated*. One of the adaptable descriptions is provided by David Prideaux (2003), who states that "the curriculum represents the expression of educational ideas in practice" (p. 268). In simplistic terms, a curriculum serves to outline *a plan* (Toombs & Teirney, 1993) of educational goals and how those goals will be achieved. The word *plan* is italicized because most educators and research indicate that there are unplanned components of any curriculum as well.

The act of structuring and sequencing the curriculum elements is the *design* aspect, and it is both art and science. The beneficiaries of a well-designed curriculum are students, faculty, other stakeholders, the profession as a whole, and society. Ultimately, the quality of health care is largely dependent on a solid educational foundation.

ELEMENTS OF CURRICULA

The challenges of designing or revising a curriculum can be overwhelming. There is no "cookbook" for designing curricula, although there are guides or models. Commonly, educators focus very narrowly on the individual components (i.e., courses) and forget about the larger picture or the varied perspectives of different stakeholders. Therefore, it is important to remember the following elements of a curriculum: (a) educational content, (b) teaching and learning strategies, (c) assessment processes, and (d) evaluations (Prideaux, 2003). These elements must be considered throughout the design process and woven together into an effective curriculum. For example, the content affects delivery, which affects assessment, and so on. In fact, constructing curriculum maps (see Chapter 4) is a method of demonstrating how these elements are indeed interconnected.

MODELS OF CURRICULA

In 1910, the Carnegie Foundation for the Advancement of Teaching published Abraham Flexner's review of 155 medical schools in the United States and Canada (Cooke, Irby, Sullivan, & Ludmerer, 2006). Referred to as the "Flexner Report," it described the "2 + 2" curriculum standard used in medical education. Following 2 years of emphasis in basic science concepts, students go on to complete 2 years of clinical education. Although this curriculum is popular, decades of use demonstrated the fragmented nature of this curriculum in which a separation exists between basic science and clinical practice. A *New England Journal of Medicine* article in 2006 (Cooke et al., 2006) reviewed and summarized medical education since the Flexner Report, stating the inadequacies of a fragmented curriculum and describing the need for "fundamental restructuring of medical education" (Cooke et al., 2006, p. 1343).

This was the evolution of the model called the *integrated curriculum*, which was designed to improve connections between basic science and clinical science to retain knowledge and develop clinical skills (Brauer & Ferguson, 2015). Pedagogical models reflecting this integration include problem-based learning (PBL) or the use of case studies, skills labs and simulations, team-based learning, and capstone projects (Schwartz et al., 2014). This integration within a curriculum can occur horizontally, vertically, or spirally.

- Horizontal integration connects or combines disciplines within the same educational level. Material is organized over a finite time, not necessarily throughout the entire curriculum. An example might involve connecting concepts from different courses during a semester using PBL.
- Vertical integration encompasses progressive integration over the length of the program to improve knowledge and skills. Moving from one level to the next typically encompasses the entire duration of a curriculum or program.
- Spiral integration is a hybrid model with increasing complexity at various stages (Schwartz et al., 2014). Students learn the anatomy and pathophysiology of the heart in one course, learn normal findings followed by "abnormals" in another, and then hear both normal and abnormal sounds in a patient (or simulator). Progressing into the next phase (i.e., clinical

rotations) would require students to identify an abnormal finding, which leads to clinical decisions and treatment plans, all the while reflecting on the science behind the clinical component. One of the keys to the spiral integration model is that the widest part of the spiral (imagine a tornado) focuses on the domains of Bloom's taxonomy (Bloom, 1956), including knowledge, skills, and attitudes (Brauer & Ferguson, 2015), so that these domains remain a focus throughout (see "Forming Instructional Objectives" and "Syllabi").

The "hidden curriculum refers to the unspoken or implicit values, behaviors, and norms that exist in the education setting" (Alsubaie, 2015, p. 125). It is important to be aware of the hidden curriculum, as it can have both positive and negative consequences. Dewey (1938) first described the hidden curriculum in *Experience and Education*, "Perhaps the greatest of all pedagogical fallacies is the notion that a person learns only the particular thing he is studying at the time. Collateral learning in the way of formation of enduring attitudes, of likes and dislikes, may be and often is much more important than the spelling lesson or lesson in geography or history that is learned" (p. 20). Nearly a century later, the hidden curriculum is still an important factor in the socialization of health professions students (Chen, 2015; Martimianakis & Hafferty, 2016). It is beyond the scope of this chapter to explore the hidden curriculum in detail. However, readers are cautioned to cultivate awareness of and consider this unintentional curriculum as they develop the curriculum. It can be used to positive advantage, or may have negative consequences (Alsubaie, 2015; Martimianakis & Hafferty, 2016).

THE CURRICULUM DESIGN PROCESS

Curriculum design should be approached in a systematic manner, with the end goals in mind throughout the process. One of the most commonly used models among the variety of approaches is the "ADDIE Model." This model, first published in 1975 by the U.S. Department of Defense to aid in military training, was then applied to both industry and education (Battles, 2006). The model has five phases, originally conceived to progress in a stepwise fashion: analysis, design, development, implementation, and evaluation. The model, as shown in Figure 2.1, has now developed into a more dynamic structure in which phases are interconnected.

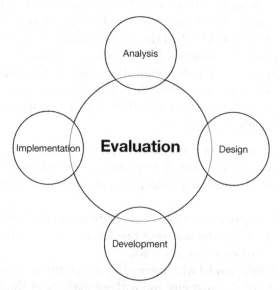

FIGURE 2.1 The ADDIE Model of curriculum design.
ADDIE, analysis, design, development, implementation, and evaluation.

Analysis

Analysis focuses on obtaining and gathering information necessary to design an effective curriculum. This phase is often hurried and taken for granted, but it is critical to determining how to move forward. Factors to consider during this phase include current and future needs, target audience, goals and outcomes of the curriculum, accreditation standards, and logistics.

Needs Assessment

One of the most essential aspects of any design is a needs assessment, a systematic and ongoing process used to collect and evaluate data about what the end goals are and how these goals are currently being met or unmet. Conducting a needs assessment ensures that time and resources are utilized effectively during the planning process, and that energies are focused on appropriate outcomes. Initiating a needs assessment requires the gathering of both objective and subjective data. Consider surveying faculty and students, stakeholders, institutional leaders, and professionals in the field. Look for common themes or identify gaps that need to be addressed. A gap analysis can identify program and curriculum strengths as well as areas in need of improvement. Currently, curriculum mapping is one method used to determine gaps and overlaps in content (see Chapter 3).

Exploring comparable curriculum designs is helpful in the analysis phase. Evaluate similarities and differences, talk with other program leaders, and identify available resources that have proved to be effective or even validated. Identifying what has worked well and what has failed is an opportunity to collaborate with fellow educators. Keep in mind that evaluating another program provides a foundation of ideas, but the needs of your program are ultimately the deciding factor when making design decisions.

Target Audience

Learners, or the target audience, drive the curriculum design, thereby affecting delivery options, timelines, learning theories, and so forth. The level of education should guide the curriculum design and lead the planning process. Undergraduate students have different needs than do graduate students. You should also consider the entrance experience or prerequisite courses required of learners. If work experience or introductory courses are part of the admission requirements, then coursework could begin at a higher level. If work experience is not required, introductory courses should be offered early in the curriculum. Although developing knowledge requires students to adapt to different learning styles, considering these differences in the planning process can influence the success of the student.

Goals and Outcomes

Once a needs assessment is completed and the target audience has been identified, goals and outcomes are identified. A goal is a broad statement of what should be included in the curriculum; goals will eventually guide course design. Goals should be realistic, attainable, and measurable. Curriculum goals should align with program and institutional aspects, such as aim, vision, and mission statement. In addition, this is the time to identify the desired approach to learning, which may affect the curriculum structure. For instance, is it the goal to have a teacher-centered or a learner-centered framework (see Chapter 1)? If learner-centered, you may consider options such as PBL or outcome-based learning, for which there is supportive evidence (see Part II). Once the goals have been recognized, more specific learning objectives can be assigned to the curriculum and to specific courses.

Accreditation Standards

When revising or designing a new curriculum, it is important to keep accreditation standards in mind. Accreditation is a process that improves the quality and consistency of higher education, ensuring that standards are continually met. What are required elements of a curriculum according to the accrediting body? Are a certain number of clinical contact hours needed, or are collaborative and interprofessional opportunities required? Accreditation standards may even go as far as to mandate necessary resources, such as student support services and financial assistance personnel. Also, consider external standards that may be required for disciplines that may differ from your own. For instance, most health professionals are required to pass a national exam upon graduation, and these requirements will differ over disciplines.

Logistical Considerations

Understanding the many logistical considerations involved when designing a curriculum can help it reach its full potential. Investigate the availability of resources for every aspect of the curriculum, including the following factors:

- Institutional requirements such as class size, start dates, and end dates
- Classroom availability, size, and layout
- Technology resources for students and faculty, and the support/maintenance needed for infrastructure
- Faculty and instructor availability: teaching loads, compensation, or effort limitations
- Interdisciplinary needs: for instance, if medical and physician assistant (PA) students share rotations together, sequencing must align
- Preceptor and clinical site availability

Design

The design phase of the curriculum process starts focusing on the details of the curriculum. Not only do decisions regarding content, pedagogical theories, and assessment methods need to be discussed, but sequencing is also an important part of the design. Learning should flow in a way that promotes the building of concepts. Think about Bloom's (1956) taxonomy and the progression from memorization of concepts to critical thinking and problem solving. In other words, teach students to crawl before they walk, and walk before they run. Other design considerations include exploring the technological resources available to incorporate a variety of teaching methods, thereby reaching more learners (see Chapter 9). Tools to help visualize the design include curriculum maps, timelines, comparison tables of current versus proposed sequencing, and even storyboards.

In addition, enlisting feedback and critiques from others is important in this step. Use both internal and external reviewers, including those completely unfamiliar with the program. Consider including current and former students, professionals in the field, and even potential applicants, as members of each of these groups can offer valuable insight. Be sure to heed the requirements of curriculum review entities at the school, institution, state, and accrediting body levels.

Development

Fine-tuning the design into a deliverable "package" occurs in the development phase of curriculum design. This involves writing detailed learning objectives, constructing syllabi and rubrics, and developing summative and formative evaluations. This phase is best approached among the team using a shared mental model, meaning there is a shared understanding of the common goal at hand. Collaboration produces a cohesive curriculum that prevents gaping holes and conversely prevents redundancies (Thomas & Kern, 2004). Piloting a curriculum or even components of the curriculum is beneficial during the development phase. Testing a rubric, module, or exam will allow you to address any problems prior to wide-scale implementation. Piloting also helps plan logistical aspects such as timing, duration, and resources, thus minimizing unforeseen issues that might otherwise have occurred. For instance, an activity that you *envisioned* taking 1 hour may end up taking much longer, which would interfere with scheduling, resource allocation, and so on.

Implementation

Implementation refers to the delivery of a developed curriculum. Refer to your timeline often, and remember to evaluate this phase continually. Take the time to observe, collect quantitative and qualitative data, judge, and critique. Throughout the implementation process, use what you may witness yourself, and the feedback received from others. Encourage feedback from others (i.e., faculty, students, and preceptors), and receive it with enthusiasm and openness to constructive criticism. Challenges and mistakes will occur, which is why implementation is followed by an evaluation process that identifies what works well and what does not and thus permits quality improvement.

Evaluation

Evaluation determines the effectiveness of the curriculum, ensuring that goals and outcomes are being achieved. This phase is not a one-time occurrence, but instead a continual process. In fact, evaluation occurs throughout each of the five phases. What is working or even worked best? What needs further development or improvement? What lessons can be learned? Soliciting feedback can take various forms: Course leaders can be asked to complete self-assessment and course assessments, student feedback via surveys and focus groups is valuable and informative, and quantitative information about student success in meeting course and program milestones (e.g., examination scores, course pass rates, skill-testing results, and certification after graduation) is invaluable. All can be used to assess the effectiveness of learning activities, the courses they comprise, and the curriculum as a whole. Again, receive feedback constructively; multiple implementation cycles may be needed before everything is "fine-tuned" and streamlined, at which time new curricular innovations may be indicated. Often, trial and error is the only true means of achieving success, and what works for one group of students at a certain time will not always serve another group as well in a different time or context. See the online supplement for Chapter 2 for additional tips and a template for course evaluation.

FORMING INSTRUCTIONAL OBJECTIVES

As educators, we are tasked with developing, refining, and assessing goals and objectives. There is often confusion surrounding the difference between goals and objectives.

A *goal* is a comprehensive statement typically describing a primary outcome. Goals are often abstract and broad; and direct learners to the intended outcome of a course or activity. An example might be, "utilize clinical data in the management of medical conditions." Now, this would be challenging for a student to tackle without more specific direction! A *learning objective* provides a learner with an expected direction and the stepping stones for acquiring knowledge or skills (Boston University School of Medicine Faculty Development Program, 2004). Although

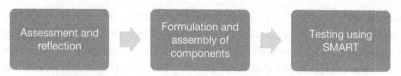

FIGURE 2.2 Steps to creating learning objectives.
SMART, specific, measurable, achievable, realistic, and time-bound.

we want our students to be self-driven and independent learners, objectives serve as a guide and define expectations in order to help them reach learning goals. You will also hear the term *instructional objective*, which focuses more on the instructor or the instructional curriculum. For instance, *in the problem-based learning case, the student will discuss a problem, identifying solutions . . .*

Developing learner or instructional objectives can be overwhelming for novice and experienced educators alike. Taking a stepwise approach may help break down the complexity (Figure 2.2).

Assessment and Reflection

The first step to developing objectives is to assess and reflect on (a) the overall goals of an activity, course, skill, and so on; (b) your learning audience; (c) Bloom's taxonomy; and (d) confounding factors.

Overall Goals

Start with the basics as objectives are derived from course goals. What is the title of this course, its course description, and goals? Stay within those constructs, keeping in mind that typically one course or activity is one piece of a much larger puzzle. Understanding the basic components helps determine how best to reach those goals using objectives.

Learning Audience

As previously mentioned, the target audience drives the curriculum design. Newly matriculated students are quite different from second- or third-year students. Distance learners may require alternative objectives than traditional in-class participants. Also remember that a given audience does not conform to one type of learning style; objectives should address a variety of styles to engage a diverse group.

Bloom's Taxonomy

The discussion of goals and objectives would be incomplete without a more detailed discussion of Bloom's taxonomy. Developed in 1956, Bloom's taxonomy is one of the most widely used classification standards and describes three learning domains: cognitive, affective, and psychomotor (Taylor & Hamdy, 2013).

- Cognitive domain: knowledge
- Affective domain: attitudes and feelings
- Psychomotor domain: manual skills

Within each of these domains are categories best described as parts of a hierarchy: a learner progresses from a lower level to a higher level of thinking over time. The *most basic level* is simple recall, whereas the *highest order level* is creating new or original work. Bloom's taxonomy has multiple variations and was even revised in the late 1990s to Bloom's taxonomy revised, or a taxonomy for learning, teaching, and assessing (Anderson et al., 2002). Figure 2.3 depicts the cognitive domain levels in Bloom's modified taxonomy. The nomenclature of the levels is in bold type; the former nomenclature is presented within parentheses. Table 2.1 provides examples of each cognitive domain as applied to the abdominal quadrants.

One role of the educator is to determine what levels a student should strive toward with the intent to build progressively by levels. Although the focus of this chapter is the cognitive domain, it is crucial for health professions educators to also include the affective and psychomotor domains. Taylor and Hamdy (2013) remind us that the practice of the health professions is related to attitudes such as lifelong learning, empathy, ethical decisions, and professionalism.

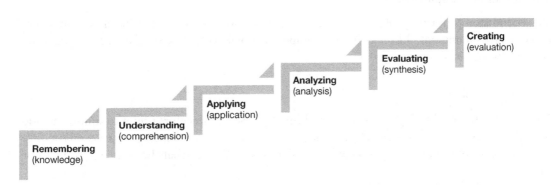

FIGURE 2.3 Bloom's modified taxonomy.

TABLE 2.1 Cognitive Domain Examples Using Bloom's Modified Taxonomy

Cognitive Level	Action Verbs	Example
Remembering Retrieve facts	Define, label, identify, name, order, recognize, recall, list, state	*Label* the quadrants of the abdomen on a diagram.
Understanding Explain concepts	Classify, describe, discuss, explain, indicate, compare, recognize, report, review, select, translate, summarize	*Describe* the components of the abdominal physical exam.
Applying Carry out or use information	Apply, choose, demonstrate, employ, illustrate, interpret, practice, perform, solve, use, execute, implement	*Perform* a focused abdominal exam in a patient presenting with right lower quadrant abdominal pain.
Analyzing Connect	Analyze, appraise, calculate, categorize, diagram, differentiate, discriminate, organize, distinguish, question	*Distinguish* between clinical exam findings associated with nonemergent abdominal pain versus acute abdomen.
Evaluating Justify	Arrange, assemble, collect, compose, construct, create, design, formulate, manage, organize, plan, prepare, propose, write, critique	*Formulate* a diagnostic plan for a patient with acute right lower quadrant pain.
Creating Produce	Argue, assess, choose, defend, estimate, judge, predict, rate, score, present, select, support, value, evaluate, generate, produce	*Present and defend* your assessment and treatment plan to your preceptor.

Confounding Factors

Do not overlook factors that may impede the creation of objectives. Have you ever written 50 objectives for a topic only to realize that those objectives cover one of 20 units in your two-unit semester course? Remember that if your objectives are serving as a guide for students, each needs to reflect your expectations of time and depth. Other factors to consider include resources available to you (as the instructor) and to your students. Objectives need to align to the recommended and required resources (e.g., textbook and manuals). Furthermore, are there resources to support your objective? For example, if you have an objective such as, *perform an intravenous catheter insertion using a simulated manikin arm*, is such a mannequin available for instruction, practice, and demonstration of the acquired skill?

Formulation of Components

The second step to forming objectives is to formulate and assemble the different components of an objective statement. Three common components of an objective statement are (a) *audience and time*, (b) *action*, and (c) *description*.

Audience and Time

Identify your intended audience and expected timeline. Some educators prefer to simply include the audience and time together: *By the end of this course, first-year nursing students will be able to. . . .* This is followed by the numbered or bulleted objectives so that the audience/time is not repeated.

Action

Identify the expected performance (via an action verb) keeping the cognitive level in mind.

Description

Specifically describe the expected action. This requires balancing too little information with too much information. Your goal is to guide students but not spoon-feed them. For example, *label the quadrants of the abdomen on a diagram* is more appropriate than *label the four quadrants of the abdomen, including the right upper, right lower, left upper, and left lower quadrants*. Table 2.1 provides action verbs and an example of a learning objective for each cognitive level.

Testing Objectives

The final step is to test your objective(s) to ensure that they are meaningful. A simple method for testing meaningfulness is to use the SMART acronym (Jung, 2007). Meaningful, SMART objectives are specific, measurable, achievable, realistic, and time-bound. See the online supplement for additional tips and a template for writing SMART objectives.

Specific

This is not the time to be vague and leave room for interpretation—be clear. Also remember that objectives are not "asked" as a question and do not end with a question mark. You can begin with an action verb and follow with descriptive content. Attempt to limit one concept per objective. If the word *and* connects two major parts of an objective, it might be better to split that objective into two objectives.

Measurable

Can you measure or assess the objective once achieved? Avoid verbs such as *know*, *understand*, and *comprehend*, which are difficult to measure. For example, this objective might be difficult to assess: *Understand the workup of abnormal uterine bleeding*. Consider rewriting to *present orally to a peer the appropriate evaluation of a postmenopausal patient with abnormal uterine bleeding*. Also remember that if you take the time to write objectives and students take the time to follow them, then students should be assessed and evaluated on those objectives. Examination questions, for instance, should be connected or linked to the concept of a written objective.

Achievable and Realistic

As discussed previously, objectives need to be achievable and realistic from both the instructor's and student's perspectives. Would we expect a student early in the training program to perform a complex procedure on an actual patient? Consider your developmental timeline and try not to set students up for failure. When you are realistic, you become aware of time and resources. If you write the objective, *assist the interventional cardiologist in a cardiac catheterization procedure*, and there is no means to do this (i.e., the hospital does not have a cardiac catheterization laboratory), the objective is not very realistic.

Time-Bound

Learners need clear expectations, and one of the important boundaries is time. This is typically accomplished by using the statement, *by the end of this unit, the student should be able to. . . .* This also reminds us to be cognizant of time in the sense of development. There is a reason why learning is progressive.

Evaluation and Refinement

Objectives should be reevaluated regularly. Suggested time points include immediately following course completion or prior to course submission for the year. Just as your course, text, and activities may change from year to year, your objectives should follow suit. Program accreditation review provides an additional opportunity for reevaluating learning objectives.

SYLLABI

Syllabi serve as a transparent means of communicating educator expectations to the learner. Educators should first consider any requirements for syllabi in the form of templates, accreditation statements, and so forth. Typically, there are departmental or school policies regarding amending or changing a syllabus once distributed. Thus, clarity and completeness are critical. After all, the syllabus communicates expectations and can be likened to a contract between the educator and the learner (Johnson, 2006). Syllabus formats vary widely, and they commonly contain the following components:

- **Course specifics:** Name and number, dates/times/location, description, and goals
- **Instructor specifics:** Name(s), role(s), and contact information; include how and when students can meet instructors or discuss issues
- **Required and recommended resources:** Texts, software, supplies, equipment, web resources, and so on
- **Plan:** Consider including a chart or outline of the schedule, dates, activities, preclass resources, in-class activities, and important milestones or due dates; learning objectives

can be embedded within the schedule or provided in combined fashion at the end of the syllabus; if applicable, consider including a statement such as *this schedule could change based on guest lecturer availability or unforeseen events*

- **Policies:** Attendance, lateness, late submissions, penalties, and remediation if available, and Title IX requirements (notice of nondiscrimination)
- **Evaluation and assessment:** Grading policies, procedures, and weight
  - Examinations: number, type, and timing parameters
  - Descriptions of assessments, rubrics
  - Rounding and curving
  - Special accommodations during testing
- **Classroom etiquette:** This may differ from general program requirements (e.g., you expect all cell phones to be left out of the anatomy lab)

CONCLUSIONS

Curricular development is the mechanism by which we express educational ideas in practice (Prideaux, 2003). Careful curriculum design is both art and science, and considers both the explicit and hidden curriculum. A well-designed curriculum benefits students, faculty, and other stakeholders such as the educational institution and accrediting bodies. Ultimately, the quality of health care is dependent on a solid educational foundation.

REFERENCES

Alsubaie, M. A. (2015). Hidden curriculum as one of current issue of curriculum. *Journal of Education and Practice, 6*(33), 125–128.

Anderson, L. W., Krathwohl, D. R., Airasian, P., Cruikshank, K., Mayer, R., Pintrich, P., . . . Wittrock, M. (2001). A taxonomy for learning, teaching and assessing: A revision of Bloom's taxonomy. New York, NY: Longman.

Artz, A. F., & Armour-Thomas, E. (1992). Development of a cognitive-metacognitive framework for protocol analysis of mathematical problem solving in small groups. *Cognition and Instruction, 9*(2), 137–175.

Battles, J. B. (2006). Improving patient safety by instructional systems design. *Quality & Safety in Health Care, 15*(Suppl. 1), i25–i29. doi:10.1136/qshc.2005.015917

Brauer, D. G., & Ferguson, K. J. (2015). The integrated curriculum in medical education. AMEE Guide No. 96. *Medical Teacher, 37*(4), 312–322. doi:10.3109/0142159X.2014.970998

Bloom, B. S. (1956). *Taxonomy of educational objectives: The classification of educational goals* (Vol. 1, pp. 20–24). New York, NY: McKay.

Boston University School of Medicine Faculty Development Program. (2004). Writing learning objectives [PowerPoint slides]. Retrieved from http://www.bumc.bu.edu/facdev-medicine/files/2012/03/Writing LearningObjectivesWebFD.pdf

Chen, R. (2015). The hidden curriculum in nursing education. *Canadian Journal of Nursing Research, 47*(3), 7–17.

Cooke, M., Irby, D. M., Sullivan, W., & Ludmerer, K. M. (2006). American medical education 100 years after the Flexner report. *New England Journal of Medicine, 355*(13), 1339–1344. doi:10.1056/NEJMra055445

Dewey, J. (1938). *Experience and education.* Indianapolis, IN: Kappa Delta Pi.

Flexner, A. (1910). *The Flexner report on medical education in the United States and Canada* (p. 58). New York, NY: Carnegie Foundation.

Jung, L. A. (2007). Writing SMART objectives and strategies that fit the ROUTINE. *Teaching Exceptional Children 39*(4), 54–58.

Johnson, C. (2006). Best practices in syllabus writing: Contents of a learner-centered syllabus. *Journal of Chiropractic Education, 20*(2), 139–144. Retrieved from https://www.ncbi.nlm.nih.gov/pmc/articles/PMC2384173/pdf/JCE-20-2-139.pdf

Martimianakis, M. A., & Hafferty, F. W. (2016). Exploring the interstitial space between the ideal and the practised: Humanism and the hidden curriculum of system reform. *Medical Education, 50*(3), 278–280.

Prideaux, D. (2003). ABC of learning and teaching in medicine: Curriculum design. *British Medical Journal, 326*(7383), 268.

Schwartz, A. H., Daugherty, K. K., O'Neil, C. K., Smith, L., Poirier, T. I., . . . Henriksen, J. A. (2014). A curriculum committee toolkit for addressing the 2013 CAPE outcomes. Retrieved from http://www .aacp.org/resources/education/cape/Documents/CurriculumSIGCAPEPaperFinalNov2014.pdf

Taylor, D. C. M., & Hamdy, H. (2013. Adult learning theories: Implications for learning and teaching in medical education: AMEE Guide No. 83. *Medical Teacher, 35*(11), e1561–e1572. doi:10.3109/01421 59X.2013.828153

Thomas, P. A., & Kern, D. E. (2004). Internet resources for curriculum development in medical education: An annotated bibliography. *Journal of General Internal Medicine, 19*(5, Pt. 2), 599–605. doi:10.1111/j .1525-1497.2004.99999.x

Toombs, W. E., & Teirney, W. G. (1993). Curriculum definitions and reference points. *Journal of Curriculum and Supervision, 8*(3), 175–195. Retrieved from http://www.ascd.org/publications/jcs/spring1993/ Curriculum-Definitions-and-Reference-Points.aspx

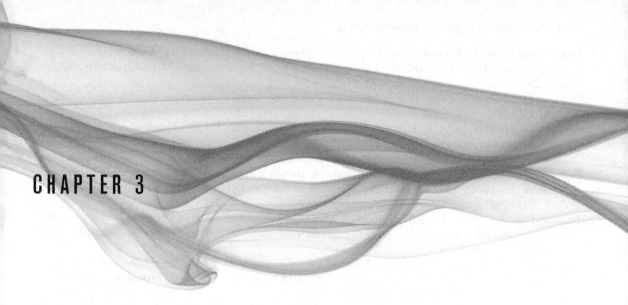

CHAPTER 3

Competencies and Milestones
Mary L. Warner

CHAPTER OBJECTIVES

- Explain key professional competencies and develop milestones for achievement during the clinical program
- Outline, develop and align competencies and milestones to program and professional goals
- Develop and use entrustable professional activities (EPAs) in health professions education

---

Quality is never an accident, it is always the result of high intention, sincere effort, intelligent direction and skillful execution; it represents the wise choice of many alternatives.

—Willa A. Foster

Perhaps the most significant paradigm shift in health professions education in the past century has been the move from curricula constrained by time and professors' desires to curricula based on learner outcomes. This approach to clinical education shifts responsibility for learning to the learners, who are expected to master minimum outcomes and who may do so at differing rates.

Renewed focus on competencies and outcomes in medical education resulted from a 1984 incident in which college freshman Libby Zion died after she was given a medication ordered by an overworked medical resident. After lawsuits ensued and were settled, sleep deprivation was identified as a major factor associated with the error, and New York State developed resident work-hour restrictions in 1987. This case forced policy makers to examine the safety of medical care provided in the United States, prompting the Institute of Medicine to publish *To Err Is Human* in 1999 (Donaldson, Corrigan, & Kohn, 2000). By the early 2000s, the Accreditation Council for Graduate Medical Education (ACGME) adopted resident competencies as the major

TABLE 3.1 A Comparison of Traditional and Competency-Based Curricula

	Traditional	Competency-Based
Focus of curriculum	Content	Outcome
Content delivery	Professor	Professor and learner
Course goals	Acquisition of facts	Knowledge application
Evaluation method	Single exam	Multiple assessments related to outcomes development

feature of the Outcomes Project (Swing, 2007) and adopted resident work-hour restrictions nationwide (ACGME and American Board of Medical Specialties, 1999). These competencies identify competence standards of the graduating resident. Taken together, the work-hour restrictions and the focus on learner quality outcomes are two major initiatives intended to improve quality of care and patient safety.

Parallel professional competencies developed in nursing when the National Organization of Nurse Practitioner Faculties (NONPF) developed and refined practice competencies for nurse practitioner (NP) graduates (NONPF, 2002). The four organizations of the physician assistant (PA) profession—American Academy of Physician Assistants (AAPA), Accreditation Review Commission on Education for the Physician Assistant (ARC-PA), Physician Assistant Education Association (PAEA), and National Commission on Certification of Physician Assistants (NCCPA)—adapted the ACGME Core Competencies to the PA profession initially in 2005 (AAPA, ARC-PA, PAEA, & NCCPA, 2012). In contrast to documents developed by nursing and medicine, *Competencies for the Physician Assistant Profession* outlines competencies of practicing PAs rather than merely those expected of new PA graduates. One of the competencies of a PA is "demonstrate commitment to excellent and ongoing professional development" (AAPA, 2005, p. 3). Although new graduates are likely interested in pursuing this competency, at the time of graduation they lack adequate experience in clinical practice to achieve it.

The evolution from traditional time and content-focused curricula to competency-based education has gained increasing favor in the past decade. Traditional curricula structured around a defined time course for all learners adopted learning goals and objectives in the latter third of the 20th century. The time required for medical training has increased since the Flexner Report (1910) because both the focus on foundational medical sciences (and their relationship to advances in molecular therapies) and clinical specialization in medicine require a broader foundation of knowledge. In the early 1970s, PA programs were 18 months in length; now the average length of this graduate degree program is more than 26 months (PAEA, 2016). Table 3.1 highlights the differences between traditional curricula and competency-based curricula (Weinberger, Pereira, Iobst, Mechaber, & Bronze, 2010). Traditional curricula impart knowledge to learners, whereas competency-based curricula evaluate learner synthesis and application of knowledge.

COMPETENCIES

For the purposes of this discussion, *competencies* are profession-specific skills or abilities. Competencies define specific behaviors that learners (and clinicians) must demonstrate when faced in various clinical encounters. Competencies represent minimum expected behaviors rather than exemplary outcomes attained by master clinicians. The term *competent* denotes that an individual has mastered one or more competencies. *Competence* is the ability to do something well;

individuals known to have competence consistently practice in a competent manner (By permission. From Merriam-Webster's Collegiate® Dictionary, 11th Edition ©2017 by Merriam-Webster, Inc. [www.Merriam-Webster.com]).

Consider this example: A common competency for a graduate-level, health professions student is to *efficiently gather an accurate patient history of present illness*. Mastery of the competency of history taking includes foundational knowledge of four elements: (a) the pathophysiology of disease and the corresponding illness scripts, (b) when to take a history and when it should not be taken, (c) ways to engage a patient to successfully gather accurate history information, and (d) the rationale for gathering a history and the anticipated potential outcomes as a result of the skill. However, knowledge of these four elements does *not* confirm that one is competent at gathering a patient's history of illness. Mastery of this competency, which is known as *competence*, requires that practitioners obtain an accurate patient history during every patient encounter. This example demonstrates that knowledge is a key ingredient for mastering a competency, but knowledge alone is not sufficient. In the traditional model of education, a student's knowledge is valued as the most important commodity, but the student's application of knowledge is not the focus and, as a result, is not always evaluated.

Beyond knowledge, other skills are needed to become competent in performing a task. Successful history taking doubtlessly requires practice to improve organization and efficiency of the encounter. New learners often struggle with guiding the patient using open-ended questioning and balancing time constraints. In the first patient interview that requires answers to social history questions that are considered socially unacceptable in conversation with strangers, the learner's voice may change inflection or the learner's neck may turn red. As experience is gained, this personal line of questioning becomes easier, and the learner's confidence builds. Time management and self-confidence are important for successful interviewing, but are only learned with experience.

Finally, as history-taking experience is gained, the experienced learner has the opportunity to reflect on successful and unsuccessful patient visits. Competent clinicians use their emotional intelligence to detect a patient's reaction to questions as a guide to the next steps. For example, a novice learner may be flummoxed by the disclosure that a patient who drinks 12 to 24 bottles of beer per day also has a history of physical abuse by his uncle. Seasoned clinicians employ their experience, remember and control their own biases, and focus on the patient's emotional needs in the moment; competent clinicians reflect on the encounter and adjust their practice through self-improvement to achieve competence.

Developing Competencies

Developing competencies for an educational program requires clarity about specific program aims (Antman et al., 2016; Slonim, Wheeler, Quinlan, & Smith, 2010). Program goals or program learning outcomes must guide the program competencies that are taught and measured. If a program goal is "effectively use a patient-centered approach in the clinical encounter to gather an accurate medical history and perform a physical examination," then consideration of measurable competencies must be developed. A few competencies that must be mastered to achieve this specific program goal might include (a) utilize patient-centered interviewing techniques as measured by the Master Interview Rating Scale (2013), (b) obtain and document an accurate medical history using the outline of the problem-oriented medical record, and (c) perform the complete physical examination and interpret abnormal exam findings. Note that these three competencies are action-oriented, measurable, and in some instances describe the specific method the learner is expected to use to demonstrate competence. Developing program-specific competencies requires contemplation of program goals and outcomes, coupled with the knowledge and skills clinicians need for safe and effective practice.

A program that has as its goal to "educate clinicians to provide care to patients from diverse backgrounds" must provide instruction about the impact of culture on health beliefs, definitions of *wellness*, and social determinants of health. To become proficient or competent at caring for patients from different backgrounds, students must also engage in multiple clinical encounters with patients from different races, ethnicities, religions, gender identities, and socioeconomic statuses. Successful competency development requires instruction that imparts knowledge and relevant clinical experiences.

Specific competencies related to the program goal of educating clinicians to provide care to a diverse patient population require learners to (a) apply adequate knowledge of health beliefs, varying definitions of wellness, and social determinants of health; (b) use proper techniques for completing a patient-centered history and physical exam; (c) use interpreter services; (d) use draping properly; (e) document clinical care of patients from diverse cultural backgrounds; and (f) document clinical care of patients from different socioeconomic backgrounds. These competencies are evaluated by faculty and preceptors based on direct observations of learners. Figure 3.1 depicts the relationship among educational goals, competencies, and measures of competency.

Competencies frame minimum expectations of learner performance in concrete terms. By their nature, competencies increase the transparency of educational outcomes, and by proxy that of professors' expectations. A student who has previous clinical experience as a paramedic, for example, may have baseline skills (knowledge and experience) related to managing hemodynamic instability. Using a competency-based approach, this paramedic may require less instruction

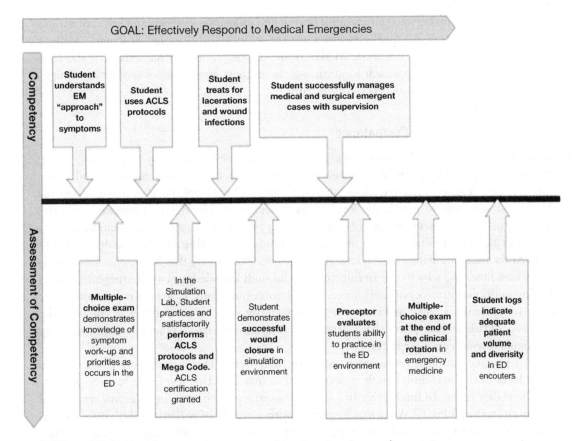

FIGURE 3.1 Relationship among program goals, competencies, and competency assessment.

ACLS, advanced cardiac life support; ED, emergency department; EM, emergency medicine.

and/or experience to demonstrate proficiency stabilizing the vital signs of a critically ill patient. Competency-based education is thus student centered—it allows students flexibility to move through the curriculum at different rates—and is focused on measurable outcomes rather than on curriculum content or faculty-centered learning objectives.

MILESTONES

Although competencies represent clear, measurable expectations of learners, they do not indicate how learners become competent. Milestones address expectations of *when* and *how* learners should demonstrate proficiency of a competency, or at least a specific element of the competency. Milestones are equally useful to professors and students because they acknowledge that most clinical competencies are not mastered on the first attempt, and that more often than not the practice of skills is needed over time. Individual milestones may be associated with multiple competencies, but all milestones are task specific.

An early milestone relating to competence of effective wound closure is "repairing dermis injured from a linear laceration using local anesthesia and simple interrupted sutures." In contrast, a more advanced milestone is "closing a complex surgical incision that includes approximation of fascia, subcutaneous tissue, and dermis." New learners who have experience closing dermal lacerations will build on their suturing expertise using simple interrupted sutures to add figure of 8, buried, and/or mattress sutures to their skill set. Beyond learning the new suture techniques, understanding the characteristics of the underlying tissue to be closed as well as the different types of suture material available makes the closure of complex wounds more challenging. This example illustrates the importance of milestone specificity to the outcome to be assessed, the relationship between curriculum timing and milestone mastery, and how milestones may relate to one another. Clinical educators use two common milestones schemata: Miller's pyramid of clinical competence and the RIME Model (reporter, interpreter, manager, and educator). Both use a stepwise approach to attaining the highest level of achievement or competence, with increasing expertise as the core feature.

Miller's Pyramid of Clinical Competence

Miller's pyramid of clinical competence (also called *Miller's pyramid of clinical assessment*) describes four sequential levels of achievement requisite for competency mastery, and it ties assessment of the learner skills to each step (Miller, 1990). This model specifies that assessments of clinical learners should match the level of their expertise. Milestones associated with the competency of "using patient-centered communication techniques to gather an accurate history and perform a physical examination" include communicating with patients who do not speak English. At the foundational (or *knows*) level, the milestone will ensure that the learner has knowledge of when, how, and why to use an interpreter, and such knowledge is most efficiently examined using multiple-choice examinations or short-answer questions. Learners move to the next level of the pyramid, known as *knows how*, by practicing with an interpreter at the bedside; achievement of this level requires that learners use their knowledge to practice communicating with patients through an interpreter.

Once a learner develops proficiency using an interpreter, the competency is assessed in the next level of the pyramid, which is designated as *shows*. In this level, the learner demonstrates the ability to use an interpreter in a simulated setting, such as in an objective structured clinical examination (OSCE). After much practice with a variety of patients and illnesses, learners achieve the *does* level, in which they use interpreters effectively in all situations in which they are required. Learner evaluation of this highest level is only possible through direct observation of learners using an interpreter repeatedly during clinical rounds (Table 3.2). Because Miller's

TABLE 3.2 Clinical Competence and Assessment

Miller's Learner Competence Level	Description of the Competence Level	Appropriate Assessment Strategies
Knows (lowest level of competence)	Learners have knowledge of when and why a particular intervention is required; learners may have learned about the skills but have not practiced them	Multiple-choice questions, essays
Knows how	Learners demonstrate success at practicing the skill, even if mastery has not yet been achieved	Multiple-choice questions, essays, oral examination
Shows	Learners show they have mastered the skill in simulated environments	Simulated assessment, OSCE, or simple bedside assessment
Does (highest level of competence)	Learners demonstrate consistent effectiveness in using the proper skill techniques in clinically appropriate situations	In situ holistic evaluation of clinical behaviors

OSCE, objective structured clinical examination.
Source: Adapted from Miller (1990).

pyramid schema primarily focuses on knowledge and skills assessments, it helps educators to ensure that clinical knowledge learners acquire is eventually applied appropriately to clinical situations.

The RIME Model

The RIME (recorder, interpreter, manager, and expert) Model utilizes a different developmental approach to clinical skills milestones (Pangaro, 1999; Sepdham, Julka, Hofmann, & Dobbie, 2007). This model conceptualizes clinical milestones as they relate to the development of clinical acumen in clinical context. This paradigm highlights that knowing how to treat a patient with pneumonia, for example, does not presume that the learner understands the intricacies or context of treating the patient lying there who has a lung infection. The RIME Model recognizes that real patient encounters require the learner to use complex clinical reasoning skills to determine whether to prescribe a macrolide alone or combination therapy; in this scenario, context considerations include comorbid illnesses, patient age, and overall renal and/or hepatic function.

A novice "clinician," or *recorder*, becomes competent in documenting an accurate medical history, a physical examination, and diagnostic data, but is unlikely to have the experience to understand the significance of the data gathered. Effective recorders apply their knowledge of anatomy, physiology, and the medical record to document the normal and abnormal findings in the patient. The second phase of the model, known as *interpreter*, involves analyzing subjective and objective findings, diagnostic test results, and formulating a differential diagnosis. *Interpreters* must organize the data, compare and contrast them with known illness scripts, and synthesize them into a list of differential diagnoses. Interpretation is a multistep, complex skill that is only mastered with time and practice.

A *manager* is a clinician who accurately gathers patient data, interprets the clinical presentation as a whole, formulates the most likely diagnosis, and develops a patient-centered treatment plan. Recognition that the most likely diagnosis may not be responding to the therapy as expected or that the patient is suffering from a comorbidity is also required of effective managers. In both scenarios, the manager may be forced to collect more information, review the data and clinical workup to date, and revise the working diagnosis or the treatment plan. Clinicians who reach the manager level are competent to safely care for patients within their scope of practice.

Similar to Miller's pyramid, the RIME Model has an *expert* or educator level. At this level, clinicians are expected to profess what they know and to mentor students and other clinicians. RIME is based on medical education pedagogy, and its straightforward framework highlights the concepts of milestones.

Developing Milestones

Although milestones are useful to learners and instructors when several intermediate steps must be mastered in order to be competent, they have limitations. Consider the competency of placing an intravenous catheter. Either a learner demonstrates competency placing the catheter, or the learner fails to do so. Although this skill doubtlessly requires practice for consistent success, once the learner practices the single skill enough, there are no additional steps that must be mastered before the learner is labeled as competent. There is limited benefit in applying the milestone paradigm to a competency that does not involve stepwise skill development. A second limitation of milestones is that they often focus attention on the baseline achievement of all students. Naturally, focusing on the minimum level of competence rather than exceptional performance fails to acknowledge students who have excelled in developing clinical acumen. Nevertheless, milestones ensure that all students meet the minimum requirements for safe and effective practice, and they help learners take ownership of their learning. Table 3.3 illustrates how milestones might be used to guide student learning by clarifying the timing of instructors' expectations.

Because milestones are stepwise intervals that correlate with increasing levels of knowledge and experience, many milestones are mastered over the course of the educational program until professional competence is achieved. To be successful, milestones must have clear outcome measures that relate to the mastery of at least one competency. Milestones are developed with consideration of both the timeline for instruction and the paradigm used for assessment, whether Miller's pyramid or the RIME Model. The time frames for meeting individual milestones depend

TABLE 3.3 Clinical Skill Development Milestones (PA Student Example)

Competency	Instruction and Practice	Time Milestone Achieved
Obtain a complete and accurate medical history	Didactic phase: first semester in lab, first semester with standardized patients, second- and third-semester clinical sessions	Beginning of second year or clinical phase
Obtain a focused and accurate medical history	Clinical phase: full-time clinical rotations	After 10 months of clinical rotations
Suture a simple laceration	Didactic phase: first semester anatomy lab, transition month suture labs, sterile technique lab Clinical phase: ED rotation, OB-GYN, general surgery, family medicine, and surgical electives	Interim didactic attainment noted on suture model; final milestone achievement by graduation
Interpret diagnostic testing	Didactic phase: clinical medicine course, practicum courses, seminar sessions Clinical phase: full-time clinical rotations	Interim didactic attainment noted during case presentations; final milestone achievement by graduation

ED, emergency department; PA, physician assistant.

on the complexity of the competency; complex competencies generally require more milestones and shorter time frames because competence is harder to achieve. As Table 3.3 indicates, some competencies lend themselves to interim milestones, whereas others do not. Finally, faculty should consider which milestone deadlines must be met in order for the learner to progress to the next educational phase in the program. As discrete units of time and behaviors, milestones help the learner develop clinical competence in a gradual and progressive manner.

ENTRUSTABLE PROFESSIONAL ACTIVITES

The concept of EPAs has been developed as a means to translate competencies into concrete elements of clinical practice. Once a student has achieved certain milestones and is deemed competent to perform a particular task, EPAs indicate that that student should be entrusted with performing it. Initially, as PA education developed in the Netherlands, EPAs were used in the clinical portions of the curriculum to delineate the responsibilities of the PA, to ensure high-quality and safe clinical education, and to identify the scope of practice of all PAs regardless of clinical setting (Mulder, Ten Cate, Daalder, & Berkvens, 2010). Entrustability occurs when learners or practicing clinicians can be trusted to perform a specific clinical activity safely, have an understanding of their own limitations, and know when to ask for help. Professional activities that can be entrusted are specific to a profession and/or to a specialty and are derived from multiple competencies required during formal education. When a student or clinician has demonstrated mastery of an EPA, the supervision required is, by definition, limited to "from a distance or postevent" only.

EPAs include activity descriptions that provide clarity to learners and faculty, specific competencies to be measured, expectations of performance (including measurement standards), and precise outcomes for assessing learner progress. The circumstances surrounding unsupervised practice and the exact number of times the activity defined in the EPA must be performed successfully before the clinician is deemed entrustable should also be made clear in the EPA. As an example, the Association of American Medical Colleges (AAMC) produced a guide for curricular outcomes to ensure that medical school graduates are prepared for their internship year. Using EPAs, the guide delineates successful behaviors of graduating medical students who can be entrusted with caring for patients as an intern (AAMC, 2014a, 2014b). The guide defines inadequate levels of competence as well. Fundamental to the concept of EPAs is the notion that both trustworthiness and self-awareness of one's abilities are required for competency and should be documented before the practitioner is permitted to perform the activity.

Developing EPAs

The use of EPAs in health professions education differs from that of milestones. The focus of EPAs is determination of competence as it relates specifically to safe practice considering a pre-designated level of minimal supervision. Learners must successfully and reliably achieve many milestones to be considered eligible for EPA determination. EPAs specify the expected proficient behavior, a specific time frame in which mastery should occur, and the definition of successful demonstration of the EPA (Ten Cate, 2005). Unlike milestones, EPAs should be standardized within specific health professions as the minimum standards required of learners to practice safely and effectively with "distant or postevent" supervision.

Relating milestones and EPAs is beneficial to learners and faculty. Achievement of the early milestone of proficient simple, interrupted suturing on a model grants the student the ability to practice laceration closure on a patient with direct supervision for several months. At one point after substantial practice, the preceptor will determine that the student has achieved the simple laceration closure milestone. Once the milestone is achieved, the health professions student is entrusted with simple wound closure while the preceptor is caring for another patient in the same room or after the wound closure is finished. Other examples of profession-wide EPAs include the AAMC guides developed for medical and surgical specialties (AAMC, 2014a) as well as pediatric medical education (Carraccio & Burke, 2010).

CONCLUSIONS

Competency-based education helps instructors and students focus on outcomes related to the development of clinical acumen. This paradigm shift has major implications for curriculum design and implementation, as well as for the evaluation of learners. Tools available to educators include implementation of learning milestones and utilization of the EPAs model to develop summative evaluations of graduating students. Use of these new approaches to health professions education will ensure improved student outcomes and greater clarity of instructors' expectations for competent performance.

REFERENCES

Accreditation Council for Graduate Medical Education and the American Board of Medical Specialties. (1999). Core competencies of physicians. Retrieved from http://www.abms.org/board-certification/a-trusted-credential/based-on-core-competencies

American Academy of Physician Assistants, Accreditation Commission on Education for the Physician Assistant, Physician Assistant Education Association and National Commission on Certification of Physician Assistants. (2012). Competencies for the physician assistant profession. Retrieved from https://www.nccpa.net/Uploads/docs/PACompetencies.pdf

Antman, K., Berman, H. A., Flotte, T. R., Flier, J., Demitri, D., & Bharel, M. (2016). Developing core competencies for the prevention and management of prescription drug misuse: A medical education collaboration in Massachusetts. *Academic Medicine, 91*(10), 1348–1351.

Association of American Medical Colleges. (2014a). Core entrustable professional activities for entering residency: A curriculum development guide. Retrieved from https://members.aamc.org/eweb/upload/Core%20EPA%20Curriculum%20Dev%20Guide.pdf

Association of American Medical Colleges. (2014b). Core entrustable professional activities for entering residency: A faculty and learner's guide. Retrieved from https://members.aamc.org/eweb/upload/Core%20EPA%20Faculty%20and%20Learner%20Guide.pdf

Carraccio, C., & Burke, A. E. (2010). Beyond competencies and milestones: Adding meaning through context. *Journal of Graduate Medical Education, 2*(3), 419–422.

Competence. (2016). *Merriam-Webster's online dictionary*. Retrieved from https://www.merriam-webster.com/dictionary/competence

Donaldson, M. S., Corrigan, J. M., & Kohn, L. T. (Eds.). (2000). *To err is human: building a safer health system* (Vol. 6). Washington, DC: National Academies Press.

Flexner, A. (1910). *Medical education in the United States and Canada: A report to the Carnegie Foundation for the Advancement of Teaching*. Boston, MA: Merrymount Press. Retrieved from http://archive.carnegiefoundation.org/pdfs/elibrary/Carnegie_Flexner_Report.pdf

Miller, G. E. (1990). The assessment of clinical skills/competence/performance. *Academic Medicine, 65*(9), s63–s67.

Mulder, H., Ten Cate, O., Daalder, R., & Berkvens, J. (2010). Building a competency-based workplace curriculum and entrustable professional activities: The case of physician assistant training. *Medical Teacher, 32*, e453–e459. doi:10.3109/0142159X.2010.513719

National Organization of Nurse Practitioner Faculties. (2002). Core competencies for nurse practitioners. Retrieved from http://c.ymcdn.com/sites/www.nonpf.org/resource/resmgr/competencies/domainsandcorecomps2002.pdf

Pangaro, L. N. (1999) A new vocabulary and other innovations for improving descriptive in-training evaluations. *Academic Medicine, 74*, 1203–1207.

Pfeiffer, C. A. (2013). *The Master Interview Rating Scale (MIRS): An instrument for faculty, students and standardized patients to use for teaching and evaluation*. Washington, DC: Association of American Medical Colleges. Retrieved from https://www.mededportal.org/icollaborative/resource/835

Physician Assistant Education Association. (2016). PAEA by the numbers: Program report 31. Retrieved from http://paeaonline.org/wp-content/uploads/2016/11/Program-Survey-31.pdf

Sepdham, D., Julka, M., Hofmann, L., & Dobbie, A. (2007). Using the RIME model for learner assessment and feedback. *Family Medicine, 39,* 161–163.

Slonim, A., Wheeler, F. C., Quinlan, K. M., & Smith, S. M. (2010). Designing competencies for chronic disease practice. *Preventing Chronic Disease,* 7(2), 1–9. Retrieved from http://www.cdc.gov/pcd/issues/2010/mar/08_0114.htm

Ten Cate, O. (2005). Entrustability of professional activities and competency-based training. *Medical Education, 39,* 1176–1177. doi:10.1111/j.1365-2929.2005.02341

Weinberger, S. E., Pereira, A. G., Iobst, W. F., Mechaber, A. J., & Bronze, M. S. (2010). Competency-based education and training in internal medicine. *Annals of Internal Medicine, 153*(11), 751–757. doi:10.7326/0003-4819-153-11-201012070-00009

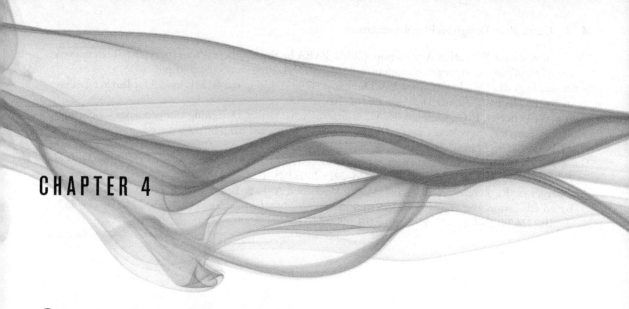

CHAPTER 4

Curriculum Mapping

Carrie A. Calloway

CHAPTER OBJECTIVE

• Map curriculum to professional competencies, milestones, and accreditation standards

I was taught the way of progress is neither swift nor easy.

—*Marie Curie*

Curriculum mapping is a process used to identify when, where, and how content is addressed across the curriculum in an effort to recognize gaps and redundancies; to ensure that content is introduced, reinforced, and assessed; to guarantee that instruction and assessment are aligned to what students are expected to learn; and to promote self-study and critical analysis. The final product, typically a matrix or searchable database, provides a snapshot of how a program is meeting its overall outcomes, milestones, and/or accreditation requirements. Curricular weaknesses, such as reliance on a single assessment method (e.g., multiple-choice questions), involuntary omission of core content, or evidence of breadth rather than depth of knowledge, can be identified and remedied through the curriculum-mapping process (Essary & Statler, 2007; Landry et al., 2011).

Whether you are developing a new curriculum or revising an existing one, curriculum mapping helps to ensure that a health professions education program is meeting its defined expectations. Predictably, there is no one-size-fits-all model for the curriculum-mapping process. Health professions education programs devise various strategies for mapping depending on multiple factors, including where they are in the curriculum development process, resource availability, and time constraints (Cottrell et al., 2016). This chapter not only explores the advantages of curriculum mapping, but also offers helpful tips for where to begin. Suggestions that can make the process a little more effective and efficient are examined, as are strategies for resolving challenges that may surface.

THE PURPOSE OF CURRICULUM MAPPING

Mapping the curriculum of a health professions education program is no easy feat. It takes the collaborative effort of faculty, administration, and staff; it takes time (and more time); and it takes dedication. As a program director, curriculum director, or dean, you will often be queried by students, faculty, accrediting bodies, and other stakeholders interested in where and how specific content is being taught, strengthened, and/or evaluated. You might know there is a course dedicated to a specific content topic or skill area, but are there other areas in the curriculum where the topic and associated skills are further defined and assessed? Aligning the curriculum to learning outcomes (see Chapter 2), in addition to specific accreditation standards, is a necessary chore in health professions education and, upon completion, can help you answer important questions about your program's curriculum. These questions include: "How well do you know what students are learning?" "How is student learning assessed within your program?" "How do you know students are meeting program learning outcomes?"

Curriculum mapping will help you understand your curriculum. It will help you identify areas of strength and weakness. It will help you evaluate the scope and sequence, ascertain whether your assessments are measuring what is being taught, and improve the overall teaching and assessment process through better organization and understanding of the overall program curriculum. The final product, a visual representation of the curriculum indicating when and in which course(s) or activities learning objectives are being introduced, reinforced, and assessed, will help you answer these important questions.

GETTING STARTED WITH CURRICULUM MAPPING

No matter what type of health professions curriculum you are mapping, the first thing to ask yourself is, "Where are we now, and where do we want to be?" In the end, you want to ensure that what is being taught at the course level satisfies the overall learning outcomes and expectations of the program (Mentkowski et al., 2016). Consequently, reviewing the course syllabus is often the first step; however, you will also want to evaluate your available resources, including human resources, monetary resources, and time, to determine the best approach. For instance, are you going to use Excel spreadsheets? What about an off-the-shelf commercial product? Electronic evaluation management systems, which are commonly used to track students' clinical progress, often include a curriculum-mapping component. Consider which course management system you use. Is there a way to maximize its purpose to accommodate curriculum mapping? In other words, can you tag content with searchable key words or phrases that will enable you to quickly locate and cross-reference where specific content is being delivered? These are all questions that must be considered early in the curriculum-mapping process.

Mapping the curriculum requires that you have a few things in place, many of which can be found in individual course syllabi: (a) program-level learning outcomes, (b) course-level learning objectives, (c) session-level learning objectives, (d) assessment methods, (e) teaching strategies, and (f) resources. As with nearly all activities in health professions education, curriculum mapping requires a collaborative effort among administration, faculty, and staff. Strategies for engaging faculty to supply necessary data are key for successful mapping initiatives. Professional development activities designed to educate faculty about the importance of well-stated learning objectives that contribute to the overall fulfillment of program expectations, including the emphasis on competency in more areas than medical knowledge alone, are a key component of a successful mapping project (see Chapter 2).

The curriculum-mapping process can be split into multiple phases or stages of progress, each requiring varying time frames to complete based on the quality of the current curriculum design. In this context, quality means clear course and lecture- or activity-level learning objectives that are specific and measurable. These are the statements that establish the expectations and direction of the course, as well as inform students about the level of understanding expected for specific content domains or competencies (see Chapter 2). These statements, or learning objectives, should also map to the overall learning outcomes of the program of study. Naturally, one of the first things to consider is alignment—alignment between what is being taught and what is being assessed (assessment to course-level mapping) and how what is being taught relates to the overall goals of the program (course-to-program-level mapping). As such, all lecture and activity objectives should correlate with course objectives, assessments, and teaching strategies. Furthermore, course learning objectives must be linked to program learning objectives, accreditation standards, milestones, and/or core entrustable professional activities (EPAs). EPAs are "mapped" to critical competencies based on milestones established for the pre-entrustable and entrustable learner for each competency. The EPA concept permits competency-based decisions regarding the level of supervision required by learners at each level of the health professions program (Cate, 2013).

One way to commence the alignment process is to create a matrix that provides a rough idea of where each program-level objective is being taught across the curriculum. This simple matrix of Xs and Os (or whatever other convention you wish to use) will provide a broad snapshot of the curriculum and will offer quick clues as to where you should focus your attention. The matrix in Exhibit 4.1 provides an example of the alignment of one physician assistant (PA) program's second semester (didactic curriculum) with competencies adapted from the National Commission on Certification of Physician Assistants (NCCPA). As can be seen, Xs represent the competencies being taught and/or assessed for each course. This matrix could be extended to include program-defined curriculum threads, accreditation standards, EPAs and other topics of interest.

It is not enough to simply indicate in which courses, program-defined expectations, competencies, EPAs, or specific content are delivered. Taking the mapping process a step further requires understanding *how* the content is being delivered and assessed. Various instructional strategies, resources, and assessment methods are often used to ensure student achievement. Once you have roughly indicated where particular competencies, milestones, EPAs, and accreditation standards are addressed, the next step in curriculum mapping is to understand how your program currently confirms achievement of program learning outcomes. Questions to answer include: "What instructional methods are currently used to deliver content?" "How are students assessed?" "Are multiple instructional strategies used?" "If not, where do you think nontraditional methods can be implemented?" If your program is not using multiple methods of assessment, the curriculum map will help you isolate those areas in need of improvement. A key point to remember: Competency reveals itself in more ways than multiple-choice questions (Angelo & Cross, 1993).

Creating a simple rubric that can be used by all faculty to detail what they expect students to learn, how they teach it, how they measure it, and how they refine it is often a crucial step in the process. This method can provide a visual pathway from activity-level instruction to overall program outcome. Starting broad and sequentially narrowing in on the requirements helps to not overwhelm faculty. A one-page form that faculty complete (whether on paper or through an electronic means, such as Google forms) for each learning activity (e.g., lecture, lab, team-based learning activity, simulation lab session, and so forth) will help gather the basic information needed. Additionally, this reflection on how each lecture contributes to the overall program expectations can help jump-start the mapping process. An abbreviated sample template for collecting data from faculty is shown in Table 4.1. When adapted to an electronic format, such as Word or Excel, this form can be completed without adding excessive workload, and triggers the consideration of important factors during the development of lectures, assessments, and

EXHIBIT 4.1 Curriculum Map Matrix for Sample Second-Semester Physician Assistant Program

	Neurology	Endocrine	Cardio	Biostatistics & Evidence-Based Medicine	Applied Therapeutics	Health Policy & Professional Practice I	Advanced Clinical Skills	Respiratory	Simulation Lab	Clinical Problem Solving I & Clinical Call
MK1	X	X	X					X	X	X
MK2	X	X	X					X	X	X
MK3	X	X	X					X	X	X
MK4	X	X	X		X			X	X	X
MK5										
MK6										
MK7										
MK8										
MK9									X	X
MK10									X	X
I&CS1										
I&CS2									X	
I&CS3									X	X
I&CS4										
I&CS5										
I&CS6										
I&CS7									X	
PC1										X
PC2									X	X
PC3									X	X
PC4										
PC5									X	X
PC6									X	X
PC7										
PC8									X	X

(continued)

EXHIBIT 4.1 Curriculum Map Matrix for Sample Second-Semester Physician Assistant Program (*continued*)

	Neurology	Endocrine	Cardio	Biostatistics & Evidence-Based Medicine	Applied Therapeutics	Health Policy & Professional Practice I	Advanced Clinical Skills	Respiratory	Simulation Lab	Clinical Problem Solving I & Clinical Call
PROF1						X				
PROF2						X				X
PROF3										
PROF4										
PROF5										
PROF6						X				
PROF7										
PROF8						X				
PBL&I1									X	
PBL&I2				X						X
PBL&I3				X						
PBL&I4				X						
PBL&I5				X						X
PBL&I6				X					X	X
PBL&I7										
SBP1						X				
SBP2						X				X
SBP3										
SBP4										
SBP5						X				
SBP6									X	X
SBP7										
SBP8									X	X
SBP9										

I & CS, interpersonal & communication skills; MK, medical knowledge; PC, patient care; PROF, professionalism; PBL & I, practice-based learning & improvement; SBP, systems-based practice.

TABLE 4.1 Abbreviated Sample Template for Data Gathering From Faculty

Course:	Instructor:	Session #	Date:
Competencies addressed: (Circle all that apply.)	1. Medical knowledge 2. Interpersonal and communication skills 3. Patient care 4. Professionalism 5. Practice-based learning and improvement 6. Systems-based practice		
Session learning objectives (Write clear learning objectives for the session.)	At the end of this session, students will be able to: 1. 2. 3. 4. 5. *Add or remove depending on the number of objectives covered during an individual session.*		
What resources were used to facilitate this session? (Circle all that apply.)	Case studies Simulation Standardized patients Cadaver Web-based resources		
How will you assess each of the learning objectives? (Circle all that apply.)	Multiple-choice exam Simulation Oral presentation Narrative evaluation Portfolio reflection Observation Rubric OTHER: _____		
What content key words or curriculum threads describe what was taught in this session? (Circle all that apply.)	Anatomy . . . . behavioral science . . . . biochemistry . . . . biostatistics . . . . cardio . . . . cell biology . . . . community health . . . . cultural competence . . . . diagnostic imaging . . . . domestic abuse . . . . . . genetics . . . . health disparities . . . . nutrition . . . . oral health . . . . substance abuse **(Include all key words you want to track.)**		

learning objectives. The data collected can be assembled into a matrix where faculty can cross-check their efforts and ensure that specific courses are supporting the core knowledge and skills needed to meet program-defined expectations.

A sample curriculum map linking overall program learning outcomes to a specific course objective is illustrated in Figure 4.1. This format can be used for each course objective and can also be used for each learning activity and assessment within courses.

Programs with an established curriculum may wish to begin by first assessing faculty understanding of learning objectives and ensuring that your current curriculum syllabi clearly state the intended learning objectives of each course. If this is accurate and reflective of the true "being taught" and "being assessed" curriculum, then you are halfway there. If not, redirect focus to the purpose of each course and its overall contribution to the program outcomes. Ask faculty to articulate this in their syllabi and provide professional developments as needed.

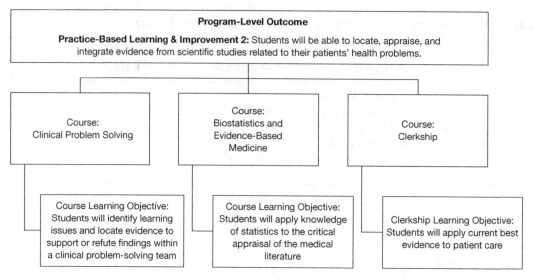

FIGURE 4.1 Sample mapping from program-level outcome to course objective.

Another strategy to ensure you are mapping the curriculum to relevant data is to use the results of benchmarked exams that break down score reports by subject area. These identified content areas provide a framework for identifying and benchmarking program outcomes and content. Through mapping initiatives, weak areas can be more easily identified and strengthened. This approach will also support the self-study and critical analysis process by providing clear data for reflection and focus for program improvement initiatives.

CHALLENGES OF CURRICULUM MAPPING

Curriculum mapping is a process and requires a series of steps to perform. In this process, many challenges can and will emerge. The noteworthy challenges to curriculum-mapping initiatives include, but are not limited to faculty buy-in, the ever-evolving curriculum, and cost (predominantly time). Each of these potential hurdles is explored, along with possible resolutions.

Faculty Buy-In

Because curriculum mapping is a large-scale endeavor, engaging faculty in the process is key; however, be prepared to be met with the "why fix it if it ain't broken" mind-set. Often citing above-average pass rates on high-stakes exams as evidence that the curriculum design and implementation is working, some faculty can be reluctant to the time investment necessary to effectively map the curriculum. Getting faculty compliance when it comes to the process of linking, and in some cases writing (depending on where you are in the curriculum development process) clear and specific learning objectives for each lecture, as well as demonstration that each assessment activity can be traced back to the learning objective, is a challenge. Compounding this challenge is the need for professional development activities in academic medicine topics to bridge the gap in their own understanding. Hosting a series of workshops dedicated to curriculum improvement is a start. The workshops should be brief, but regular. They should be structured and provide adequate time for practice and feedback. A mentorship program or a promotion and tenure incentive to participate may help in gaining faculty interest and compliance.

In addition, the institution of a subcommittee of the curriculum committee charged with the oversight and continued momentum of a mapping project may prove useful. In collaboration with faculty and administrative leadership (i.e., dean of curriculum or director of assessment), involving students in the committee can be a helpful approach. The students are living the curricular experience and can help confirm or counter whether specific learning objectives are being addressed.

Evolving Curriculum

The curriculum is always adjusting to new demands, whether internal or external. In fact, the well-known saying that "half of what is learned in medical school is wrong, we just don't know which half yet" provides even more incentive to monitor and revise the curriculum as needed. Not only do accreditation standards spell out specific curriculum topics that must be addressed, but local, national, and global topics of interest may find their way into the fold as a curriculum thread that must also be documented and monitored. The curriculum map will allow faculty and administration to clearly see where topics are taught and assessed so that they may be easily isolated when the need for revision surfaces.

Cost in Time

The challenge of time can present in many forms. For one, time is very limited among health professions educators. With clinical evaluations, patient rounds, and teaching, little time remains to reflect meaningfully on what exactly students are learning and how their learning is documented and measured. Furthermore, consolidating all the needed information to embark on the mapping process can take a considerable amount of time. Take baby steps and set goals. For example, you may want to get started by first determining where your program objectives are being addressed across the curriculum. Later, you may opt to drill down to specific lectures or activities. Do not take on more than you can handle. Expect the process to take at least a year to pull together—and do not forget—because of the evolving curriculum, the project will never actually be complete. It will become a living and breathing document needing regular upkeep.

Of all the challenges, by far the greatest is attacking this project alone. Assemble a committee to help review the current curriculum and to monitor not only that accreditation standards are being met, but also that content coverage and alignment are evident.

BENEFITS OF CURRICULUM MAPPING

A successful curriculum-mapping project has many advantages. It allows for the identification of gaps and overlaps in content, and also provides clear evidence that content is being introduced, reinforced, and assessed, thereby identifying curricular strengths and weaknesses. The notable benefits of curriculum mapping include enhanced collaboration among faculty, administration, and staff; identification of content redundancies and omissions; graphical presentation of alignment between what is being taught and assessed; demonstration of compliance; and a tool for data reporting and continuous program improvement.

Promotes Collaboration

The curriculum-mapping process can bring faculty together. Uchiyama and Radin (2009) reported "an increase in collaboration and collegiality among faculty . . . as an unintended outcome" (p. 271) of a curriculum-mapping project. In addition, the open communication that results facilitates a deeper understanding of the purpose and process than simply requesting information from faculty. As mentioned previously, faculty buy-in is often a challenge; however, with a support network in place, the rewards outweigh the burdens.

Helps to Bridge the Gaps and Dissolve the Overlaps

Curriculum mapping can help isolate gaps and overlaps in the curriculum. No one can deny the importance of revisiting important concepts in the curriculum; however, the reintroduction should further understanding by expanding the depth of knowledge, not merely repeating it. When redundancies surface, they can be used to create solid discussion points for faculty meetings. Identification and revision of repetition is one outcome of a successful mapping process. Similarly, the curriculum map can make it easier to identify topics that are not being covered or not adequately covered.

Visualizes Alignment

The curriculum map typically looks like a matrix with the expected program-level objectives, milestones, EPAs, and/or accreditation standards presented down the first column and a list of courses or activities across the top of a spreadsheet (or vice versa). Where the cells meet, an X or O or other combination of letters, numbers, or colors can be entered to indicate the presence of the competency, standards, EPAs, or milestones in that particular course or activity (see Table 4.1). The product of curriculum mapping can deliver evidence that assessments reflect instruction, that learning goals are being met, and that content coverage is comprehensive.

Assures Compliance With Accreditation Standards

The curriculum map can demonstrate to accrediting bodies that the curriculum meets the required expectations, particularly when it comes to showing where specific program-level learning objectives, milestones, or EPAs are being covered throughout the curriculum. It is recommended that those mapping the curriculum develop a system to highlight where specific accreditation standards related to content are being met. Using the Xs and Os convention mentioned previously, you could expand this practice to use A (for accreditation standard), M (for milestones), and E (for EPAs). The specific abbreviations do not matter, as long as they are understood by faculty, administration, and staff. When the program comes up for an accreditation review, you will be prepared to demonstrate compliance with specific standards and present clear evidence for how the program documents and tracks when, where, and how content is taught and assessed.

Demonstrates Relevance

A detailed curriculum map clearly summarizes what is being learned, where it is being learned, and how it is being assessed. Consequently, it can help students understand the relevance of the topics covered in the curriculum, particularly if connections are made to accreditation standards, program learning outcomes, and EPAs. As previously mentioned, involving students in the mapping process has its benefits. Students have lived the curriculum experience and can help to confirm coverage of content and alignment with assessment. Involving students also permits them to understand the reasoning behind the curriculum's structure and function.

Supports in Data Reporting

The curriculum map can help program directors and curriculum deans easily prepare reports related to the content areas addressed, the amount of time dedicated to specific topics, and where specific competencies and skills are introduced and reinforced. Curriculum maps and resulting reports can also be shared with faculty to illustrate the instructional strategies and assessment methods used to meet program requirements and evaluate student progress. Resulting reports often prompt faculty to rethink or adjust the ways in which they approach assessment. For instance, a transition to team-based and problem-based learning strategies is often a by-product of curriculum-mapping endeavors.

Promotes Program Self-Study

Accrediting agencies mandate that programs provide a narrative on how the curriculum not only meets standards, but also how it meets the overall program-defined expectations. In order to identify their strengths and weaknesses, programs use enormous amounts of data, ranging from examination of course evaluations to analysis of score reports on national benchmark exams. The addition of the curriculum map to the dossier can help to further facilitate self-study, thus helping in continuous program improvement and data-driven curricular revision.

CONCLUSIONS

Curriculum mapping, though not a simple activity, is an effective strategy for ensuring depth and breadth of core content coverage and skill development. Finding a strategy that works according to your program's resources is the first step. Remember, the purpose is to help the program ensure a comprehensive curriculum that prepares students for professional practice. Tracking when, where, and how content is delivered and assessed can get complicated, but following a few of the strategies presented in this chapter will assist the process.

REFERENCES

Angelo, T. A., & Cross, P. K. (1993). *Classroom assessment techniques: A handbook for college teachers* (2nd ed.). New York, NY: Jossey-Bass.

Cate, O. T. (2013). Nuts and bolts of entrustable professional activities. *Journal of Graduate Medical Education, 5*(1), 157–158.

Cottrell, S., Hedrick, J. S., Lama, A., Chen, B., West, C. A., Graham, L., . . . Wright, M. (2016). Curriculum mapping: A comparative analysis of two medical school models. *Medical Science Educator, 26*(1), 169–174.

Essary, A., & Statler, M. (2007). Using a curriculum map to link the competencies for the PA profession with assessment tools in PA education. *Journal of Physician Assistant Education, 18*(1), 22–28. Retrieved from http://www2.paeaonline.org/index.php?ht=action/GetDocumentAction/i/25268

Landry, L. G., Alameida, M. D., Orsolini-Hain, L., Boyle, A. R., Privé, A., Chien, A., . . . Leong, A. (2011). Responding to demands to change nursing education: Use of curriculum mapping to assess curricular content. *Journal of Nursing Education, 50*(10), 587–590.

Mentkowski, M., Abromeit, J., Mernitz, H., Talley, K., Knuteson, C., Rickards, W. H., . . . Mente, S. (2016). Assessing student learning outcomes across a curriculum. In *Assessing competence in professional performance across disciplines and professions* (pp. 141–157). New York, NY: Springer Publishing.

Uchiyama, K. P., & Radin, J. L. (2009). Curriculum mapping in higher education: A vehicle for collaboration. *Innovative Higher Education, 33*(4), 271–280.

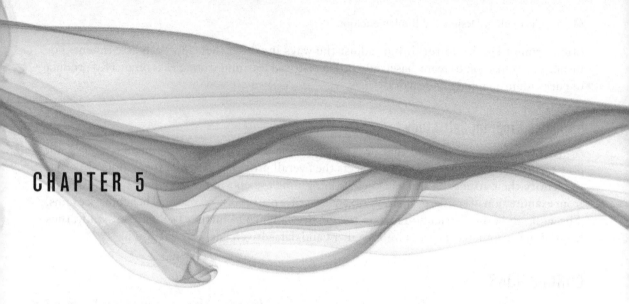

CHAPTER 5

Interprofessional Education: What, Why, When, and How?

Kevin Lohenry, Désirée Lie, Ashley Halle, and Sae Byul (Sarah) Ma

---

CHAPTER OBJECTIVES

- Define interprofessional education (IPE) and expected competencies for students
- Describe different levels of learning and curricula for IPE
- Recognize key resources and steps for implementing IPE curricula
- Choose appropriate evaluation tools for students and the IPE curriculum

---

I can do things you cannot, you can do things I cannot; together we can do great things.

—*Mother Teresa*

According to the World Health Organization (WHO; 2010), interprofessional education (IPE) "occurs when two or more professions learn about, from and with each other to enable effective collaboration and improve health outcomes" (p. 10). IPE is now recommended or required among accrediting bodies of many health professions (Zorek & Raehl, 2013). Although curricular recommendations exist, systematic implementation among universities has been variable, at best (Roger & Hoffman, 2010). IPE is considered a foundation for future team-based care, which in turn is linked to improved patient and health care quality outcomes (Reeves, Perrier, Goldman, Freeth, & Zwarenstein, 2013; Reeves et al., 2010; Zwarenstein, Goldman, & Reeves, 2009). Although competencies have been described by different organizations (Association of American Medical Colleges [AAMC], 2011; Barr & Low, 2011; Orchard et al., 2010; WHO, 2010), there is general agreement about the core components of IPE that can be taught, learned, and applied

TABLE 5.1 Core Competencies for Interprofessional Collaborative Practice

World Health Organization	Interprofessional Education Collaborative	Canadian Interprofessional Health Collaborative Working Group
1. Acquisition of the knowledge and skills linked to interprofessional education	1. Values/ethics for interprofessional practice	1. Interprofessional communication
2. Understanding the roles and responsibilities of other professionals	2. Roles/responsibilities	2. Patient-/client-centered care
3. Development of teamwork skills	3. Interprofessional communication	3. Role clarification
4. Ethics/attitudes	4. Teams and teamwork	4. Team functioning
5. The patient		5. Collaborative leadership
6. Learning/reflection		6. Interprofessional conflict resolution

Source: Adapted from Interprofessional Education Collaborative (2011) and Thistlethwaite et al. (2014).

to practice (AAMC, 2011; Interprofessional Education Collaborative [IPEC], 2011). The most commonly listed competencies (Table 5.1) are understanding the roles and responsibilities of other professions, teamwork skills, communication and collaboration, patient-centered care, reflection, and ethics and values of interprofessionalism (AAMC, 2011; Orchard et al., 2010; Thistlethwaite et al., 2014). These competencies encompass knowledge, attitude, and skills, which in turn must be assessed.

In this chapter, we focus on the framework for designing and executing IPE curricula. The logistics of bringing together faculty and students from two or more professions to prepare for future collaborative practice can be daunting. An early team-building approach that includes colleagues from other health professions schools or programs can set a strong foundation for addressing multiple administrative challenges, such as scheduling and timing. Other challenges include synchronizing course content, recognizing faculty expertise, establishing a shared system of credits among the involved programs (Barnsteiner et al., 2007), potential turf wars, issues relating to financial support, power disparities among faculty members, and recruiting appropriate clinical sites. IPE curricula should be designed by interprofessional teams whose members reflect the core values of team-based care and are familiar with the learning needs of their students and of students from other professions.

TYPES OF IPE CURRICULA

We categorize IPE curricula as (a) foundational or *didactic* (involving knowledge and patient simulations) and (b) *clinical* (involving application to actual practice and real patients). Didactic curricula are grounded in the acquisition of knowledge and attitudes, whereas clinical curricula add experiential learning to apply knowledge and attitudes to team skills concerning patient management. For example, the competency "roles and responsibilities" could be associated with the following knowledge objectives: *identify roles and responsibilities of the physician, nurse, social worker, and dietician in the care of patients* and *describe ways in which the care of a patient is shared by the physician, nurse, and dietician in the care of patients with diabetes.* Objectives that involve clinical team skill acquisition might include the following: *distinguish roles of the advanced practice registered nurse,*

nurse practitioner, pharmacist, physician assistant, and physician when prescribing for the hospitalized patient and *communicate one's own role in relation to other professions when caring for a patient.*

To guide educators reading this chapter, we provide examples that include sample learning objectives, competencies addressed, suggested teaching method(s), potential evaluation strategies, and faculty development approaches for each curriculum type (didactic vs. clinical). We recommend that IPE be integrated and show developmental progression across the training continuum, so that graduating students understand that the IPE competencies apply in all areas of their future team practice.

THE ROLE OF FACULTY DEVELOPMENT IN IPE CURRICULA

Faculty development is critical to the delivery of successful and effective IPE curricula, especially as faculty members from different health professions have diverse opinions and backgrounds in educational theory and methods. Allocating time for faculty members to create common ground for teaching, facilitation, and student and team assessment before implementing an IPE curriculum for students will set the stage for a successful IPE experience. It is crucial that participating faculty members be inclusive and respectful toward those from other professions, particularly when explaining the benefits of interprofessionality to students. Students may enter programs with negative stereotypes of other health care professions that influence their future work behaviors (Rudland & Mires, 2005), and it has been suggested that these stereotypes may be propagated and reinforced by faculty members (Ponzer et al., 2004). Sufficient training must be provided prior to teaching encounters to avoid spreading the silo effect among health professions students. This is central to the tenet of learning to understand each other's unique contributions to the health outcomes of patients so we avoid staying in our own professionally centric silos.

EARLY STEPS IN IPE CURRICULUM DEVELOPMENT

In programs without known or preexisting IPE curricula, an educator may begin with a needs assessment to identify "hidden" curricula in which IPE may already be unintentionally addressed. For example, it is possible that in some clinical settings, such as a rehabilitation or senior center, multiprofessional teams are already working together, and students are being exposed to several professions. Students may have also been exposed to a multiprofessional panel presentation on scopes of practice. Once curricular opportunities and areas of deficit are recognized, an educator could then reach out to other interested professional schools with the goal of finding common ground to build IPE curricula. Ample preparation time should be allocated for addressing the logistical challenges of limited resources and aligning multiple schedules to accomplish interprofessional experiences. Efforts should be made to design, pilot, and then refine longitudinal curricula and experiences that build on prior learning and that culminate in the demonstration of desired IPE competencies. Such efforts require careful attention to the selection of teaching strategies and evaluation tools.

CREATING DIDACTIC IPE CURRICULA

The main challenge during the didactic phase is limited scheduling time and logistical conflicts. Thus, didactic educational models often begin with a one-time interprofessional activity. Holding more regular didactic IPE sessions depends on the geographic proximity between professional schools and the availability of time slots in each curriculum. With a top-down approach, deans or provosts from different professional schools/programs may be able to agree to set aside curricular time to offer a weekly or monthly IPE course that instructs students from all health professions on campus. This top-down approach, which occurs when institutional leaders issue the directive to implement IPE curricula across programs and professions, may possess greater resources. We next present one example of creating didactic curricula using a "bottom-up" (faculty-initiated) approach.

Exemplar: A Didactic (Bottom-Up) Curriculum

The bottom-up approach occurs when faculty and/or programs/schools seek to meet their own accreditation standards around IPE and develop their own work group without distinct executive direction from the institution's leaders.

Situation

You are a new junior member of the occupational therapy faculty and your program director asks you to create IPE activities for students that align with new IPE accreditation requirements.

Basics

You begin by conducting a needs assessment, which reveals that your institution has an IPE committee organized by university librarians that meets quarterly. When you attend one of their meetings to learn more, you discover that the only interprofessional events held in the past have involved lectures with panels of guest speakers from different professions. You and your director agree that this activity is not enough to meet your accreditation standards. Because you seek more interactive and meaningful experiences, you contact the National Center for Interprofessional Practice and Education (NEXUS®, 2017) to gather ideas and resources, and consider developing an interprofessional event using a case study approach.

Assembling an Education Team

The next step is to reach out to colleagues on the IPE committee to create an interprofessional event. Faculty members from six professions express interest, but the logistics of scheduling a day and time that work for all of them proves insurmountable. You decide to choose the time selected by four professions: occupational therapy (yourself), nursing, pharmacy, and physician assistant (PA) programs, leaving out medicine and dentistry for now. You initiate a new planning subcommittee representing these four professions, and you are selected as the leader by the other professions. Each member commits to weekly meetings or conference calls over the next 3 months.

Preparing for Your First Team Meeting

You prepare for the first face-to-face meeting by gathering important resources (such as published IPE competencies) and composing an action-oriented agenda addressing IPE competencies, logistics, and faculty development.

A Sample Agenda

1. Introduce the team and discuss the clinical roles and the educational background of the professions represented; conduct an icebreaker activity.
2. Confirm date/time, location, and duration of the next IPE event; select faculty development date/time and location.
3. Determine the pertinent IPE competencies.
4. Design case studies to meet the needs of all four professions.
5. Consider faculty development: needs assessment, objectives, and activities.

6. Identify the best evaluation strategies for the IPE event.
7. Outline action items for each subcommittee member.

One icebreaker activity to get the first meeting of the IPE subcommittee underway is "two truths and a lie," in which each member lists three statements about his or her profession: one that is a lie or misconception and two that are true.

After the subcommittee confirms date and time for a 4-hour IPE event, the pharmacy faculty member volunteers to take charge of the logistics of student and faculty room/group assignments, food for the event, and the faculty development session, with assistance from a support staff member to help prevent faculty burnout. All members will recruit faculty from their own profession to participate in the IPE event.

The subcommittee then identifies competencies to be addressed for this IPE event (e.g., competencies from IPEC [2011], Thistlethwaite et al. [2014], and WHO [2010]). Your subcommittee agrees to select *roles/responsibilities* and *teamwork* as the core competencies.

The subcommittee next identifies appropriate instructional objectives followed by the subject for a case study. The PA faculty member volunteers to take the lead and write up the case for review. The case involves a 75-year-old male with a postfall subdural hematoma, which allows each team to integrate its respective foci of this case. The PA faculty member will focus on the medical care of and decision making concerning the intracranial hemorrhage, the pharmacy faculty member focuses on the pharmacological principles, the RN faculty member on the specific nursing documentation and care items, and the occupational therapy faculty member on rehabilitative principles. The nursing faculty member, who has experience with faculty development, takes on the task of designing the 4-hour faculty development training.

Finally, the subcommittee agrees to an evaluations strategy based on the previous research experiences of the pharmacy and PA faculty members. It will consist of an online postsurvey of students and faculty concerning the event and whether its objectives were met. You volunteer to prepare the event evaluations for the subcommittee's review.

Future conference calls are planned for discussing the tasks identified. A 3-month timeline is detailed. You discuss budget estimates for expenses related to the event (e.g., food, drink, and transportation). Your subcommittee acknowledges that programs will not be sustainable without financial support, and so the subcommittee agrees that each profession will begin meeting with its respective leadership to get buy-in. The subcommittee agrees to weight the financial contributions based on a percentage that reflects the number of students in each program.

Preparing for the Next Event: Continuation and Follow-Through

The event timeline not only supports facilitation of a smooth event, but also serves to remind subcommittee members of the next steps as the date approaches. Each subcommittee member emails pertinent documents to all other members to allow all to review the others' work, facilitating decision making at the next meeting. The nursing faculty organizes a faculty development session after the case is designed and faculty members are recruited. Feedback from the faculty is unanimously positive; all are grateful to learn of one another's scopes of practice and to receive a preview of the case study.

Day of the Event

The pharmacy faculty member arranges for transportation of off-site students and faculty members to the event, for 20 rooms for groups of 24 students and two faculty each, and for event ushers and refreshments for a postevent social. All faculty facilitators meet to review the syllabus before proceeding to the interprofessional small groups. Ahead of the event, the PA faculty member will send out syllabus materials and agendas to students. The subcommittee members act as observers and rotate through the small groups to serve as problem solvers and maintain quality control. Following the event, you send out an email to students and faculty with a link to the postevent survey.

PostEvent Wrap-Up and Debriefing

After the event, the subcommittee holds a debriefing meeting to discuss the event, including its challenges and successes, and to review the evaluations. Faculty members from the two professions that were not able to participate are invited to the debriefing to help plan the next step. During the debriefing, the PA faculty member generates the idea of including interprofessional simulations as a logical next step to build on the first IPE event. The subcommittee agrees to investigate this activity further as an option for the following year.

You have helped to create the first IPE event as a building block for adding future teaching opportunities.

Didactic (Top-Down) Curricula

The top-down approach occurs when institutional leaders intentionally collaborate regarding accreditation standards that specifically require IPE. The leaders (deans and provosts) meet and then charge the programs within their professions to create curricular slots to address IPE specifically. This approach provides more abundant administrative resources to implement new IPE teaching. The role of individual educators is to participate in actively designing, implementing, and evaluating curricula.

Summary of Didactic IPE Curriculum Development

IPE core competencies provide a clear framework for designing and implementing didactic curricula. However, certain details—identifying which professions should be involved in each educational event, selecting instructional objectives and best teaching strategies, scheduling faculty training, and choosing types of evaluation—are left to the participating educators. The case study chosen should be both topical and inclusive of all professions participating. The work involved demands teamwork among faculties from diverse professions and should break down existing silos across professions. Faculty teams working on IPE curricula should incorporate reflection in their process, view IPE curriculum development as a continuous work in progress, and hold themselves accountable for learning outcomes for their students.

CREATING CLINICAL IPE CURRICULA

Clinical curricula help apply learned classroom knowledge in the clinical setting or practice. The purpose of clinical curricula is to prepare students for practice. The steps for the design and implementation of IPE clinical curricula include (a) conducting a needs assessment, (b) selecting an ideal IPE site, (c) determining the best possible learning objectives and competencies, (d) creating and implementing effective teaching strategies to achieve the objectives, and (e) identifying and applying tools for evaluating students. We recommend a subcommittee or team approach to designing clinical IPE curricula similar to a team approach to didactic courses.

Conducting a Needs Assessment and Selecting an Ideal IPE Site

Just as for didactic curricula, the first step in planning clinical IPE curricula is a needs assessment. The goals are to identify the availability of clinical sites, preceptors, and IPE throughout the community; to determine where IPE is welcome; to provide training so that preceptors understand inclusive language for interprofessional care; and to consider the potential contributions of each profession to the health care team. Seek sites that have the interest and space to accommodate interprofessional teams.

Next, determine which students from each program have already received IPE training, and what learning gaps remain. Here, an IPE subcommittee or team can be tasked with obtaining information about the needs of clinical-phase students from each profession.

Other subcommittee members can take on the task of identifying the best clinical settings for IPE learning. An ideal IPE setting includes teams with students, faculty, and administrators at times the IPE teams can meet and learn together. In compliance with the various professional regulations, the faculty member who will play the role of the supervising clinical provider must be from one of the students' professions (Bridges, Davidson, Odegard, Maki, & Tomkowiak, 2011; D'amour & Oandasan, 2005). Other faculty members are needed to support the teaching role, and coprecepting among different faculty members is an excellent model to use in clinical settings. For example, within an ambulatory care clinical site, the students involved may be from pharmacy, advanced practice registered nurse programs, and medicine programs. The faculty members involved might be a physician and a registered nurse who also plays a role of a nurse clinic manager. The nurse manager can provide teaching opportunities of the policy, procedures and administrative functions of the clinical site, as well as coordinate the scheduling for the IPE team. The nurse clinic manager can provide regular scheduled times and space for the IPE team to see patients and to meet to reflect, discuss, and review the roles and responsibilities of the various disciplines.

Determining the Learning Objectives and Competencies

The IPE clinical subcommittee can communicate with the clerkship/rotation directors of each profession involved and negotiate the addition of IPE objectives not currently met in the programs. After a thorough review of existing learning objectives, the IPE clinical subcommittee can offer to meet to fill gaps in IPE learning by creating new IPE experiences to fit the clerkship involved.

Developing and Implementing Effective Teaching Strategies

The following material includes some examples of aspects of an IPE clinical curriculum.

Purpose

To provide a real-time, collaborative practice learning experience to develop competencies concerning *roles and responsibilities, patient-centered care*, and *teamwork* in preparation for future interprofessional collaborative practice.

LEARNING OBJECTIVES

- Recognize the roles and responsibilities of members of the interprofessional team.
- Establish collaborative professional relationships with members of the interprofessional team.
- Establish collaborative professional provider–patient relationships.
- Demonstrate effective communication skills with patients and interprofessional teams in the planning, collaboration, coordination, delegation, and delivery of patient care.

Participants

Include students from three or four different health professions (maximum of five to six students from each profession to address space and time limits).

Description and Timeline

Each team is assigned 60 to 70 minutes to conduct a prehuddle, a patient interview, a physical examination, and a posthuddle, and then present the patient to the preceptor/clinical instructor. During the prehuddle, all students will share their profession's scope of practice, and their respective roles and responsibilities. The student team will assign roles for the patient encounter. During the patient encounter, students will fulfill their respective responsibilities to elicit pertinent clinical information. At the posthuddle, the student team will collaborate to create an assessment and a plan for best care, and to agree on how to present their findings to the preceptor. The preceptor will then give feedback and see the patient with the team. Ten minutes is allocated for team reflection and feedback at the end of the activity.

Evaluation of Clinical Activity

As with other educational activities, the IPE activity may be assessed by a postactivity survey or through written reflections by students and faculty, as well as through faculty assessments of both student and team performance using existing tools or scales (see "Additional Resources").

An ideal IPE site allows interprofessional teams to work together with interprofessional preceptors to provide care for patients. Once the setting is identified, a curriculum subcommittee can be charged with creating appropriate learning objectives and evaluation strategies for IPE curricula. Ideally, institutions would have access to quality IPE clinical settings, but in some instances—because of the challenges of patient privacy, the economics of patient care and patient preference, and inadequate faculty preparation—ideal IPE sites may be limited. An alternative strategy for student teams is to learn to use simulated patients in team objective structured clinical examination (TOSCE), standardized patients, or simulated settings.

SELECTING TOOLS FOR EVALUATING STUDENTS

A variety of evaluation tools that measure individual attitudes and performance may be used in IPE curricula (www.nexusipe.org; www.ipe.utoronto.ca/curriculum/facilitators/tools-resources; www.mededportal.org/collections/ipe). Many are self-reported attitude measures with only a few objective and observer-based scales. Which tools are ultimately used depends on the focus of the educational strategy, but several examples of evaluation tools are available for consideration, including ones assessing attitudes and other skills.

The Collaborative Healthcare Interdisciplinary Relationship Planning (CHIRP) scale is a 14-item questionnaire that is focused on assessing student attitudes about interdisciplinary team learning. This tool includes seven specific subscales (dominance, empathy, interdependence, organizational climate, recognition, respect, and sharing). According to Havyer and colleagues (2016), this tool provides excellent validity for content, factor analysis, internal structure, and relationships to other variables, but it is limited to a classroom setting and lacks generalizability.

The 19-item Readiness for Interprofessional Learning Scale (RIPLS) consists of four subscales that include teamwork and collaboration, negative professional identity, positive professional identity, and roles and responsibilities. This scale is designed for students in earlier stages of training and is thus less appropriate for use in clinical settings (Lie, Fung, Trial, & Lohenry, 2013), but it may be ideal for health professions across multiple institutions (Havyer et al., 2016). The RIPLS still lacks studies that examine the impact of teams in addressing the health care needs of patients and populations.

A tool used to assess team skills is the modified McMaster–Ottawa Scale, which is observer based and assesses the competencies of communication, collaboration, roles and responsibilities, conflict management, patient- and family-centeredness, and team function (Lie et al., 2015). A faculty video is available to standardize ratings (Forest, Lie, & Ma, 2016).

The Communication and Teamwork Skills (CATS) assessment is a tool that utilizes trained observers to assess 18 teamwork behaviors; it provides weighted scoring according to the quality of the behavior across four areas: communication, cooperation, coordination, and situational awareness (Havyer et al., 2016). Because this tool involves direct observation of teams and their communication skills, it has been well received and shown to have high interrater reliability; however, its requirement of trained observers limits its feasibility (Havyer et al., 2016). In addition to assessing students, IPE curricula will benefit from overall program evaluation strategies that address the effectiveness of different approaches for different health professions.

CONCLUSIONS

Designing IPE curricula may be initiated from either a "top-down" or a "bottom-up" approach; decisions are often dependent on accreditation requirements for the health professions involved. Whether the decision comes from senior leadership or as a groundswell of IPE, interest among faculty may ultimately influence the speed of curriculum development but should not significantly influence the curriculum itself. Effective IPE curricula require well-trained faculty members who support team-based care and use the inclusive language of interprofessionality. Such curricula often include a needs assessment, the participation of students from the same level of learning, and icebreakers and/or social settings to facilitate discussion. Well-planned sessions are based on the needs assessment and subsequent instructional objectives. Successful IPE experiences should include instructional objectives based on specific competencies from the WHO or the Interprofessional Educational Collaborative, plus planned reflection and feedback. Various clinical IPE experiences could have similar constructs but should occur with patient care teams whose supervised clinical experiences may involve a variety of health professions and include clinical faculty members who have been trained to teach learners from other health professions (Lie, Forest, Kysh, & Sinclair, 2016).

REFERENCES

Association of American Medical Colleges. (2011). *Core competencies for interprofessional collaborative practice: Report of an expert panel*. Washington, DC: Interprofessional Education Collaborative. Retrieved from https://members.aamc.org/eweb/upload/Core%20Competencies%20for%20Interprofessional%20 Collaborative%20Practice_Revised.pdf

Barnsteiner, J. H., Disch, J. M., Hall, L., Mayer, D., & Moore, S. M. (2007). Promoting interprofessional education. *Nursing Outlook, 55*(3), 144–150. doi:10.1016/j.outlook.2007.03.003

Barr, H., & Low, H. (2011). Centre for the Advancement of Interprofessional Education (CAIPE): The definition and principles of interprofessional education. Retrieved from http://caipe.org.uk/about-us/the-definition-and-principles-of-interprofessional-education

Bridges, D. R., Davidson, R. A., Odegard, P. S., Maki, I. V., & Tomkowiak, J. (2011). Interprofessional collaboration: Three best practice models of interprofessional education. *Medical Education Online, 16*(1), 1–10. doi:10.3402/meo.v16i0.6035

D'amour, D., & Oandasan, I. (2005). Interprofessionality as the field of interprofessional practice and interprofessional education: An emerging concept. *Journal of Interprofessional Care, 19*(Suppl. 1), 8–20.

Forest, C. P., Lie, D. A., & Ma, S. B. (2016). Evaluating interprofessional team performance: A faculty rater tool. *MedEdPortal, 12*, 10447. doi:10.15766/mep_2374-8265.10447

Havyer, R. D., Nelson, D. R., Wingo, M. T., Comfere, N. I., Halvorsen, A. J., McDonald, F. S., & Reed, D. A. (2016). Addressing the interprofessional collaboration competencies of the Association of

American Medical Colleges: A systematic review of assessment instruments in undergraduate medical education. *Academic Medicine, 91*(6), 865–888.

Interprofessional Education Collaborative. (2011). Core competencies for interprofessional collaborative practice. Retrieved from http://www.aacn.nche.edu/education-resources/ipecreport.pdf

Lie, D., Forest, C. P., Kysh, L., & Sinclair, L. (2016). Interprofessional education and practice guide no. 5: Interprofessional teaching for prequalification students in clinical settings. *Journal of Interprofessional Care, 30*(3), 324–330.

Lie, D., Fung, C., Trial, J., & Lohenry, K. (2013). A comparison of two scales for assessing health professional students' attitude toward interprofessional learning. *Medical Education Online, 18*. doi:10.3402/meo.v18i0.21885

Lie, D., May, W., Richter-Lagha, R., Forest, C., Banzali, Y., & Lohenry, K. (2015). Adapting the McMaster–Ottawa scale and developing behavioral anchors for assessing performance in an interprofessional team observed structured clinical encounter. *Medical Education Online, 20*. doi:10.3402/meo.v20.26691

NEXUS. (2017). Retrieved from https://nexusipe.org/advancing/assessment-evaluation

Orchard, C., Bainbridge, L., Bassendowski, S., Stevenson, K., Wagner, S. J., Weinberg, L., . . . Sawatsky-Girling, B. (2010). A national interprofessional competency framework. Retrieved from www.cihc.ca/files/CIHC_IPCompetencies_Feb1210.pdf

Ponzer, S., Hylin, U., Kisoffsky, A., Lauffs, M., Lonka, K., Mattiasson, A. C., & Nordstrom, G. (2004). Interprofessional training in the context of clinical practice: Goals and students' perceptions on clinical education wards. *Medical Education, 38*, 727–736. doi:10.1002/9780470776438

Reeves, S., Perrier, L., Goldman, J., Freeth, D., & Zwarenstein, M. (2013). Interprofessional education: Effects on professional practice and healthcare outcomes (update). *Cochrane Database of Systematic Reviews, 2013*(3), 1–47. doi:10.1002/14651858.CD002213.pub3

Reeves, S., Zwarenstein, M., Goldman, J., Barr, H., Freeth, D., Koppel, I., & Hammick, M. (2010). The effectiveness of interprofessional education: Key findings from a new systematic review. *Journal of Interprofessional Care, 24*(30), 230–241.

Rodger, S., J. Hoffman, S., & World Health Organization Study Group on Interprofessional Education and Collaborative Practice. (2010). Where in the world is interprofessional education? A global environmental scan. *Journal of Interprofessional Care, 24*(5), 479–491.

Rudland, J. R., & Mires, G. J. (2005). Characteristics of doctors and nurses as perceived by students entering medical school: Implications for shared teaching. *Medical Education, 34*, 448–455.

Thistlethwaite, J. E., Forman, D., Matthews, L. R., Rogers, G. D., Steketee, C., & Yassine, T. (2014). Competencies and frameworks in interprofessional education: A comparative analysis. *Academic Medicine, 89*(6), 869–875.

World Health Organization. (2010). Framework for action on interprofessional education and collaborative practice. Retrieved from http://www.who.int/hrh/resources/framework_action/en

Zorek, J., & Raehl, C. (2013). Interprofessional education accreditation standards in the USA: A comparative analysis. *Journal of Interprofessional Care, 27*(2), 123–130.

Zwarenstein, M., Goldman, J., & Reeves, S. (2009). Interprofessional collaboration: Effects of practice-based interventions on professional practice and healthcare outcomes. *Cochrane Database of Systematic Reviews,* (3), CD000072. doi:10.1002/14651858.CD000072.pub2

PART II
Active Teaching–Learning Methodologies

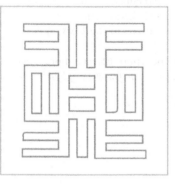

NEA ONNIM NO SUA A, OHU
"He who does not know can know
from learning."

*This is a symbol of knowledge, lifelong education, and
a continued quest for knowledge.*

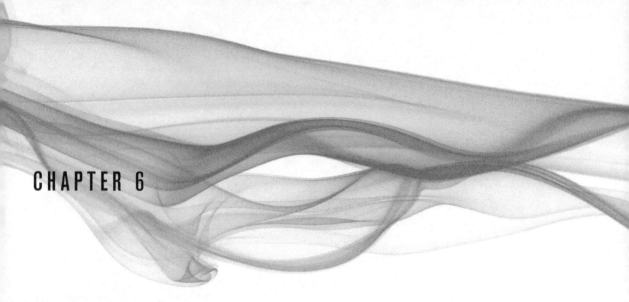

CHAPTER 6

Problem-Based Learning

Susan Hawkins, Judy Truscott, and Alyssa Abebe

CHAPTER OBJECTIVES

- Use problem-based learning to increase active learning
- Recognize common barriers and how to overcome them

A learning method based on the principle of using problems as a starting point for the acquisition and integration of new knowledge.

—*H.S. Barrows*

Curricular change towards problem-based learning is becoming a feature of professional education where the demands of universities and employers are requiring that professionals of the future can adapt to changing climates.

—*Maggi Savin-Baden*

Problem-based learning (PBL) is an instructional, active method of teaching in which students direct their own learning. Students working in small groups investigate cases/problems through research and use critical thinking and problem-solving skills while being facilitated by an instructor (hereafter called *facilitator*). Open-ended questions drive the learning from initial presentation to resolution. Students challenge their own and the group's knowledge to solve a case together, thus learning new information as the case unfolds. This promotes team and communications skills within the small groups. Cases are chosen to allow students to explore different approaches to each patient's clinical presentation, and patient cases should increase in complexity over the course of the curriculum as students become more medically sophisticated.

Cases are "located" in a specific medical setting so that students learn the difference in approach between acute and chronic care settings. Cases are based on actual patients, and the facilitator's level of questioning can be basic or more detailed depending on when in the curriculum the case is located. PBL promotes the development of critical thinking skills and enhances problem-solving skills (Barrows & Tamblyn, 1980). Students learn to apply their past and current knowledge to actual cases and situations. Students' motivation is thought to be increased when they apply their knowledge in real-life situations rather than memorize facts for future applications. Students must also be aware of whether or not their individual knowledge base is sufficient to care for the patient adequately. The ability to comprehend and acknowledge medical concepts helps students learn and teach others more effectively, thus enhancing the team's learning and confidence level. As students learn to research the information needed to care for the patient and teach this information to groupmates, the team's confidence level and aggregate knowledge increase (Barrows & Wee Keng Neo, 2010; Center for Teaching and Learning, Stanford University, 2001).

HISTORY AND FORMAT OF PBL

PBL was first introduced into the medical school curriculum in the late 1960s at McMaster University in Canada. The curricular committee adapted the concept from Harry Shoemaker, who was using active learning to teach electronic maintenance for U.S. Army Signal Corps members. By giving his students real-life problems and having them learn to find the solutions on their own, Shoemaker was able to accomplish his learning objectives in a more effective and positive way, leading him to discontinue lectures and lab demonstrations. McMaster incorporated PBL into first-year medical education to prepare students for the clinical year when they worked directly with patients. PBL has since been implemented in a variety of educational settings (Barrows, 1994; Neufeld & Barrows, 1974).

Four components separate the different models and approaches to PBL (Barrows & Wee Keng Neo, 2010):

- Extent of facilitator direction
- Problem design and structure
- Problem sequence
- Acquisition of patient information

In the academic setting, the amount of facilitator involvement distinguishes the models and approaches. Facilitators may gently guide students toward problem solution or may remain completely neutral during the process. Problems can be very complex or simple, sequenced in an organ system progression, organized by age groups, or organized randomly. Programs can decide whether or not students may have access to resources, such as notes, journal articles, or textbooks, while working through the problem. Some programs may not allow students to have access to resources during the session. When students fail to request a necessary piece of patient information, facilitators may provide the information at that time or may wait until the end of the case. As in real life, students learn from their errors. If they fail to ask for a vital piece of information and thus delay correct diagnosis, they learn the importance of thorough questioning. Thus, the pedagogy of PBL more directly mimics professional and workplace demands as compared to a lecture-based curriculum.

PBL ADVANTAGES AND DISADVANTAGES

From the student perspective, PBL appears to improve clinical reasoning and the ability to integrate knowledge across multiple disciplines (Fischer-Tenhagen, Heuwieser, & Arlt, 2016;

McCannon, Robertson, Caldwell, Juwah, & Elfessi, 2005; Wijnen, Loyens, & Schaap, 2016). Students begin to develop a reasoning process and expand the problem to different areas of health care (basic science, pathophysiology, anatomy, clinical practice, and so forth). They are taught to treat a patient as a whole, across all areas of that patient's life, including social aspects (finances, family situation, and so on). In a lecture-based program, these skills are typically taught in different classes rather than integrated as a whole. Students also self-direct their learning, training themselves to become lifelong learners while they are in school and transition into clinical practice. Students are trained to critically evaluate themselves and their teammates, challenging each other to become better medical providers. Because PBL is team based, acquiring team skills allows students to work effectively and efficiently together toward the goal, teaching each other throughout the process and in turn developing better study habits. Multiple studies have also shown that students find PBL enjoyable and motivating (Walsh, 2005). Students are more enthusiastic to learn, which may account for the increased job satisfaction for the facilitator (Ribeiro, 2001). Students within a PBL Model have enhanced interpersonal skills, which are difficult to teach in lecture format. Despite these advantages, it has been noted in some cases that PBL students do not have in-depth basic science knowledge as compared to lecture-based learning (LBL) students (Solomon, 2005). PBL students are slower than LBL students to apply a forward reasoning process (pattern recognition). PBL students are trained to use hypothetical deductive skills to solve a particular problem, also known as *backward reasoning*. On certifying standardized tests, there is no significant difference found in students' scores between PBL or LBL curricula.

CONTRASTING PBL WITH SIMILAR PEDAGOGIES

In order to comprehend PBL, it is important to discuss other similar types of active learning such as case-based learning (CBL), team-based learning (TBL), and flipped classrooms. With PBL, the students have no prior knowledge of information and learning is acquired while the case is occurring, with the case driving the learning. CBL, much like PBL, is self-directed as students work through a case or problem. However, with CBL, students have received curricular content prior to the case and use that knowledge to solve the particular case. Students use knowledge from either previously solved cases, prior clinical experience, or material that was covered in class (Williams, 2005).

TBL is similar to PBL and CBL in that students work together as a group, although they do not solve a particular problem or case. TBL uses a three-step approach to teaching (Michelson, Knight, & Fink, 2004):

- Students have prior reading or complete an out-of-class activity before class
- A readiness assurance test (RAT) is administered individually and then again in a small group
- After the RAT, there is an application-focused exercise done in class

The "grade" is determined by the individual's RAT score plus the group's RAT score. A class exercise is done after the RATs to emphasize both the material prepared ahead of time and the performance on the RAT (Brame, 2016).

Flipped classrooms are similar to PBL in that they require students to engage in an activity that is completed in class with the help of the instructor. It takes the traditional style of lecture followed by homework and "flips" it. Students prepare ahead of time by watching a video, reading, or doing an assignment; then the "case" is completed during the class. Students are engaged in the classroom setting as a result of knowledge acquired beforehand (Lage, Platt, & Treglia, 2000).

BASIC PRINCIPLES OF PBL

The basic principles of a PBL session include the following (Barrows &Wee Keng Neo, 2010):

- Introduction of the group members
- Climate setting to establish the "rules" of PBL
- Identification of goals by students
- Directions to set up elements of the PBL process
- Introduction of the case
- Development of a differential diagnosis
- Facilitator questioning students as the case progresses (Exhibit 6.1)
- Setting up a knowledge abstraction template (Exhibit 6.2 and Figures 6.1 and 6.2)

EXHIBIT 6.1 Useful Phrases to Use When Probing for Student Information

How do you know that?	Where is that located?
How does that happen?	What causes that?
Why does that happen?	What do you need to ask to rule that out?
When does that happen?	What does a PA need to know about that?
What do the rest of you think?	How will that help you take care of this patient?
Is that always true?	What do you think?
Does everyone agree with that?	Are you sure about that?
How does that work?	Do you think you know it, or do you know you know it?
How are those related?	
What makes you think that?	
What do you need to know to take care of this patient?	**When You Are Otherwise Stumped as to Where to Go:**
Why do you ask that question?	Let's review the idea list
How would that help you arrive at a diagnosis?	Could someone summarize the problem?
Can someone draw that?	
Do those things always occur together?	

EXHIBIT 6.2 Knowledge Abstraction Grid

Differential Diagnosis	Epidemiology/Etiology	Symptoms/Signs	Treatment/Patient Education
Otitis Media			
Otitis Externa			
Mastoiditis			

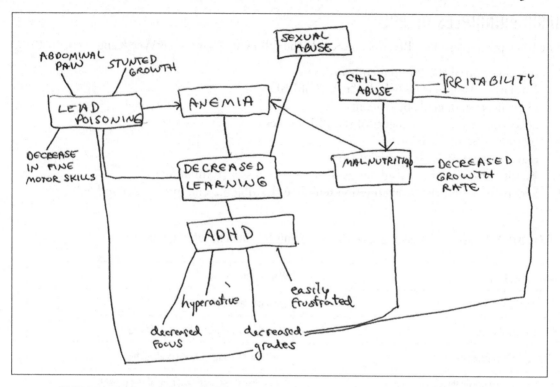

FIGURE 6.1 Decreased learning is the concept based on the patient's complaint. ADHD, attention deficit/hyperactivity disorder.

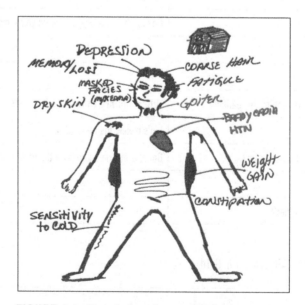

FIGURE 6.2 Knowledge abstraction body mapping.

Introductions occur at the initial meeting of a new group. The facilitator introduces himself or herself first, including a "fun fact" with the introduction. This will often have students adding "fun facts" about themselves as they model the facilitator. The inclusion of the fun fact creates a more relaxed environment and establishes the role of the facilitator as guide rather than a teacher.

Climate Setting

Climate setting occurs in the first session of each new group. Walsh (2005) describes climate setting as creating "a safe, conducive environment for self-directed learning" (p. 11). During this portion of the session, the facilitator provides information about the process, what is expected of students, and what students should expect of the facilitator. The facilitator advises students that he or she will ask questions rather than provide information. Questions are meant to help students determine what they know and do not know. Individuals may feel uncomfortable questioning statements made by group members who have strong personalities or a great deal of medical experience. This is important because students learn to respectfully disagree with each other, a valuable skill when working as part of a health care team.

Goals

Goals should be developed to identify what students hope to accomplish both in each session and during the course. Goals are best documented on a large sheet of paper so that they may be posted on the wall during each session and are easily visible to the group members and facilitator. These may be either individual or group goals, but it is essential that goals are measurable. Typically, a group new to the process of PBL will make goals about the process, such as "learn about PBL," "meet the group," and so forth. The facilitator helps the group develop more content-specific and behavioral goals. These should be reviewed on an ongoing basis and may change as students receive feedback about behaviors, communication, team skills, participation, self-directed learning, clinical reasoning, and so forth (Barrows & Wee Keng Neo, 2010).

Patient Encounter

The patient's chief complaint is presented to the group with the group generating a differential-diagnosis list. This list is created during a brainstorming session and all students' ideas should be documented. Students may feel that more information is necessary to generate ideas, but the facilitator encourages a robust list that encompasses multiple organ systems. At this point, students are not required to justify their ideas, just to list them. Once a robust differential-diagnosis list is developed, students begin to gather information about the patient. Documentation occurs continually by recording patient information as students receive it. Further patient information is obtained through direct patient questioning, formulating a question as if asking a patient. The goal is to prepare students for clinical rotations by training them to interact verbally with a patient. The facilitator's role during this portion is to test students' clinical reasoning, probe their knowledge, and push for learning issues. Students have multiple opportunities to present the case as if to a preceptor, receiving feedback from both group members and the facilitator, allowing the development of presentation skills for clinical experiences (Barrows & Wee Keng Neo, 2010).

Learning Issues

Students declare a learning issue when they do not possess sufficient knowledge in order to adequately care for the patient. Students research this information outside of the PBL session. Learning issues are not democratic group decisions. Any student may list a learning issue both during and at the end of the session. Students choose which learning issues they wish to research. If, at the end of the class session, the group is no longer interested in a particular learning issue, they may eliminate it from the list. The facilitator questions the students regarding their knowledge related to the case. The facilitator looks for signs of confusion or disagreement among group members and, if noted, asks questions to generate discussion. If the group cannot achieve consensus, this generates a learning issue to be clarified. Allowing some silence in the room after posing a question gives students time to state that they do not understand. Questioning should probe students on many different areas important to the care of the patient: symptoms, signs, pathophysiology, treatment, mechanism of action of medications, patient access to care, cultural variabilities in caring for patients, and so forth. During subsequent sessions with the same case, the facilitator may question resources used by students, which reinforces their use of evidence-based medicine. As the case progresses, questions become more focused based on the information students have acquired through self-directed learning (Barrows & Wee Keng Neo, 2010).

Closing the Case

Once students have gathered all information, completed a physical examination, and ordered any diagnostic tests, they must develop a diagnosis and treatment plan. Requiring (all students must do this) students to "role-play" the health professions student in a clinical setting as well as the patient gives practice in patient education. Students should be given the opportunity to give difficult information to the "patient" and his or her "family members" when consistent with the case outcome. Students are then told the actual "outcome" of the case, which could include the following:

- A patient leaves the hospital against medical advice
- A patient fails to follow instructions
- A patient dies
- A patient's outcome is positive

Students are questioned about how their treatment plan differed from the case outcome in order to generate more discussion and opportunity for education. Students also review what they learned and how they might have approached the problem differently if they had to do it over again. Students choose an overarching area to prepare for a subsequent session during which the facilitator may ask more general questions about disease process, anatomy, treatment, or any other aspect of the clinical area chosen. This process is called *knowledge abstraction*, as students move from the specifics of the case to the more abstract disease process or pathophysiology of diseases within an organ system (Barrows & Wee Keng Neo, 2010). Examples of student-generated knowledge abstractions can be found in Figures 6.1 and 6.2.

Assessment

Once students reach the end of the defined unit, assessment takes place via multiple-choice examination, a written case examination, an oral examination, an objective structured clinical examination (OSCE), a performance evaluation, or a combination of any of these. The performance evaluations given to students during the unit and postunit are important assessments of the students' ability to understand and explain the material, work as a team, use appropriate clinical reasoning to navigate through a problem, and speak to the level of a patient or clinician. Each program can choose assessment methods appropriate to its curriculum and usage of PBL (Barrows & Wee Keng Neo, 2010).

Feedback

In PBL, feedback is an integral component of the learning process. The actual mechanics of giving and receiving feedback are easily incorporated. The facilitator is a role model for giving and receiving feedback and thus is not only an observer but an active participant as well. Feedback should occur often enough for students to be able to demonstrate improvement, ideally at least twice during any unit of group work. Students evaluate themselves first, and then receive feedback from each group member and then from the facilitator. Next, the facilitator self-evaluates and students then give feedback to the facilitator, allowing the students to observe appropriate feedback responses. It is important that the facilitator self-evaluates as this parallels the student process (Barrows & Wee Keng Neo, 2010).

Criteria for feedback are established at the beginning of the course and appear in the course syllabus. Criteria chosen should reflect values of the program and can contain both content items and behavioral items. An operational definition and a rubric for each criterion are helpful to promote consistent feedback. Student evaluation measures can include:

- Clinical reasoning
- Self-directed learning
- Knowledge integration
- Participation
- Team skills
- Feedback
- Communication skills

Faculty evaluation criteria can include:

- Climate setting
- Direction
- Goals
- Confrontation
- Feedback
- Knowledge integration

Management of the Process

Managing the personalities in the group may be a difficult task for the facilitator. Overbearing group members may need tools to help them participate less. Similarly, quiet group members may need encouragement and/or methods to initiate participation in a more verbose group. If at times the group seems to be overwhelmed with information, periodically review of the ideas list or asking someone to summarize the case may help to refocus the group. At the end of the PBL session, the facilitator asks each group member to state the most likely diagnosis, which directs the students' planning for the next session. Each student must commit to one diagnosis, which encourages the student to use clinical judgment even though the case may be incomplete. Students choose which learning issues they would like to research prior to the next session. The facilitator should encourage students to select learning issues that are interesting to them so they are motivated to learn the material. At the end of a case, students develop a diagnosis and treatment plan. Students present this information along with patient education. This can be accomplished by writing the diagnosis and treatment plan on the board and by role-playing the patient education (Barrows & Wee Keng Neo, 2010).

When the curriculum runs over months to years, Barrows and Wee Keng Neo (2010) recommend that it should be split into units. Group members and facilitators should change with each unit. A group of seven students is considered an ideal number of participants, but groups can range from five to 10 members. If students do not change groups, they tend to become set in their roles within the group, and the group forms fixed expectations and opinions of each other. By changing groups, students have the opportunity to establish new roles and improve interpersonal skills. Students experience different group dynamics and facilitator styles, which helps them prepare for changing rotation sites and various preceptors. The length of the particular unit may depend on the number of facilitators who are available, the overall length of the didactic curriculum, or the university calendar. With a typical semester of approximately 14 weeks, a logical breakdown might be 4 to 5 weeks per unit or 7 weeks per unit depending on the didactic length. Units then can be differentiated by body systems (one or more) or another way that makes logical sense for a program's curriculum. There may be some advantages to modeling unit length to be consistent with rotation length so that students are used to changing settings periodically prior to the clinical year.

If a program uses multiple PBL groups, some system for supervision of the facilitator ensures that students receive the core knowledge required for each unit and that the process is similar no matter who facilitates. Faculty can observe each other giving feedback similar to the student feedback process.

INTEGRATING PBL INTO A LECTURE-BASED CURRICULUM

PBL can be incorporated successfully into a lecture-based curriculum provided that faculty are trained in student-centered techniques and their roles are clearly delineated. The role of the facilitator must be defined for students when doing PBL; otherwise, students might think that the facilitator is withholding information. Similarly, it is preferable to begin PBL early in the curriculum rather than waiting for the end of the didactic year. Later in the program, students may expect faculty to always provide answers and may become resentful when faculty do not (Barrows & Wee Keng Neo, 2010).

Courses in which clinical thinking and critical analysis are natural components of the material, such as Clinical Medicine and Clinical Problem Solving, are best for incorporating PBL into an existing lecture-based curriculum. Introduce the clinical case and have the lectures accompany or follow the case. The desire to solve the case drives the desire to learn the material.

CONCLUSIONS

PBL, either as an entire curriculum pedagogy or part of a lecture-based curriculum, can develop clinical reasoning and problem-solving skills as well as professional behavior and team skills. Students who learn via patient scenarios may be better prepared for rotations and clinical practice, although studies have not confirmed this. Solving the clinical case becomes its own motivation to learn, and evidence-based practice skills are an everyday component of their education. Students develop the ability to be life-long learners, a critical skill given the ever-changing knowledge base required for clinical practice.

REFERENCES

Barrows, H. (1994). *Practice-based learning: Problem-based learning applied to medical education.* Carbondale, IL: Southern Illinois University School of Medicine.

Barrows, H., & Tamblyn, R. (1980). *Problem-based learning: An approach to medical education.* New York, NY, Springer Publishing.

Barrows, H., & Wee Keng Neo, L. (2010). *Principles and practice of PBL* (Rev. ed.). Carbondale, IL: Southern Illinois University School of Medicine.

Brame, C. J. (2016). Team-based learning. Retrieved from https://cft.vanderbilt.edu/guides-sub-pages/team-based-l

Center for Teaching and Learning, Stanford University. (2001). Problem-based learning. *Speaking of Teaching, 11*(1). Retrieved from http://web.stanford.edu/dept/CTL/Newsletter/problem_based_learning.pdf

Fischer-Tenhagen, C., Heuwieser, W., & Arlt, S. (2016). Creative learning methods and open choice of topics facilitate self-directed learning and motivation of veterinary students. *Creative Education, 7,* 1906–1912.

Lage, M., Platt, G., & Treglia, M. (2000). Inverting the classroom: A gateway to creating an inclusive learning environment. *Journal of Economic Education, 31*(1), 30–43.

McCannon, R., Robertson, E., Caldwell, J., Juwah, C., & Elfessi, A. (2005). Students' perceptions of their acquired knowledge during a problem-based learning case study. *Occupational Therapy in Health Care, 18*(4), 13–28.

Michelson, L. K., Knight, A. B., & Fink, D. (2004). *Team-based learning: A transformative use of small groups in college teaching.* Sterling, VA: Stylus.

Neufeld, V. R., & Barrows, H. S. (1974). The "McMaster philosophy": An approach to medical education. *Journal of Medical Education, 49*(11), 1040–1050.

Ribeiro, L. (2001). The pros and cons of problem-based learning from the teacher's standpoint. *Journal of University Teaching and Learning Practice, 8*(4). Retrieved from http://files.eric.ed.gov/fulltext/EJ940100.pdf

Solomon, P. (2005). Problem-based learning: A review of current issues relevant to physiotherapy education. *Physiotherapy Theory and Practice, 21*(1), 37–49. doi:10.1080/09593980590911499

Van Rhee, J., Wardle, S., Hutchinson, C., Applegate, E. B., Vangsnes, E. H., Meyer, J. M., . . . Fenn, W. H. (2003). Problem-based learning in physician assistant education: Establishing a basis for a comparative study. *Perspective on Physician Assistant Education, 14*(4), 242–248. Retrieved from http://journals.lww.com/jpae/Abstract/2003/14040/Problem_based_Learning_in_Physician_Assistant.8.aspx

Walsh, A. (2005). *The tutor in problem-based learning: A novice's guide.* Hamilton, ON: McMaster University, Faculty of Health Sciences. Retrieved from http://fhs.mcmaster.ca/facdev/documents/tutorPBL.pdf

Wijnen, M., Loyens, S. M. M., & Schaap, L. (2016). Experimental evidence of the relative effectiveness of problem-based learning for knowledge acquisition and retention. *Interactive Learning Environments, 24*(8), 1907–1921.

Williams, B. (2005). Case-based learning: A review of literature: is there scope for this educational paradigm in prehospital education? *Emergency Medicine Journal, 22*, 577–581. doi:10.1136/emj.2004.022707

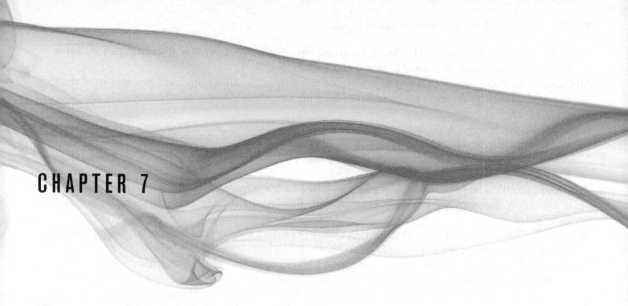

CHAPTER 7

Team-Based Learning

Victoria Wallace and Lisa Walker

CHAPTER OBJECTIVES

- Use team-based learning to increase active learning
- Recognize common barriers and how to overcome them

Why is it, in spite of the fact that teaching by pouring in, learning by passive absorption, are universally condemned, that they are still so entrenched in practice?

—*John Dewey* (1916, p. 46)

ORIGIN OF TEAM-BASED LEARNING PEDAGOGY AND ITS APPLICATION IN HEALTH PROFESSIONS EDUCATION

Although team-based learning (TBL) has been an active learning strategy for several decades in business schools, it is a relatively new approach to teaching in health professions. Before discussing why and how TBL can be implemented into health professions education, it will help to understand where TBL began and how it has evolved. First, let us review TBL's history and how it was created.

Larry Michaelsen, then professor of management at the University of Oklahoma's Business School, originated TBL in 1979. Michaelsen originally taught an undergraduate class of around 40 students using a case-based, Socratic teaching style. Students were able to demonstrate deep learning and problem-solving skills by applying concepts rather than just memorizing them. Michaelsen's class eventually grew from 40 to 120 students. For him, several key challenges needed to be resolved: student engagement, accountability, and preparation. He wrestled with how he could maintain the same level of engagement and learning in a large class, while also keeping individual students accountable. He also needed to find a way that he could ensure each individual students would come to class prepared to work on the learning activities (Michaelsen, Knight, & Fink, 2004; Sibley & Ostafichuk, 2014).

Over time, Michaelsen devised several critical strategies that today make up the structure of TBL. Readiness assurance tests (RATs), given early in the class, hold each student accountable for his or her work, individually and within the team. They also ensure that students come to class prepared for the day's activities. Well-structured application activities help with management and facilitation challenges. The "4S" framework (significant problem, same problem, specific choice, simultaneous report) structures the activities so that large numbers of small teams can all work simultaneously to problem solve and collaboratively make decisions. Data collection and analysis provided evidence that the strategies were working (Michaelsen et al., 2004).

Undergraduate faculty outside of the University of Oklahoma discovered TBL through Michaelsen's publications and workshops. Faculty attending the TBL workshops were especially interested in seeing how this method could improve student learning in their own courses. Faculty teaching accounting, microbial physiology, organization/communication, and organic chemistry were some of the first to try out TBL and experience positive results (Dinan & Frydrychowski, 1995; Lancaster & Strand, 2003; McInerney & Fink, 2003, Roebuck, 1998). Medical educators were next to try TBL.

Although many health professions educators had already embraced problem-based learning (PBL), this methodology required several trained facilitators in a single course (Searle et al., 2003). Facing curriculum changes and fewer faculty resources, many health professions educators needed another strategy to keep large classes of students engaged in high levels of learning (Searle et al., 2003). Unlike PBL, TBL required only one instructor. After attending a Michaelsen workshop, Baylor Medical College faculty were motivated to integrate elements of TBL into their teaching and TBL quickly expanded across Baylor (Haidet, O'Malley, & Richards, 2002). A few years later, Baylor Medical College obtained a grant to train and support faculty in TBL implementation and evaluation at 10 different medical schools (Searle et al., 2003; Sibley & Parmelee, 2008).

TBL continued to spread through health care education. Through trial and error, refinements have made over the years in an effort to improve TBL. Although TBL has evolved, the foundation of TBL remains focused on student engagement/collaboration, preparation, and structured problem-solving activities.

THE PROCESS OF TBL

Although TBL follows a fairly prescriptive process and TBL sessions require more time to prepare than a typical lecture, it also allows for a great deal of creativity. And engaging in a well-designed TBL class is so much more rewarding than lecturing—for both instructors and students. As stated earlier, TBL addresses the PBL resource challenges. Where PBL teams meet separately with individual faculty facilitators and often have assigned projects outside of class time, TBL teams work together in one large classroom with a single faculty member during a scheduled class period. This allows one faculty member to teach the whole class. This also prevents another PBL challenge: out-of-class teamwork for which a small number of students do the work, but the whole team gets the credit. The TBL process is diagrammed in Figure 7.1 (Michaelsen, Knight, & Fink, 2004; Sibley & Ostafichuk, 2014).

Creating Teams

The creation of teams should be done at the very beginning of a TBL course. In order to provide students a rich learning environment, student teams should be no more than five to seven

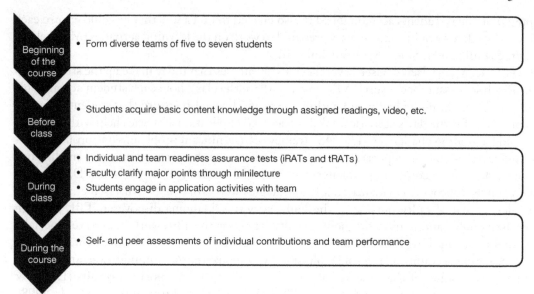

Beginning of the course
- Form diverse teams of five to seven students

Before class
- Students acquire basic content knowledge through assigned readings, video, etc.

During class
- Individual and team readiness assurance tests (iRATs and tRATs)
- Faculty clarify major points through minilecture
- Students engage in application activities with team

During the course
- Self- and peer assessments of individual contributions and team performance

FIGURE 7.1 The team-based learning process.

members and the composition of each team should be as diverse as possible. A team composed of students with similar undergraduate grade point averages (GPAs), work experience, race/ethnicity, age, gender, and so forth will diminish the team's efficacy and opportunities for each member of the team to both contribute to and benefit from his or her teammates' knowledge and experience (Michaelsen & Sweet, 2012). The simplest way to create a diverse team is to use a survey tool that will aggregate data. There are several free, online survey tools that will do the work of creating diverse teams and allow faculty to customize the survey questions if there are other student characteristics to include. A listing of recommended TBL resources may be found in the online supplement (Chapter 7 Exemplar). For example, faculty may want to include factors such as number of years in the workforce, leadership style preference, and learning style preference, to name a few (Michaelsen, 1992).

In addition to diversity, it is important that the team-formation process be transparent to students to avoid any appearance of faculty manipulation or planning in designing teams. It is also essential that teams remain together for an extended period of time (through a module, course, semester, or academic year). This allows teams to experience the ups and downs of working together and resolving issues and conflicts (Michaelsen et al., 2004).

Student Preparation for Class

A TBL class is a version of the flipped classroom, where students are expected to acquire basic content knowledge prior to the class session. Using a variety of faculty-selected assignments, such as reading textbook chapters and journal articles, listening to podcasts, audio or video recordings, voice-over presentations, presentations with supporting notes, or any combination of these, students can work at their own pace and determine the amount of time they need to invest in their learning. Using a variety of media helps engage students at many levels during this independent learning. For a single class session, an outline or a handful of very specific learning objectives can help students focus on critical content. Students should expect to spend one to two times the amount of class time in preparation (i.e., a 2-hour class = 2–4 hours of preparation) and readings should not exceed 40 to 50 pages (Michaelsen & Sweet, 2009).

In-Class Readiness Assurance Process

A two-part in-class readiness assurance process is used. First, an individual test containing 10 to 25 multiple-choice questions (MCQs), also known as an *individual readiness assurance test (iRAT)*, is based on the preparation assignment given at the beginning of the class session. The iRAT serves two important purposes. First, it builds in individual accountability for the prep work. Students are far less likely to default to their team members to do the heavy lifting if part of their course grade relies on the effort they put forth in preparing for class. Second, it gives faculty an opportunity to identify individual students at risk (Michaelsen & Sweet, 2009).

Immediately following the individual quiz, students take the same MCQ test with their team (team readiness assurance test, or tRAT). Students should not have access to their grade on the individual quiz until the team quiz is completed. This ensures a rich discussion when students have a difference of opinion on any given question. The opportunity for students to elaborate what they have learned during the tRAT process is one of the true benefits of TBL; elaboration moves information into the brain's hard drive, improving retention and recall (Michaelsen et al., 2004). The use of commercially available scratch-off answer cards provides teams and faculty with immediate feedback and is strongly recommended.

The Minilecture

At the conclusion of the readiness assurance process, there is often a 10- to 15-minute lecture to either highlight the major take-home points from the preparation materials or to clarify any points of confusion identified from the results of the iRAT and tRAT. Another way to do this is to ask each team to write down any lingering questions members have about the material and assign those questions to other teams. Teams work together to craft a clear answer to their assigned question, with faculty input and guidance, and then present their answers to the class (Michaelsen et al., 2004).

Application Activities

Collaborating with teammates to address real-life situations and problems is at the heart of the TBL process, and it offers many benefits. A well-crafted application activity will challenge and engage all members in the activity, mobilizing the strengths and assets of each member of the team while building capacity, knowledge, and skills across the entire team. In a traditional TBL session, each application activity should incorporate the "4S" framework, as previously mentioned. The assignment should be based on a significant, real-life problem, each team should be working on the same problem at the same time, teams should have to make a specific choice from a series of options (MCQ, a list of drugs or possible diagnoses, and so forth), and teams should report their answers simultaneously. To illustrate how this might work in a health professions class, one might assign a patient or client case that requires students to decide the best treatment or next steps. This is an example of a problem that has significance to the students. All teams, in one large classroom, work on the case at the same time. Faculty provide the teams with options to choose from and reveal team answers all at the same time. Some of the tools used for teams to reveal answers are small dry-erase boards or laminated cards with A, B, C, and so on for MCQ responses. After revealing answers, faculty lead the whole class in discussion of the case and responses. Especially rich discussions can ensure when a case is challenging and teams reveal conflicting responses (Michaelsen & Sweet, 2009).

Other types of application activities that do not strictly follow the "4S" rule can be equally effective. One example is a variation of PBL, called the *Gallery Walk* (Allen, Larmer, & Bayer, 2013). This active learning strategy can be integrated into a TBL activity or the traditional classroom. To implement the Gallery Walk, give each team the same case and allow the teams to develop a complex treatment plan. Post the treatment plans on flip-chart paper around the classroom. Have all the teams review other teams' proposed plans and have students use sticky notes to support or disagree with the various treatments posted. This Gallery Walk is an active learning strategy and can be integrated into a TBL or traditional classroom. Follow the Gallery Walk activity with a large-class discussion on why teams chose particular plans and what points they agreed or disagreed on.

Self- and Peer Assessments

One of the major benefits of TBL for health professions students is the opportunity to learn to work closely and effectively with a diverse group of classmates. The skills they acquire in conflict resolution, giving and receiving feedback, and team processes will be crucial to their success as members of interprofessional health care teams in the future. As tensions arise within diverse student teams, the process of self- and peer assessments can help students identify areas of conflict and routes to resolution. It is also one of the most challenging aspects of TBL to implement and manage. Students are often resistant to the idea of giving teammates a "grade" or providing honest feedback to those who are overbearing or not contributing. So if there is resistance, why do it? Most teams, given enough time, will eventually experience conflict. That conflict can interfere with students' learning and their willingness to contribute to the work of the team. Providing an opportunity to share concerns, respond to positive and critical feedback from peers, and strategize for improving team function helps in the development of important interpersonal skills (Michaelsen et al., 2004; Michaelsen & Sweet, 2009).

To help facilitate the self- and peer-assessment process, several free online survey products exist that can be administered anonymously or with identifiers. Students evaluate themselves and their teammates regarding contribution to the work. They also assess the team's performance as a whole. Most of these products aggregate the data and provide students with a report comparing their self-assessment to their team's responses. The reports are also available to faculty and provide insight into issues or conflicts within the team and even between individual members on a team. In addition to a survey or formal evaluation, face-to-face meetings facilitated by faculty, counseling, or academic support personnel can help teams work through interpersonal conflict and identify strategies for working more effectively together.

Grading in TBL Courses

The iRAT, tRAT, and self- and peer assessments need to be graded and factored into the students' overall grade in a course. Faculty should also balance the value of the team's successes (RAT, application activities) with the need to adequately assess each individual student's acquisition of the learning outcomes for the course. Whether or not to grade the in-class application activities is an individual faculty choice (Michaelsen et al., 2004). The authors have not graded application activities and have found that students' efforts, enthusiasm, and engagement have persisted across the entire academic year despite the absence of a grade as motivator.

LEARNING THEORIES AND OUTCOMES

Research has shown that TBL improves critical thinking and long-term retention (McInerney & Fink, 2003). It improves student engagement (Chung, Rhee, Baik, & A, 2009; Clark, Nguyen, Bray, & Levine, 2008; Kelly et al., 2005; Levine et al., 2004), problem-solving skills (Hunt, Haidet, Coverdale, & Richards, 2003; Kelly et al., 2005), and communication and teamwork (O'Malley et al., 2003; Thompson et al., 2007). Perhaps that is why TBL health care students perform better than non-TBL students (Grady, 2011; Kamei, Cook, Puthucheary, & Starmer, 2012; Koles,

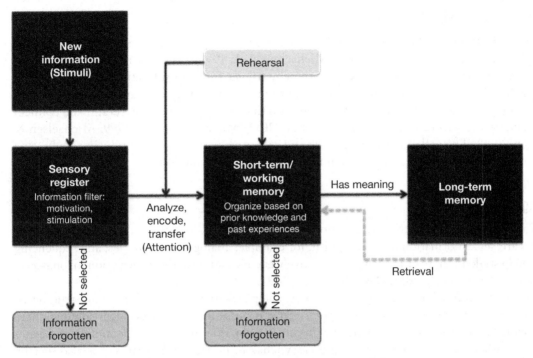

FIGURE 7.2 Information-processing model.

Nelson, Stolfi, Parmelee, & Destephen, 2005; Koles, Stolfi, Borges, Nelson, & Parmelee, 2010; Letassy, Fugate, Medina, Stroup, & Britton, 2008; Persky, 2012; Thomas & Bowen, 2011; Zingone et al., 2010).

Cognitive learning theory (CLT) and constructivism can help explain why TBL, as an instructional strategy, has been so successful. CLTs, also referred to as *cognitivism* or *cognitive information processing*, are based on arguments that people mentally process new information that is presented to them, rather than previous beliefs by behaviorists that people just simply respond to stimuli. Simply put, CLT focuses on how people learn related to attention, information processing, and memory (Davis & Arend, 2013). Figure 7.2 illustrates an information-processing model based on how cognitive processes work.

Information processing can be viewed as a means by which new information becomes embedded in short- or long-term memory and is retrieved for use. The process involves sensory register, short-term (working) memory, and long-term memory (Davis & Arend, 2013).

Sensory Register

When information is first presented, it enters our sensory register. The information is filtered based on student motivation or stimulation. In TBL, an authentic problem requiring higher order learning is typically presented. Real-world problems resonate with students, whereas the complexity requires students to engage and think more deeply (Brown, Roediger, & McDaniel, 2014; Michaelsen & Sweet, 2009). Correctly developed application exercises do not necessarily have a right or wrong answer, and therefore students experience a mental conflict. This tension keeps them mentally engaged and motivated to solve the problem—if not, the information may not attach to memory and be forgotten (Michaelsen, Black, & Fink, 1999). The information is analyzed, encoded, and transferred to short-term memory.

Short-Term/Working Memory

Depth of learning is enhanced when TBL activities conflict with students' existing knowledge in long-term memory (Brown et al., 2014; Michaelsen et al., 1999). Students' minds are challenged to clarify information through rehearsal, thereby trigger further exploration of ideas, improving learning. Information presented multiple times, with appropriate variation and immediate, timely feedback, leads to a greater likelihood that students will learn, retain, and connect information to future problems (Brown et al., 2014; Michaelsen et al., 1999; Michaelsen & Sweet, 2009). The collaborative teamwork and repetitive nature of content during application exercises and tests in TBL are important in supporting this function.

Long-Term Memory

Creating TBL activities that are appropriate for developing students' knowledge and transfer skills are key. Information organized with, for example, analogies, summaries, and sequencing will help students more efficiently and effectively encode and store the information in long-term memory (Brown et al., 2014; Davis & Arend, 2013).

Evolving from CLT, constructivism can also help explain why TBL works. Constructivists, such as Dewey (1933), view learning as an active process focused on problem solving where individuals construct new knowledge by linking information to prior understanding and experience, rather than passively acquiring it (Hrynchak & Batty, 2012). Learning is also socially constructed where meaning-making happens through shared perspectives and experiences in communities of practice (Hrynchak & Batty, 2012; Lave & Wenger, 1991; Vygotsky, 1978). TBL is a unique pedagogical method that aligns with both cognitive learning and constructivism views where students are active participants and activities are focused on experience, collaboration, and reflective thinking. To best structure TBL learning opportunities, instructors should ask themselves the following questions:

- How can I create TBL content and application exercises that will motivate and engage students (connect to prior knowledge and experience) but not overload their cognitive capacity?
- How should I create TBL materials so that students can efficiently and effectively process the new information? (analogies, mnemonic devices, summaries, etc.)
- How do I indicate and help facilitate the information that is important for students to remember?

CREATING A QUALITY TBL SESSION USING BACKWARD DESIGN

Any quality, instructionally sound course aligns goals and objectives with learning activities and assessments. TBL courses are no different. TBL will likely require faculty to completely redesign an existing course. *Backward design*, a term coined by Wiggins and McTighe (1998), is a process for designing instruction that focuses a course on what a student should be able to *do*, rather than what an instructor should teach (Figure 7.3). Although most instructional design models have a similar approach, backward design is the model currently followed in most academic institutions. In all practicality, faculty should first learn about backward design before implementing TBL (Wiggins & McTighe, 2005).

The backward design process begins by asking, "What are my big ideas? What do I want my students to look like after they complete my course?" These should be big and broad. In a three-credit course, it is typical to see two to four big ideas—these are the course goals. In order for students to achieve these course goals, smaller measurable, observable tasks should be defined. For each goal, faculty should ask, "What will students *do* to show that they have

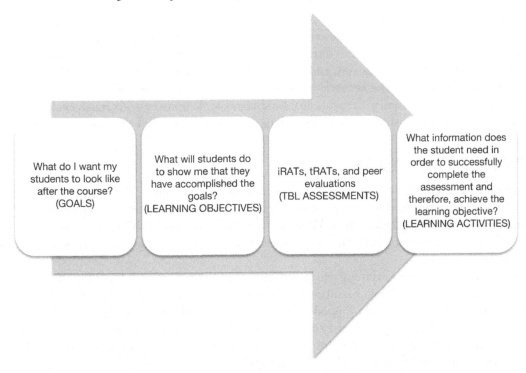

FIGURE 7.3 Schematic model of backward design.
iRATs, individual readiness assurance tests; TBL, team-based learning;
tRATs, team readiness assurance tests.

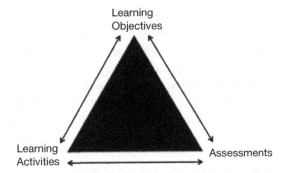

FIGURE 7.4 Alignment of learning objectives, learning activities, and assessments.

achieved this goal?" One to several tasks—or objectives—will be required in order to achieve a single goal. These are the learning objectives. The learning objectives must be observable and measurable so that students are able to demonstrate their ability to achieve them. How they demonstrate proficiency will vary.

Next, faculty need to determine how students will be assessed and what learning activities will be needed. In TBL, students are assessed through iRATs, tRATs, scored application exercises, and peer evaluations. Learning activities are designed by asking, "What information does the student need in order to successfully complete the assessment and, therefore, achieve the learning objective?" TBL learning activities typically include prework completed outside of class, minilectures, and application activities during class. The prework can take on many forms: readings, narrated minilectures, minicases, and so forth. The key requirement to all activities is that they align and support both the assessments and learning objectives (Figure 7.4).

Alignment of these curricular elements enables students to demonstrate—through evidence—that they are able to successfully achieve the learning objectives and, thus, the course goals.

PREPARING FACULTY FOR TBL

In addition to knowing how to design an instructionally sound course, there are several key factors faculty should understand before implementing TBL. First and foremost, faculty should experience TBL before implementing it. Whether observing a colleague's TBL course or attending a workshop, experiencing it firsthand provides an understanding that cannot be gained by only reading literature.

TBL is an active learning strategy where activities are learner centered. It is a big shift from traditional lecture-style teaching. Faculty must resist the urge to use long lectures as a means of "teaching content" and embrace a flipped-style of teaching in which students learn outside of class. The role of faculty shifts to facilitator, guide, and listener. Didactic learning happens outside the classroom with materials that are prepared in advance. In class, the majority of faculty time is spent administering RATs and facilitating application exercises.

Faculty and administrators also need to be prepared for a greater investment of time in preparing TBL sessions. Transforming faculty expertise into a 2- or 3-hour lecture takes far less effort and time than identifying quality preclass assignments, writing readiness assurance process (RAP) questions, and designing complex and engaging application activities. Although faculty will update lectures from year to year, transforming a course from traditional lecture to TBL and refining those TBL classes over time will require a commitment by both the faculty and the academic leadership.

Taking shortcuts by trying out various aspects of TBL that seem appealing or easy is rarely successful. TBL should be embraced in its entirety. The various elements of TBL are included to address accountability, fairness, and team equity. Implementing only portions of TBL may result in ineffective teams and class management challenges.

Last, developing and administering application exercises is one of the greatest challenges for new TBL instructors. Designing the activities requires not only deep knowledge of the content but also creative ideas about tasks that can be developed into meaningful, authentic application exercises. Several resources provide more detail on creating application exercises (Hawkins, 2014; Michaelsen, 1992; Michaelsen, Fink, & Knight, 1997; Michaelsen & Sweet, 2009). MedEdPORTAL has a library of free, peer-reviewed cases designed for TBL classrooms (www.mededportal.org) and the TBL Collaborative (www.teambasedlearning.org) is a membership-based organization with many excellent resources. During class, faculty need to be prepared to make on-the-fly adjustments when an activity takes longer (or shorter) than estimated. If some of the teams complete an activity before others are ready, having a follow-up question or a way for students to take a problem to another level of analysis will keep the quick teams actively engaged while others finish up the original problem.

PREPARING STUDENTS FOR TBL

TBL is a huge paradigm shift not only for faculty, but for students as well. It is not uncommon for students who expect passive forms of learning to express frustration with TBL. Students will be surprised by how much effort it takes to engage and problem solve. Advance planning and effective communication are key to successful implementation. Faculty must be explicit about why TBL was chosen for the class format and what students will gain from the experience. Students may need to be educated about how different learning strategies accomplish different levels of learning. For instance, although lectures are an acceptable strategy for sharing didactic content where students need only recall information, TBL will develop students' ability to think critically, analyze information, and solve problems.

CONCLUSIONS

In summary, TBL is an active learning strategy that can be successfully implemented in large classrooms with one faculty facilitator. In addition to the benefits of active learning, TBL incorporates accountability to the team. Students are developing teamwork and interpersonal conflict resolution skills not practiced in a classroom focused on individual student performance or even performance in small group work where accountability is not enforced or assessed. Although making the leap from lecture to TBL has its challenges, early evidence suggests that it will have a positive impact on health professions graduates' ability to be critical thinkers working effectively in high-functioning health care teams.

REFERENCES

Allen, C., Larmer, J., & Bayer, L. (2013, September 11). Hang out with BIE: An introduction to gallery walks [Video file]. Produced by Buck Institute for Education. Retrieved from https://www.youtube.com/watch?v=rQlHu1Tb3IA&feature=youtu.be

Brown, P. C., Roediger, H. L., & McDaniel, M. A. (2014). *Make it stick*. Cambridge, MA: Harvard University Press.

Chung, E. K., Rhee, J. A., Baik, Y. H., & A, O. S. (2009). The effect of team-based learning in medical ethics education. *Medical Teacher, 31*(11), 1013–1017. doi:10.3109/01421590802590553

Clark, M. C., Nguyen, H. T., Bray, C., & Levine, R. E. (2008). Team-based learning in an undergraduate nursing course. *Journal of Nursing Education, 47*(3), 111–117. doi:10.3928/01484834-20080301-02

Davis, J. R., & Arend, B. D. (2013). *Facilitating seven ways of learning: A resource for more purposeful, effective, and enjoyable college teaching*. Sterling, VA: Stylus.

Dewey, J. (1916). *Democracy and education: An introduction to the philosophy of education*. New York, NY: Macmillan.

Dewey, J. (1933). *How we think*. New York, NY: D.C. Heath.

Dinan, F. J., & Frydrychowski, V. A. (1995). A team learning method for organic chemistry. *Journal of Chemical Education, 72*(5), 429. doi:10.1021/ed072p429

Grady, S. E. (2011). Team-based learning in pharmacotherapeutics. *American Journal of Pharmaceutical Education, 75*(7), 136. doi:10.5688/ajpe757136

Haidet, P., O'Malley, K. J., & Richards, B. (2002). An initial experience with "team learning" in medical education. *Academic Medicine, 77*(1), 40–44. Retrieved from http://ovidsp.tx.ovid.com

Hawkins, D. (2014). *A team-based learning guide in the health professions*. Bloomington, IN: AuthorHouse.

Hrynchak, P., & Batty, H. (2012). The educational theory basis of team-based learning. *Medical Teacher, 34*(10), 796–801. doi:10.3109/0142159X.2012.687120

Hunt, D. P., Haidet, P., Coverdale, J. H., & Richards, B. (2003). The effect of using team learning in an evidence-based medicine course for medical students. *Teaching and Learning in Medicine, 15*(2), 131–139. doi:10.1207/S15328015TLM1502_11

Kamei, R. K., Cook, S., Puthucheary, J., & Starmer, C. F. (2012). 21st century learning in medicine: Traditional teaching versus team-based learning. *Medical Science Educator, 22*(2), 57–64. doi:10.1007/BF03341758

Kelly, P. A., Haidet, P., Schneider, V., Searle, N., Seidel, C. L., & Richards, B. F. (2005). A comparison of in-class learner engagement across lecture, problem-based learning, and team learning using the

STROBE classroom observation tool. *Teaching and Learning in Medicine, 17*(2), 112–118. doi:10.1207/ s15328015tlm1702_4

Koles, P., Nelson, S., Stolfi, A., Parmelee, D., & Destephen, D. (2005). Active learning in a year 2 pathology curriculum. *Medical Education, 39*(10), 1045–1055. doi:10.1111/j.1365-2929.2005.02248.x

Koles, P. G., Stolfi, A., Borges, N. J., Nelson, S., & Parmelee, D. X. (2010). The impact of team-based learning on medical students' academic performance. *Academic Medicine: Journal of the Association of American Medical Colleges, 85*(11), 1739–1745. doi:10.1097/ACM.0b013e3181f52bed

Lancaster, K. A., & Strand, C. A. (2001). Using the team-learning model in a managerial accounting class: An experiment in cooperative learning. *Issues in Accounting Education, 16*(4), 549–567. doi:10.2308/ iace.2001.16.4.549

Lave, J., & Wenger, E. (1991). *Situated learning: Legitimate peripheral participation.* New York, NY: Cambridge University Press.

Letassy, N. A., Fugate, S. E., Medina, M. S., Stroup, J. S., & Britton, M. L. (2008). Using team-based learning in an endocrine module taught across two campuses. *American Journal of Pharmaceutical Education, 72*(5), 103. doi:10.5688/aj7205103

Levine, R. E., O'Boyle, M., Haidet, P., Lynn, D. J., Stone, M. M., Wolf, D. V., & Paniagua, F. A. (2004). Transforming a clinical clerkship with team learning. *Teaching and Learning in Medicine, 16*(3), 270–275. doi:10.1207/s15328015tlm1603_9

McInerney, M. J., & Fink, L. D. (2003). Team-based learning enhances long-term retention and critical thinking in an undergraduate microbial physiology course. *Microbiology Education, 4*, 3–12. doi:10.1128/ 154288103X14285806229759

Michaelsen, L. K. (1992). Team learning: A comprehensive approach for harnessing the power of small groups in higher education. In *To improve the academy* (Vol. 11, pp. 106–122). San Francisco, CA: Jossey-Bass (Original work published 1992). Retrieved from http://digitalcommons.unl.edu/podim proveacad/249

Michaelsen, L. K., Black, R. H., & Fink, L. D. (1999). Problems with learning groups: An ounce of prevention. *Journal of Legal Studies Education, 17*(1–2), 91–115. doi:10.1111/j.1744-1722.1999.tb00305.x

Michaelsen, L. K., Fink, L. D., & Knight, A. (1997). Designing effective group activities: Lessons for classroom teaching and faculty development. In *To improve the academy* (Vol. 16, pp. 373–397). Retrieved from http://digitalcommons.unl.edu/podimproveacad/385

Michaelsen, L. K., Knight, A. B., & Fink, L. D. (2004). *Team-based learning: A transformative use of small groups in higher education.* Sterling, VA: Stylus Publishing.

Michaelsen, L. K., & Sweet, M. (2009). The essential elements of team-based learning. In L. Michaelsen, M. Sweet, & D. Parmelee (Eds.), *Team-based learning: Small group learning's next big step. New directions in teaching and learning* (Vol. 116, pp. 7–27). San Francisco, CA: Jossey-Bass.

Michaelsen, L. K., & Sweet, M. (2012). Creating effective team assignments. In L. K. Michaelsen, D. X. Parmelee, K. K. McMahon, & R. E. Levine (Eds.), *Team-based learning for health professions education* (pp. 35–59). Sterling, VA: Stylus.

O'Malley, K. J., Moran, B. J., Haidet, P., Seidel, C. L., Schneider, V., Morgan, R. O., . . . Richards, B. (2003). Validation of an observation instrument for measuring student engagement in health professions settings. *Evaluation and the Health Professions, 26*(1), 86–103. doi:10.1177/016327870225009

Persky, A. (2012). The impact of team-based learning on a foundational pharmacokinetics course. *American Journal of Pharmaceutical Education, 76*(2), 1–10. doi:10.5688/ajpe76231

Roebuck, D. B. (1998). Using team learning in business and organizational communication classes. *Business Communication Quarterly, 61*(3), 35–49. doi:10.1177/108056999806100304

Searle, N. S., Haidet, P., Kelly, P. A., Schneider, V. F., Seidel, C. L., & Richards, B. F. (2003). Team learning in medical education: Initial experiences at ten institutions. *Academic Medicine, 78*(10), S55–S58. Retrieved from http://ovidsp.tx.ovid.com.

Sibley, J., & Ostafichuk, P. (2014). *Getting started with team-based learning.* Sterling, VA: Stylus Publishing.

Sibley, J., & Parmelee, D. X. (2008). Knowledge is no longer enough: Enhancing professional education with team-based learning. *New Directions for Teaching and Learning, 2008*(116), 41–53. doi:10.1002/ tl.332

Thomas, P. A., & Bowen, C. W. (2011). A controlled trial of team-based learning in an ambulatory medicine clerkship for medical students. *Teaching and Learning in Medicine, 23*(1), 31–6. doi:10.1080/10401 334.2011.536888

Thompson, B. M., Schneider, V. F., Haidet, P., Levine, R. E., McMahon, K. K., Perkowski, L. C., & Richards, B. F. (2007). Team-based learning at ten medical schools: Two years later. *Medical Education, 41*(3), 250–257. doi:10.1111/j.1365-2929.2006.02684.x

Vygotsky, L. S. (1978). *Mind in society: The development of higher psychological processes.* Cambridge, MA: Harvard University Press.

Wiggins, G. P., & McTighe, J. (2005). *Understanding by design* (2nd ed.). Alexandria, VA: Association for Supervision and Curriculum Development.

Zingone, M. M., Franks, A. S., Guirguis, A. B., George, C. M., Howard-Thompson, A., & Heidel, R. E. (2010). Comparing team-based and mixed active-learning methods in an ambulatory care elective course. *American Journal of Pharmaceutical Education, 74*(9), 160. doi:10.5688/aj7409160

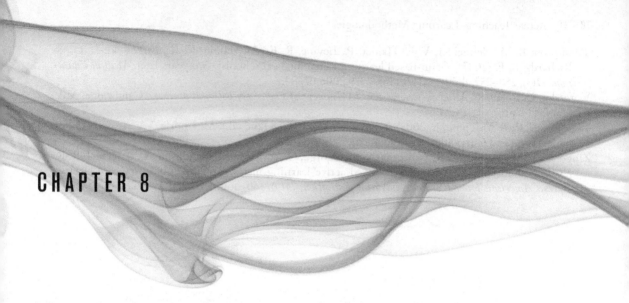

CHAPTER 8

Flipping the Classroom Without Tears

Amy A. Nichols

CHAPTER OBJECTIVES

- Use the "flipped classroom" to increase active learning
- Recognize common barriers and how to overcome them

The flipped classroom has many benefits for students—but, students will not always understand those benefits automatically. Communicate regularly with students about why you are flipping and how it will benefit students both now and later.

—*Robert Talbert,* Four Things I Wish I Had Known About the Flipped Classroom

WHAT IS ALL THIS TALK ABOUT THE FLIPPED CLASSROOM?

As we all know, educational trends come and go. The flipped classroom is perceived to be the latest trend in the educational world. Is this really a new innovative approach to teaching or a modification of a method used long ago? Flipping the classroom really refers to trading lecture time for practice time, and changing learning from passive to active. Evidence indicates that flipping a classroom has been around for quite some time, but the current momentum began in the early 2000s when the concept was first mentioned in the *Journal of Economics Education* as the inverted classroom (Lage, Platt, & Treglia, 2000). What has been recharged is the way that the idea is being applied, which is gaining traction and, most of the time, much approval. Many say that reversing the content delivery and practice is a decade's-old practice (Kachka, 2012). So, if it is not something new in education, why all the excitement and why try this strategy in the classroom?

Benefits and Concerns of Lecturing Versus Flipping the Classroom

Lecture as a teaching technique is not going away, as the state of finances in academia today dictates that class size will not decrease to lower the student-to-instructor ratio (Kachka, 2012). Therefore, lecturing makes fiscal sense. Flipping and moving the lecture to preclass assignments saves application and group work for the classroom experience. This change in from the lecture model increases both learner and teacher productivity. Implementing a flipped classroom enables more focused analysis and synthesis takes place in the classroom (Berrett, 2012; Bishop & Verleger, 2013).

Effectively flipping a classroom generates numerous benefits. Flipping uses technology to move passive, one-way lecturing as the only means of teaching, to active learning. Flipping creates a new space in the classroom where the instructor and students can interact. The increase in teacher–student interaction during class time is what characterizes its success (White, 2012). Flipping the classroom also makes differentiating instruction based on students' needs easier because everyone does not necessarily need to do the same task in class (Liles, 2012). Simply looking at the perceived and real benefits of flipping as well as the amount of research recently done should be an incentive to consider flipping the classroom as a wonderful way to reach students and approach mastery of content (Bishop & Verleger, 2013; Honeycutt, 2012b).

Some of the early adopters of the flipped classroom in science and health professions education include two chemistry teachers from Colorado, Bergmann and Sams (2008), who recognized its success in their classroom and disseminated their observations to other educators. Flipped classrooms have been shown to foster increased learning for students in various health professions courses (Billings & Halstead, 2015; McLaughlin et al., 2014; Nguyen, Wong, & Pham, 2016; Smith, 2014).

Although the flipped classroom is gaining traction and being implemented, simply flipping the classroom alone does not increase student success. The instructor must capture the opportunity in the right place at the right time to guide and interact with students. Looking at this new definition of preassignment in a flipped classroom, there are many details to consider, which sometimes makes flipping a daunting task.

The prework or preclass preparation can take on many forms. Reading, case studies, videos, voice-over PowerPoints are just a few examples of such preparation. It is also worth considering that the lecture does not have to be a lecture at all. Preclass assignments that have been used for many traditional lecture-based classes may be readily adapted. How the prework is used in the flipped classroom is where all the magic occurs (Alvarez, 2011).

What about common concerns regarding the flipped classroom process? What if a student fails to do the prework? If there has been homework, there have been students who fail to complete preparation and simply show up for class unprepared. Although this is an understandably valid concern, failure of some to complete the work should not be the reason to dismiss the flipped classroom concept. Another concern revolves around faculty competence in flipping the classroom. What if my flipping moments fail? What if I seem like I do not know what I am doing in front of the students? Also, there are comments like, "It takes too much time to flip my classroom, or it takes too much time to prepare all of the prework content and I do not have time to devise so many new teaching strategies." Trends come and go in education. Flipping a classroom is not a new concept to education. If the concept is good enough to exist for years and years, updating it for 21st-century learning seems to be a good idea. It does take a little work, but planning, implementing, and revising are all doable tasks and each effort builds a block upon which the next term can be built.

THOUGHTS TO CONSIDER BEFORE YOU FLIP

Fight the Urge to Flip Everything

Faculty interested in the flipped classroom get very motivated about the flipped classroom and want to change all their classes. They modify it all; flip every lesson, every assignment, every task. And they get burned out. The first way to save time is to back away from a course and identify its flippable moments; this will help you choose what, when, and how to flip. Know where to spend your time and energy so everyone, students and faculty, can avoid feeling overwhelmed (November, 2012).

Small Steps

Once you decide what to flip in the class, it is important to focus on one lesson at a time. If there are 10 classes in a course, begin with one. Choose one that you are the most comfortable with in terms of the content and your expertise. Start by reviewing the learning outcomes for the class and then chose where to flip. Try one flipped strategy during the lesson. If you are just beginning, start with a simple strategy, to see how it feels. Flipped classrooms do not have to be all or nothing; you can flip parts of a lecture or an assignment and leave the rest unchanged (Honeycutt, 2016).

Building Space in Your Teaching Day

Once you look at which lessons to flip, build space into the teaching plans. Anticipate that it will take double the time that it normally takes to have questions asked and answered. For example, if it takes you 5 minutes to solve a problem in a lesson, plan for your students to take 10 minutes to discuss and answer that same issue. If you are trying out new technology in a lesson, plan for it not to work the first time. If you are introducing a new activity, allot enough time to explain the process three times. Build leeway into your class time to stay in control and avoid getting overly stressed and feeling insecure in a dynamic learning environment (November, 2012).

Redefining Time in the Classroom

Redefining how you spend time in the classroom is essential. If you think that you will just add flipped activities into the classes that you have been teaching for a while, you must rethink how your time is defined. It takes time to plan activities for the flipped classroom, but it also takes time to prepare a lecture. With practice, you will be creating your lesson plan and at the same time think, "I could flip the class at this point with an activity or case study." Remember in your flipped classroom, time will be spent walking around, talking with students, helping them synthesize, and being dynamically passive (November, 2012).

Refrain From Jamming It All In

Many faculty who implement a flipped classroom do so by adding this onto an already established class without reevaluating and revising their plans. In doing less and accomplishing more with this strategy, faculty will be surprised by the power of a flipped classroom (Hyatt, 2015). Sometimes, we think we must "cover" everything on a syllabus. We must assign more homework, require more reading, add more writing, work more problems, and give more examples. Such overload for faculty and students leads to burnout. When it comes to the flipped classroom model, you do not have to use a new flipped approach every single day for every single class. Not every assignment needs redesigning. By flipping only what needs flipping, by stepping back and doing less, your students will accomplish more (Houston & Lin, 2012).

HOW DO I START FLIPPING MY CLASSROOM?

What Skills Do I Need to Be Successful to Flip My Classroom?

Flipped learning environments require careful planning and design, but the plan is only part of the equation. The instructor's skill and attitude are critical to making the flipped approach successful. Instructors must consider not only the components of a flipped classroom or a flipped lesson plan, but also the professional development and training necessary to create a successful flipped learning experience for themselves and their students. Often the discussion about instructor training and education often gets missed, and much of the focus is about the lesson plan and how to flip the class. Flipping the instructor must be considered at the same time.

Most faculty members assume that instructors already know their material and how to teach in their discipline. However, the instructor's role is different in a flipped classroom. The structure of the flipped classroom is often very difficult for faculty to grasp; and learning to let go of control in the classroom is an opportunity that is challenging. The "sage on the stage," who tells students what they are going to learn, lectures to them, and tests them with a final exam needs to be eliminated so that faculty and learners alike will think in a new way. The faculty role requires a new set of skills and attitudes about what the learning process involves. Faculty are now the "guide on the side"; they ask what students need to be able to do or accomplish with the course material and then support students as they learn. Instructors might consider the process of flipping an opportunity for self-evaluation, in which to determine their strengths, challenges, and teaching behaviors. For example, a flipped classroom can be an interactive and messy place. Are you comfortable with this kind of learning environment? Are you able to manage the environment and keep students on task, moving toward the goals of the class, without lecture and without stress? Are you comfortable letting go of some of the control? Can you let the class waver from the main objectives and steer the class back on task? These are important questions to ponder, as the answers will help you decide how and when you will be flipping content in the class.

Faculty need to be comfortable thinking on their feet, to address questions without always giving away the answer, and be prepared to change direction if things are not going as planned. Lastly, adaptability is critical in the flipped classroom. Reading the classroom's current state is crucial to determining whether students are learning or getting overwhelmed. There is a lot of energy in flipped classrooms and a balance between freedom and flexibility and maintaining control is essential. Without planning, the class can turn into a confused place where only frustration occurs for both the faculty and students. Faculty who integrate active learning into their courses need to create opportunities to interact with students, both individually and in groups.

Even though flipped classrooms are dynamic settings, it is still important for instructors to consider that they must maintain a balance of control and be able to let go of the learning environment. They are still the leaders of the class, and have the responsibility to keep students moving toward learning goals. Instructors using flipped lessons must anticipate and be prepared to harness and control the energy generated during class while still creating a welcoming and inclusive space for students to practice and learn from each other.

Prior to flipping a class, faculty should ask themselves a few questions and reflect on their teaching style to determine whether they are ready for the new approach (Honeycutt, 2016). Ask questions such as: "Am I prepared to ask a range of questions?" "Would I be comfortable letting go of the control in my classroom?" "Am I willing to take risks in the classroom?" "Am I willing to learn new things about my teaching and from the students?"

Despite the growing popularity of student-centered learning, not everyone understands or appreciates the role of the flipped classroom as an approach to shift away from instructor-focused classrooms. Instructors should also carefully consider the culture of their departments, schools, colleges, or universities before implementing a new approach (Honeycutt, 2016). Although flipping is gaining traction on campuses across the country, not all are embracing it with the same enthusiasm or in the same ways. Teaching in a flipped classroom does not look like traditional teaching, and those who are unfamiliar with it might not understand or appreciate it. This is particularly important when students evaluate the course and their faculty scores are used to determine faculty advancement. The department should be aware that flipping the class is exciting as well as risky, and students' evaluations may reflect positives and negatives that are very different from past evaluation scores.

Students Who Come to Class Unprepared

Unprepared students are another challenge facing all educators in classrooms today, but this is a recurring area of concern in the flipped classroom. Instructors need to consider how those students will affect the learning environment and create strategies to enhance motivation. The consequences related to unprepared students in a flipped classroom are different from those in a lecture-centered one. Because in-class activities are essential to the prior-to-class activities, it is critical that students come to class prepared to participate. In the active learning environment, it is nearly impossible for students to achieve the learning outcomes unless they have completed the prior-to-class work. If too many students are unprepared, the entire pace of the lesson can be derailed and prepared students will become increasingly frustrated with this approach.

To address these challenges, it is important to consider integrating formative assessment strategies or informal assessment activities into the class. Students could complete a quiz during the first 5 minutes of the class time. Groups can also prove to be a powerful motivator. If students must come to class and work together, peers will hold one another accountable for the success of their team. However, the instructor must create this culture early in the semester and continuously cultivate it over the entire course. Some educators also recommend creating lesson plan alternatives to accommodate the unprepared students and the high-achieving students who want to go further than the boundaries of the lesson plan.

The challenge of unprepared students is not a new phenomenon, and is an area of concern for many educators who are choosing an alternative course design. Many educators who are flipping their classes or using alternatives to the lecture find that students are increasingly motivated and eager to succeed in these learning environments (Honeycutt, 2016).

Steps to Creating a Flipped Classroom Experience

Planning and preparation are the most important parts of flipping a classroom. Even for a seasoned instructor, this type of planning and preparation can be overwhelming and, if overlooked, will break a flipped classroom. To avoid tears and becoming overwhelmed with the thought of trying something new, follow the next four steps to create a class lesson plan that will ultimately decrease anxiety and increase success. In their white paper, titled "The Flipped Approach to a Learner-Centered Class," Honeycutt and Garrett (2013) describe the four steps to creating a flipped classroom experience: (a) the purpose, (b) the prior-to-class activities, (c) the in-class activities, and (d) the closing. It is important to plan learning outcomes and strategies for each part of the lesson plan to create an integrated learning experience for students. It is not enough to simply record a lecture and put it online for students to watch. The purpose must be linked to the prior-to-class, in-class activities, and the closing. When the four parts of the flipped lesson plan are fully integrated in this way, students will recognize the learning experience as a process from beginning to end, and they will see the connections between the out-of-class activities and the active learning experiences they participate in during class.

Purpose

The purpose is the goal of the lesson. Another way is to ask what are the learning objectives of the class. The learning objectives drive the class activities. All activities, discussions, and assignments should be designed to help students achieve the goal. The purpose should answer this question: "What should students be able to do with the course material at the end of the class?" It is not enough to think about what students should know, define, or understand; what students should be able to *do* is most important. Objectives should be specific, measurable, and observable. The objectives should be dynamic and challenging for students to achieve. If the lesson plan itself is well designed and executed, and students are supported throughout the process, then they can reach, or possibly exceed, the learning goal.

Prior-to-Class Activities

Prior-to-class activities should be connected to the objectives, and each activity should have at least one learning outcome for students to achieve before they come to class. The more specific the learning outcome, the more likely students will complete the task before they come to class.

In-Class Activities

Instructors can then design in-class activities to hold students accountable for the prior-to-class work. This will also reinforce the learning outcomes and connect back to the overall purpose of the lesson. It is imperative that instructors define learning outcomes and learning activities prior to class so that they clearly articulate what students are supposed to do and learn. If instructors cannot articulate what students need to be able to do with the material, they cannot convey those expectations to students. Clearly communicating the tasks and expectations allows instructors to hold students accountable for achieving the prior-to-class learning objectives. If students are unable to figure out what to do because the objectives were not clearly stated, it will be difficult for the instructor to assess whether students learned what was intended. Finally, there would be no continuity between the prior-to-class activities and the in-class activities. This sacrifices a valuable connection because in-class activities help reinforce the learning process.

Closing

The end of class allows instructors to revisit what was learned and set the stage for what comes next. Because the end of class can serve as a link between the current class and the next one, instructors need to plan an effective closing. As faculty design lesson plans and develop in-class and out-of-class activities, closing brings these experiences together in ways that prepare students for the next step. In the flipped learning environment, the in-class activities should focus on higher level learning outcomes because class time is when instructors are available to guide students through more difficult and challenging materials. During class, students are engaging in learning experiences that allow them to evaluate, critique, judge, or create new knowledge. The end of class should be designed to ensure learning occurred and students are now prepared to move to work on the next class assignment.

CONCLUSIONS

For the 21st-century learner, educators must be prepared to engage in digital classrooms that are highly connected and flipped. Health professions students are lifelong learners, so flipping their classrooms provides an opportunity to nurture self-directed learning and ongoing self-improvement. Flipping the classroom can be an exciting, exhausting, and rejuvenating process.

The effort and rewards outweigh the risks and struggles and, with practice, will free time and space for true significant learning in the classroom.

REFERENCES

Alvarez, B. (2011). *Flipping the classroom: Homework in class, lessons at home*. Washington, DC: National Education Association. Retrieved from http://learningfirst.org/success-story/flipping-classroom-homework-class-lessons-home

Bergmann, J., & Sams, A. (2008). Remixing chemistry class. *Learning and Leading with Technology, 36*(4), 24–27.

Berrett, D. (2012). How "flipping" the classroom can improve the traditional lecture. *The Education Digest, 78*(1), 36. Retrieved from http://chronicle.com/article/How-Flipping-the-Classroom/130857

Billings, D. M., & Halstead, J. A. (2015). *Teaching in nursing: A guide for faculty*. Philadelphia, PA: Elsevier Health Sciences.

Bishop, J. L., & Verleger, M. A. (2013, June). The flipped classroom: A survey of the research. *ASEE National Conference Proceedings, 30*(9), 1–18.

Honeycutt, B. (2012a, April 16). A syllabus tip: Embed big questions. *Faculty Focus*. Retrieved from http://www.facultyfocus.com/articles/instructional-design/a-syllabus-tip-embed-big-question

Honeycutt, B. (2012b, April 16). Flipping is about more than videos! *Faculty Focus*. Retrieved from http://barbihoneycutt.com/flipping-is-about-more-than-videos

Honeycutt, B. (2016). *Flipping the college classroom: Practical advice from faculty*. Madison, WI: Magna.

Honeycutt, B., & Garrett, J., (2013). The flipped approach to a learner-centered class. Madison, WI: Magna.

Houston, M., & Lin, L. (2012, March). *Humanizing the classroom by flipping the homework versus lecture equation*. Paper presented at Society for Information Technology & Teacher Education International Conference, Austin, TX.

Hyatt, M. (2015). *Shave 10 hours off your work week*. Aurora, CO: Wolgemuth & Hyatt.

Kachka, P. (2012). *Understanding the flipped classroom: Part 1*. Madison, WI: Magna.

Lage, M., Platt, G., & Treglia, M. (2000). Inverting the classroom: A gateway to creating an inclusive learning environment. *Journal of Economic Education, 31*(1), 30–43.

Liles, M. (2012, April 10). Flip your classroom with discovery education [Web log message]. Retrieved from http://blog.discoveryeducation.com/blog/2012/04/10/flip-your-classroom-with-discovery-education

McLaughlin, J. E., Roth, M. T., Glatt, D. M., Gharkholonarehe, N., Davidson, C. A., Griffin, L. M., . . . Mumper, R. J. (2014). The flipped classroom: A course redesign to foster learning and engagement in a health professions school. *Academic Medicine, 89*(2), 236–243.

Nguyen, T., Wong, E., & Pham, A. (2016). Incorporating team-based learning into a physician assistant clinical pharmacology course. *Journal of Physician Assistant Education, 27*(1), 28–31.

November, A. (2012). Flipped learning: A response to five common criticisms. Retrieved from http://novemberlearning.com/resources/archive-of-articles/flipped-learning-a-response-to-five-common-criticisms

Smith, J. S. (2014). Active learning strategies in the physician assistant classroom: The critical piece to a successful flipped classroom. *Journal of Physician Assistant Education, 25*(2), 46–49.

White, D. (2012). [Literature justification for blended/reverse instruction.] Unpublished raw data.

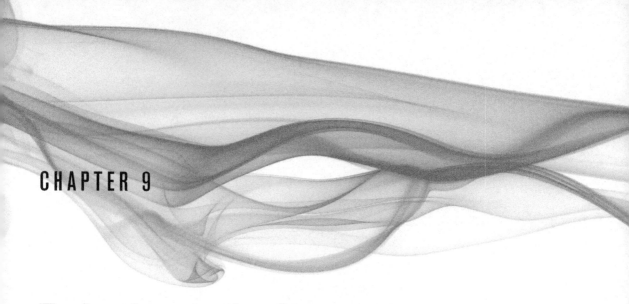

CHAPTER 9

Technology in the Classroom

Nina Multak

CHAPTER OBJECTIVE

- Use technology to promote active learning in the classroom, including screen-capture video software, wikis, social media, learning management systems, adaptive learning programs, and more

Tell me and I forget, teach me and I remember, involve me and I learn.

—*Benjamin Franklin*

Technology, and educational technology in particular, involves the practical application of current knowledge. Educational technologies may be harnessed to achieve the overarching goal of health professions education—better health of patients, better patient experience, and lower costs. New educational modalities are currently replacing the traditional lecture. The teaching–learning process is no longer bound by geography or conventional time constraints. Educational innovators are seeking new ways to construct curricula, courses, and content and test new technologies to enhance both individual and team-based learning. The power of educational technologies to transform our health professions education system lies in its potential (Robin et al., 2011).

USING TECHNOLOGY IN THE CLASSROOM

Technology is becoming more and more integrated into our society, and it makes sense for faculty to use the most current software and devices to support learning in the classroom and in clinical environments (National League of Nursing Board of Governors, 2015). Smartphones are commonly used, tablets are replacing computers and laptops, and social media use has become a daily pastime for many individuals. The rapid and widespread adoption of these technological innovations has completely changed the way we conduct our daily lives, including how knowledge is acquired and taught in our classrooms. Integrating technology into classroom practice can be a great way to strengthen engagement by linking students to a global audience and helping them practice collaboration skills that will prepare them for the future (Bennett et al., 2008).

We define educational technologies as materials and devices used for training, learner assessment, or education administration (Cook et al., 2011). Maintaining a broad view of educational technologies helps us put into proper perspective current trends and suggests that online learning and high-fidelity manikins may eventually be replaced by newer, more fashionable technologies (Cook, 2006). These relatively new developments include a diverse range of Internet-based software, mobile devices, computer-based applications, high-fidelity simulators, 3D virtual reality programs, and more.

Some of the benefits of using educational technology in a course include:

- **Technology can keep students focused for longer periods of time:** The use of computers, tablets, and smartphones to look up information/data saves time, especially when used to access a comprehensive resource to conduct research. This time-saving aspect can keep students focused on a project, perhaps neglecting the information that they find as "low-hanging fruit" and develop learning through developing skills of exploration and research.
- **Technology promotes active learning and makes students excited to learn:** When technology is integrated into courses, learners are more likely to be interested in, focused on, and excited about the subjects they are studying. Subjects that might be difficult or less interesting for some students can become more interesting as they engage with the information through additional virtual lectures, interactive games, and educational videos.
- **Technology enables students to learn at their own pace:** With the integration of technology, students are able to get focused and individualized instruction from the technology used. This allows students to engage with the information at times that are most convenient for them and helps them become more self-directed in the learning process.
- **Technology prepares students for the future:** By learning to use technology in the classroom, both faculty and students will develop critical thinking and workplace skills they will need to be successful in their futures. Education is no longer just about learning and memorizing facts and figures; it is about collaborating with others, solving complex problems, developing different forms of communication and leadership skills, and improving motivation and productivity.

There are also some perceived negative aspects to using technology in the classroom. However, in most cases, the pros largely outweigh the cons. The best way to guard against any negative effects of technology integration and implementation is to make sure teachers and students are trained on the proper use and etiquette of the resources. Faculty should be trained in the effective use of technology and should always understand how and why each device is being used.

Technology-enhanced learning strategies will support both the initial phases of education as well as lifelong learning (Yavner et al., 2015). Blended learning and asynchronous strategies will facilitate career transitions by enabling students to learn while working (Garrison & Kanuka, 2004). Simulation technologies will enable students to engage in deliberate practice as individuals and in interprofessional teams, tackling progressively challenging situations in a safe environment, free from concerns about harming patients (Cook et al., 2013; Ericcson, 2004; Motola et al., 2013).

TECHNOLOGY INTEGRATION

Before we can discuss how to shift our pedagogy or the role of the faculty in a classroom that is integrating technology, it is important to first define what *technology integration* actually means. *Integration* refers to students using technology daily, while also having access to a variety of tools that match the task at hand and provide the opportunity to build a deeper understanding of content. But how we *define* technology integration can also depend on the kinds of technology available, how much access one has to technology, and who is using the technology. Willingness to embrace change is also a major requirement for successful technology integration. Technology is continuously and rapidly evolving. It is an ongoing process that demands continual learning.

Effective technology integration must occur across the curriculum in ways that research shows deepen and enhance the learning process. In particular, it must support four key components of learning: active engagement, participation in groups, frequent interaction and feedback, and connection to real-world experts. Effective technology integration is achieved when the use of technology is routine and when technology supports curricular goals.

Learning through projects while equipped with technology tools allows students to be intellectually challenged while providing them with a realistic snapshot of what the modern office looks like. Through projects, students acquire and refine their analysis and problem-solving skills as they work individually and in teams to find, process, and synthesize information they have found online.

The plethora of online resources can provide each course with interesting, diverse, and current learning materials. Addressing the critical role of faculty in identifying, evaluating, and adapting technologies for education is an important issue. There is no question that we need to be identifying educational technologies that can maximize lifelong learning for students, graduate trainees, faculty members, clinicians, and patients (Harden, 2005). We also need to focus on making sure that faculty are supported so that they can become comfortable with the new technology, which will expand their impact and efficiency. Technology should be used to bridge the gap between education and clinical experiences, enhancing collaboration and interprofessional teamwork between and among faculty and students from different health professions and facilitate partnerships with patients and their families (Djukic, 2012). Table 9.1 lists a representative selection of several key technologies and issues related to their use in health professions education. These innovations, which have helped countless people during regular daily activities, can also impact learning.

IMPLEMENTING TECHNOLOGY IN THE ONLINE AND FACE-TO-FACE CLASSROOM

Employment of best practices in online and face-to-face instruction helps to ensure successful implementation of instructional technology. Various options for integrating technology using commonly available software and devices are summarized next.

Presentation Software

Presentation software enables instructors to embed high-resolution photographs, diagrams, videos, and sound files to augment text and verbal lecture content. Tablets can be linked to

TABLE 9.1 Representative Educational Technologies Used in Health Professions Education*

Technology	Examples in Health Professions Education
Technologies for face-to-face instruction	
Audience response systems	Students may use ARS to provide immediate feedback on interactive quizzes.
Electronic whiteboards ("SmartBoards")	Used to augment live lectures that broadcast the instructors' "chalkboard" drawings to remote learning sites.
Generative learning activities	Students in a problem-based learning course collaboratively authored wikis to teach each other in small groups.
Technologies for online instruction	
Augmented reality and virtual learning environments	Augmented reality devices have been used during basic science lectures to enhance the experience with clinic-based patient interviews and exam findings.
Learning management systems	HPE programs use a variety of commercially available products to support both live and online course administration.
Learning objects and course materials	Many HPE schools use online learning modules and supplemental online course materials.
Massive open online course	Health professions educators have created MOOCs on various health care–related topics.
Medical visualizations	3D anatomy simulators are used to teach complex anatomic and dynamic physiologic topics in new ways.
Mobile devices and apps	Several HPE schools are issuing mobile devices to learners; both faculty and students are developing apps and resources for teaching and assessment.
Technologies for simulation-based instruction	
Manikins	Lifelike full-body and torso models of a complete human are in broad use for clinical education in all HPE.
Part-task trainers and workstations	Anatomical physical models that simulate a portion of the body or simulators used to train specific clinical tasks (e.g., interventional cardiology, laparoscopic surgery).
Virtual hospitals	Some hospitals maintain simulated clinical spaces, such as operating and emergency rooms, in which learners can practice teamwork, communication, and clinical workflows.
Virtual patients	Virtual patients are developed through a collaboration involving a nonprofit organization and national education organizations.
Virtual reality simulators	VR simulators, which provide an immersive sensory experience that simulates a physical place, have been used to practice teamwork and emergency incident response.
Technologies for assessment, evaluation, and administration	
Curriculum-mapping tools	Schools are increasingly using these tools to support "mapping" a curriculum. Doing so helps identify redundancies, gaps, common themes, and other opportunities for improvement across classes and program years. Mapping also facilitates connecting course objectives to competencies and milestones.

(continued)

TABLE 9.1 Representative Educational Technologies Used in Health Professions Education (*continued*)

Technology	Examples in Health Professions Education
Computer-aided assessment	In broad use across HPE, these strategies include computer-based quizzes, exams, and assessments. Advantages include automated grading, instant feedback, multimedia and interactive questions, enhanced security, and automated analytics.
Learning analytics	Analytics are being used to answer complex questions about effective teaching and learning, and to render suggestions to optimize education for both individual students and educational programs.
Learner portfolios and coaching systems	Many schools are using portfolios to facilitate the assessment of, and reflection on, information about learners' educational achievements, performance, and progress.
Technologies that integrate with clinical practice	
Bedside clinical technologies	Clinical technologies are being used by HPE learners to collect data in real time from patients at the bedside. Learning how to accurately capture and interpret clinical data will enhance patient-centered education.
Point-of-care learning	Academic medical centers are leveraging EMRs, clinical decisions support systems, and computerized provider order entry systems to not only deliver care, but also to teach learners about systems, populations, and health care quality.

ARS, audience response systems; EMRs, electronic medical records; HPE, health professions education; MOOC, massive open online course; VR, virtual reality.
Source: Modified from Stuart and Triola (2015, Table 1).

computers, projectors, and the cloud so that students and instructors can communicate through text, drawings, and diagrams. Advantages include:

- Displaying lecture outlines, visual examples (photos, graphs, diagrams, videos), and/or instructions for classroom activities
- Displaying sample test questions or concept questions to check student understanding (possibly used with personal response systems)
- Creating opportunities for students to organize content and present to peers as part of a lecture
- Providing "skeletal" outlines that facilitate student note taking
- Providing a resource that guides students' review of lecture material (alone or in connection with audio/video recordings of lecture)
- Examples: Microsoft PowerPoint, Apple Keynote, Google Slides, Prezi

Clickers and Smartphones

Clickers and smartphones are a quick and easy way to survey students during class. This is great for instant polling, which can quickly assess students' understanding and help instructors adjust pace and content. Advantages include:

- Assessing students' prior knowledge and identifying misconceptions before introducing a new subject
- Checking students' understanding of new material
- Starting class discussion on difficult topics
- Using peer instruction and other active learning techniques
- Administering tests and quizzes during lecture
- Gathering feedback on teaching
- Recording class attendance and participation

Assessment Software

Assessment software enables instructors to effectively evaluate students' learning needs, mastery of course material, and learner outcomes (Amin et al., 2011). Advantages include:

- Checking prior knowledge and interest with pretest
- Helping students keep up with material with online quizzes
- Communicating grades quickly and confidentially using an online grade book
- Developing individualized remediation plans

Course Management Tools

Learning management systems allow faculty to organize all the resources students and faculty need for a class (e.g., syllabi, assignments, readings, online quizzes); provide valuable grading tools; and create spaces for discussion, document sharing, and video and audio commentary.

Lecture-Capture Tools

Lecture-capture tools allow instructors to record lectures directly from their computer, without elaborate or additional classroom equipment. Consider recording your lectures as you give them and then upload them for students to rewatch. Studies show that posting recorded lectures *does not* diminish attendance and students really appreciate the opportunity to review lectures at their own pace. Advantages include:

- Allowing students to review content that they found difficult to understand during lecture
- Creating recordings to be used for future students to prepare for class
- Archiving lectures and classroom activities for course planning
- Providing an alternative for students who miss class
- Providing lectures for interdisciplinary courses from other departments
- Examples of technology used: Camtasia Relay, Podcast Recordings, iTunes, Classroom Recording Services

Online Collaboration Tools

Online collaboration tools allow students and instructors to share documents online, edit them in real time, and project them on a screen. This gives students a collaborative platform in which to brainstorm ideas and document their work using text and images.

Online Discussions

Online discussions create a virtual active learning environment in which students and faculty can engage in synchronous and/or asynchronous dialogue. Advantages include:

- Enabling whole-class or small-group discussion of class materials
- Reading responses
- Promoting online debates

- Brainstorming and prioritizing ideas
- Offering online Q&A about class material and/or course logistics
- Engaging in discussion with the wider community
- Enabling students to collect, share, and discuss relevant resources with each other

Online Videoconferencing

Online videoconferencing provides flexibility in content delivery and engages multiple learning styles, including auditory and visual. Advantages include:

- Offering office hours to off-campus students
- Facilitating group interaction or conduct student meetings
- Teaching class while out of town (e.g., attending academic conferences)
- Team teaching with instructors at another university
- Connecting students to native speakers in language classes
- Interviewing experts/guests
- Collaborating with classes at other universities
- Offering virtual field trips
- Examples: Skype, Google+ Hangouts, Apple FaceTime, Zoom, Adobe Connect

Online Writing Tools

Online writing tools provide flexible strategies for learners to engage in writing exercises, give and receive feedback, and develop team skills in writing projects. Advantages include:

- Allowing individual or group writing assignments of any length
- Enabling peer review of writing assignments
- Offering metacognitive reflection on writing
- Allowing for collaborative note taking and writing projects
- Facilitating writing for the wider community
- Enabling individual reflective journals or portfolios
- Examples: Google Drive, Blogs such as Blogger and Wordpress, Wikis such as PBWiki

Resource and File Sharing

Resource and file sharing software enables real-time sharing of course materials between instructors and learners and fosters collaborative learning. Advantages include:

- Sharing of course materials
- Sharing of videos
- Providing online space for collaboration
- Examples: Google Drive, Dropbox, iTunes

Screencasting

Screencasting also enables real-time sharing of course materials between instructors and learners and fosters collaborative learning. Advantages include:

- Providing feedback on student work
- Responding to classroom assessments of student learning
- Modeling problem-solving and other expert skills
- Creating opportunities for active learning
- Creating tutorials and other supports for students
- Examples: Jing, Camtasia

CONCLUSIONS

If used incorrectly, technology can cause more harm than good, and can widen educational disparities. However, appropriate use of technology can improve student focus, promote active learning, and let students learn at their own pace. Today's learners have become increasingly digitized and find technology very conducive to learning (Ruiz, 2006). In addition, the increased use of online teaching and learning modalities requires greater familiarity with technology. Educators therefore have to adapt and use technology in the classroom to meet the needs of diverse learning styles.

REFERENCES

Amin, Z., Boulet, J. R., Cook, D. A., Ellaway, R., Fahal, A., Kneebone, R., . . . Ziv, A. (2011). Technology-enabled assessment of health professions education: Consensus statement and recommendations from the Ottawa 2010 conference. *Medical Teacher, 33*(5), 364–369.

Bennett, S., Maton, K., & Kervin, L. (2008). The "digital natives" debate: A critical review of the evidence. *British Journal of Educational Technology, 39*(5), 775–786.

Cook, D. A. (2006). Where are we with Web-based learning in medical education? *Medical Teacher, 28*(7), 594–598.

Cook, D. A., Brydges, R., Zendejas, B., Hamstra, S. J., & Hatala, R. (2013). Mastery learning for health professionals using technology-enhanced simulation: A systematic review and meta-analysis. *Academic Medicine, 88*(8), 1178–1186.

Cook, D. A., Hatala, R., Brydges, R., Zendejas, B., Szostek, J. H., Wang, A. T., . . . Hamstra, S. J. (2011). Technology-enhanced simulation for health professions education: A systematic review and meta-analysis. *Journal of the American Medical Association, 306*, 978–988.

Djukic, M., Fulmer, T., Adams, J. G., Lee, S., & Triola, M. M. (2012). NYU3T: Teaching, technology, teamwork: A model for interprofessional education scalability and sustainability. *Nursing Clinics of North America, 47*(3), 333–346.

Ericsson, K. A. (2004). Deliberate practice and the acquisition and maintenance of expert performance in medicine and related domains. *Academic Medicine, 79*(Suppl. 10), S70–S81.

Garrison, D. R., & Kanuka, H. (2004). Blended learning: Uncovering its transformative potential in higher education. *Internet and Higher Education, 7*, 95–105.

Harden, R. M. (2005). A new vision for distance learning and continuing medical education. *Journal of Continuing Education in the Health Professions, 25*(1), 43–51.

Motola, I., Devine, L. A., Chung, H. S., Sullivan, J. E., & Issenberg, S. B. (2013). Simulation in healthcare education: A best evidence practical guide. *Medical Teacher, 35*(10), e1511–e1530.

National League for Nursing Board of Governors. (2015). *A vision for the changing faculty role: Preparing Students for the technological world of health care.* Washington, DC: National League for Nursing Press.

Robin, B. R., McNeil, S. G., Cook, D. A., Agarwal, K. L., & Singhal, G. R. (2011). Preparing for the changing role of instructional technologies in medical education. *Academic Medicine, 86*(4), 435–439.

Ruiz, J. G., Mintzer, M., & Leipzig, R. M. (2006). The impact of e-learning in medical education. *Academic Medicine, 81*(3), 207–212.

Stuart, G., & Triola, M. (2015). *Enhancing health professions education through technology: Building a continuously learning health system.* New York, NY: Josiah Macy Jr. Foundation. Retrieved from http://macy foundation.org/publications/publication/enhancing-health-professions-education-through-technology

Yavner, S. D., Pusic, M. V., Kalet, A. L., Song, H. S., Hopkins, M. A., Nick, M. W., & Ellaway, R. H. (2015). Twelve tips for improving the effectiveness of web-based multimedia instruction for clinical learners. *Medical Teacher, 37*(3), 239–244.

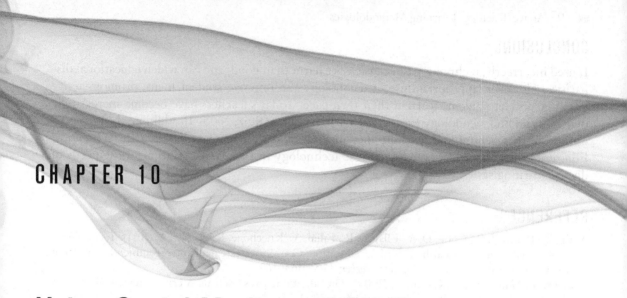

CHAPTER 10

Using Social Media and Big Data to Facilitate Teaching and Learning in Health Professions

Bianca Belcher and Jessica Duff

CHAPTER OBJECTIVES

- Integrate big data and social media analytics in the teaching enterprise
- Use social media and big data in clinical education
- Summarize university/program policies and recommendations

The world is being re-shaped by the convergence of social, mobile, cloud, big data, community and other powerful forces. The combination of these technologies unlocks an incredible opportunity to connect everything together in a new way and is dramatically transforming the way we live and work.

—Marc Benioff, Chairman and CEO, Salesforce

INTEGRATION OF BIG DATA AND SOCIAL MEDIA ANALYTICS INTO HEALTH PROFESSIONS EDUCATION PROGRAMS

The big data movement and social media have already significantly impacted a diverse number of industries, such as marketing, aviation, and health care, and hold the potential to significantly impact graduate health professions education as well. *Big data*, defined as a large volume of structured and unstructured data, has revolutionized the way that marketers market. The collection, analysis, and use of this data have changed the health care industry in areas of price optimization, customer engagement/insight, and geo-analytics (Columbus, 2016). Southwest Airlines, for example, has been utilizing big data to collect and analyze speech during live-recorded customer service conversations to extract deeper and more meaningful information about how people feel (Rijmenam, 2016). The health care industry has begun to integrate big data analysis to find disease trends and better understand patient behavior. This chapter defines big data and social media and discusses opportunities for their integration into health professions educational programs. The main objectives are to give readers a basic understanding of both big data and social media, provide examples of how each is being integrated in various industries, and provide the resources that readers need to start utilizing big data and social media in graduate health professions programs curricula and to enhance program recognition.

BIG DATA

Big data is a relatively new term that gained conceptual momentum in a research report published by Doug Laney, a distinguished data analyst, in 2001, describing the three Vs of big data: volume, velocity, and variety (Laney, 2001). *Volume* is defined as a large amount of data collected and stored. The volume of data generally exceeds the analyzing capacity of many information systems in existence. It is estimated that 2.5 quintillion bytes of data are being created daily by numerous electronic transactions such as consumer purchasing, web searches, GPS locating, and social media interactions. That amount of data would fill 10 million Blu-ray discs, and if those discs were stacked, the Blu-ray tower would be the equivalent of four Eiffel Towers (Walker, 2015). To further put this into perspective, Wal-Mart collects approximately 2.5 million gigabytes of data per hour on its customer transactions, which is the equivalent of 50 million file cabinets worth of text (McAfee & Brynjolfsson, 2012). It is not just the volume of data, but the velocity at which it is being created that is impressive. Social media and mobile technology are constantly creating active and passive data streams of locations, activities, and preferences. Lastly, variety is the type and configuration, both structured and unstructured, of data being collected. It is being gathered from a variety of sources such as GPS, video postings, social media engagement, and wearable devices. Consumer companies have been utilizing data to better understand their customers' needs. There is an opportunity for health professions programs to do the same.

Big data has changed our ability to understand human behavior and learning. In his 2016 article published in the *International Journal of Market Research*, Colin Strong described that our lives are increasingly being played out online and we are leaving behind data trails that track our behaviors with an unprecedented level of granularity (Strong, 2016). The most well-known example of big data tracking of human behavior in the health care arena occurred when Google created a real-time model that predicted flu spread in 2009. Historically, the Centers for Disease Control and Prevention (CDC) tracked viral spread by utilizing medical chart reviews, direct reporting, and flu swab results. The CDC correlated the numbers once a week, which often led to a 1- to 2-week lag in results reporting. This lag left some public health groups unprepared for outbreaks in their area. Google took another approach. It analyzed 50 million of the most common search terms used during flu season for 2003 to 2008 and then cross-referenced those terms with the areas of the country most heavily affected by the flu during those years. In the end, Google developed a mathematical algorithm using 45 search terms that produced results similar to the official CDC results but in real time, thus eliminating the 1- to 2-week lag (Mayer-Schönberger & Cukier, 2013). In the context of academia, analysts can utilize millions of data points to gain a better understanding of student learning preferences. Spotify[1] and researchers at the University of Cambridge discovered that cognitive styles were a strong predictor of musical preference (Greenberg, Baron-Cohen, Stillwell, Kosinski, & Rentfrow, 2015). Perhaps, this research could be extrapolated to benefit academia by examining whether cognitive styles could be a predictor of learning outcomes. Might a program have the ability to predict which students will excel in problem-based learning (PBL) versus lecture-dominant learning based on big data and social media analytics?

When considering the integration of big data into health professions education, careful attention must be paid to data collection, data analysis, and the visualization and application of the information (Daniel, 2015). First, data collection must be purposeful, relevant, and stored in a usable format. For example, grading a simple multiple-choice test for 1,000 students on an online learning management platform, such as Blackboard, is relatively simple. Once the exam is created, the learning management tool does most of the work by giving each student a percentage grade and allows the instructor to run a test analysis to determine question difficulty, discrimination, and reliability. All of the input and output is the same (structured) and is easily comparable, making it easy to see trends. A singular academic program would not produce enough data to be considered big data, but if it collects data in a manner that can be easily aggregated with several other programs, the resulting data could be valuable. On the other hand, grading 1,000 essay-based exams or video blog assignments is labor intensive because the output is unstructured and more difficult to correlate. Essays, for example, potentially have many unstructured components, such as the varied content, hyperlinks, embedded photos, multiple student contributors, and so forth. Once usable data is collected, it must be analyzed in a manner that will help generate action. Revisiting the original goals of the data collection will prevent the mere linking of data points and correlation of data sets, and help with meaningful application to the goal. After collecting and analyzing data, it must be presentable and interpretable in order to guide decision making. The collection and analysis of information are largely quantitative, algorithmic, and computer based. A crucial step in the process is repurposing the findings in a manner that can be understood by the program or institutional decision makers.

A real-world example of the integration of data collection and analysis into education is found in the AltSchool. The AltSchool has pioneered the concepts of collecting, analyzing, and utilizing big data in and around the classroom since 2014 (Ventilla, 2014). The AltSchool consists of a group of private schools started by Max Ventilla, former Google executive, designed to provide students with a technology-enabled network that connects them, their parents, and their teachers to deliver personalized education. They use software to personalize a series of assignments for each student. Similar to the process that Netflix uses to analyze viewing preferences to generate a list of recommended programs, the AltSchool has a team of 50 engineers analyzing student learning patterns and content preferences to generate a "playlist" of lessons and assignments due each week (Simon, 2016). They extrapolated this technique to a group of graduate medical learners to give students the customized edge they need to more quickly master key concepts.

SOCIAL MEDIA ANALYTICS

The first mention of social interaction over a computer network was published in a series of memos written by J. C. R. Licklider in 1962 (Leiner et al., 2016). The concept of social interaction was eventually developed into the Internet. Web 1.0, the first version of the Internet, consisted primarily of static sites that could only be created with coding and did not promote social engagement or permit user impact. In the second stage of development, the Internet transitioned from static, noninteractive sites to dynamic sites that allowed user-generated content and interaction. This shift occurred in the late 1990s/early 2000s and was called Web 2.0 (O'Reilly, 2005). Web 2.0 laid the groundwork for the social networking explosion. *Social media* is defined as websites and/or applications that enable users to create and share content or participate in networking. Social networks are "web-based services that allow individuals to (a) construct a public or semipublic profile within a bounded system, (b) articulate a list of other users with whom they share a connection, and (c) view and traverse their list of connections and those made by others within the system" (Boyd & Ellison, 2007, p. 211). The concept of social media started in the early 1980s with the Bulletin Board System (BBS), but really hit its stride in 2002 when the networking site Friendster was launched. Since Friendster, thousands of social media platforms have been developed, but the most popular platform to date is Facebook. Facebook was developed in 2004 by Mark Zuckerberg, who was a student studying at Harvard at the time, and it went public in 2006. Facebook has more than 1.3 billion active users today (Digital Trends Staff, 2016). Twitter, another popular platform, has roughly 313 million users, but a slightly different demographic than Facebook (Statista, 2016). Of the world's adult population, 62% are active Facebook users, whereas Twitter captures only 20% of adults. Twitter is more popular among young adults, however (Duggan, 2015). This chapter focuses on how to analyze data generated from these social media platforms and how to utilize the data in health professions education.

Data analytics is defined as the evaluation of large quantities of information with the purpose of looking for trends, patterns, correlations, and insights. Analytics tools help the user quantify and categorize information into usable data sets. Basic social media analytics are good for reviewing reach, engagement, and benchmarking. *Reach* is the number of people who saw the post, but engagement is a better indicator of the interactions with content. *Engagement* refers to interaction with a post beyond just reading it. The engagement rate is a great way to measure interest in content and is calculated as the percentage of people engaged with content based on the number of people who saw the post. A benchmarking tool compares engagement from two time periods. This is useful when trying new content-posting strategies.

Examples of Analytical Tools

Google Analytics

Google analytics is a free, expansive, and versatile data tool offered by Google that allows analytics tracking across videos, social network platforms, websites, and personal devices (Corporate author, 2016). It offers in-depth objective data on many valuable outlets and is not limited to Google-hosted sites or social media platforms. Google analytics quantifies current number of site visitors, repeat customers, site referral sources, users browser type, social media data, and much more.

Advantages

- One of the most versatile of the free applications
- Offers a free online analytics academy (Corporate author, 2016)
- Can be utilized for both website and social media platform tracking
- Offers a plug-in[2] for blog-hosting sites, such as Wordpress

Disadvantages

- Creation of custom reports is limited, though likely sufficient for most health professions programs
- The upgraded version (Google Analytics Premium) is expensive
- Frequent upgrades to the free version require one to refamiliarize oneself with the interface and tools

Facebook Insights

Insights is a free analytics tool offered by Facebook to provide objective data on shared content and followers (Vahl, 2015). Basic Insights is ideal for reviewing post reach, engagement, and benchmarks. Insights also offers a downloadable version that delivers more in-depth information. The download provides an Excel spreadsheet with a significant amount of data. There are several categories of data that are available by download only, one of which is website clicks.

Advantages

- Free service
- Data is exportable to Excel
- In-depth analytics
- Real-time data

Disadvantages

- Data limited to Facebook
- Basic Insights engagement values are only available for a limited time (must be downloaded to be kept indefinitely)
- Downloadable Insights are limited by time and/or number of historical posts
- Cannot easily correlate data with exported data from other social media platforms

Twitter Analytics

Twitter is a social media platform that began in 2006 and users produce more than 500 million daily Tweets (Statista, 2016; Corporate author, 2016a). A *tweet* is a posting on Twitter, which can contain 140 characters or less. Twitter business analytics is a free tool offered by Twitter to provide objective data on shared content and followers (Corporate author, 2016b). Each *Twitter handle*, or user name (@username), has its own analytics page. The home page is described as the "report card" for each handle. It has monthly statistical tracking, a spotlight of the top-performing Tweets[3], and attempts to connect you to popular users within your network. On the Tweet activity dashboard, metrics of individual Tweets are tracked, such as *views*, *Retweets*, and *likes*. The audience insight dashboard reveals followers and their demographics.

Advantages

- Free service
- Analytics are exportable to Excel
- Real-time data
- Easy to navigate

Disadvantages

- Data limited to Twitter
- Cannot easily correlate data with exported data from other social media platforms
- If you have a popular Twitter account, there could be a lot of data to sort through

Social Media Management Dashboard

A social media management dashboard, such as Hootsuite, allows the user to manage and collect analytics on multiple platforms and profiles from a single interface. In short, these dashboards simplify tracking and posting on multiple social media accounts. For example, content can be composed once and posted on multiple platforms at the same time. Users also have the ability to schedule posts to go live in the future giving the illusion that a site is constantly active. The social media manager can create and schedule content for the next month in a single day. The dashboard does offer limited content suggestions as well.

Advantages

- May offer a free limited service account
- Can post to multiple outlets and track analytics from one interface
- Allows the user to schedule posts in advance
- Real-time data
- Allows you to see analytics from multiple social media accounts

Disadvantages

- Free services usually include a limited number of social media accounts and basic analytics
- Has a learning curve
- May not be able to export data freely with free version

INTEGRATION OPPORTUNITIES FOR THE HEALTH PROFESSIONS PROGRAM

Building an Interdisciplinary Team

First and foremost, building an interdisciplinary team is a crucial step to integrating large-scale big data into an academic program. It is unlikely that a single program will have the necessary resources to undertake this daunting task alone. Success is more likely to favor a multidisciplinary team with full support from the university or college's resources. As discussed previously, significant planning and computer expertise are required to properly collect, analyze, and use data. An interdisciplinary team should minimally include a project manager, data scientist, a data engineer, and content experts from all of the involved departments. The project manager serves as the team leader and keeps the project organized and moving in the right direction. Most important, the team leader should look to assemble a group dedicated to data-driven decision making and continuous data collection and utilization improvement techniques. The data scientist cleans and organizes data, collects data sets, mines data sets for patterns, and refines algorithms. The data engineer prepares and manages the big data infrastructure and produces reports for the data scientist to convert raw data into actionable items. Finally, the content experts work closely with the data scientist to interpret the data and ensure that the actionable items are logical in context.

The University of Otago, founded in 1869 and located in New Zealand, is well known for its work in research and teaching. In 2013, the university began an institutional collaborative project called *University of Otago Technology-Enhanced Analytics* (UO-TEA), which involved building an interdisciplinary team to explore the potential of data analytics in academia (Daniel & Butson, 2013). As Daniel describes, at the conclusion of their research, the "UO-TEA Framework describes a wide range of administrative and operational data gathering processes aimed at assessing institutional performance and progress in order to predict future performance and identifies potential issues related to academic programming, research, teaching, and learning" (Daniel, 2015, p. 8). The framework consisted of four major analytics categories: (a) institutional analytics, (b) information technology analytics, (c) academic/program analytics, and (d) learning analytics (see Table 10.1).

Institutional and information technology analytics are considerations for a large university- or college-wide big data initiative, whereas academic/program and learning analytics are manageable projects for individual programs.

Online Learning Management Platform Analytics

Online learning management platform analytics allow instructors to track and analyze student engagement. Statistics tracking allows the user to see the number of student views for a

TABLE 10.1 University of Otago Technology-Enhanced Analytics Framework

Institutional analytics	Analysis of operational data that can help make effective decisions at an institutional, department, or program level
Information technology analytics	Analysis of data from various sources (i.e., student information, learning management systems, alumni databases, and potentially social media) with the goal of developing and implementing new technology and data tools as needed
Academic/program analytics	Program-specific analysis provides data support for strategic decision making as well as benchmarking for comparisons with other similar institutions
Learning analytics	Analysis of data surrounding learners with the goal of optimizing and/or customizing learning and the learning environment

particular test item; item analysis allows the user to analyze exam questions for discrimination and difficulty; and course report provides a view of student activity and behavior by tracking hours spent, clicks on a certain area, and time of day/week/month of activity. Many platform analytics tools allow the user to track student behavior and time dedicated to retention of concepts. The collection of this data over time may have predictive value in the near future.

Health Educational Management Tools

A health care education management tool, such as E*Value, streamlines several aspects of health professions education such as coursework, scheduling, clinical site management, and evaluations (MedHub, 2016). Data sets have the potential to help educators gain a broader understanding of site availability and volume as well as student and preceptor evaluation trends, both of which could go a long way to shaping clinical-year placements. The data could also be used in demonstrating compliance and meeting the needs of accreditation bodies. The analysis could inform decision making in cases of requests for increases in enrollment or the opening of an additional school in the immediate area.

In a more granular example, students log their clinical case experiences within these management tools. Case-log analysis demonstrates a clinical site's case volume and variety and could help clinical coordinators better align student strengths and weakness with the clinical site. The end-of-rotation evaluations (completed by both the student and the preceptor) could be assessed for early trends that could (a) help educators catch students and/or sites that are in need of remediation and (b) help programs uncover deficiencies in the didactic curriculum. For example, if all preceptors over the past 3 years rated "student oral presentations skills" at an average of 3.4 out of 10, then an opportunity has presented itself for curriculum changes or additions to better prepare students to deliver oral presentations in the future. The postcurriculum change preceptor ratings can be compared to the baseline to evaluate the effectiveness of the change.

Personalized Modules

Many health professions programs already utilize comprehensive exams at some point in the curriculum to compare their students with other students nationally. For example, nearly 90% of physician assistant (PA) programs use the Physician Assistant Clinical Knowledge Rating and Assessment Tool (PACKRAT) to compare their students with the national average and obtain a moderate correlation of how students may perform on the Physician Assistant National Certifying Exam (PANCE; Physician Assistant Education Association [PAEA], 2016). PACKRAT results are released in a detailed performance report that shows the percentage of correct questions within a given subject such as cardiology or hematology, but the questions themselves are not released. The concept of personalized modules takes "result and compare" one step further by assigning learning modules to students based on their comparative results. For example, a second-year PA student scores 47.7% correct in cardiology, but the national average for all participating second-year students is 64.5%. Data and test analysis could be used to not only *show* students the area of weakness, but also to assign them online learning modules targeting their *specific* weakness (i.e., recognition of ventricular arrhythmias on EKG or medication side effects of beta-blockers) within the subject of cardiology.

USE OF SOCIAL MEDIA FOR PROGRAM BRANDING

Social Media Spotlighting

Spotlights are short (3–5 sentences) advertisements on students, alumni, or faculty that highlight them or their accomplishments and should include a photo. How can spotlighting help drive brand recognition for your program?

- It highlights a person who embodies the best qualities of the program.
- It increases engagement. It encourages individuals to tag themselves and/or share a post on their own social media platforms. This drives reach and engagement because individuals are not only creating a rewarding post, but are also putting that post in front of a social media audience with a personal connection to the story.
- It demonstrates program impact. If current students, alumni, or faculty are succeeding in the community or profession, then the program is succeeding.

Tailored Marketing Campaigns

By tracking social media platform analytics, a program can gain a better understanding of the demographic profile of visitors, what times of day are best to post new content, and post types that receive the highest engagement ratings. With this information, a program could be more strategic about when and how to introduce program highlights or alumni donation campaigns on social media platforms in order to gain the most traction. For example, if data analytics show that post engagement by viewers in the annual income bracket of more than $75,000 is the highest when posts contain a photograph and go live between 5 p.m. and 8 p.m., that program might pair a student spotlight post with a donation request during that time period.

CHALLENGES TO INTEGRATION

Although much of this chapter is dedicated to highlighting the advantages of using big data and social media analytics, there are some clear challenges that should be briefly mentioned:

- **Cost:** Unlike social media platforms, there is a large expense associated with big data collection, storage, and processing. If the intention is full-scale integration, full institutional support is recommended.
- **Differentiating correlation and causation:** This is a well-known challenge of interpreting and integrating big data. The Google flu case presented earlier in the chapter is a good example of correlation, not causation. The Google algorithm is based solely on search queries, meaning that the flu and people googling the flu tend to happen at the same time, but one does not *cause* the other. There is a clear benefit in the Google flu case, but the limitations of correlation must be recognized.

- **Institution policy:** This is usually more of a consideration than a challenge. Most higher education institutions have strict social media policies that include the use of logo, school colors and font, and platforms supported. Prior to creating a program page, it would be wise to seek out the institution's social media director for guidance.
- **Privacy:** Similar to the Health Insurance Portability and Accountability Act (HIPAA) for patient protection, there is the Family Educational Rights and Privacy Act (FERPA) for students. Some programs ask students to sign photo privacy waivers that include language specific to social media posting. It is recommended that this be discussed with the campus social media director and/or campus legal counsel.

CONCLUSIONS

In conclusion, the use of big data holds great potential in health professions education. Careful attention must be paid to collection, analysis, and use of the information to ensure that it matches with predetermined goals. Although it is recommended that an interdisciplinary team approach be implemented for large-scale plans of integration, tracking social media analytics on the program level can be implemented quickly and with minimal cost.

NOTES

1. **Spotify:** An online music and podcast streaming service that originated in Sweden and is available in more than 50 languages.
2. **Plug-in:** Computer software that adds specific features onto an existing program, also known as an *add-on*.
3. **Tweet:** A post on Twitter that can contain text, links, videos, and/or photos but is limited to 140 characters.
4. **Retweet:** A reposted or forwarded Tweet, a method to share content created by other Twitter users.

REFERENCES

Boyd, D. E., & Ellison, N. B. (2007). Social network sites: Definition, history, and scholarship. *Journal of Computer-Mediated Communication, 13*(1), 210–230.

Columbus, L. (2016). Ten ways big data is revolutionizing marketing and sales. Retrieved from https://www.forbes.com/sites/louiscolumbus/2016/05/09/ten-ways-big-data-is-revolutionizing-marketing-and-sales/#47c2bea621cf

Corporate author. (2016). Retrieved from https://analyticsacademy.withgoogle.com

Corporate author. (2016). Retrieved from https://www.google.com/analytics/standard

Corporate author. (2016a). Twitter: About. Retrieved from https://about.twitter.com/company

Corporate author. (2016b). Twitter business analytics. Retrieved from https://business.twitter.com/en/analytics.html

Daniel, B. (2015). Big data and analytics in higher education: Opportunities and challenges. *British Journal of Educational Technology, 46*(5), 904–920.

Daniel, B. K., & Butson, R. (2013, November–December). *Technology enhanced analytics (TEA) in higher education*. Paper presented at the International Conference on Educational Technologies, Kuala Lumpur, Malaysia.

Digital Trends Staff. (2016). The history of social networking. Retrieved from http://www.digitaltrends.com/features/the-history-of-social-networking

Duggan, M. (2015). The demographics of social media users. Retrieved from http://www.pewinternet.org/2015/08/19/the-demographics-of-social-media-users

Greenberg, D. M., Baron-Cohen, S., Stillwell, D. J., Kosinski, M., & Rentfrow, P. J. (2015). Musical preferences are linked to cognitive styles. *PLOS ONE, 10*(7), e0131151.

Laney, D. (2001). 3D data management: Controlling data volume, velocity, and variety. *META Group Research Note, 6*, 70.

Leiner, B. M., Cerf, V. G., Clark, D. D., Kahn, R. E., Kleinrock, L., Lynch, D. C., . . . Wolff, S. (2016). Brief history of the Internet. Retrieved from http://www.internetsociety.org/internet/what-internet/history-internet/brief-history-internet

Mayer-Schönberger, V., & Cukier, K. N. (2013). *Big data: A revolution that will transform how we live, work, and think*. Boston, MA: Houghton Mifflin Harcourt.

McAfee, A., & Brynjolfsson, E. (2012, October). Big data: The management revolution. *Harvard Business Review*. Retrieved from https://hbr.org/2012/10/big-data-the-management-revolution

MedHub. (2016). E*Value: For healthcare education. Retrieved from http://www.medhub.com

O'Reilly, T. (2005). What is WEB 2.0? Design patterns and business models for the next generation of software. Retrieved from http://www.oreilly.com/pub/a/web2/archive/what-is-web-20.html

Physician Assistant Education Association. (2016). PAEA PACKRAT. Retrieved from http://packratexam.org

Rijmenam, M. V. (2016). Southwest Airlines uses big data to deliver excellent customer service. Retrieved from https://datafloq.com/read/southwest-airlines-uses-big-data-deliver-excellent/371

Simon, D. (2016, April 15). Is personalized learning the future of school? *CNN*. Retrieved from http://www.cnn.com/2016/04/15/health/altschool-personalized-education

Statista. (2016). Number of monthly active Twitter users worldwide from 1st quarter 2010 to 2nd quarter 2016 (in millions). Retrieved from https://www.statista.com/statistics/282087/number-of-monthly-active-twitter-users

Strong, C. (2016). The big opportunity in Big Data. *International Journal of Market Research*, *58*(4), 499–501.

Vahl, A. (2015). How to use Facebook insights to improve engagement. Retrieved from http://www.socialmediaexaminer.com/how-to-use-facebook-insights-to-improve-engagement

Ventilla, M. (2014). AltSchool. Retrieved from https://www.altschool.com

Walker, B. (2015). Every day big data statistics—2.5 quintillion bytes of data created daily. Retrieved from http://www.vcloudnews.com/every-day-big-data-statistics-2-5-quintillion-bytes-of-data-created-daily

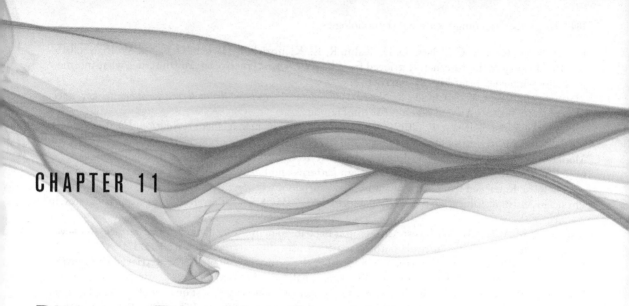

CHAPTER 11

Distance Education Strategies
Susan E. White

CHAPTER OBJECTIVE

- Design, implement, and evaluate an online learning community, including telelearning, interactive videoconferencing, and synchronous and asynchronous activities

---

Medical education is not just a program for building knowledge and skills in its recipients . . . it is also an experience which creates attitudes and expectations.

—Abraham Flexner

HISTORY OF DISTANCE EDUCATION

Educating students who are at a distance from a campus or school has long been a challenge. In 1858, using the available technology of the postal service, the University of London established an external program (now called the *international program*) to conduct courses using mail correspondence, thus effectively establishing the first distance education (DE) program. Correspondence schools offered flexibility in terms of time and location and were popular in Europe and the United States in the 1800s. The model was used for primary and later secondary education in Australia when the Western Australia Correspondence School (now the Schools of Isolated and Distance Education [SIDE]) was founded in 1918. When radio was added in 1940 to broadcast lessons to students, it was an example of using the available technology to provide education.

As technologies have developed, education has taken advantage of the ability to connect students at a distance and to offer them education through different technological modalities (Exhibit 11.1). These technologies encompass a wide variety of video, audio, and interactive

---

EXHIBIT 11.1 Definitions

Asynchronous distance education: This refers to a process in which one or more cohorts of students receive the same content but at different times.

Blended or **hybrid education:** This method uses a combination of in-person classroom and online or virtual education, with 30% to 79% of the educational content delivered online (Friesen, 2012). There are four models of blended education—rotational, flex, self-blending, and enriched virtual.

Distance education: Education that occurs in geographically distant sites. This includes synchronous and asynchronous methods; courses may include traditional, web-assisted, blended, or online education.

LMS: This refers to *learning management systems*, which is software accessible online that provides learning materials. An LMS may be as simple as a shared drive or may include the ability to create quizzes, discussion boards, wikis, journals, and other features.

MOOCs: Massive open online courses (MOOCs) offer educational content on an Internet platform. They may be self-paced or instructor paced.

Online education: This is education in which more than 80% of the content is delivered online. There are usually very few or no classroom meetings (Friesen, 2012).

Self-paced: This refers to a method in which students access the material on their own time and at their own pace.

Synchronous distance education: This is a process in which one or more cohorts of students receive the same content simultaneously in real time.

Telelearning: The Greek word *tele* means far off. Collis, in 1998, defined *telelearning* as "using telematics for learning-related purposes," which may be geographically near or far (Collis, 1998). It is also called *eLearning*.

Traditional education: This refers to educational content that is delivered face to face in a classroom without any use of technology (Friesen, 2012).

Videoconferencing: This is the use of video and audio together in a real-time interactive meeting.

Web-assisted education: This refers to education in which 1% to 29% of the content is delivered online (Friesen, 2012).

---

options that can be used alone or together to provide educational content. The rapidly evolving nature and technology of DE creates both opportunities and challenges for educators. On one hand, there is the opportunity to educate students at distant sites and to use innovative teaching techniques; on the other hand, best practices are still being developed.

DE has been used in whole or in part for primary, secondary, undergraduate, and graduate education. A study of full-time virtual schools and blended-learning schools for precollege education in the United States showed 447 full-time virtual schools with 262,000 students and 87 blended schools with 26,155 students in 2013 to 2014 (Miron & Gulosino, 2016). Although this represents a small portion of the public school children in the United States, students are being exposed to virtual education at younger ages. In their 2013 paper, Allen and Seaman (2013) noted that 32% of all students report taking at least one online course and that a total of 6.7 million students have taken at least one online course since 2003. This means that students entering a graduate or health professions program probably have some previous experience with online learning.

USES OF TECHNOLOGY IN EDUCATION

As technology has developed and grown, so, too, has the use of technology to deliver educational content. The ability to educate students outside a physical classroom is appealing on many levels for educators, colleges, and students. Classroom size, availability of students and instructors, and other physical boundaries may not apply to online courses. For students, the ability to take courses at home or on their own time may be an advantage to those who work or for whom travel to a campus is difficult. This has led to a rise in innovative web-based education, which takes many different forms.

Courses may be thought of as traditional, web-facilitated, blended (sometimes called *hybrid*), or online based on the percentage of course material delivered online. In addition, the ability to connect classrooms via video over long distances has also transformed education and is termed *DE* (see Exhibit 11.1). Courses that are taught using synchronous or asynchronous education may be traditional, web-facilitated, blended, or online. These types of courses are popular in health sciences education and are covered in this chapter.

The percentage of course material delivered online determines whether the course is traditional (0% online), web-facilitated (1%–29% online), blended (30%–79% online), and online (>80% online; Allen & Seaman, 2013, 2016). Web-facilitated courses typically use a learning management system (LMS), such as Moodle or Blackboard, a website or shared drive to post items such as a syllabus or assignments, whereas the course content is delivered face to face in a classroom. Blended courses have a much larger percentage of online content and may use videos, prerecorded lectures, wikis, journals, papers, quizzes, and discussion boards. There is still an in-classroom component; however, the number of face-to-face in-class encounters is reduced when compared to traditional or web-facilitated courses. Online courses offer at least 80% of the educational content online and have few, if any, face-to-face meetings in a classroom. Massive open online courses (MOOCs) are a good example of an online course in which all the content—including lectures, discussions, assignments, and assessments—is delivered online through an LMS (Coursera Inc.; edX Inc.). Online courses may be synchronous but are more often asynchronous, with each student progressing through the course with a set timeline.

ONLINE COURSES

In higher education, MOOCs have led the way in online courses, the percentage of higher education institutions offering them increased from 2.6% in 2012 to 8% in 2014 (Allen & Seaman, 2016). MOOCs differ from other types of online learning in that students do not typically register, pay tuition, or receive credit. Therefore, in this chapter, we exclude MOOCs from our discussion of online courses.

In the fall of 2014, individuals using exclusively DE accounted for 14% of all higher education students, which represents an increase from 12% in 2013 (Allen & Seaman, 2016). Forty-eight percent of these students were enrolled at a public institution (Allen & Seaman, 2016). Among graduate students, the number of students enrolled in all DE (733,152) was about 3 times higher than those enrolled in some DE courses (233,155) in 2014 (Allen & Seaman, 2016). It is interesting to note that Allen and Seaman found that DE students are highly concentrated, close to two thirds of the DE enrollments occur in only 10% of all higher education institutions (Allen & Seaman, 2016). This data has some interesting implications for graduate health care education. It indicates increased accessibility for students and therefore may increase opportunities for a diverse range of students. The high concentration of DE in a small number of institutions means that students have a cohort of similarly trained colleagues. Allen and Seaman (2016) also note that the high concentration means that the decisions of a relatively few educators have a large impact on students, health care education, and DE.

Learning outcomes for online education have been difficult to assess. Reviewing the literature, there are a large number of reports of learning with a specific outcome of a narrowly focused educational objective—for example, video podcasting for clinical skills in nursing, an online course in hospice care, and a blended course in a surgical clerkship (Hurst, 2016; Liebert, Mazer, Bereknyei, Lin, & Lau, 2016; Tse & Ellman, 2016). In their 2015 report, Allen and Seaman showed the number of chief academic officers who rated online education as good as or better than face-to-face instruction has increased from 57.2% in 2003 to 71.4% in 2015 (Allen & Seaman, 2016). It is important to note that there has been a lack of studies comparing online education to in-person education and that the study relied on the attitudes of provosts.

Faculty preparation for teaching an online course varies and requires knowledge and training in use of the LMS and other software required to teach a course. In addition, software knowledge needs to include not only instruction in the mechanics of its use, but also how it may be used pedagogically to engage students. Switching from a traditional lecture-based course to an online or blended course can require significant faculty time. In 2013, 41.4% of academic leaders believed that it takes more faculty time and effort to teach online, whereas 9.7% disagreed and 45.7% were neutral (Allen & Seaman, 2013).

Assessment in online courses may use the traditional methods of testing, such as quizzes, exams, or assignments (see Chapter 18). Although classroom participation is absent, online discussion boards have an advantage over classroom participation in that they contain documentation of participation. In that sense, it is possible to grade students not only by participation but also on the quality of their comments and to do so during any point of the class. This can encourage more participation and thoughtful commentary if done at several points during the course. Online discussion also promotes diversity in that it draws out students who may be reluctant to speak out in a classroom setting.

BLENDED COURSES

In comparison to online courses, it appears that a larger number of students are educated using blended courses, although the exact percentages are not available. Although precise definitions may differ, Allen and Seaman define a *blended course* as offering 30% to 70% of the educational content online with few in-person meetings (Allen & Seaman, 2016). In "Report: Defining Blended Learning," Friesen states, "blended learning designates the range of possibilities presented by combining Internet and digital media with established classroom forms that require the physical co-presence of teacher and students" (Friesen, 2012, p. 1). Blended courses offer a wide range of possibilities in terms of technology and pedagogy. This would include courses using the flipped classroom model (see Chapter 8) as well as self-study modules, online discussion boards, wikis, quizzes, assignments (both individual and group), and assessments. Blended courses also offer the ability to connect with students in the classroom and to do hands-on activities there. Blended courses can be offered in synchronous or asynchronous format using various technologies such as videoconferencing.

Various models of blended learning have been proposed by Staker and Horn in their 2012 report on primary and secondary schools' use of blended courses—the rotational model, flex model, self-blending model, and the enriched virtual model (Staker & Horn, 2012; Figure 11.1). Each of the models is considered with some thoughts for its application to health professions education.

In the rotational model, online education is combined or embedded in a range of in-classroom instructions in a cyclical manner. Students are moved through a series of learning activities, including at least one online and one in-class activity. This rotation can be determined by a fixed schedule or is based on learners' needs. One advantage of this model is that it can facilitate learning at different paces using a variety of pedagogical strategies to meet learners' needs. An example might be videos or podcasts of a lecture, or groups of students working together on a concept or project. The in-classroom component may be used to ensure progress of the entire class (see Figure 11.1).

With the flex model, students receive primarily online education under the instructor's supervision in the classroom with both the students and the instructor physically present in the classroom. This model was thought to be more appropriate to elementary education in which

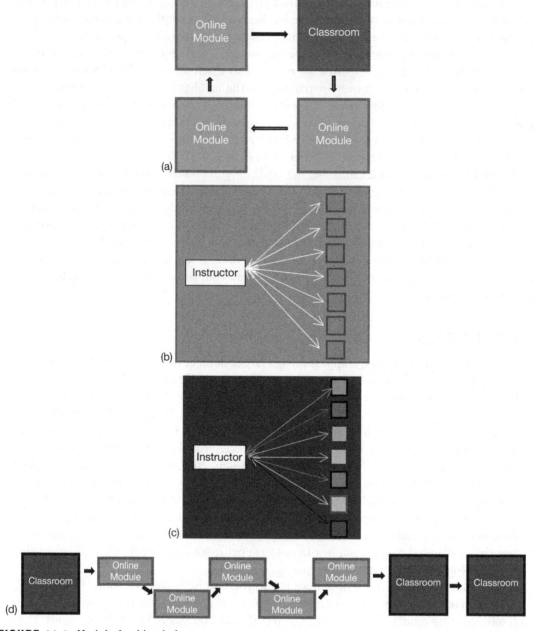

FIGURE 11.1 Models for blended courses.

(a) Rotational model—the course rotates from online to traditional classroom in cyclic fashion, with students completing at least one online module.

(b) Flex model—there is one instructor and students following the same online module in a physical classroom.

(c) Self-blending model—the instructor and students are located in the classroom with students following different online modules.

(d) Enriched virtual model—instruction is mostly provided online with few classroom meetings.

one instructor has the ability to monitor student progress and distractibility of students might be an issue (Friesen, 2012; Staker & Horn, 2012). In health care education, students are adults so this may not be a good venue for this model. One exception might be in teaching procedures or skills testing in which students could view online modules and then demonstrate the skill for instructors in the classroom (see Figure 11.1).

The self-blending model consists of students in a classroom with an instructor with all students taking different courses independently online. This model, like the flex model, is thought to be more applicable to elementary education, where direct supervision is needed (Friesen, 2012; Staker & Horn, 2012; see Figure 11.1).

The enriched virtual model consists mostly of online education and occasional in-class face-to-face meetings that enrich the online material. The number and type of classroom meetings may vary and may include the instructor meeting with the whole class or with separate cohorts. The course may meet at any number of times and may vary in frequency. This model is thought to be most applicable to higher education (Staker & Horn, 2012) and has been widely adopted in graduate nursing education (McAfooes, 2015). Examples might include a research course with one in-class meeting at the start, followed by online learning modules and projects, and student presentations during several classroom meetings at the end; or a course in counseling or physical exam skills might contain online modules with counseling techniques or physical exam skills that might be followed by face-to-face practice sessions with the instructor (see Figure 11.1). Options for assessment of student knowledge include pre- and postmodule quizzes, examinations, projects, presentations, essay, or papers. As in online course discussion boards, discussion may be evaluated for participation as well as quality of comments.

Little is known about the work involved for faculty to prepare blended courses. However, it is likely that similar to online courses, preparation of blended courses may require more time compared to traditional teaching methods. Meeting with small cohorts or individual students can also increase time for faculty, especially if travel is required. Monitoring and managing discussion boards are also time-consuming. Blended courses can also be used with videoconferencing software for the in-class portion or to meet with students individually or in groups. Blended courses offer flexibility and adaptability for online and in-person instruction.

SYNCRHONOUS AND ASYNCHRONOUS DE

DE involves the use of videoconferencing software to connect one or more classrooms so that instruction can occur in all classrooms no matter the distance. Instruction can be synchronous or asynchronous and both have advantages and disadvantages that are worth considering. In synchronous DE, the classroom where the teaching occurs is replicated in one or more other classrooms in real time. Using video and audio links, the podium presentation and the instructor appear in all the classrooms at once. One of the advantages of synchronous DE is that all students receive the same instruction no matter where they are located, thus ensuring educational equality. Using video and audio techniques, students and the lecturer may interact with each other, and thus best mimics the traditional in-classroom experience for both the lecturer and students.

Asynchronous DE involves the use of video to capture the lecture or lesson, which is then viewed by students at various times. It may be viewed by students together in a classroom or individually at home, but not while the classroom session is occurring. Students receive the same information, albeit at different times, and therefore receive equal educational material. However, there is not an option to ask questions or interact with the instructor for those viewing the recorded video. One option to mimic the in-classroom experience at the distant campus is to have students view the video as a group at the distant site. This would allow student-to-student interaction and possible instructor interaction via video. Both groups would receive the same content and would be able to interact with each other; however, the experience for each classroom would be slightly different.

Another option for asynchronous DE is for learners to view the video individually at their convenience. Although the content may be the same presentation, the in-classroom experience is different from the one experienced by the student who views the video. Asynchronous DE does offer the advantage of convenience for the student, particularly if the video is watched individually and may therefore be an advantage for teaching across time zones or for students who work. Individual learners are able to decide when and where they learn best, which may also be an advantage for them.

Before we address the technological and curricular challenges of DE, it should be noted that there are subtle differences for the student in both the recorded classrooms and in the distance classrooms. For the learners in the classroom where the lecture is recorded, the instructor may behave slightly differently during a recording than during a live lecture. Movement may be restricted to remain on camera and use of a microphone may change tone or intonation. Instructors may also be self-conscious about being videoed. Although both cohorts of learners would be exposed to the same changes in the instructor, it may mean that the experience of the class or course is different when it is recorded than when it is live. Studies by Massey, Lee, White, and Goldsmith (2012) and Goldsmith and colleagues (2009a) looked at depression and anxiety in students in two health professions accelerated programs (pharmacy and physician assistant [PA]) and found that students in both distant and in-person cohorts experience the same increasing level of anxiety and depression over the semester. The same authors also evaluated academic achievement and found no difference between the distance and in-person cohorts (Goldsmith et al., 2009a, 2009b; Massey et al., 2012).

TECHNOLOGY AND DE

The challenges of DE are both technological and educational. The technological challenges of linking video and audio to more than one classroom, often at geographically distant sites, can be daunting and is subject to loss of connection. Programs offering synchronous DE must have a backup plan in case of disconnection, and it is suggested that classes be recorded so that if disconnection occurs, it will be possible to have an asynchronous session using the recorded presentation.

The physical design of the classroom and placement of screens, cameras, and microphones are important and require an expert who understands not only audio and video equipment, but also acoustics, recording, and Internet capabilities. Often the equipment company will also offer design services, which is helpful for the technological aspects covered. It is important to carefully consider the various pedagogical approaches to be used, and faculty who will be teaching in the DE classrooms should be involved in the planning. Setting up the classroom for a lecture-based course is very different than setting it up for a course that depends heavily on classroom discussion. Input from faculty allows designers to understand how their system will be used and should result in a design that is flexible and functional (Figure 11.2).

The basics concepts of the DE classroom include unobstructed views of the presentation and the ability to hear the instructor. Cameras are generally mounted on the ceiling, which prevents obstruction of the view and makes them inconspicuous. Both the teaching and distant classroom(s) should have the ability to adjust lights and volume separately. This allows all the classrooms to optimize the learning environment. In all classrooms, the other students and the instructor should be visible. This allows both the instructor and students to feel connected to each other. In the distant classroom, a flat panel screen or projection of the instructor should be placed where an instructor normally stands and be approximately life sized. If the projection is too large or too small, it diminishes the virtual reality of the instructor and it may be uncomfortable and unnatural for students. Likewise, the instructor in the teaching classroom should be able to view the students in the distant classroom. Often the distant classroom(s) are viewed on screens behind the live students, which gives the effect of a large lecture hall. Students in the distant classroom should be able to view those in other classroom(s).

Options for microphones are varied and should take into consideration how the instruction will be given. Handheld microphones are awkward for the presenter to juggle and the quality

Teaching Classroom	Distant Classroom(s)
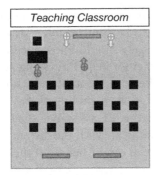	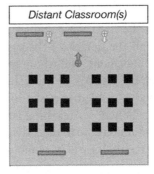

In the teaching classroom, cameras focus on the instructor and the students in the classroom. The distant classroom is projected on the screens at the back of the room. This allows the instructor and students in the teaching classroom to see students in the distant classroom when they are speaking. A presentation projector shows the presentation on the front screen. In the distant classroom(s), the instructor is shown on the screen to the left of the classroom and the presentation is on the center screen. Two screens in the back of the distant classroom show the students in the teaching classroom, which permits them to be seen by distant students. The ability of participants to see each other enhances interaction across classrooms.

- ■ Student
- ■ Instructor
- ▭ Projection screen
- ⚙ Camera (arrow indicates direction)
- ⚙ Presentation projector (arrow indicates direction)

FIGURE 11.2 Distance education classroom setup.

of speech may vary depending on how the microphone is held. Podium microphones fix the presenter to the podium and also may cause variations in the quality of speech. Wireless microphones affixed to a shirt or a headset offer the best voice quality and the most flexibility in movement and are therefore recommended.

Communication from the teaching to distant classroom(s) allows students in both classrooms to ask questions and participate in the class. Microphone options include ceiling microphones, desk microphones, or wireless handheld microphones. Ceiling microphones are inconspicuous and may be set up so that the whole classroom may be heard, which mimics a small- to medium-sized traditional classroom in terms of students being heard by the instructor in the teaching classroom. The disadvantage of ceiling microphones is that they can pick up ambient noise such as paper shuffling, students talking, and even keyboard typing. The ambient noise from the distant classroom can be heard in the teaching classroom, which is distracting. On occasion, microphones can amplify the noise from the distant classroom as it is picked up in the teaching classroom, which can result in both classrooms experiencing a high level of background noise. Careful placement of microphones and consultation with audio engineers can avoid such a situation.

Desk microphones offer the ability to turn on or off the microphone at will and therefore decrease the issue of ambient noise. They do require the student to turn on the microphone, which can have the effect of decreasing the number of questions from the distant classroom. In addition, if the microphones are all off, students in the distant classroom could be disruptive to the session without the instructor realizing it. Handheld wireless microphones are subject to the difficulty of reaching the person who has a question, variation in voice quality, and damage from frequent passing. Other options for communication between the teaching and distant classrooms include email or texting to ask questions during class.

Orientation of instructors to the system and classroom is crucial as familiarity with the equipment allows both the instructor and students to be comfortable. Although instructors may not need to know all the details of the system, they should know the basics of adjusting lights, volume, slide advancement, and whom to contact for help. Pretesting presentations with videos, audience-participation slides, or links should be done ahead of time. Informational technological (IT) assistance is needed to assist instructors in including theses educational tools and for troubleshooting. Whenever teaching is occurring, IT assistance should be available for potential issues. One should be able to directly communicate with the distant classroom, which does not depend on the technology (e.g., a phone), which can be helpful if there is partial loss of a connection.

The experience of teaching in synchronous DE is different from that of teaching in a live classroom or simply being recorded. Depending on the course, modifications may be needed to deliver content and engage students. For instructors, it is helpful to have the experience first-hand of being in both the teaching and distant classroom to understand the differences between the two learning environments. Although it is easier to engage the live students seated in the classroom, this can lead to students in the distant classroom feeling ignored. Learning to look into the camera that projects the image of the instructor to the distant classroom allows the distant class to have eye contact with the instructor and to feel included. However, doing so requires knowing which camera to use and then remembering to look from the live students to the distant ones. Usually, this can be done with a subtle change of gaze; over time, this becomes a learned behavior for instructors. Likewise, learning to wait for sound delays in questions or comments from the distant classroom is a behavior that must be developed. For this reason, instructors who have participated and experienced a class in both the teaching and distant classrooms will have a better understanding of the challenges and environment of both classrooms.

CURRICULUM AND DE

Courses that are taught using DE need to consider the DE method (synchronous or asynchronous), available audiovisual (AV) equipment and its limitations, as well as class sizes, and the presence or absence of faculty in the distant classroom(s). Because technology may not work at any given time, one needs a clear backup plan. Providing students with clear expectations for classroom behavior, participation, and backup plans for technology issues will decrease their anxiety and prevent frustration. Clear communication on a regular basis with faculty located at different sites encourages collegiality and understanding of the issues. Often, distant sites are set up with a smaller number of students and faculty and consideration must be given to providing support for the distant site(s) to prevent them from feeling unwanted or unimportant. Students and faculty at the distant site should have equal access to instructors, library resources, and laboratory facilities.

Although studies have demonstrated that both cohorts of students perform equally well in DE programs, the physical separation of students and faculty at distant sites can make each cohort wary of the other. Interaction between faculty and students occurs at many levels outside of the classroom and can be either formal or informal. Office hours and time before and after class are often formal interactions based on a student's needs. Informal interaction occurs in the halls, parking lots, and around campus. The challenge of having students at a distant site(s) is providing these opportunities for both formal and informal interactions. Video technology can be used to solve some of these problems; holding office hours over Skype or video-conferencing the distant students into meetings are some examples. Students on both campuses can work together on projects using Google Drive and therefore get to know each other. If the sites are not too geographically distant, having instructors occasionally visit the distant classroom and perhaps even teach from there increases the human connection between faculty and students. Having one or two students from each campus spend a day on the other campus as an "ambassador" also increases the understanding and communication between the cohorts. Social gatherings can also serve to increase the communication between the cohorts.

For asynchronous DE, student isolation is more acute as students are learning on their own. Although this method does allow students flexibility around scheduling their learning, it does mean that they do not have a cohort of students or faculty that they see on a daily basis. For students, asynchronous education at home can permit them to advance educationally without relocation. When students gather to view an asynchronous video together, discussion and interaction can occur; however, because the video is recorded, students may well question the value in viewing it in a classroom versus online at home. Faculty interaction with individual students learning online at home is challenging.

Pedagogical approaches for DE classrooms can range from traditional lecture to audience participation devices (clickers) to flipped classroom with discussions. Just like the traditional classroom, student engagement is important. As noted earlier in this chapter, students at distant sites need to feel that they are included in the classroom. Eye contact from the instructor, audio connection for questions, and virtual presence in the teaching classroom are all important tools. Just as in the traditional classroom, the importance of engaging the students in the material cannot be underestimated. Methods for doing this in a DE classroom are still being developed and often require new ways of thinking about existing technology while also keeping an eye out for developing technology and apps.

Studies have shown that knowledge retention is better with frequent testing, and audience response systems (clickers) allow frequent quizzing within an eLearning presentation to engage students with the material (DelSignore, Wolbrink, Zurakowski, & Burns, 2016). Because DE classrooms mimic eLearning, similar findings might be expected in DE. More recently, the flipped classroom has become an important tool in education. In this model, students view or read material before coming to class and spend class time applying the material by, for example, doing case studies or working on problems together. Rather than lecture, the instructor serves as a facilitator during the classroom work.

Using some of the techniques listed in Figure 11.2, flipped classrooms can be used by DE classes. To prevent noise from becoming a distraction, the microphones can be turned off while students are working together and then groups on both campuses can share their work. In some video systems, it may be possible to turn cameras to the classrooms that are facing each other. This is an interesting technique for a class discussion or debate. Ground rules for speaking need to be developed for audio delay; formal debate rules work especially well.

PRACTICAL TEACHING TIPS AND BEST PRACTICES

Just as teaching in a traditional classroom requires preparation, so, too, does teaching in the DE classroom when there is a camera involved. We have discussed the use of microphones, but there are other considerations to keep in mind. Table 11.1 describes some problems and solutions for DE classrooms. Items for consideration include clothing, motion, speech, and humor. The physics of light and sound and the medium of video require some thinking and adjustments that are not needed in the traditional classroom. As noted previously, audio is delayed and one must learn to factor that into discussions and questions.

Humor is often a welcome break during class and certainly DE classrooms are not an exception. Visual humor via cartoons or pictures tends to work better than auditory jokes since both groups of students see the joke at the same time. Given the slower transmission of sound, auditory humor often results in the teaching classroom laughing and drowning out the punch lines for the distant classroom(s), which creates frustration.

TABLE 11.1 Common Problems and Solutions in Distance Education

Problem	Teaching Classroom	Distant Classroom
Sound		
Ambient noise too loud	Check for background noise, consult audio engineer, consider using tablets rather than keyboards	
	Increase sound insulation in room	
	Have faculty in classroom to assess issue	
Instructor not audible in distant classroom	Check microphone and battery	Check system
Video		
Instructor blurry	Review clothing suggestions	
Video halting with motion	Check for shiny objects on clothing and remove	Check projector
Instructor off camera	Mark movement limits on floor	Check camera and projector
Not working	Check camera and projector	Check camera and projector
Classroom participation		
Students not participating	Call on students by name.	
	Think—Pair—Share	
	Engage in small-group work with microphones off, then share.	
	Use audience participation clickers and make this competitive by setting up teams across the two classrooms.	
	Have faculty in classroom to interact with students.	
Discussion not robust	Engage in small-group work on each campus with microphones off, then meet to present and discuss.	
	Turning off microphones and having faculty in each classroom facilitates discussion. Students share major points across the two campuses with microphones on.	
	Have a debate—turn cameras or arrange classroom so both groups of students are facing each other and use formal debate rules.	
Case study participation low	Break each campus into small groups and give each group a paper with large letters A to E printed (corresponding to MCQ answers) on it. All groups answer the same questions projected on screen. After time for discussion, each group raises the paper to give the answer. Groups can be called on to defend their choice.	
	Use texting or email to have students answer the questions. Having a second person to manage the email/texts is helpful.	
	Use clickers to elicit answers. Ask students to defend their answer. See previous suggestions.	

MCQ, multiple-choice question.

Movement around the classroom is possible if the camera is able to follow the instructor. If not, then the limits of the visual range of the camera should be clearly delineated to avoid the instructor moving off camera in the distant classroom, which makes the instructor sound like a disembodied presence. Two types of clothing are to be avoided—red and large overt patterns. With motion, both red and patterned clothing tend to blur, creating an odd and distracting image. Likewise, large earrings and jewelry sometimes are subject to blur artifact as well. Wearing clothing that matches the background of the projected image often makes the instructor appear to be a talking head and therefore should be avoided.

Nervous tics, such as visual expressions and voicing of fillers such as um, seem to get exaggerated in DE, especially in the distant classroom. If possible, record a short segment of the lecture ahead of time and view it; this allows faculty to become aware of these issues. Although the temptation is to raise one's voice to be heard in the distant classroom, speaking at a slow to moderate speed in a medium tone works best. Very rapid speech is difficult to hear in the distant classroom.

CONCLUSIONS

Online learning and videoconferencing technologies offer the ability to teach students in geographically distant locations, thus opening health care education to a wide range of students. Programs in graduate health care education often use blended courses with 30% to 70% of the education delivered online. Two models of blended courses, the rotational model and the enriched virtual model, are well suited to graduate education. In-classroom material may be delivered using videoconferencing technology to allow the instructor to teach in several classrooms on distant campuses, either synchronously or asynchronously. This method allows for educational equivalency and presents some unique challenges.

REFERENCES

Allen, I. E., & Seaman, J. (2013, January). *Changing course: Ten years of tracking online education in the United States*. Babson Park, MA: Babson Survey Research Group. Retrieved from http://www.onlinelearningsurvey.com/reports/changingcourse.pdf

Allen, I. E., & Seaman, J. (2016). *Online report card: Tracking online education in the United States*. Babson Park, MA: Babson Survey Research Group and Quahog Research Group. Retrieved from https://onlinelearningconsortium.org/read/online-report-card-tracking-online-education-united-states-2015

Collis, B. A. (1998). New wine and old bottles? Tele-learning, telematics, and the University of Twente. In M. F. Verdejo & G. Davies (Eds.), *The virtual campus: Trends for higher education and training* (pp. 3–16). London, UK: Chapman & Hall.

DelSignore, L. A., Wolbrink, T. A., Zurakowski, D., & Burns, J. P. (2016). Test-enhanced e-learning strategies in postgraduate medical education: A randomized cohort study. *Journal of Medical Internet Research, 18*(11), e299. Retrieved from http://www.jmir.org/2016/11/e299

Friesen, N. (2012). Report: Defining blended learning. Retrieved from http://learningspaces.org/papers/Defining_Blended_Learning_NF.pdf

Goldsmith, C. W., Miller, K. E., Lee, L., Moreau, T., White, S. E., & Massey, S. L. (2009a). The effects of synchronized distance education (SDE) on anxiety, depression and academic achievement in a physician assistant studies program. *International Journal of Instructional Technology and Distance Learning, 6*, 1–9. Retrieved from http://www.itdl.org/Journal/May_09/article02.htm

Goldsmith, C. W., Miller, K. E., Lee, L., Moreau, T., White, S. E., & Massey, S. L. (2009b). The effects of synchronized distance education on academic achievement in a physician assistant program. *Journal of Physician Assistant Education, 20*, 17–21. Retrieved from http://journals.lww.com/jpae/Abstract/2009/20020/The_Effects_of_Synchronized_Distance_Education_on.5.aspx

Hurst, K. M. (2016). Using video podcasting to enhance the learning of clinical skill: A qualitative study of physiotherapy students' experiences. *Nurse Education Today, 45*, 206–211. Retrieved from doi:10.1016/j.nedt.2016.08.011

Liebert, C. A., Mazer, L., Bereknyei, M. S., Lin, D. T., & Lau, J. N. (2016). Student perceptions of a simulation-based flipped classroom for the surgery clerkship: A mixed-methods study. *Surgery, 160*(3), 591–598. doi:10.1016/j.surg.2016.03.034

Massey, S., Lee, L., White, S. E., & Goldsmith, C. W. (2012). The effects of synchronized distance education (SDE) on anxiety, depression, and academic achievement in first year doctor of pharmacy students in an accelerated curriculum. *Currents in Pharmacy Teaching and Learning, 4*, 285–291. doi:10.1016/j.cptl.2012.05.005

McAfooes, J. (2015). Teaching and learning in online learning communities. In D. M. Billings & J. A. Halstead (Eds.), *Teaching in nursing: A guide for faculty* (pp. 401–421). St. Louis, MO: Elsevier Health Sciences.

Miron, G., & Gulosino, C. (2016). Virtual schools report 2016: Directory and performance review. Retrieved from http://nepc.colorado.edu/publication/virtual-schools-annual-2016

Schools of Isolated and Distance Education. Heritage: The SIDE story. Retrieved from http://primaryside.wa.edu.au/Heritage/history.html

Staker, H., & Horn, M. B. (2012). Classifying K-12 blended learning. Retrieved from http://www.inacol.org/resource/classifying-k-12-blended-learning

Tse, C. S., & Ellman, M. S. (2016). Development, implementation and evaluation of a terminal and hospice care educational online module for preclinical students. *BMJ Supportive and Palliative Care, 7*(1), 73–80. doi:10.1136/bmjspcare-2015-000952

PART III
Clinical
Education

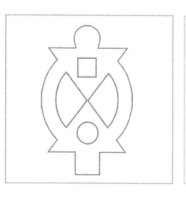

BOA ME NA ME MMOA WO
"Help me and let me help you."

Symbol of cooperation and interdependence

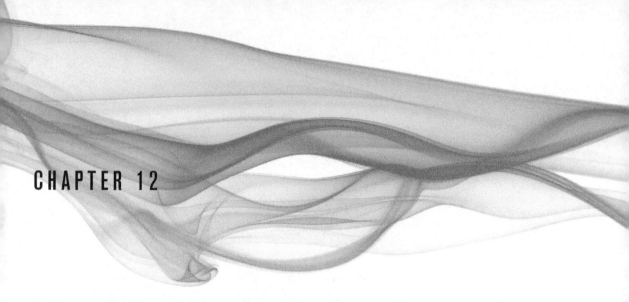

CHAPTER 12

Recruiting and Maintaining Clinical Training Sites

Andrew P. Chastain

CHAPTER OBJECTIVE

- Use strategies to develop and maintain clinical training sites, including methods for overcoming challenges

---

He who studies medicine without books sails an uncharted sea, but he who studies medicine without patients does not go to sea at all.

—William Osler

Performing the duties of a clinical coordinator of a health care training program takes much skill and effort. First comes all the preparation: obtaining qualified preceptors, reaching educational affiliation agreements, and conducting student health and background screening; then this intricate puzzle of moving parts that is the clinical curriculum for health care students can be set in motion.

Creating such a masterpiece can be one of the most rewarding activities within a practitioner-training program. The participation in and completion of fruitful clinical rotations allows students to test the knowledge they attained during the didactic portion of their training, and to gain knowledge, skills, and confidence that are unattainable in the classroom. But creating such a curriculum is not easy; it can be fraught with unforeseen obstacles and bogged down by system failures or delays. Unfortunately, some students will develop health or personal issues, providers will change practice, and personnel of health systems/facilities will change allegiance.

The key to success as a clinical coordinator is to have in place alternatives that allow students' clinical experience to continue without delaying their matriculation.

Clearly, being highly organized is the key to success for professionals considering a position as a clinical coordinator, or for those already serving as clinical coordinators. It is imperative that such professionals have at the outset a clear understanding of the all the duties expected of them. The expectations of the training program and of other faculty or staff concerning the clinical coordinator's responsibilities must also be clear. Other key questions to contemplate, preferably before accepting a position as a clinical coordinator, include the following:

- Will teaching responsibilities be required with this position (during either the didactic or the clinical phase)? If so, what percentage of time will be devoted to each aspect of the position?
- What type and amount of administrative assistance will be provided?
- With whom does the program have established relationships in providing clinical experiences/rotations?
- Who are the key players in hiring graduates of the program?
- What type of support might the university's/college's legal department provide in negotiating educational agreements?
- Will this position be coordinating clinical clerkships as part of a team involving multiple disciplines (e.g., RN/nurse practitioner [NP]/physician assistant [PA]/doctor of pharmacy [PharmD]) or only a single discipline?
- What standards for accreditation must be met by students matriculating through the clinical portion of training?

In addition to being highly organized, clinical coordinators should be adept at communicating professionally with potential preceptors of all kinds and designations, medical staffing officers, legal support personnel, members of the faculty, and, most important, students. Clinical coordinators also need to understand the objectives for each of the clinical rotations that will be coordinated. The goal should be to match correctly the personalities of students and providers while successfully exposing learners to clinical situations that allow them to complete the required objectives. Because careful attention to detail and the ability to communicate within a health care team are essential for effective clinical coordinators, health care education programs often employ successful clinicians who are transitioning into the world of academia for these positions. Those who have been successful in providing excellent care to patients while navigating an increasingly complex health care delivery system can be extremely important assets in arranging outstanding clinical rotations.

SITE ACQUISITION

Obtaining and retaining appropriate clinical rotation sites are essential duties of clinical coordinators, and procuring, developing, and maintaining the relationships involved in these processes can be challenging. For programs that are embedded within a school of medicine, a school of allied health science, or a school of nursing, rotations may exist within the university's health care delivery system. For those working within an institution of higher learning that is not affiliated with a health care system, developing these clerkships may be more challenging. Schools that have multiple degree-granting programs that include clinical training often create a centralized office that coordinates the assignment of students from all disciplines. To "share" sites between programs and universities more effectively, some programs are creating clearinghouses for preceptor utilization (Accreditation Review Commission on Education for the Physician Assistant, 2016). Regardless of a program's status or affiliation, acquiring the right type of preceptors to provide clinical experiences for students is of primary concern.

Identifying the "right" preceptors requires a great deal of effort, so clinical coordinators must work with each provider to ensure he or she understands the objectives of the rotation he or she will be teaching. Because it is important for clinical coordinators to understand the level of the students who will be joining them, many programs use graduates of the program. Once they have gained adequate experience and a strong footing in their own professional practice, program graduates are often a great and willing resource of excellent preceptors.

Before entering a clinical office/hospital rotation, the background and educational experience of each student must be considered. Students must understand the program's expectations concerning the number of patients they will see during a daily shift. Ideally, clinical coordinators should visit practice sites to obtain this information and develop a relationship with the clinicians and staff there. The coordinator should learn about the type of experiences students can expect to have during this rotation. The use of a preceptor form (see Exhibit 12.1), which documents the details of a provider's practice, can help achieve these tasks and produce an accurate record of each of a program's preceptors as well as to assess clinical sites.

The collection of this data informs coordinators about the type of practices through which students will be rotating. Many programs compile a database of clinical site demographics, such as inner city, urban, suburban, rural, and underserved. This information is invaluable to a program when applying for educational grants and accurately representing itself within the community. The collection of this data must also investigate the current status of each preceptor's health care license. All states, as part of the public record, allow license verification of health care providers, and the license of that provider must disclose any previous or pending action.

After all the parties agree they would like to pursue a relationship in educating the program's students, the next issue is whether an educational affiliation agreement is needed. Many solo practitioners choose to enter into this relationship without a formal agreement as long as they are provided copies of the students' certificates of insurability. Many larger institutions, such as hospitals and health care corporations, require a negotiated and formally executed affiliation agreement before any student can participate. That this can be an arduous process lasting months is perhaps one of the largest sources of discouragement for clinical coordinators. Many times, great preceptors with interest in providing a superlative educational experience will be identified, only to be rebuffed when the legal department and the university cannot reach an acceptable agreement or cannot agree in a timely manner. Developing a strong relationship with your institution's legal department is essential to making this process move quickly and efficiently.

Clinical coordinators must also continually assess the quality of each rotation. This not only ensures ongoing quality control among clinical sites, but is often an accreditation standard, as is the case for Standard C4.01 of the Accreditation Review Commission on Education for the Physician Assistant (Gerstner, 2016). Such assessments can be accomplished in multiple ways, including clinical faculty in-person site visits, visits via electronic means, and student evaluations of preceptors. Because of the massive workload that can be involved, processes that delineate how often these visits/inquiries will be made and who will be conducting them must be put in place. The manpower needed to complete this task thoroughly can be tremendous. To improve quality and clarify learning objectives, clinical programs often produce a dedicated preceptor manual. Individual health care disciplines may also produce similar manuals. Physician Assistant Education Association (2012) produces a preceptor orientation handbook: *Preceptor Orientation Handbook: Tips, Tools, and Guidance for Physician Assistant Preceptors.*

SCHEDULING

Scheduling students into required rotations is the next piece of the puzzle in clinical coordination. Each school has its own way of scheduling students to ensure they meet the program/accreditation standards for their discipline. Most schools begin with a query of each of the preceptorship sites

EXHIBIT 12.1 Form for Assessment of Clinical Sites

Preceptor Form

Primary preceptor: MD, DO, NP, PA who will take responsibility for the majority of the student's clinical instructions and whose practice is in primary care medicine.

Supplemental preceptor: MD, DO, NP, PA whose practice supplies required learning experiences that are not sufficiently provided by the primary preceptor (e.g., pediatrics, women's health).

Facility: (Check whether the student will be precepting at a facility such as multispecialty clinic, hospital, and so on; see Practice Speciality.)

Student name:	Faculty advisor:
Desired clinic/rotation start date:	Site visitor:
Days able to work with student: Monday Tuesday Wednesday Thursday Friday Saturday/Sunday	

1. Preceptor Information

Preceptor name: State license #:		
	MD/DO	Primary
	NP	Supplemental
	PA	Asst. preceptor
	Board Certified	
Clinic name:		
Address:		
City: State/Zip:		County:
Tel:	Fax:	
*Email:	Cell:	
Please add email address for the student evaluations as we send them to your email account		

Practice specialty:			Surgery
General practice	Pediatrics	Behavior Med/Psych	Inpatient
Internal medicine	GYN	Orthopedics	Emerg. Department
Family practice	OB	Other_____	Trauma

(*continued*)

EXHIBIT 12.1 Form for Assessment of Clinical Sites (*continued*)

Precepting experience:			
Have you previously precepted a PA student?		Yes	No
If "yes" please provide student's name:			
Current hospital staff privileges			
	Location (City):	Hospital staff status:	
Facility:			
Facility:			

6. Signatures

I agree to:

- provide student training and supervision in accordance with state law
- provide for a variety of patient encounters necessary for an appropriate learning experience
- review regularly the student's objectives to identify the focus of his or her studies and assure that the clinical experience meets the student's learning goals
- review regularly the student's objectives to identify the focus of his or her studies and ensure that the clinical experience meets the student's learning goals
- provide the agreed-upon hours of experience required for the student's training
- ensure that the student does not practice beyond his or her competency or legal authority
- review and countersign every student's medical record within 24 hours
- provide feedback to the student and program regarding student performance; this includes quarterly written evaluations and/or end-of-rotation evaluations
- notify the student's faculty advisor and site visitor at the earliest sign of a problem to ensure timely resolution
- acknowledge that the student will be providing the program with a written evaluation of the preceptorship at the end of the preceptorship or rotation

Signature:	MD/DO		Primary
	NP		Supplemental
	PA		Asst. preceptor
Print Name:		Date:	

Approved by

Faculty advisor:	Date:
Site visitor:	Date:
Program:	Date:

DO, doctor of osteopathic medicine; NP, nurse practitioner; PA, physician assistant.

to ascertain how many students will be accepted to that rotation over a clinical year. This helps them build a matrix of available rotations over the upcoming clinical period, with especially close attention to school closures such as holidays and breaks between terms. It is also essential to identify preceptors' planned vacations, conferences, and release time for research. During this process, schools may also opt to present a list of possible rotations/preceptors to their students so that they may indicate their preferences among the offered rotations.

After the lists of both preceptors' and students' preferences are compiled, the intense and, sometimes, days-long process of matching begins. Clinical coordinators must consider all the options/availabilities for each rotation. They should consider each student's request while matching each with opportunities and providers who will both challenge them and allow ample growth over time. Careful judgment is needed to match the personalities and styles of students and preceptors. This process is usually completed 3 months in advance of the clinical year.

Once the matching process for rotations is complete, students are then notified of their clinical rotation schedule for the upcoming year. Next, students must complete onboarding with the medical staff offices at the rotations' facilities. Most programs provide students a list of medical staff officers for the respective clinical sites where rotations are assigned. Some programs, however, package this onboarding for the facility in an effort to retain key clinical sites. First, the program obtains a complete file of all the paperwork students need to complete onboarding at that health care facility, including various types of screening such as drug screening; tuberculosis screening; criminal background checks; online, computer-based modules for training in patient privacy; Health Insurance Portability and Accountability Act (HIPAA) materials; bloodborne pathogen screening; and specific training on the electronic medical record (EMR). Then, the program sends each student who will be working within this facility a packet of paperwork to complete. Once all students complete the paperwork for the rotation site, the program bundles the paperwork and sends it directly to the facility's medical staff office for bulk processing. Although this can be an onerous task for the education program's staff, it ensures that all components of the onboarding process will be completed in a timely fashion for each student. It also reduces the probability that unforeseen events delay the matriculation of one or more students at this site. This process enables students to appear to the human resources department to receive a badge on their first day of the rotation with all requirements completed, and thus meaningful learning can begin right away.

ASSESSMENTS

Once clinical coordinators have created a harmonious clinical learning environment, they must then evaluate students, preceptors, and the clinical site. The clinical team must track students' schedules, the types of patients seen, and the procedures experienced. Most programs accomplish these goals by using electronic web-based interfaces that can be accessed remotely by students, preceptors, medical facilities, staff, and program faculty. Current notable stakeholders in this realm include eMedley by AllofE (www.emedley.com), MedHub's product E*Value (www.medhub.com/evalue), and Typhon Group (www.typhongroup.com), which are paid services that can be customized to suit the needs of your students and your program. Each of these companies provide services and products that can meet the needs of clinical coordinators for evaluating clinical clerkship sites and their preceptors while compiling data on each student's experiences in clinical rotations. In addition, these companies provide a myriad of other services, including curriculum mapping, assessment and testing, scheduling, student information databases, preceptor information, clinical site information, contract and agreement databases, and documentation associated with student onboarding/credentialing.

Selecting a platform to facilitate these functions is extremely important and should be made at a program/department level with input from key users. When evaluating these products, consider the user interface that students, preceptors, staff, and faculty will be navigating. Look for features that allow concise and timely documentation by all players involved in the process, and consider maximizing utility by using as few platforms as possible.

Evaluating students' clinical experiences is often accomplished through an electronically delivered evaluation tool based on a modified Likert-type scaling system. The goal is to create a tool that concisely and accurately reflects the opinion(s) of each evaluator. An example is presented in Exhibit 12.2. These evaluations must be sent to preceptors in a timely fashion so that they can be completed before the end of the educational term. Often, these evaluations must be complete and report acceptable performance before the end of rotation (EOR) exams.

The goal of EOR exams is to test students' knowledge of the topics/objectives of the rotation in which they just participated. Some PA programs use "home-grown" exams to assess the knowledge of their students to this end. More than 100 PA programs across the United States use the Physician Assistant Education Association (PAEA) EOR exams. These exams, based on the same blueprint and topic list as the Physician Assistant National Certifying Exam (PANCE), are delivered via a web-based format. "Each End of Rotation exam consists of 120 multiple-choice questions (MCQs). One hundred of these questions are scored, and the other 20 questions are unscored pre-test items which are used to gather statistics. The exam is divided into two sections of 60 questions each" (Physician Assistant Education Association, 2016).

Currently, peer-reviewed, statistically validated EOR exams are available for the following rotations: emergency medicine, family medicine, general surgery, internal medicine, pediatrics, psychiatry and behavioral health, and women's health. Each exam currently costs $30 and requires the presence of a proctor during testing. Of note, the PAEA does not assign passing scores for exams; instead, each program must analyze national and class data to determine what scores merit which grades. Many programs choose to use the data to create a Z-score regression that ultimately decides the grade on each exam. Although these exams are costly—$10,500 yearly for a class of 50 (assuming no failures), the feedback obtained by both the program and the students makes these exams a must.

RETAINING PRECEPTORS

A hot topic among many health care training programs is: "What are we going to do to keep these wonderful preceptors?" There are many ways to recognize these providers for the invaluable experience and tutelage they provide students. Some programs give providers university- or program-branded gifts or apparel. Many programs offer certificates of appreciation suitable for hanging in the clinician's office/reception area. Others recognize outstanding preceptors with teaching awards at white-coat or graduation ceremonies.

A particularly valuable commodity to preceptors is continuing medical education (CME) credit. For many years, PAs could claim hour-for-hour credit for all activities related to training students. In 2014, in an effort to increase the number of preceptors and ultimately grow the profession (American Academy of Physician Assistants [AAPA], 2016), AAPA and the PAEA agreed to provide Category 1 CME for student preceptorship. Although this reward is meager compared to clinicians' efforts to train students, it is a move in the right direction. This CME can only be granted by approved PA programs that have paid a nominal fee to participate in this CME-granting program. Note that a maximum of 10 Category 1 CME credits per calendar year may be awarded to each preceptor (American Academy of Physician Assistants, 2016).

Although being awarded Category 1 and/or Category 2 CME is a sure reward, some hospitals and health care corporations have begun recognizing the teaching of health care students as an important role in creating the next generation of providers. As such, many have created clinical ladder programs that reward current clinicians for various professional and scholarly activities. These programs are often incentivized by promotion or increased compensation. Some

> **EXHIBIT 12.2** Sample of a Standard Form for Preceptor Evaluation of Students

Preceptor Evaluation of Student

Subject (name of student): _____

Evaluator: _____

Site: _____

Period: _____

Dates of activity: _____

Activity:	Family practice	Internal medicine	Pediatrics
	Gynecology	Obstetrics	Surgery
	Inpatient	Emergency medicine	Women's health

Please rate student performance from 1 to 5 (1 = Poor, 2 = Needs improvement, 3 = Competent, 4 = Skilled, 5 = Excellent) in the following areas. You may also include comments related to the student's strengths and areas for improvement.

Minimum passing score is 3. Please provide comments for any score below 3.

Student attended as contracted (Question 1 of 8—Mandatory)

Yes   No

Techniques (Question 2 of 8—Mandatory)

Competence area	1 = Poor	2 = Needs improvement	3 = Competent	4 = Skilled	5 = Excellent	Not Applicable
Medical interview						
Physical examination						
Oral case presentation						
Written patient record						
Clinical procedures						

Techniques comments (Question 3 of 8)

Clinical knowledge (Question 4 of 8—Mandatory)

Competence area	1 = Poor	2 = Needs improvement	3 = Competent	4 = Skilled	5 = Excellent	Not Applicable
Factual knowledge and concepts						
Problem solving/critical thinking						
Assessment/Differential diagnosis						

(continued)

EXHIBIT 12.2 Sample of a Standard Form for Preceptor Evaluation of Students (*continued*)

Ability to form management plan						
Patient education						
Patient follow-up						
Preceptor evaluation of student						

Clinical knowledge comments (Question 5 of 8)

Professionalism (Question 6 of 8—Mandatory)

Competence area	1 = Poor	2 = Needs improvement	3 = Competent	4 = Skilled	5 = Excellent	Not Applicable
Relating to patients						
Relating to colleagues						
Responsiveness to feedback						
Understanding role of physician assistant (PA)						
Confidence and motivation						
Reliability and dependability						
Overall professionalism						

Professionalism comments (Question 7 of 8)

(Question 8 of 8—Confidential)

Dear Preceptors—Please know that students can view in E*value your ratings and comments for them in the evaluation sections included here. If you have any comments or concerns that you would rather not have a student read verbatim but would still like to share with our program, then please include them in the confidential comments box included. This will allow the student's faculty advisor to address with the student any concerns that you may have as well as discuss strategies to help the students improve.

programs may also offer adjunct clinical faculty appointments as an incentive to clinicians who fulfill extensive and ongoing clerkship roles.

Finally, a topic of heated debate is whether programs should widely adopt a system that pays preceptors to provide clinical experience. Many are slow to adopt this trend and continue to follow the historic precedent of counting on the altruistic nature of volunteer preceptors. An increasing trend, however, favors a model in which payment is rendered for this service. According to a recent PAEA annual report, 21.1% of all programs indicated that they had allocated funds to pay preceptors (PAEA, 2013). The Association of American Medical Colleges (AAMC) PAEA clerkship study indicates that 21.7% of PA program survey respondents are paying for supervised clinical training, with a range of payments from $100 to $450 per student per week (PAEA Board of Directors, 2013).

CONCLUSIONS

A day in the life of a clinical coordinator can be demanding. At any given moment, a clinical coordinator can be asked to be a teaching faculty member, a budding legal advisor reviewing affiliation agreements, a liaison to the local community hospital, and the administrator/proctor for EOR exams. And although this position can be extremely demanding, it can also be one of the most rewarding experiences possible. To have placed students in a wonderfully fulfilling clinical rotation in which they can realize their full potential as budding providers can sometimes feel overwhelmingly rewarding. Without a doubt, the clinical coordinator fills one of the most important positions within a medical training program. Without the opportunities to practice on patients that clinical coordinators help provide, students could never become clinicians.

REFERENCES

Accreditation Review Commission on Education for the Physician Assistant. (2016). *Accreditation standards for physician assistant education* (4th ed.). Johns Creek, GA: Author. Retrieved from http://www.arc-pa.org/wp-content/uploads/2016/11/AccredManual-4th-edition.Nov2016.pdf

American Academy of Physician Assistants. (2016). Category 1 CME for preceptors. Retrieved from https://www.aapa.org/wp-content/uploads/2016/12/Category-1-CME-for-Preceptors-Guide.pdf

Gerstner, L. (2016, May 3). Get to know your clinical education neighbors. Retrieved from http://paea online.org/get-to-know-your-clinical-education-neighbors-2

Physician Assistant Education Association. (2012). Preceptor orientation handbook: Tips, tools, and guidance for physician assistant preceptors. Retrieved from http://paeaonline.org/publications/preceptor -handbook

Physician Assistant Education Association. (2013). The quest for clinical training sites. Retrieved from http://paeaonline.org/research/clinical-training-sites

Physician Assistant Education Association. (2016). PAEA End of Rotation™ exams: Exam details. Retrieved from http://www.endofrotation.org/exams/exam-format

Physician Assistant Education Association Board of Directors. (2013). *PAEA clerkship site survey* (pp. 1–3). Alexandria, VA: Physician Assistant Education Association.

ADDITIONAL ONLINE RESOURCES

Association of American Medical Colleges. Learning from Teaching. Retrieved from www.aamc.org/initiatives/cei/learning

National Organization of Nurse Practitioner Faculties. Preceptor Portal. Retrieved from www.nonpf.org/?page=PreceptorPortal_Main&hhSearchTerms=%22preceptor%22

Physician Assistant Education Association. (2016, September 29). *PAEA Clinical Educators Handbook*. Retrieved from http://paeaonline.org/publications/clinical-educator-handbook

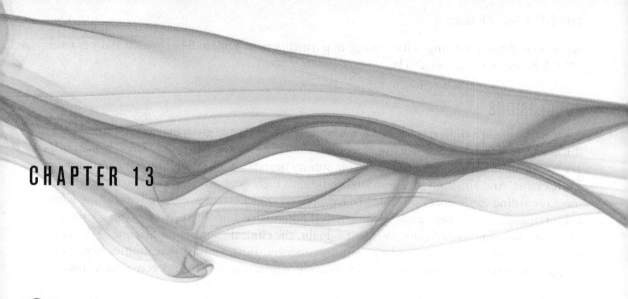

CHAPTER 13

Simulation in Clinical Education
Natalie Walkup, Carolina Wishner, and April Gardner

CHAPTER OBJECTIVES

- Use practical strategies to implement low- to high-fidelity simulation
- Recognize common pitfalls and how to avoid them

The best places to learn are not always the most convenient places to teach.

—Helen McIlvain

Clinical simulation is an instructional design that substitutes real patient encounters with artificial models, live actors, or virtual-reality patients. Simulation in health professions curriculum allows trainees to experience realistic patient situations without exposing patients to risks associated with trainee inexperience (Gaba, 2004). It can be a valuable tool for teaching both clinical skills and clinical interprofessional collaboration. Through simulation, learners can develop confidence, and the skills acquired in simulated settings can be transferred to real patient encounters. Simulation consists of both low-fidelity and high-fidelity simulations. Low-fidelity simulation involves using a manikin or task trainer, but no input or feedback response is present. High-fidelity simulation allows for input and response to students (Donkers, Truscott, Garrubba, & DeLong, 2016).

The benefits of simulation are vast. Research shows that incorporating simulation into health professions curriculum increases students' knowledge and skills more than traditional lecture or clinical experience (Alluri, Tsing, Lee, & Napolitano, 2016). This applies to a broad range of professions, including nurses, doctors, respiratory therapists, physical therapists, and physician assistants (PAs; Curl, Smith, Chisholm, McGee, & Das, 2016). Our experiences also suggest that students learn more about their own competencies and abilities to work as part of a team.

This learning can be further enhanced when students from different professions collaborate in simulation. When students work with learners outside of their own field, they also gain better understanding of their own role and expertise within the team environment, as well as gain respect for other students' knowledge and professions (Kyrkjebo, Brattebo, & Smith-Strom, 2006).

EXAMPLES OF WHERE SIMULATION CAN BE INCORPORATED INTO THE CURRICULUM

Simulation can be incorporated into the clinical curriculum in many places; examples include disaster preparedness, response to emergency situations, clinical procedures, surgical preparation, OB/GYN education, history taking and physical exam skills, and objective structured clinical examinations (OSCEs) and remediation.

Disaster Preparedness

Preparedness for serious, unanticipated disasters, such as a disease outbreak, terrorist attack, trauma, fire, hurricanes, and other natural disasters, is a critical need. Through disaster simulation, we can analyze risks; improve coordination, communication, triage, treatment, decontamination, and evacuation; and do other things (Larson, Metzger, & Cahn, 2006).

Learning to Respond to Emergency Situations

Simulation training can be a vital component of emergency medicine modules. Simulation can be incorporated in the curriculum to enhance students' clinical experiences in assisting with codes and help them better understand the process. Basic life support (BLS) and advanced cardiac life support (ACLS) training practice and simulation application will boost their confidence in real-life situations (Durham & Alden, 2008).

Learning Procedures

With the shortage of clinical training sites, along with the increasing numbers of trainees and the increased scrutiny about patient safety and issues of malpractice, teaching and learning procedures in a clinical setting are becoming a daunting task. Clinical skills, such as urethral catheterization, venous access, arterial puncture, and blood gas sampling, can be taught efficiently through simulation experiences. Simulation will replicate patient case scenarios in a realistic environment for the purpose of skill practice, training, feedback, and assessment. It will provide predictable, consistent, standardized, safe, and reproducible training to students (Sahu & Lata, 2010).

Surgical Preparation

In a surgery setting, simulation provides trainees with hands-on training in a "safe" environment without compromising patient safety (Kunkler, 2006). It provides opportunities for repetitive practice to master a given skill and also provides ongoing training opportunities and improves the educational experience (Okuda et al., 2009). Clinicians working in the outpatient surgical setting can improve on many diagnostic and therapeutic procedures through simulation practice such as wound care, laceration repair, and abscess incision and drainage. They can also practice procedural sedation, regional block anesthesia, arthrocentesis, lumbar puncture, and thoracentesis.

OB/GYN Education

Through the use of manikins and trainers, simulations can be used to practice deliveries, tend to childbirth, and manage OB/GYN emergencies such as preeclampsia and postpartum hemorrhage.

History-Taking and Physical Exam Skills

Simulation can be used to teach how to take a patient history, interviewing and communication skills, as well as how to effectively perform a physical exam. In addition to peer-to-peer learning, trainees work with artificial models, live actors, or virtual-reality scenarios to practice history-taking and physical exam skills. This is generally a less intimidating environment, which allows the beginner to develop confidence before going to the real world of patient care. For the educator, simulation platforms provide a controlled environment where teaching scenarios can be standardized. The simulated environment also allows repetitive practice with feedback and the ability to alter the difficulty level. Simulation will also provide exposure to uncommon events and the opportunity to assess learners without any risk to patients (Durham & Alden, 2008).

OSCE and Remediation

In OSCEs, simulations can assess multiple competencies for health professions. Furthermore, simulations provide a unique opportunity for clinical skill remediation. Very often, clinical programs receive reports from preceptors that a student does not meet expectations. Educators can then use simulation to recreate a realistic clinical environment to assess and remediate that particular learner in a safe and controlled manner.

EXAMPLES OF HOW AN INTERPROFESSIONAL SIMULATION EXERCISE CAN BE IMPLEMENTED

First, seek out faculty from other professions who may be interested in helping build an interprofessional simulation program. Those who are inspired and excited about being involved from the beginning can help carry some of the workload and shape the program. After appropriate faculty are identified, it is important to create scenarios. These simulation scenarios must appropriately incorporate the professions that are present. It is important to let faculty from each profession provide input regarding their students' roles in the scenario. After selection of the scenarios, take time as an interprofessional faculty group to run a mock simulation. This allows the faculty to identify issues in the scenario that need to be changed in order to encourage creative thinking and collaboration among the students. In addition, it allows for the faculty to feel confident about the scenario and the overall expected learning outcomes.

Providing the students some time on the simulators for training is an important part of introducing students to interprofessional simulation. It is helpful to increase students' confidence and participation if they have already been trained on how the simulator works and how they should perform their evaluation. When students are more confident about their own role and abilities during the simulation, they are more likely to interact with students from other professions thus creating a more vibrant simulation experience.

Debriefing is vital to any interprofessional simulation. There are multiple models used for simulation debriefing, such as using an algorithm or a laissez-faire approach (Nystrom, Dahlberg, Edelbring, Hult, & Dahlgren, 2016). However, the distinguishing feature between simulation debriefing and interprofessional simulation debriefing is the discussion of how the team and collaboration work. This often does not naturally come up in a debriefing session. However, it is important that the interprofessional collaboration is discussed in a manner that does not single out any one person or profession. Instead, stay focused on the teamwork approach and what the students learned about working together and the skills that other students displayed during the simulation that were specific to their profession.

Interprofessional Simulation Scenario

The University of California, Davis, nurse practitioner (NP) and physician assistant (PA) programs use simulation and change to *Integrative Case-Based Learning*© (see Chapter 21) in their course, Preparation for Clinical Practice. In this course, the use of simulation provides a safe, controlled environment in which to teach patient care, care transitions, and interprofessional teamwork. This 10-week course blends low- to high-fidelity simulations in which small groups of NP and PA students apply social determinants of health through an unfolding case study. A common medical condition with diverse demographics is provided to each group as they follow a patient through a variety of simulated health care settings.

Simulation scenarios are enacted in the emergency department; operating room; postanesthesia care unit; as well as inpatient, skilled nursing, home health, office, and telemedicine environments. An interdisciplinary team of faculty that includes physicians, NPs, PAs, pharmacists, and nurses facilitates the simulation scenarios. Each week, presimulation learning is provided to students through flipped-classroom pedagogy (see Chapter 8). An in-class discussion prior to the simulation lab enhances student preparation and confidence. Using *Integrative Case-Based Learning* in the simulations, practical learning in cultural competency is tied to the varying socio-eco-geographic resources in the cases. Students are responsible for assessment, management of care transitions, procedures, preceptor presentations, orders, and documentation of visits. Team-based care is emphasized with interprofessional faculty and student teams. Real-time feedback and coaching enhances student learning.

The active-learning strategies used in this course allow students to integrate and apply concepts from the entire didactic year. By the end of this 10-week course, students are able to:

• Demonstrate person-centered care
• Be able to describe their role in various clinical settings
• Demonstrate proficiency in oral presentation, differential diagnosis, critical thinking and problem solving, and documentation of encounters
• Explain how the context of care affects clinical decision making
• Demonstrate the ability to work and communicate with various members of the health care team, including transitions of care

COMMON CHALLENGES AND PRACTICAL SUGGESTIONS

Many programs struggle with offering simulation because of budget issues, as simulators can be very expensive in terms of initial cost, ongoing maintenance, and user expertise. However, it is important to remember that through combined resources, it is possible to provide valuable experiences for students without high-cost simulators. Alternatives to high-fidelity manikins include standardized patients, partial-task trainers, screen-based computer simulators, and virtual-reality simulators (Loftin, Garner, Eames, & West, 2016). A standardized patient is person who has been trained to portray, in a consistent, standardized manner, a patient in a medical situation.

Standardized patients are used to teach and evaluate students. Partial-task trainers are simulators that permit learners to practice a specific psychomotor skill (e.g., venous cannulation or suturing). They do not incorporate "patient" feedback, such as pain from the procedure. Screen-based computer provided a model or scenario that can be executed by the student either pre-class or as an in-class activity. Computer simulation in health professions education is typically interactive, often in the form of a branching scenario. Students' scenario output can then be analyzed by the instructor.

Virtual reality simulation generates 3D objects and environments to create interactive scenarios that immerse students in the learning experience. The principle of virtual reality e-learning is to instruct, practice, and assess learners' knowledge using real-to-life situations.

Simulation can be intimidating, especially for faculty who have not incorporated simulation into their curriculum previously. In this case, it may be better for the faculty member to start his or her teaching with a method that she or he is most comfortable with. For example, a lecture on patient assessment could be followed by a simulation experience in which students assess a patient (high-fidelity or standardized patient) and document their findings. Simulation instruction can be even more intimidating when learners come from different backgrounds or disciplines, such as in interprofessional education. Boet, Bould, Burn, and Reeves (2014) identified 12 tips to help faculty members with high-fidelity interprofessional simulation:

1. Focus on the interprofessional component. It is important to remember that the interprofessional component is a vital part of the simulation that has its own learning curve and challenges. The interprofessional component is just as important as the medical knowledge.
2. Anticipate logistical challenges. Scheduling, faculty availability and resources, and finding common learning objectives can be challenging and time-consuming. It is important to find institutional leaders who are supportive and will help facilitate faculty collaboration.
3. Find interprofessional simulation champions. Each profession needs to have a designated person who is excited about the simulation process. This helps establish equity between professions and helps with recruitment and student feedback.
4. Balance diversity with equity. Schedule students with a balance across professions, and make sure that no profession is privileged throughout the process.
5. Develop scenarios relevant to all professions. It is important to consider simulation scenarios in which all professions that are present play an important role. Each student needs to feel that he or she is a vital part of the team.
6. Be mindful of sociological fidelity. The strong history of hierarchical medicine cannot be ignored. It is important that simulation scenarios foster an environment of teamwork and do not create power struggles throughout the simulation.
7. All professors need to be "on the same page." It is important that a prebriefing takes place between faculty to establish clear rules and specific goals of the interprofessional experience.
8. Beware of interprofessional debriefing challenges. Although students should be allowed to share their views during the debriefing, faculty need to make sure that blame is not placed on other professions or individuals. If the simulation did not go well, the focus should be on the errors in the system, and not the individuals involved.
9. Use simulation to add value to the curriculum. Interprofessional simulation cannot stand alone in the curriculum. It is important that other interprofessional opportunities are available for students to interact outside of simulation. This helps to foster collaboration among students and strengthens the simulation experience.
10. Focus the assessment on the team. Select an assessment modality as a collaborative faculty to ensure that the learners are learning what needs to be covered. Consider both qualitative and quantitative approaches to team assessment to measure not only medical skills, but also crisis management, attitude, respect, and stereotype transformation.
11. Support the interprofessional simulation educators. Take time to collaborate with other faculty and offer training sessions so that everyone feels appreciated and confident about the experience. This enhances the educator's ability to identify teaching moments throughout the simulation experience.

12. Take advantage of the research opportunity. More research is needed for interprofessional simulation in order to have a better understanding of what does and does not work well. This is a key time for educators to share information they have learned through interprofessional simulation with faculty outside of their institution.

CONCLUSIONS

Simulation has endless possibilities for faculty, students, and practitioners in the health professions. It creates realistic clinical situations through which learners can develop confidence and acquire practical skills without exposing patients to risks associated with trainee inexperience. Simulation can be used to supplement various aspects of the curriculum, such as teaching emergency preparedness, surgical training, and OB/GYN procedures. It can be used as a platform for competency assessment and remediation. Simulation is an effective tool in providing interprofessional education, but success depends on the quality of collaboration and planning done by the faculty.

Despite various benefits associated with simulation, there are a number of challenges in implementing an effective simulation program. The cost of equipment and lack of skilled manpower are major limiting factors. It is important that faculty take time to be trained on simulators, create goals and objectives for students, and create scenarios that foster positive collegial interaction among students. For interprofessional simulation, all faculty need to share a similar vision for their students in order to encourage teamwork.

It is important to incorporate debriefing and feedback in each simulation exercise. Student feedback is important to the assessment process, both qualitative and quantitative, to ensure that course goals and objectives are being met and to follow student progress over time. Finally, faculty may share their experiences and assessments through publication and contribute to the growing body of literature on simulation. Overall, more research is needed to understand the best practices of simulation and to address challenges of inconsistent outcome measurement.

REFERENCES

Alluri, R. K., Tsing, P., Lee, E., & Napolitano, J. (2016). A randomized controlled trial of high-fidelity simulation versus lecture-based education in preclinical medical students. *Medical Teacher, 38*, 404–409.

Boet, S., Bould, M. D., Burn, C. L., & Reeves, S. (2014). Twelve tips for a successful interprofessional team-based high-fidelity simulation education session. *Medical Teacher, 36*, 853–857.

Curl, E. D., Smith, S., Chisholm, L. A., McGee, L. A., & Das, K. (2016). Effectiveness of integrated simulation and clinical experiences compared to traditional clinical experiences for nursing students. *Nursing Education Perspectives, 37*(2), 72–77.

Donkers, K., Truscott, J., Garrubba, C., & DeLong, D. (2016). High-fidelity simulation use in preparation of physician assistant students for neonatal and obstetric care. *Journal of Physician Assistant Education, 27*(2), 68–72.

Durham, C. F., & Alden, K. R. (2008). Enhancing patient safety in nursing education through patient simulation. In R. G. Hughes (Ed.), *Patient safety and quality: An evidence-based handbook for nurses* (pp. 1364–1403). Rockville, MD: Agency for Healthcare Research and Quality.

Gaba, D. M. (2004). The future vision of simulation in health care. *Quality and Safety in Health Care, 13*(Suppl. 1), i2–i10.

Kunkler, K. (2006). The role of medical simulation: An overview. *International Journal of Medical Robotics, 2*(3), 203–210.

Kyrkjebo, J. M., Brattebo, G., & Smith-Strom, H. (2006). Improving patient safety by using interprofessional simulation training in health professional education. *Journal of Interprofessional Care, 20*(5), 507–516.

Larson, R. C., Metzger, M. D. & Cahn, M. F. (2006). Responding to emergencies: Lessons learned and the need for analysis. *Interfaces, 36*(6), 486–501.

Loftin, C., Garner, K., Eames, J., & West, H. (2016). Use of Harvey the cardiopulmonary patient simulator in physician assistant training. *Journal of Physician Assistant Education*, 27(1), 32–39.

Nystrom, S., Dahlberg, J., Edelbring, S., Hult, H., & Dahlgren, M. A. (2016). Debriefing practices in interprofessional simulation with students: A sociomaterial perspective. *BioMed Central Medical Education*, 16,148.

Okuda, Y., Bryson, E. O., DeMaria, S., Jacobson, L., Jr., Quinones, J., Shen, B., & Levine, A. I. (2009). The utility of simulation in medical education: What is the evidence? *Mount Sinai Journal of Medicine*, 76(4), 330–343.

Sahu, S., & Lata, I. (2010). Simulation in resuscitation teaching and training: An evidence-based practice review. *Journal of Emergencies, Trauma and Shock*, 3(4), 378–384.

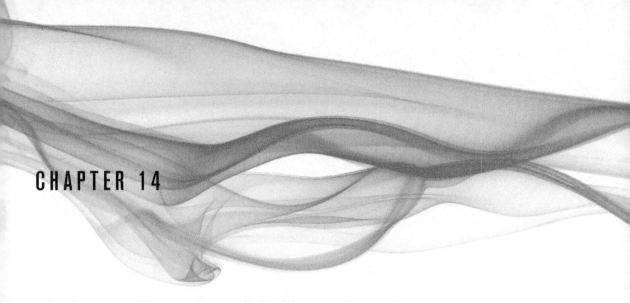

CHAPTER 14

Interprofessional Education in the Clinical Setting

Angel K. Chen, Tamatha Arms, Barbara L. Jones, Jeffrey Okamoto, Noell Rowan, and Evaon C. Wong-Kim

---

CHAPTER OBJECTIVES

- Use clinical teaching strategies, including micro-skills for effective preceptors and preceptor development
- Provide effective clinical teaching in interprofessional and interdisciplinary teams

---

The value of experience is not in seeing much, but in seeing wisely.

—*William Osler*

CLINICAL TEACHING

Learning in the clinical setting is the foundation by which health professions learners practice their skills and shape their professional identity. Faculty must prepare the clinical environment, learners, and preceptors/field instructors who support learners to thrive in the clinical environment. Although this has traditionally been done within one's own profession, the health care environment has shifted to follow an interprofessional collaborative care model to provide high-quality and safe patient-centered care; thus support of the environment, learners, and preceptors/instructors must also transition to an interprofessional model (see Chapter 5). Learners report that there is a gap between the classroom and clinical environment in regard to interprofessional collaborative practice; thus, faculty must create environments that are more suitable for interprofessional collaborative practice as health professionals have traditionally been trained within their own professional silos. In this chapter, we provide guiding principles for the preparation of the clinical environment, learners, and preceptors/field instructors for interprofessional clinical teaching, as well as exemplars from our institutions highlighting key strategies.

Preparing the Environment

Clinical environments must be supportive of all the health professions learners who rotate through the sites, including identification of their names, programs, and rotation schedules. All learners should be represented within the environment as this allows learners and team members to know the individuals who are on their team as well as their roles and responsibilities. Additional measures may be taken to best facilitate the team and teaching huddles, such as creating space for the team to gather in the clinical setting to have discussions, and creating time in the schedule for the team to have huddles and face-to-face team discussions. Exemplar A highlights University of California, San Francisco's (UCSF) experience in implementing teaching huddles in the Veterans Affairs Center and Education in Patient-Aligned Care Teams (EdPACT) program. The environment can also be designed for informal teaching discussions for all learners across professions in the clinical setting, regardless of the formal team formation.

Preparing the Learner

Knowledge

Learners are guided by interprofessional collaborative practice core competencies (Interprofessional Education Collaborative [IPEC], 2011, 2016) as well as their own professional clinical competencies to prepare them to function within the roles and scope of practice in the clinical setting. In designing the learners' clinical experience, the faculty must incorporate didactic content to build learners' knowledge base around interprofessional collaboration, and complement this with actual skill application in a simulated or real clinical environment. In addition, students must also learn the roles and responsibilities and scope of practice of those professions they learn *from*, *with*, and *about* in the clinical environment (World Health Organization, 2010).

Skills

Essential skills to enhance interprofessional collaboration include clear communication and conflict-management skills. Their "toolbox" should include a variety of communication strategies, such as the ISBAR (introduction, situation, background, assessment, and recommendation) mnemonic or check-back process (Agency for Healthcare Research and Quality [AHRQ], 2014), and a range of conflict-management response styles and collaborative language and reframing skills. In addition to didactic knowledge, learners benefit from having an opportunity to practice communication and negotiation skills with team members prior to collaborating in the clinical environment. Exemplar B highlights University of North Carolina, Wilmington's experience in implementing interprofessional simulation exercises with the learners.

Attitude/Culture

Another essential element to prepare learners is the ability to recognize unconscious bias. Cultural and societal cues are deeply rooted from birth, thus everyone carries unconscious bias with him or her. These unconscious biases may even play a role in one's choice of health care profession and in how one interacts with other health care professionals and patients. Developing awareness of one's own thoughts, beliefs, and behaviors is a starting point to recognizing uncon-scious bias through reflective practice. One tool to use to assess and measure one's attitudes and beliefs is the Implicit Association Test (Project Implicit, 2017). Once recognized, the health care professional can then work toward preventing bias from influencing his or her behavior and deci-sion making in the clinical setting.

Furthermore, training health care professionals to work collaboratively to support patients requires commitment and compassion. Providing meaningful care to patients can create tre-mendous compassion fatigue and provider distress. Therefore, it is essential to create opportu-nities for health care providers to share their authentic reactions to the intensity of their clinical experiences, which is demonstrated in Exemplar C, the Dell Children's Medical Center, Austin, Texas experience in implementing Schwartz Rounds. Social workers are well trained in leading interprofessional rounds given that their education includes specific skills in group develop-ment, collaboration, and facilitation, and they intently focus education on the micro, mezzo, and macro aspects of care (Jones & Phillips, 2016; Schwartz Center for Compassionate Care, 2017).

Preparing the Faculty/Preceptor/Field Instructor

Clinical Micro-Skills

Faculty, preceptors, and/or field instructors (depending on profession) all require preparation in supporting learners in the clinical setting. Traditional clinical micro-skills include the use of the One-Minute Preceptor (OMP; Gallagher, Tweed, Hanna, Winter, & Hoare, 2012), which is a five-step strategy that supports efficient and targeted clinical teaching. This model allows the learner to make a commitment to his or her understanding with the use of supportive evidence, and allows the faculty/preceptor/field instructor to teach a general rule related to the current case as well as reinforce what was done right by the learner and what can be improved. Another framework for the faculty/preceptor to use with learners is the SNAPPS Model (summarize, narrow, analyze, probe, plan, select; Wolpaw, Papp, & Bordage, 2009), in which learners can present clinical information in a systematic way that narrows down their thinking and allows for targeted questioning of the faculty/preceptor with a focused area to explore further. Both of these models support time-efficient teaching in the clinical setting.

Feedback for Clinical Performance

Providing feedback regarding clinical performance to the learner is a key component of clinical teaching. The art of giving feedback is knowing when and how to offer feedback to the learner as well as how to elicit feedback from the learner. Feedback, if not given properly, may be over-whelming for the learner and/or be received incorrectly. Faculty may adopt a variety of models, including **ask** (self-assessment)–**tell** (preceptor assessment)–**ask** (impact of feedback) or **keep** (reinforce)–**stop** (corrective), **start** (next steps). These models allow the learner to first do a self-assessment prior to the faculty's input, after which the faculty provides positive reinforcement as well as specific corrective feedback on the learner's behavior and future plans. Exemplar D demonstrates the University of Hawaii's experience in implementing the interprofessional Pono Clinic, which formally includes a feedback component for learners.

In simulation exercises, feedback is provided through debriefing sessions in which learners are asked about their own assessments, followed by how they would have done things differ-ently or how the exercise impacted their future actions. Learners who participate in clinical sim-ulations also receive feedback of their interactions within the simulation, from faculty who observed the interactions, or directly from the standardized patients in the simulation. With the use of recorded simulation sessions, learners can review the encounter and provide critical self-reflections of their behavior in the simulation.

Assessment/Evaluation

Assessment and evaluation of learner performance may be done in a variety of ways. One evaluation tool used in medicine is the Recorder–Interpreter–Manager–Educator (RIME) Model (Pangaro, 1999). This is an evidence-based and valid synthetic model used to effectively describe and assess a learner's progress through the stages of health education. Another assessment used is the Brief Structured Clinical Observation (BSCO; Pierce, Noronha, Collins, & Fancovic, 2013), which allows faculty to efficiently assess a learner's skills in the clinical setting.

A number of evaluation tools have been designed for use in interprofessional simulation, such as the Interprofessional Collaborative Competencies Attainment Survey (ICCAS; Archibald, Trumpower, & MacDonald, 2014). The ICCAS is a 20-question Likert scale questionnaire that can be used for assessment/evaluation of learners to measure pre- and postevaluation of skills in interprofessional communication, collaboration, team functioning, patient/family-centered approach, and conflict management as set forth in the domains of this survey.

Interprofessional Clinical Teaching Skills

Previous clinical training has typically focused on a single profession; however, the evidence suggests that interprofessional collaborative practice provides safer patient care of increased quality. Health professionals are now expected to be trained in interprofessional collaborative settings. This means that faculty/preceptors/field instructors also need to meet IPEC competencies for interprofessional collaborative practice, and share the same knowledge and skill set as do the learners from different professions in the clinical setting. Faculty/preceptors/field instructors can approach clinical teaching using the following five steps (Chen, Rivera, Rotter, Green, & Kools, 2016; Lie, Forest, Kysh, & Sinclair, 2016; see Exhibit 14.1)

Faculty Development

Faculty/preceptor/field instructor development remains a vital, yet often missed, part of clinical teaching (Chen et al., 2016). Resources have been created through the National Center for

---

EXHIBIT 14.1 Five-Step Guide to Interprofessional Clinical Teaching

1. **Set the stage**
   a. Introduce interprofessional education (IPE)/interprofessional collaborative practice (IPCP) and culture of inclusiveness.
   b. Set ground rules on professionalism, respect, team culture, and clear expectations.
   c. Know professional identity and biases; explore hierarchy and power issues.

2. **Engage all learners**
   a. Know your learners' roles and responsibilities, scope of practice, and learning needs.
   b. Provide time and space for learners to work together; provide clinical and teaching huddle.

3. **Apply teaching tools**—Modify traditional clinical teaching tools—such as One Minute Preceptor (OMP)
   a. Reinforce the good, and correct mistakes.
   b. Assign homework and report back.

4. **Be a role model**—Model effective communication and conflict management
   a. Challenge assumptions.
   b. Avoid use of jargon from a single profession.
   c. Acknowledge expertise of other professionals.

5. **Debrief and reflect**—Reflect and summarize
   a. Gather reflections of both the facilitator and the learners.
   b. Provide timely feedback to and from learners and faculty.
   c. Consider teaching observations.

Interprofessional Practice and Education (NEXUS®) with an Interprofessional Preceptor Toolbox (NEXUS, 2015). Challenges in implementing faculty/preceptor/field instructor development programs include finding time and place for the training. In lieu of a formal development program, peer-teaching observation may be a simple and quick alternative to providing constructive feedback to new and established faculty/preceptors/field instructors on their clinical teaching style with their learners. In addition, this can build the community of clinical educators and provide a peer-support mechanism for further development.

EXEMPLARS

Exemplar A: Teaching Huddles as Key to Clinical Teaching—University of California, San Francisco and Veterans Affairs Center and EdPACT

The Veterans Affairs Center and EdPACT designed workforce education to train practicing teams for collaborative care models involving interprofessional primary care training for MD and nurse practitioner (NP) learners. San Francisco VA Health Care System was one of five centers of excellence across the United States to receive the 5-year funding, in collaboration with the UCSF School of Nursing, School of Medicine, and Office of Medical Education.

The guiding principles within the EdPACT program included interprofessional collaboration, patient-centered communication and shared decision making, a sustained relationship, and performance improvement. Patients were managed by interprofessional teamlets, each composed of an NP student and two second-year medicine residents, along with health care professionals from dietetics, pharmacy, psychiatry, social work, and psychology. The curriculum for the trainees included six didactic conferences per week, 3½ days of clinic per week as experiential workplace reinforcement, and time and place for critical reflection (U.S. Department of Veterans Affairs, 2016). Specific curricular content is listed in Exhibit 14.2. Additional resources are listed at the end of the chapter.

EXHIBIT 14.2 University of California, San Francisco and Veterans Affairs Center and Education in Patient-Aligned Care Teams Curriculum

---

1. Didactic content via interactive small-group seminar
   a. Huddling
   b. Team member roles
   c. Handoff communication
   d. Feedback
   e. Conflict resolution
   f. Debriefing
2. Workplace reinforcement
   a. Huddling
   b. Huddle coaches
   c. Preceptors reinforce skills and provide feedback during huddles
   d. Teams engage in formative assessment processes
3. Reflection via half-day retreat
   a. Team building
   b. Opportunities to reflect
   c. Identify similarities and differences

Full project information is available at the following website: www.va.gov/oaa/coepce/sanfrancisco.asp

Huddle

An interprofessional team huddle plays an important role in the success of this collaborative care model. The purpose of the huddle is to provide quality patient care through structured opportunities for team members to communicate and collectively strategize about daily schedule and workflow, patients' special needs and preferences, and previsit planning. The huddle also offers a time and place for team members to safely voice their concerns and to work together to problem solve and strategize around conflicts and barriers. Huddles provide a time for team members to teach, model, and reinforce teamwork competencies and build relationships with each other.

To implement the huddle, interventions were needed at three levels:

1. **Structural/organizational:** The structure of the huddle process included learner integration considerations, optimal scheduling, huddle location, and leadership support for huddle coaches.
2. **Procedural:** Train huddle coaches to help facilitate huddle groups, design a huddle checklist, and implement a preceptor huddle. The huddle coaches' role is to monitor that all members attend and that huddles take place, that individuals model the appropriate skills and techniques to lead huddles, that they motivate and foster team spirit and collaboration, that they guide and support by providing information when no other team member can, that they teach and ask the team to practice appropriate skills, and that they provide feedback on relational and process factors.
3. **Relational:** Implement the team retreat, communication training, and debriefing meetings.

Faculty/Preceptor Development

Faculty and preceptors received training on TeamSTEPPS® 2.0 (AHRQ, 2016), giving/receiving feedback, conflict management, and clinical communication tools. They also trained huddle coaches and participated in monthly curricular standing meetings as well as preceptor huddles.

Through this model of patient-centered interprofessional training, future health care providers can adopt principles and a skill set to optimize their ability to work together in the clinical setting to deliver high-quality and safe patient care.

Exemplar B: Interprofessional Simulation Exercise—University of North Carolina, Wilmington

Interprofessional collaboration is a necessity in the clinical area for overall health care improvement. Studies have shown that beliefs, attitudes, and a lack of understanding and respect of other's roles are barriers to interprofessional collaboration. This exemplar involves the use of an interprofessional simulation with social work, nursing, and recreation therapy students collaborating together on a typical clinical case involving an older adult farmer and his family in a a simulated apartment setting. The students experience participating in an interprofessional team meeting in which the patient and family are present and involved.

Learners

Learners from social work (undergraduate and graduate level), nursing (undergraduate level), and recreation therapy (undergraduate level) participated, with a total of 191 students included over two occurrences.

Simulation Design

A simulation design template (National League for Nursing, 2010) was used to conceptualize the simulation details and as a teaching tool for all social work, nursing, and recreation therapy courses (see scenario and template in Exhibit 14.3, online supplement). Learners worked in pairs to demonstrate their assessment, and provided a report to the next pair of learners in another profession. Once this process was completed, the entire team met with the standardized patient to have a team meeting. The simulation is video-recorded and streamed live into a classroom for the rest of the students in all three professions in each class to observe together, after which they are debriefed with evaluation.

Prebrief

A prebrief process is structured to give the standardized patients the scenario and to do a few practice run-throughs ahead of time with the script so they are ready to work with learners in a simulated environment. Learners also review the scenario and then are provided one-on-one mentoring with their own faculty prior to the simulation exercise.

Debrief

Once the clinical simulation in the rehabilitation setting has ended with the interprofessional team meeting, a debriefing session takes place in a large classroom with all of the standardized patients and interprofessional teams of learners and faculty, to provide feedback and reflections.

Evaluation and Feedback

Immediate feedback is provided by faculty involved in the simulation as well as from the larger group in the debriefing session stated previously. Students are also given the ICCAS (Archibald et al., 2014) to assess knowledge and growth in interprofessional team skills. Last, social work learners complete simulation critique exercises to demonstrate critical reflection (see critique questions in Exhibit 14.4, online supplement).

Impact

Providing learners with this type of interprofessional training and simulation enhances their understanding of each other's roles and responsibilities as well as more clearly defines their own role. Through enhanced understanding, a greater respect for each profession emerges, thus improving communication among all professions for the patient and family's benefit. Learners are more prepared to enter the clinical workforce and work within interprofessional teams.

Exemplar C: Schwartz Rounds™—Dell Children's Medical Center, Austin, Texas

Schwartz Rounds™, founded in 1995 in Boston, is a model of caregiver support that is now used in more than 400 health care organizations in the United States and Canada and in more than 120 health care organizations in the United Kingdom (Lown & Manning, 2010). Schwartz Rounds offers health care providers a regularly scheduled time during their fast-paced worklives to openly and honestly discuss the social and emotional issues they face in caring for patients and families. In contrast to traditional medical rounds, the focus is on the human dimension of medicine. Caregivers have an opportunity to share their experiences, thoughts, and feelings on thought-provoking topics drawn from actual patient cases. The premise is that caregivers are better able to make personal connections with patients and colleagues when they have greater insight into their own responses and feelings. A hallmark of the program is interprofessional dialogue. Panelists from diverse professions participate in the sessions, including physicians, nurses, social workers, psychologists, allied health professionals, and chaplains. After listening to a panel's brief presentation on an identified case or topic, caregivers in the audience are invited to share their own perspectives on the case and broader related issues.

These rounds offer caregivers from a variety of professions the chance to develop reflective practice and to strengthen interprofessional relationships. A recent evaluation of the project in six sites showed improvement in teamwork and in the appreciation of interprofessional roles and contributions (Lown & Manning, 2010). Participants also reported decreases in perceived stress and improvements in the ability to cope with the psychosocial demands of care (Lown & Manning, 2010).

Dell Children's Medical Center in Austin, Texas, began implementing Schwartz Rounds in September 2014 facilitated by a chaplain and a social worker. This program was championed by Dr. Craig Hurwitz, medical director of the Dell Children's Pediatric Palliative Care Program. Along with colleagues Richard Lawlor, program manager; Krista Gregory, chaplain and director of the Resilience Center; and Barbara Jones, professor of social work and associate dean at UT Austin, School of Social Work; Dell Children's has hosted 12 Schwartz Rounds averaging 250 participants from various disciplines, including medicine, nursing, social work, psychology, child life, physician assistant, therapists (occupational and physical), pharmacy, security, and others. Topics have included transitioning youth to adult care, delivering difficult news, and supporting children and families when they have conflicting goals of care, among many other topics.

Participants in this program report that the Schwartz Rounds allowed them to discuss challenging social and emotional aspects of patient care and gave them new insights into the perspectives and experiences of colleagues and patients and families. Participants also report that as a result of the discussions they feel less isolated in their work and better prepared to handle tough and sensitive patient situations. Participants feel better able to express thoughts, feelings, and questions about patient care with their colleagues. More information can be found on the center's website (www.theschwartzcenter.org).

Exemplar D: Pono Clinic, University of Hawaii

Hawaii has had an interprofessional training program since 1994, funded by the Maternal and Child Health (MCH) Bureau, U.S. Department of Health and Human Services, Health Resources and Services Administration. This program is one of 52 Leadership Education in Neurodevelopmental and Related Disabilities (LEND) programs in 44 states. The program is designed to emphasize graduate-level training within an interprofessional environment to prepare trainees to later improve the health of children and teens with neurodevelopmental disabilities, such as autism and intellectual disabilities. The training consists of multiple activities, including clinical exposure, leadership training and experiences, and interdisciplinary team building.

Participants

The interprofessional team in Hawaii consisted of learners from the following professions: audiology, speech–language pathology, medicine (developmental–behavioral and general pediatrics), health administration, nursing, social work, law, dentistry, dental hygiene, and psychology. Twenty-five to 40 learners and faculty (2:1 ratio) in the Hawaii LEND participated in the year-long program each school year. The LEND core team negotiated with administrators to have faculty from multiple schools and departments participate, and to recruit learners prior to the start of each academic year.

Clinic Design

The clinical experience in the advanced clinical practicum portion of the program took place within the Pono Clinic. The Pono Clinic was unique because it was an interprofessional training environment where the learners from multiple disciplines had support from faculty from multiple disciplines while seeing actual patients in real time.

The word *pono* in Hawaiian has many meanings including: Goodness, uprightness, morality, moral qualities, correct or proper procedure, excellence, well-being, prosperity, welfare, benefit, behalf, equity, sake, true condition or nature, duty; moral, fitting, proper, righteous, right, upright, just, virtuous, fair, beneficial, successful, in perfect order, accurate, correct, eased, relieved; should, ought, must, necessary ("Pono", 2004).

This clinic had two main goals: (a) to provide exemplary family-centered care to children with neurodevelopmental disabilities and their families, and (b) to support an interprofessional training environment for present and future leaders to improve systems of care for children and families. Patients seen in the Pono Clinic had a variety of diagnoses, and represented Hawaii's diverse group of ethnicities and cultures. Learners appreciated how these cultures influenced child health and families' perceptions of disability. Learners participated in both clinical and didactic sessions throughout the program (see Exhibit 14.5 for an example of a Pono Clinic schedule, online supplement).

Preparation of the Environment

The University of Hawaii School of Medicine Department of Pediatrics provided the clinic space. The Pono Clinic began with an "arena" assessment setup, where the child and family met with the entire team at the same time in a large conference room. This was often found to be stressful for the child and family. Thus, changes were made for the patient and family to meet with each team (consisted only of two to three learners) for their specific assessment, in an exam room with a one-way mirror and an audio setup so that the team members who were not in the room could still observe the session. For each clinic session, the patient and family participated in a series of assessments, each lasting about 90 minutes. Although the new setup was not as overwhelming as the "arena" arrangement, it still caused some confusion in families, which may meet up to 10 learners and faculty in one clinic session.

Preparation of Learners

Learners prepared for Pono Clinic by reviewing a vignette related to the patient prepared by the faculty. Families provided consent for the medical record to be reviewed. Teams of learners participated in the interprofessional group discussions to prepare for the 90-minute assessment with the patient and family. They reviewed questions raised by outside clinical teams caring for the patient, as well as planned steps for workups (including selection of assessment tools) and recommendations (see Exhibit 14.6 for sample discussion questions, online supplement).

Faculty Role

Faculty members were responsible for selecting appropriate patients for the Pono Clinic experience. Faculty participated in the interprofessional team discussions prior to the team assessment as well as met separately from the learners to discuss their performance and ways to optimize the progression of their professional, leadership, and team skills. Faculty can focus on challenges that the learners have in meeting competencies in interpersonal relationships, team dynamics, and leadership roles. Faculty are expected to mentor and support learners from within and outside their profession, and have an opportunity to better understand expectations for learners in other professions in this interprofessional model.

Interprofessional Clinical Teaching

Learners in the Pono Clinic are expected to perform assessments, including history taking, physical examination, psychological and language assessments, clinical feeding and swallow assessments, occupational and physical therapy assessments, and naturalistic observations of the child playing or doing some task. A lead learner is designated for each patient. The lead learner needs to have an understanding of the professions available, their roles and responsibilities related to the patient's condition, and any role overlap to avoid duplication of assessments and efforts. Critical information to solve the problem often was uncovered by having the appropriate profession identify key information about a situation; for example, the behavioral overlay over a swallowing deficit in someone with cerebral palsy or understanding the social situation behind non-compliance with treatment. If a profession, such as nursing, was selected to be one of the teams directly interfacing with the patient and family, nursing faculty can directly mentor the learners in particular strategies and assessment tools. Interprofessional learners are able to learn *with*, *from*, and *about* each other through observation of an assessment performed by a member of a different profession.

Interprofessional team discussions included talking about the differences between the various disciplines roles and responsibilities and scope of practice. For instance, what are the differences and similarities between the roles of a psychologist and a social worker in a clinical situation? Also, there were discussions regarding how explicit the articulation of the boundaries between patients and professionals are, depending on the profession; the availability of, and the referral process to different types of professionals; how the social support, school, medical, and family systems intersect; and the importance of the interprofessional team approach in providing quality clinical care.

Feedback

Faculty provide feedback to learners throughout the academic year in a variety of ways, including during debriefings following the clinic sessions, in individual learner meetings, during LEND class group discussions, or through individual written feedback (see Exhibit 14.7 for "Evaluation of Trainee Performance," online supplement). The feedback includes positive reinforcement of things done well, or constructive criticism discussing improvements that can be made by individual learners or the team in general. Lastly, learners complete an evaluation of the Pono Clinic in a final course evaluation (see Exhibit 14.8 for "Trainee Evaluation", online supplement).

Impact

The following are some of the outstanding elements of this interprofessional clinical training model.

1. Opportunities exist for learners and faculty to meet IPEC competencies, to understand another profession's roles and responsibilities and scope of practice in providing real-life clinical care.
2. Opportunities exist for each profession to advance the skill set of its multilevel learners in the Pono Clinic through exposure to a variety of assessment tools and strategies.
3. Learners actively participate in interprofessional teams in the clinical setting to better understand differences among professions and participate in problem-solving and conflict-management tasks for care of complex patients.
4. There is a structured time and place for interprofessional learners and faculty to participate in group discussions, debriefings, and critical reflections outside of the clinical setting, yet still within the structure of a formal academic curriculum.
5. Pono Clinic patient cases are used for case-based learning within the training program.
6. Learners trained in the LEND program were more prepared for interprofessional collaborative practice than others who were not exposed to the interprofessional approach during their training.

CONCLUSIONS

This chapter serves as a guide to support interprofessional clinical teaching in a variety of settings with a range of health professions learners. The four exemplars provide different approaches and aspects of interprofessional clinical teaching, including how faculty can prepare the environment, learners, and faculty/preceptors/field instructors to support interprofessional education and practice. Using these foundational guidelines and resources, including the five-step guide to interprofessional clinical teaching outlined in Exhibit 14.1, faculty will prepare and support health professions learners who have the skill set to function effectively in today's health care environment to provide collaborative, compassionate, and safe patient-centered care.

REFERENCES

Agency for Healthcare Research and Quality. (2014). *Pocket guide: TeamSTEPPS®*. Rockville, MD: Author. Retrieved from http://www.ahrq.gov/teamstepps/instructor/essentials/pocketguide.html

Agency for Healthcare Research and Quality. (2016). *TeamSTEPPS® 2.0*. Rockville, MD: Author. Retrieved from http://www.ahrq.gov/teamstepps/instructor/index.html.

Archibald, D., Trumpower, D., & MacDonald, C. J. (2014). Validation of the interprofessional collaborative competency attainment survey. *Journal of Interprofessional Care, 28*(6), 553–558. doi:10.3109/13561 820.2014.917407

Chen, A. K., Rivera, J., Rotter, N., Green, E., & Kools, S. (2016). Interprofessional education in the clinical setting: A qualitative look at the preceptor's perspective in training advanced practice nursing students. *Nurse Education in Practice, 21,* 29–36. doi:10.1016/j.nepr.2016.09.006

Gallagher, P., Tweed, M., Hanna, S., Winter, H., & Hoare, K. (2012). Developing the one minute preceptor. *Clinical Teacher, 9*(6), 358–362. doi:10.1111/j.1743-498X.2012.00596.x

Interprofessional Education Collaborative. (2011). *Core competencies for interprofessional collaborative practice: Report of an expert panel*. Washington, DC: Author.

Interprofessional Education Collaborative. (2016). *Core competencies for interprofessional collaborative practice: 2016 update*. Washington, DC: Author. Retrieved from http://www.aacn.nche.edu/education -resources/IPEC-2016-Updated-Core-Competencies-Report.pdf

Jones, B., & Phillips, F. (2016). Social work leadership in interprofessional education in health care. *Journal of Social Work Education,52*(1), 18–29.

Lie, D. A., Forest, C. P., Kysh, L., & Sinclair, L. (2016). Interprofessional education and practice guide No. 5: Interprofessional teaching for prequalification students in clinical settings. *Journal of Interprofessional Care, 30*(3), 324–330. doi:10.3109/13561820.2016.1141752

Lown, B. A., & Manning, C. F. (2010). The Schwartz Center Rounds: Evaluation of an interdisciplinary approach to enhancing patient-centered communication, teamwork, and provider support. *Academic Medicine, 85*(6), 1073–1081. doi:10.1097/ACM.0b013e3181dbf741

National Center for Interprofessional Practice and Education. (2015). Preceptors in the Nexus Toolkit. Retrieved from https://nexusipe.org/engaging/learning-system/preceptors-nexus-toolkit

National League for Nursing. (2010). *Simulation in nursing education: From conceptualization to evaluation*. New York, NY: Author.

Pangaro, L. (1999). A new vocabulary and other innovations for improving descriptive in-training evaluations. *Academic Medicine, 74*(11), 1203–1207.

Pono. (2004). Retrieved from http://wehewehe.org/gsdl2.85/cgi-bin/hdict?e=d-11000-00---off-0hdict --00-1----0-10-0---0---0direct-10-ED--4-------0-1lp0--11-en-Zz-1---Zz-1-home-pono--00-3-1- 00-0---4----0-0-11-00-0utfZz-8-00&d=D18537&l=haw

Pierce, R., Noronha, L., Collins, N. P., & Fancovic, E. (2013). Brief structured observation of medical student hospital visits. *Education and Health Journal, 26,* 188–191. doi:10.4103/1357-6283.126003

Project Implicit. (2017). Implicit association test. Retrieved from https://implicit.harvard.edu

Schwartz Center for Compassionate Care. (2017, March). Schwartz Rounds. Retrieved from http://www .theschwartzcenter.org/supporting-caregivers/schwartz-center-rounds

U.S. Department of Veterans Affairs. (2016, October). Center of excellence in primary care education. Retrieved from http://www.va.gov/oaa/coepce/sanfrancisco.asp

Wolpaw, T., Papp, K., & Bordage, G. (2009). Using SNAPPS to facilitate the expression of clinical reasoning and uncertainties: A randomized comparison group trial. *Academic Medicine, 84*(4), 517–524. doi:10.1097/ACM.0b013e31819a8cbf

World Health Organization. (2010). *Framework for action on interprofessional education & collaborative practice.* Geneva, Switzerland: Author. Retrieved from http://apps.who.int/iris/bitstream/10665/70185/1/WHO_HRH_HPN_10.3_eng.pdf

ADDITIONAL RESOURCES

Education in Patient Aligned Care Teams (EdPACT): www.sanfrancisco.va.gov/education/edpact.asp

Huddle video: https://edpact.wordpress.com/huddle-video

Huddle checklist: www.edpact.files.wordpress.com/2016/04/huddle-checklist-for-edpact-trainees-v8-24-2015.pdf

Huddle scenarios: www.suzannecgordon.com/wp-content/uploads/2015/09/Select-Huddle-Scenarios-for-Website-Resource-9-25-2015.pdf

Huddle coaching:

Shunk, R. (2014). Coaching the huddle. In S. Gordon, D. L. Feldman, & M. Leonard (Eds.), *Collaborative Caring: Stories and reflections on teamwork in healthcare.* Ithica, NY: Cornell University Press. Retrieved from http://www.suzannecgordon.com/wp-content/uploads/2015/10/How-to-Huddle-Shunk.pdf

Shunk, R., Dulay, M., Chou, C. L., Janson, S., & O'Brien, B. C. (2014). Huddle-coaching: A dynamic intervention for trainees and staff to support team-based care. *Academic Medicine, 89*(2), 244–250. doi:10.1097/ACM.0000000000000104

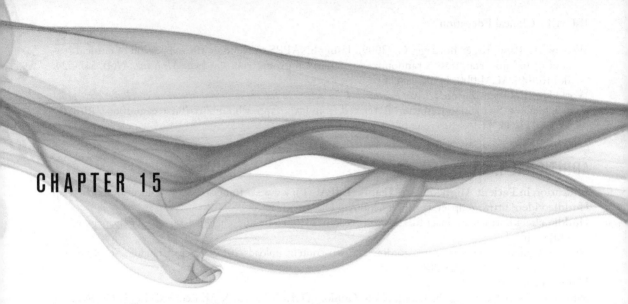

CHAPTER 15

International Clinical Education

Nicholas M. Hudak, Dennis Clements, and Michael V. Relf

CHAPTER OBJECTIVE

- Create partnerships for effective international learning experiences, including rotation design, implementation and evaluation, ethical issues, and avoiding potential pitfalls

---

We shall not cease from exploration, and the end of all our exploring will be to arrive where we started and know the place for the first time.

—*T. S. Eliot*

INTERNATIONAL CLINICAL EDUCATION AS PART OF HEALTH PROFESSIONS EDUCATION

The purpose of this chapter is to describe factors to consider when designing, implementing, and evaluating international clinical education (ICE) for learners in health professions education programs. ICE involves supervised learning in clinical settings outside the home country of a health professions education program. In a globalized world, many health professions educators believe that licensed providers should have the skills to care for diverse patients and populations in their home country and abroad. Over the past several years, increasing numbers of health professions learners have been participating in ICE, often referred to as *international rotations* or *clerkships*, and service learning and similar outreach experiences (Matheson, Walson, Pfeiffer, & Holmes, 2014). ICE is reported to impact learners' knowledge, attitude, and skills positively, as well as to foster cultural sensitivity and influence where participants choose to work (Jeffrey, Dumont, Kim, & Kuo, 2011). Despite these benefits, the quality of learner, program, and clinical site experiences varies by institution, and best-practice guidelines are

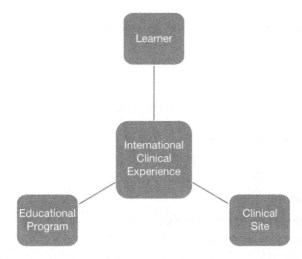

FIGURE 15.1 Conceptual framework of program, site, and learners.

lacking (Jeffrey et al., 2011). This chapter describes the "nuts and bolts" that educators should address, particularly around the three main stakeholders (i.e., educational program, clinical site, learners), which allow for ICE to be mutually beneficial for all involved (Figure 15.1). This chapter also provides "how to" recommendations to inform educators' approach and decision making when designing ICE. Although recommendations from the literature and the authors are valuable, educators must consider contextual elements such as program and institutional policies, curriculum and accreditation standards, laws related to international travel, unique qualities of the international site and community, and the expectations of learners and learning outcomes.

Ethical Considerations

It is important to keep ethical considerations at the forefront of ICE design, implementation, and evaluation as opportunities for learners to participate in ICE proliferate (Peluso, Encandela, Hafler, & Margolis, 2012). ICE has been scrutinized by educators, health care providers, and researchers for posing risks to international clinical sites and the international community, particularly in low-resource settings, as well as learners and programs (Exhibit 15.1). Risks to clinical sites may include the burden of hosting learners for a short period of time, often described as *medical tourism*, which can be disruptive to the clinical environment. Also, resources, such as medical supplies and medications that are provided for learners, are often only temporary (Bozinoff et al., 2014). Examples of risk to learners may include illness or injury, inadequate supervision in clinical settings, and lack of preparation to be able to fully participate in clinical and cultural learning (Logar, Le, Harrison, & Glass, 2015). Program risks may include liability associated with risks to learners, financial and effort costs for faculty and staff, and the inability to evaluate learning outcomes. Given these and other potential risks, a guiding principle for educators is to have knowledge of potential risks and then mitigate those risks to ensure that the ICE partnership is sustainable and beneficial to the clinical site and the community in addition to the program and its learners (Adams, Wagner, Nutt, & Binagwaho, 2016; Crump & Sugarman, 2008; Wallace & Webb, 2014). Conceptual models for partnership and sustainability in global health have been described in the literature (Leffers & Mitchell, 2011). Other barriers to successful ICE include safety concerns during travel, lack of consistent funding, limited faculty experience, and inadequate resources to support learners during ICE experiences (Jeffrey et al., 2011). These barriers underscore the imperative of proper planning, implementation, and evaluation that is guided by health professions educators.

EXHIBIT 15.1 Challenges and Risks of International Clinical Education

Program

- Liability associated with risks to learners
- Cost of time and effort for educators to design, implement, and evaluate international clinical education experiences
- Difficulty evaluating learning outcomes
- Failure of learner to achieve learning objectives
- Nonsustainable partnership

International clinical site

- Burden of hosting learners for a short period of time
- Temporary supply of medical resources may arrive with learners
- Disruption of patient care
- Disruption of education of domestic health professions learners
- Nonsustainable partnership

Learner

- Illness or injury
- Inadequate supervision in clinical settings
- Lack of preparation to fully participate in clinical and cultural learning
- Cost of participation
- Failure to achieve learning objectives

Although not within the scope of this chapter, there is a growing demand for ICE to involve bidirectional exchanges in which learners from both international partner institutions participate in clinical learning at each other's site (Bozinoff et al., 2014; Kulbok, Mitchell, Glick, & Greiner, 2012; Peluso et al., 2012; Pitt, Gladding, Majinge, & Butteris, 2016). Although this chapter cannot address every factor related to hosting international learners, the content within this chapter may provide valuable information for educators involved designing and implementing these experiences.

THE THREE MAIN STAKEHOLDERS

The three main stakeholders in ICE are the education program and its sponsoring institution, the international clinical site and its community, and the learners who participate in the course. Educators involved with ICE have the responsibility of addressing a great number of factors unique to international experiences, in addition to customary tasks for domestic clinical sites. Therefore, this chapter is organized to describe key factors for each stakeholder in three sections: program factors, clinical site factors, and learner factors. Each stakeholder is equally important and the sections of this chapter are sequenced to facilitate a comprehensive understanding of ICE with regard to the order of course design.

Program Factors

Programmatic factors—a descriptor representing the health professions education program, the sponsoring institution or school, and program faculty and staff—are critical in ensuring ICE success. The rationale for offering ICE must be defined early and align with the program mission. Faculty and staff time and effort must be allocated to meet the responsibilities involved in the design, implementation, and evaluation of ICE. Upon that foundation, the program must ensure that appropriate policies are in place and affiliations are established with the international clinical site. Within the framework of policy and the program curriculum, course objectives and methods of assessment can be developed and then continually evaluated.

Mission, Policies, Affiliation

Mission

The mission of a program and its institution is an important determinant of establishing and maintaining ICE. The first step in establishing ICE opportunities is to consider how this type of learning experience aligns with the institution's mission and the program's expected outcomes for learners upon completion of the program. Leadership at both the institutional and program levels plays integral roles in initiating and sustaining support for ICE. Therefore, educators should involve appropriate leadership throughout the process, which may include the dean, academic dean, clinical dean, department chair, program director, curriculum committee, and other faculty, as well as legal counsel and risk management. Educators in some programs may have to advocate for the establishment of ICE. However, less advocacy may be needed if a program or institutional mission has international priorities or if other programs within the institution offer ICE experiences. In any circumstance, it is imperative for the program to understand and present the purpose of providing ICE and how such an offering contributes to the broader mission (Walker, Campbell, & Egede, 2014). Examples of program goals include increasing learner opportunities for developing cultural competency, promoting recruitment of program applicants, and having clinical sites where learners can practice other language skills (Exhibit 15.2). Equally important, educators should understand and present risks associated with ICE and the resources necessary for design, implementation, and evaluation to ensure that leadership and program faculty are aware of what such a commitment entails.

EXHIBIT 15.2 Goals and Benefits of International Clinical Education

Program

- Provide unique learning opportunities for learners
- Recruit learners
- Foster educational partnerships
- Reduce burden of domestic clinical placements

International clinical site

- Financial benefit
- Awareness of international visitors
- Need for a long-term partnership
- Reciprocal education
- Experience of diverse learners

Learner

- Impacts learners' knowledge, attitude, and skills based on course objectives
- Fosters cultural competency
- May influence where participants choose to work (community/rural setting, underserved populations)

Policies

Program policies are essential to informing and guiding the design, implementation, and evaluation of ICE. Policies should focus on promoting learning outcomes and mitigating risks to the program, clinical site, and learners. Topical categories include the affiliation process; course requirements; risk management; and financial responsibilities to the program, clinical site, and learners (Exhibit 15.3). Given the priority for learners' health and safety while abroad, a well-defined safety and security plan should be created to mitigate risk (Hansoti et al., 2013). Educators should determine which established policies pertain to ICE so they are not duplicating policies when making necessary revisions. For example, established program policies related to immunization requirements for clinical education at domestic sites may be sufficient for international sites. In many cases, educators will have to develop new policies that pertain to ICE. For example, policies may need to be developed for a pretravel health evaluation, dress code, and recommendations for use of technology such as using social media during the ICE experience. Polices should be developed with regard to the program, the larger institution, accreditation standards, U.S. Department of State guidelines, and national and international laws. Given the variety of topics and sources of information available, educators should involve appropriate members of their institution, ranging from leadership to risk management, when reviewing, revising, and drafting new policies. It is also important for educators to recognize that the ongoing evaluation of ICE at the program, clinical site, and learner levels informs subsequent policy revisions.

Affiliation

A formal clinical affiliation agreement or a memorandum of understanding is customarily established between the program and the clinical training sites both domestically and abroad to outline the responsibilities of each partner. Although programs should have standard affiliation agreements with domestic clinical sites, there are unique factors involved with ICE that may require revision of standard affiliation agreements or creation of agreements specifically for ICE. During the initial discussions between the program and the clinical site, it is recommended that the purpose, scope, and type of agreement be discussed to ensure clear communication and develop trust given that such agreements may not be utilized in all countries. Furthermore, processing these types of documents frequently takes longer than execution of domestic agreements, so anticipatory planning is essential. Regardless of the document used, the agreement

---

EXHIBIT 15.3 Program Policies: Common Topics

- Restricted regions for sites
- Affiliation process
- Health and safety requirements of learners
- Professional behavior and attire of learners
- Course requirements in regard to objectives and evaluation
- Risk management and indemnity release
- Protocol for academic and nonacademic issues
- Financial responsibilities to the learners, program, and site
- Use of technology
- Safety and security plan

should define the responsibilities of each partner and should address elements of governance, funding arrangements, duration of experience, clinical supervision, logistical support, and mechanisms for conflict mediation and unexpected incidences (Peluso et al., 2012). Legal counsel and risk management should be aware if not involved in the affiliation process. These units can help negotiate issues related to malpractice, liability insurance, and contractual arrangements. Furthermore, laws and regulations related to foreigners studying, volunteering, or engaging in clinical care must always be considered.

Curriculum, Learning and Evaluation, Coordination

Curriculum

Educators must carefully consider how ICE fits into the program curriculum with regard to the expected learning outcomes and reference to the accreditation standards. Similar to other clinical education courses, educators must address standard requirements for courses such as course goals and objectives, instructional methods, methods of evaluation, as well as which faculty and staff will be involved in the course. Educators should reference their profession's accreditation standards for educational programs to ensure compliance with those standards with regard to ICE. Accreditation standards may or may not have specific items related to ICE. Even when there are no directly related standards, there may be standards that indirectly relate. For example, an accreditation standard about the evaluation of clinical training sites would pertain to both domestic and international sites. Educators may benefit from consulting with other programs from their profession involved with ICE to learn their experience regarding compliance with accreditation standards. In addition, educators can reference ICE resources provided by professional organizations. Important curricular questions include whether the ICE course should be required or elective, whether ICE hours count toward hours required for program completion, whether there is a separate course for each clinical site or a single course with several sites, when the ICE course should be scheduled during the clinical training, and how to determine course goals and methods of evaluation. Such curricular decisions are best made by the collective faculty and program leadership through established approaches, such as a curriculum committee or council.

Learning and Evaluation

The learning objectives for ICE should define expected outcomes for learners; resonate with reasons why ICE is offered; and describe the knowledge, skills, or attitudes that will be evaluated. A 2013 systematic review reported 22 educational objectives consistent across several institutions, and these objectives were categorized as preelective, intraelective, and postelective (Cherniak, Drain, & Brewer, 2013). Objectives from the authors' respective programs are also consistent (Exhibit 15.4). Understanding health equity and being able to effectively work within interdisciplinary teams are two more recently cited objectives for ICE (Adams et al., 2016; Peluso et al., 2012). Whether an ICE experience is required or elective may impact the course objectives and requirements. Instructional methods in the clinical setting include the actual clinical experience as well as other activities such as language training, educational lectures, and other cultural learning activities. Objectives for preparticipation and postparticipation activities may also be included with the course objectives. As with all other educational interventions, learning objectives should be assessed at the individual learner level and across cohorts as part of broader evaluation of the entire ICE course. Methods of evaluation may include exams, clinical instructor evaluation of learner performance, learner projects or presentations, self-assessment, reflective writing, and learners' feedback about the experience. Methods for evaluating clinical sites and learners are described in subsequent sections of this chapter.

EXHIBIT 15.4 Common Learning Objectives

- Gain knowledge of common conditions and diseases that are endemic to unique regions outside of the home country
- Develop an understanding of patient assessment and treatment in an international setting
- Recognize cultural, social, economic, and political determinants of health and health care in an international setting
- Discuss the benefits and challenges of providing health care in an international community
- Demonstrate the ability to learn and prepare for clinical learning in an international setting
- Reflect on the professional and personal learning outcomes of an international clinical experience

---

Coordination

The ICE course should have at least one dedicated faculty coordinator as well as sufficient administrative staff support to ensure success from early planning through ongoing evaluation. Delineation of roles and responsibilities can facilitate completion of the many required tasks at the program, site, and learner levels. Although a single educator or perhaps a few educators may be involved with coordinating ICE experiences, there is certainly value in involving a program's entire faculty to ensure their understanding of the ICE goals, learner participation and experiences, learning outcomes, as well as benefit to the program and site. Other educators within the program or institution may also contribute to the course through involvement in learner selection, site evaluation, predeparture training, as well as evaluation of learners and the ICE course. It is imperative for program and administrative leadership to understand that the design, implementation, and evaluation of ICE requires a significant amount of time and effort for the faculty coordinator and support staff to address the multitude of factors described in this chapter. Therefore, careful consideration should be made to determine workload and that workload should be reassessed over time. Program leadership should also be cognizant of other financial and nonfinancial resources that the course coordinator may need access to, including but not limited to other institutional resources such an international office and financial support for travel to evaluate clinical sites or to supervise learners.

Clinical Site Factors

The second set of factors that need to be addressed to ensure successful ICE are clinical site factors. The use of the words *clinical site* in this section is a descriptor representing the international clinical sites, the in-country clinical instructors/preceptors and administrative staff, as well as the local community and host country. Identification of international clinical sites is the first step that leads to initial evaluation of the clinical site and community that involves bilateral exchange of information. Once a clinical site is affiliated with the program, the process of ongoing evaluation begins to ensure that a positive, equitable, and sustainable partnership is developed (Peluso et al., 2012; Walker et al., 2014). Four key factors for successful global health partnerships described by researchers also apply for educators and include (a) mutual respect and benefit, (b) trust, (c) good communication, and (d) clear partner roles and expectations (John, Ayodo, & Musoke, 2016).

The Faculty Ambassador

Because both programs and sites have a significant number of individuals in various roles, at the program level it is important to determine which faculty member or members are responsible for site identification and evaluation, as well as whether evaluation will be in-person or conducted by telecommunications. The relationship between the faculty member and the clinical site is key to any success that might occur, so it can be strategic to have the faculty coordinator of the ICE course be responsible for both initial and ongoing evaluation of the site. It is very sensible for the faculty member most knowledgeable about the ICE course and learners to also be the expert on the clinical sites. Because partnerships take a significant amount of time to develop and may last for several years, the continuity of having a single or small number of faculty "ambassadors" provides continuity and trust in the relationship.

Site Identification

When preparing to identify a site, the program should first establish criteria for site selection with regard to program mission, course goals, global regions of interest, travel restrictions, learners' interests, safety considerations, and the health care system. Another consideration is language and whether the learner visitor will be suitably prepared to communicate in the language that is needed. Some health professions will need to assess whether or not their respective professions or similar professions exist in certain countries, such as physician assistants (PAs), nurse practitioners (NPs), and physical therapists (PTs). The absence of an identical or similar profession may not preclude the establishment of an ICE partner, but may be a consideration and can guide information-sharing about professions. Once these factors are addressed, focus turns to identifying clinical sites that are willing to host international learners and to provide supervised clinical learning experiences. As part of this process, the program also needs to assess communities' receptivity to hosting international learners.

A program or its institution may identify clinical sites through its relationships with international partners, often for research or clinical purposes. An educator may also identify sites by reaching out to other educators within or outside his or her own institution to solicit recommendations for potential partners. Other ways to identify sites are via Internet searches, through professional or national associations, and networking at conferences. It is also possible to partner with other institutions or nongovernmental organizations that have global partners.

Regardless of the means by which a site is identified, it is imperative that the faculty coordinator have a high level of knowledge about the site and community, as well as trusting relationships with providers and administration at the site. It is extremely important to understand the expectations of the individual partners for the success of the learner experience and to ensure continuation of such experiences. All prospective collaborations, especially new sites that have not hosted international learners, warrant careful scrutiny beginning with site identification and through initial evaluation.

Initial Evaluation

The process for initial and ongoing evaluation of an international clinical site should be determined early in the development of an ICE course. The program needs to decide how the approach will be similar to evaluation of domestic clinical sites as well as what additional information may need to be assessed. Factors unique to international sites may include language requirements, housing options, and expectations for learner involvement in patient care (e.g., direct or observational), ensuring appropriate clinical supervision, ICE placement fees, and safety assessment (Exhibit 15.5). Initial evaluation of the clinical site is the first step in bilateral exchange of information between the program and the site. This exchange of information is, in many ways, frontloaded during the initial evaluation, and very much continues throughout the duration of the partnership.

The faculty coordinator also needs to determine who at the international clinical site should be involved with both initial and ongoing evaluation of the ICE partnership. At the program level, the faculty coordinator should also consider involving institutional or program leadership in certain conversations and communications, particularly when establishing a partnership. Most

---

EXHIBIT 15.5 Tasks for Initial Site Evaluation

Information to provide to clinical site

- Information on program, role of practitioner (DO, MD, NP, PA, PT, RN, SW, etc.)
- Course/clinical/learning objectives
- Methods of learner evaluation
- Learner role/scope
- Requirements of supervisor/preceptor
- Affiliation process
- Method of learner evaluation and site experience
- Contact information
- Process for scheduling learners

Information to gain from clinical site

- Clinical settings where training will take place
- Clinicians will provide supervision
- Common medical problems
- Staff designated as learner point of contact
- Housing options
- Information about community
- Documentation/immigration/practice requirements of the site and country
- Associated fees

DO, doctor of osteopathic medicine; MD, doctor of medicine; NP, nurse practitioner; PA, physician assistant; PT, physical therapist; SW, social worker.

---

early correspondences are by electronic or telecommunications to query for feasibility and interest in partnering with ICE. If the response is affirmative, further exchange of information should detail the expectations for both the program and the clinical site. At that point, conversations can begin to define and clarify both expectations and responsibilities as well as explore issues of concern (Walker et al., 2014). It is important in these early conversations for faculty to understand how the site will benefit from hosting international learners and to confirm that the presence of international learners will not disrupt the supervising providers' delivery of patient care or the education of other learners training at the clinical site.

Once there is sufficient exchange of information and conversations for the program to establish a partnership, the program needs to determine whether an in-person evaluation of the clinical site and community is indicated. An in-person evaluation is the most thorough method to gain information about the clinical site, provide information about the program, and form trusting relationships with individuals at the clinical site. An in-person visit also provides a solid foundation for future conversations that will occur as part of ongoing site evaluation. Site evaluation should be conducted in person before the first learner placement as it allows for interaction between the educator and the local community as well as facilitates a better understanding of the environment in which the learner will be placed. In addition, firsthand evaluation of the site better prepares the faculty coordinator to design predeparture training.

Ongoing Evaluation

Although the largest amount of knowledge may be acquired during initial evaluation, ongoing evaluation is the means by which the partnership is assessed for mutual benefit and the relationship is maintained (Peluso et al., 2012; Walker et al., 2014). Feedback from the site is also important so that it is clear that learners benefit and are not disruptive to health care delivery or culturally inappropriate. Ongoing evaluation should be conducted routinely with respect to program policy and with reference to accreditation standards. Routine distance evaluation by telecommunications should be scheduled at least annually and can also be acquired by other means such as a survey. Routine in-person evaluation should be conducted at a frequency determined by the program and clinical site necessary to maintain the partnership, which is often every few years. Both distant and in-person evaluations demonstrate continued commitment to understanding how the process is affecting the site and offer opportunity for continued discussion about how to improve the experience for both partners.

Learner Factors

The third set of factors to address to ensure successful ICE are learner factors. Although learners meet most of the learning objectives during the experience, there are several preparticipation and postparticipation activities that facilitate achievement of those objectives. Key preparticipation events include the application and selection process as well as predeparture training. Key postparticipation tasks include evaluation of learner outcomes, including assignments and projects, as well as surveying the learners about their ICE experience.

Selection

Selection of learners who will succeed in ICE is a critical task. Most ICE courses are elective rather than required for learners. Therefore, educators must determine how learners will be informed about ICE opportunities and the process by which learners will be selected to participate. These tasks should be scheduled in advance, often by more than 1 year, to ensure sufficient time for the selection process as well as to schedule learners in coordination with the clinical site. Like other aspects of their education, learners should receive ample information about ICE to ensure that they are making an informed choice when requesting to participate in the course.

Key information needed to inform learner decision making includes course objectives and methods of evaluation, course requirements and policies, details about the clinical site and country, potential risks of participation, health- and medical-related requirements, financial costs, and details about the experiences of prior learners who have participated in the course. Several of the factors described earlier are discussed in this section. In regard to financial costs, it is important for learners to understand what expenses are involved with ICE, what expenses they are responsible for, and what options may be available for financing the experience. Expenses may include airfare, in-country transportation, lodging, clinical site fees, entry Visas, cost of postexposure prophylactic medications, immunizations, pretravel medical evaluation, and evacuation insurance. Options for financing experiences may include scholarships and increasing education loan amounts. Educators should consult their institution's office of financial aid for rules regarding educational loans.

Learners should also be informed about the selection process, which may include an application, essays, interviews, and letters of recommendation. It is also beneficial to inform learners about selection criteria, which can inform their decision to request participation based on whether or not they meet those criteria. Common selection criteria include proficiency in a specific language, prior travel experience, professionalism, academic standing, and the individual's goals for the ICE experience. When determining these criteria, fundamental questions for educators to ask are whether or not the learner is capable of achieving course objectives, is culturally sensitive and competent, adaptable, and able to be a professional representative of the program, profession, and home country. Educators also need to determine who should be involved in the selection process, which may include the faculty coordinator, faculty advisors of the applicants, other clinical faculty, program leadership, alumni, as well as representatives from the host clinical site.

Predeparture Training

Predeparture training is essential to preparing learners to engage in both the clinical setting and community (Cherniak et al., 2013; Purkey & Hollaar, 2016; Walker et al., 2014; Wallace & Webb, 2014). Tasks for predeparture training may be put into one of two categories, those related to the logistics of preparing for the experience and content that facilitates learning during the experience. The list of logistical tasks is extensive and may include application to the clinical site, obtaining passport and other travel documentation to enter and exit the country, scheduling air and ground transportation, arranging lodging, having a pretravel medical evaluation, registering travel plans with the U.S. Department of State, paying fees associated with the experience, and securing related travel insurance, including health insurance (Exhibit 15.6). It should be noted that several of these tasks are very typical of what any individual should do when traveling abroad for any purpose. Scheduling an appointment with a travel clinic is particularly important to ensure that the learner has received appropriate immunizations, medications, and postexposure prophylactic therapies. Learners benefit from receiving this list of tasks several months prior to departure and having access to the faculty coordinator to address any questions or concerns.

Because many ICE experiences are relatively short in duration, predeparture training should also provide learners with information about what they are likely to encounter in the clinical site and community so that they can maximize their time while abroad and participate within their scope as a learner. Similar to logistical tasks, the list of content to cover is substantial (Exhibit 15.7). Educators should consider providing information about the course policies and procedures, methods of evaluation, background on the clinical site and health care system, learning strategies, guidelines for adjusting to foreign culture and travel, health issues and diseases endemic to the community, as well as the culture and languages of the host country. Information on culture may include lifestyle, economy, population demographics, attire, religion, gender roles, arts, media, food and drink, geography, wildlife, and plants. Predeparture training should also educate learners about relevant ethical issues and provide a framework for participating within the context of ethical dilemmas that may be experienced while abroad (Logar et al., 2015). Learning a foreign language or even common phrases may be perceived

---

EXHIBIT 15.6 Logistical Tasks for Learner Preparation

- Participation agreement/indemnity release
- Letter of introduction to learner from program clinical site
- Site application/registration
- Travel documentation
- Transportation: air, ground
- Housing
- Pretravel medical evaluation
- Registration with U.S. Department of State
- Health insurance and travel insurance
- Update emergency contact information

EXHIBIT 15.7 Topics to Include in Predeparture Training

- Review of course policies and procedures, objectives, components of evaluation, and logistical preparation
- Review and practice work flow at international location, including how to get help when needed
- Discuss various components of host country/region culture, including lifestyle, economy, population demographics, dress/attire, religion, gender roles, arts, media, food and drink, geography, wildlife, and plants; review recent history of the host country, as well as the current political structure and political events
- Discuss strategies to avoid ethnocentrism and promote cultural humility/respect
- Describe common pathological conditions unique to populations in the host country/region
- Demonstrate foreign language communication skills with basic medical and travel-related phrases
- Be aware of health- and medical-related research priorities in the host country
- Clinical site and health system—describe each host country's health system, including structure, providers, and payer system, as well as recent events and issues
- Consider ethics and privacy—including four principles of ethics in global health and culture: Discuss how learners can positively and negatively impact others with regard to ethical principles; describe domains of privacy and related components; review guidelines for respecting privacy as a learner and the initial process for reporting potential privacy violations
- Practical travel preparation—present recommendations and strategies for preparing for international travel
- Adjusting to foreign cultures and travel—explain how to prepare for the impact of an international experience, manage expectations and involvement in clinical and cultural experiences, and strategies to adjust to challenges and culture shock

---

positively by the site and community. Learners should also be given guidance on how to behave as a learner in an international setting. For example, in many countries learners do not customarily ask questions of their supervisors in clinical settings. Content for predeparture training should also include information and recommendations from prior learners who have been to the clinical site given the value of firsthand experience.

Instructional methods for predeparture training content may include lecture, group discussion, required or recommended readings, journal club, self-directed modules, and case-based simulation. Learners may also be evaluated based on their participation in and contribution to predeparture training. Educators may assess learners' readiness prior to their departure as well as their perceptions of the predeparture training after their experience abroad. Content resources for predeparture training may include the health professions education literature, the course coordinator and other faculty familiar with the clinical site, providers at the clinical site who supervise learners, prior learners who have participated in the experience, the U.S. Department of State, and web-based resources from professional organizations. Partners at the clinical site may also provide resources for predeparture training. Because predeparture training is so involved, educators must allow sufficient time for the content to be provided and learners to be evaluated prior to their departure. Many programs begin their predeparture training 6 to 12 months in advance of student departure to the site.

Clinical Learning

Successful learning in the clinical setting is contingent upon a learner having an appropriate amount of supervision and sufficient interactions with patients and the health care team. Although participating in clinical learning, learners should always have at least one or two points of contact with providers or staff who are available to address questions or concerns with or related to clinical learning or other logistical matters. It is the responsibility of the faculty coordinator to identify in advance who these individuals are and to facilitate introductions between those individuals and the learner.

Another important source of support for a learner could be other learners from his or her own program as well as learners from other domestic or international health professions education programs. Many programs are deliberate in assigning at least two or more learners from their own program to a single site during a specific time frame as a type of "buddy system." Learners should also be encouraged to maintain contact with family and friends as a source of social support. In many instances, learners will travel with their own faculty to the international clinical site. In such circumstances, the faculty member may be providing care at the clinical site or present to assist in the supervision of learners.

When faculty do not join learners while abroad, the faculty coordinator or other designee should readily be accessible to learners to address urgent and nonurgent questions and concerns. Although learners may confer with the faculty coordinator on an as-needed basis, they may also schedule routine communication by email or teleconference to discuss the experience. A key message to relate to learners is to have a very low threshold for presenting questions, concerns, and potential emergencies to program faculty and designees at the clinical site.

It may be helpful for learners to have an algorithm to follow to address specific types of concerns (Hansoti et al., 2013). For example, learners should always know what steps to take in the event of a personal illness or blood or body fluids exposure. It is important to note that not all concerns may be related to learners' own health, but that learners might need assistance in making sure they can optimize their learning experiences and achieve learning objectives in a culturally appropriate manner. Last, learners should be encouraged to express gratitude to the clinical site and community in a manner that is culturally appropriate and customary for international visitors.

EVALUATION

Although the requirements and assessment methods for ICE courses will typically be similar to other clinical courses, international clinical rotations may have unique learning objectives and evaluation methods. All learners should be evaluated based on course objectives and requirements, which may include evaluation of clinical skills from supervising providers, a written exam to assess knowledge, surveys to share their perceptions of the experience, projects to disseminate learning outcomes of their experiences, and logging data about the clinical experiences (Cherniak et al., 2013). If learners will be evaluated by supervising providers at the clinical site, both the learners and providers at the clinical site should be aware of this responsibility and how evaluations should be both obtained and completed. In some cases, evaluation forms may need to be modified in regard to content or language to ensure accurate evaluation of learners' performance. It is important for the faculty coordinator to be familiar with how domestic learners at the clinical site are customarily evaluated and to inform the providers about methods used for the partnering program. Data acquired through evaluation are essential in determining whether the learners achieved their course objectives. Similar to other clinical sites, data from learners' experiences and their perception of the experience can be shared with the clinical site to improve experiences for future learners. In some instances, this data may help a program determine that a clinical site should no longer be utilized. In addition to obtaining data for the purpose of course evaluation, data from evaluation of outcomes is also the source of information for scholarly work related to ICE.

Postreturn Debriefing

Learners should also participate in postreturn debriefing with the faculty coordinator, which may be conducted in an individual or group format. This may be considered a component of evaluation depending on the purpose and other elements of evaluation. Key topics may include evaluation of the elective, including positive and negative experiences, review of health and safety, reintegration, and discussion of impact of experience on future practice (Cherniak et al., 2013; Purkey & Hollaar, 2016). Similar to some elements of predeparture training, educators should schedule the postreturn debriefing in close proximity to the learners' return from the ICE experience. A postreturn debriefing also provide the faculty coordinator with a firsthand account of the experience and information that may be useful for future learner experiences.

CONCLUSIONS

ICE can have a positive impact on learners' knowledge, attitude, and skills. Programs that choose to offer ICE have a duty to provide well-designed course and experiences that are driven by mission, objectives, and desired learning outcomes. In order for ICE to be successful, the following factors have to be given high priority: ethical considerations, stakeholder involvement, well-defined objectives, and evaluation. Another requirement for the success of ICE is a robust orientation process and a mechanism to debrief both learners and international clinical partners. In addition, program designers should ensure appropriate matching of participants to host destinations. That is, international clinical experiences are not "one size fits all." Taken altogether, ICE offers numerous opportunities to foster cultural sensitivity and may be one way to reduce global health disparities and prepare health professionals of the 21st century to provide care to diverse, global communities.

REFERENCES

Adams, L. V., Wagner, C. M., Nutt, C. T., & Binagwaho, A. (2016). The future of global health education: Training for equity in global health. *BMC Medical Education, 16*(1), 296–302.

Bozinoff, N., Dorman, K. P., Kerr, D., Roebbelen, E., Rogers, E., Hunter, A., . . . Kraeker, C. (2014). Toward reciprocity: Host supervisor perspectives on international medical electives. *Medical Education, 48*(4), 397–404.

Cherniak, W. A., Drain, P. K., & Brewer, T. F. (2013). Educational objectives of international medical electives: A narrative literature review. *Academic Medicine: Journal of the Association of American Medical Colleges, 88*(11), 1778–1781.

Crump, J. A., & Sugarman, J. (2008). Ethical considerations for short-term experiences by trainees in global health. *Journal of the American Medical Association, 300*(12), 1456–1458.

Hansoti, B., Douglass, K., Tupesis, J., Runyon, M. S., Sanson, T., Babcock, C., . . . Martin, I. B. (2013). Guidelines for safety of trainees rotating abroad: Consensus recommendations from the Global Emergency Medicine Academy of the Society for Academic Emergency Medicine, Council of Emergency Medicine Residency Directors, and the Emergency Medicine Residents' Association. *Academic Emergency Medicine, 20*(4), 413–420.

Jeffrey, J., Dumont, R. A., Kim, G. Y., & Kuo, T. (2011). Effects of international health electives on medical student learning and career choice. *Family Medicine, 43*(1), 21–28.

John, C. C., Ayodo, G., & Musoke, P. (2016). Successful global health research partnerships: What makes them work? *American Journal of Tropical Medicine and Hygiene, 94*(1), 5–7.

Kulbok, P. A., Mitchell, E. M., Glick, D. F., & Greiner, D. (2012). International experiences in nursing education: A review of the literature. *International Journal of Nursing Education Scholarship, 9*(1). doi:10.1515/1548-923X.2365

Leffers, J., & Mitchell, E. (2011). Conceptual model for partnership and sustainability in global health. *Public Health Nursing, 28*(1), 91–102.

Logar, T., Le, P., Harrison, J. D., & Glass, M. (2015). Teaching corner: "first do no harm": Teaching global health ethics to medical trainees through experiential learning. *Journal of Bioethical Inquiry, 12*(1), 69–78.

Matheson, A., Walson, J. L., Pfeiffer, J., & Holmes, K. (2014). Sustainability and growth of university global health programs: A report of the Center for Strategic & International Studies Global Health Policy Center. Washington, DC. Retrieved from http://2014cughconference.org/wp-content/uploads/2014/05/Sustainability-and-Growth-of-University-Global-Health-Programs.pdf

Peluso, M. J., Encandela, J., Hafler, J. P., & Margolis, C. Z. (2012). Guiding principles for the development of global health education curricula in undergraduate medical education. *Medical Teacher, 34*(8), 653–658. doi:10.3109/0142159X.2012.687848

Pitt, M. B., Gladding, S. P., Majinge, C. R., & Butteris, S. M. (2016). Making global health rotations a two-way street: A model for hosting international residents. *Global Pediatric Health, 3,* doi:10.177/2333794 X16630671

Purkey, E., & Hollaar, G. (2016). Developing consensus for postgraduate global health electives: Definitions, pre-departure training and post-return debriefing. *BMC Medical Education, 16*(1), 1.

Walker, R. J., Campbell, J. A., & Egede, L. E. (2014). Effective strategies for global health research, training and clinical care: A narrative review. *Global Journal of Health Science, 7*(2), 119–139.

Wallace, L. J., & Webb, A. (2014). Pre-departure training and the social accountability of international medical electives. *Education for Health, 27*(2), 143.

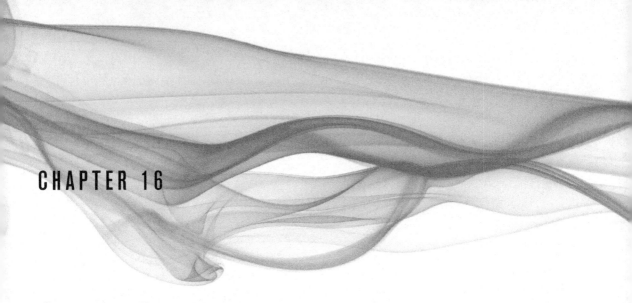

CHAPTER 16

Service Learning

Hoonani Cuadrado, Sharon E. Connor, Corinne Feldman,
and Mary Marfisee

CHAPTER OBJECTIVES

- Explain the pedagogy and benefits of service learning
- Integrate meaningful community service, civic responsibility, and social justice into the curriculum

---

What I hear, I forget. What I see, I remember. What I do, I understand.

—Xunzi (340–245 BCE)

HISTORY OF SERVICE LEARNING

The idea of student education being enriched by developing and executing service-centered activities has become popular in a variety of health professions programs. Although it may be difficult to pinpoint the exact entry of this learning method into the mainstream pedagogy, it was likely brought to the fore through the innovations of John Dewey during the era of progressive education in the early to mid-20th century (Giles & Eyler, 1994). Dewey proposed that society's ills would be improved by getting people out of the classroom and encouraged students and teachers to become intimately acquainted with the conditions of their local communities (Dewey, 1938). In 1969, returning Peace Corps volunteers, administrators, and university faculty convened in Atlanta, Georgia, to discuss linking the fervor of international service within the broader concept of education, and the term *service learning* was coined (Busch, 2016).

DEFINITION AND PEDAGOGY OF SERVICE LEARNING

Providing effective education in the health sciences can be challenging. Not only are health educators challenged with teaching up-to-date didactic medical knowledge, but they must also prepare students to understand social determinants of health, defined as the societal, environmental, personal, and situational conditions contributing to a person's health (Sørensen, et al., 2012). Traditionally, health professions education has been lecture based and instructor centered. This dominant pedagogy may prepare students academically, but does little to address the increasingly complex health care needs of a culturally diverse society. Service learning is a curricular strategy that combines community service with academic objectives (Stewart & Wubbena, 2014). The key elements to any service learning activity are (a) addressing a need in the community (Savanick, 2015; Stewart & Wubbena, 2014), (b) providing a structured educational component for students, and (c) engaging students in guided reflection about their experiences (Giles & Eyler, 2012).

BENEFITS OF SERVICE LEARNING

Service learning has the potential to benefit all participants—students, academic institutions, faculty, and their surrounding communities. With regard to students, studies have shown service learning to have a positive effect on academic, interpersonal, social awareness, and responsibility outcomes. Scholarly enhancement can be seen in improved grade point averages (GPAs), writing, and critical thinking skills (Astin, Vogelgesang, Ikeda, & Yee, 2000). Interpersonal competencies can be appreciated with students manifesting improved social skills, better goal-setting behaviors, and better cooperative/interdisciplinary skills (Eyler, Giles, Stenson, & Gray, 2001). Finally, beneficial outcomes include improved character values and responsible behaviors. As students work with underserved populations, they gain a better understanding of public health concerns in resource-poor environments (Parski & List, 2008). They learn to appreciate cultural diversity and show more tolerance of ethnic diversity (Astin et al., 2000). They begin to feel responsible for the community and are motivated to take action to benefit the community (Billig, 2000). Indeed, service learning experiences can have future significance: Students who have been involved in service learning are more likely to be actively engaged in community service after graduation as well as consider a career in public service (Astin et al., 2000).

Not only can service learning benefit academic institutions, it can also offer faculty opportunities for professional development. Offering service learning as part of a pedagogical practice within a curriculum can raise institutional visibility and attract engaged and highly motivated students to the university. Researchers have illustrated that student engagement is the greatest predictor of retention and cognitive and personal development in college students (Billig, 2000). In many instances, service learning projects support the humanistic missions of a university and strengthen campus–community relationships. In addition, service learning outside the traditional classroom can encourage a unique set of faculty leadership skills: networking, public speaking, and research. Networking can foster a collaborative spirit among other agencies, institutions, and departments within the institution for future research or public speaking engagements. Public speaking engagements can reveal additional resources for either the academic institution or the community partner.

PLANNING AND PREPARING FOR SERVICE LEARNING IN THE CURRICULUM

Planning

When planning for service learning in the curriculum, it important to consider core competencies. The Accreditation Council for Graduate Medical Education (ACGME) suggests implementing competencies involving social awareness and responsibility, interaction that incorporates contextual awareness, critical thinking, and ethical decision making for all health professionals (Joyce, 2006). Service learning is an ideal teaching method to develop these attitudes and skills. Although the benefits of initiating service learning in a curriculum may seem overwhelmingly positive, challenges reported by faculty are worth noting: They may include lack of financial support, lack of time for planning and implementing, lack of administrative support, and lack of faculty interest (Anderson & Pickeral, 1998).

Piloting service learning into an elective course may be the simplest way to begin (Frawley, 2013). Because multiple community partners are typically needed, it may be easier to begin small. When the service experience is a required component of a large teaching program, a pilot program can help identify logistical challenges and determine necessary resources. To meet health professions accreditation criteria, site visits and assessments may play a significant role.

Preparation

When preparing materials for the curriculum committee, course objectives must align with curriculum outcomes. The program and the amount of academic credit offered should be in proportion to the time spent on the activity. When deciding where the course best fits in the curriculum, it is important to consider students' base knowledge and skill level. Course objectives that are related to communication skills, cultural sensitivity, knowledge of health disparities, or enhanced awareness of social determinants of health are easily realized with service learning experiences.

Consideration should also be given to an institution's time commitment to a particular service learning project. Some community partners (both domestic and international) may offer concentrated, finite experiences to the student but long-term care to an underserved community. A domestic example of this may be a program that trains students to perform oral health risk assessment in preparation for an annual 2-day dental clinic that gives free care to thousands in the community. An international example may be a partner that offers a yearly 5-week elective clinical rotation in global medicine to a clinic that serves five villages with one health care provider. Both experiences are intensive and mutually beneficial, providing a service learning experience to the student while meeting a community need.

This type of experience is in direct contrast to longitudinal service experience, which allows students to grow more familiar with the community they are serving and to build on existing skill sets. For example, a school may offer expanding levels of multiyear community service learning elective courses. The first and second years of the course may serve to build a strong base of history taking and physical exam skills. The third and fourth years may introduce the development of managerial skills, patient education, and advocacy. Upon graduation, students are well prepared to manage an entire clinic, advocate for patient rights, and become rapid change makers when they identify communities with unmet needs (Pelletier, 2016).

Building Relationships

The key to success of any well-designed service learning program is having and maintaining solid relationships within the community (Civic Engagement and Service-Learning, University of Massachusetts Amherst, 2016). Part of the preparation for implementing service learning projects may be initiating and nurturing relationships with community agencies that have expressed a desire to partner. Understanding their needs from the beginning is the key to effective planning and long-term success. Project goals identified by the community and adopted by the educational partner have stronger potential for impact, success, and sustainable relationships. There are many potential community partners:

- Homeless shelters
- Soup kitchens/food banks
- Faith-based organizations: Catholic Charities, Lutheran Social Services
- Service organizations: Rotary, Lions, Kiwanis clubs
- Charitable organizations: Salvation Army, United Nations Children's Fund (UNICEF), Volunteers of America

Constant communication is essential to maintaining these relationships. Because the communities that are served persist and the student flow is dynamic, it is important to build foundational relationships between faculty and a designated community liaison who will remain with the program. Memoranda of understanding (MOU) are often required before providing any service, such as free health care, at a community site or church. An MOU will commonly outline the following: (a) release the community organization of any liability for the specifically outlined services rendered, (b) describe the intended services to be delivered, (c) declare who will be eligible for the services, and (d) define the requirements of the partnering organization. Most academic institutions have standard MOUs that are adaptable to the community they are serving. Including community partners in satisfaction surveys as well as sharing year-end statistics with them can be a powerful tool and asset for their fund-raising efforts as well. Not only are community partners required to report collaborative projects with their stakeholders, but sharing of data often identifies other community needs as well. Open, frank discussion can plant the seed for future collaborative projects fostering new partnerships that encourage the campus–community relationships initiated by service learning activity to thrive.

TYPES OF SERVICE LEARNING ACTIVITIES

Developing meaningful activities is mandatory for service learning. Site selection for these activities is most important to provide experiences that allow students to meet course objectives. There are four primary types of service learning activities educators can implement: direct, indirect, research, and advocacy (Colorado State University, 2016). Who is served and how the service is rendered distinguishes the different types of projects. Selecting the type of service learning activity, therefore, will depend on the course objectives and outcomes desired.

Direct

Direct service learning opportunities require contact with the person being served. It includes person-to-person, face-to-face service projects in which the students' service directly impacts individuals who receive the service from the students (University of Central Arkansas, 2016).
   Examples include:

- Offering free physical therapy to the elderly
- Assisting a physician in a rural Tanzanian clinic that serves many villages
- Demonstrating proper toothbrushing techniques to elementary-school-aged children

Indirect

Indirect service learning opportunities require students to work behind the scenes and they do not have direct contact with the community they are affecting. This includes working on broad issues, environmental projects, or community development projects that have clear benefits to the community or environment, but are not necessarily helpful to the individually identified people with whom the students are working. Indirect activities in service learning are just as valuable as the direct service provided. Indirect activities may leave behind a tool that is useful well beyond the service provided by the student (University of Central Arkansas, 2016). Examples include:

- Establishing a medication formulary for a local community center
- Developing patient education videos in American Sign Language for the hearing impaired
- Creating informational pamphlets for a free clinic

Indirect service learning projects will likely involve direct contact with the community partner in helping to guide the development of resources that are practical for the target population to use. Indirect activities may require substantial planning and collaboration between the community agencies/sites and the health professions school, and should include input from the site, preceptors, and supervisors. When developing successful indirect activities, university leadership should ensure that the activity benefits are long-lasting.

Research

Research service learning opportunities require students to collaborate with a community partner to gather information regarding a particular interest or concern. This type of research lends itself to a robust curriculum that combines authentic research, opportunity for assessment, and real-time impact on community partners (Steinberg, Bringle, & Williams, 2010). Examples include:

- Collecting food-access data from local communities
- Collecting data from health care providers about their attitudes toward human trafficking in the community
- Collecting data for a hospital to help reduce *Clostridium difficile* infections

In addition to collaborating with a faculty mentor, students will learn how to navigate through an institutional review board process, ensuring that the ethical considerations required for defined special populations are accounted for in the study design and execution.

Advocacy

Involving students in social justice advocacy was a major net effect goal of service learning promoters such as Dewey (1938). This aligns with the inherent responsibilities of health care providers to be advocates for their patients. Students are encouraged to lend their personal voices, writing abilities, and talents to impact change for patients who might otherwise not have a voice. Examples include:

- Providing additional information for a patient who is trying to decide whether or not to accept a treatment plan
- Handing out human trafficking awareness cards to fellow health care providers
- Organizing a trip to the state government to raise awareness about medical concerns in your community

STAFF DEVELOPMENT

Although service learning presents excellent opportunities for both teachers and learners to broaden their experience outside the traditional classroom, it is important to acknowledge that unfamiliar tasks commonly associated with the development of a project or course can be cause for resistance from fellow faculty and administration (LeCrom, Pelco, & Lassiter, 2016). Service learning projects and courses require development of community partnerships as well as an extensive amount of planning and preparation of curricula and creative assessment tools. In an assessment by LeCrom and colleagues (2016) regarding the faculty emotions felt during the process of service learning courses, it was apparent that the emotional gratification and witnessed success of students must be balanced with the potential for administrative tasks and burnout. Without deep departmental support, course sustainability may not last past the enthusiasm of the initial faculty course developer.

Preparation of interested staff members allows for improved planning and execution of the service learning project (Bennett, Sunderland, Barleet, & Power, 2016). It allows for potential pitfalls to be identified early and for clear student expectations to be defined prior to the project's initiation. The development of a faculty toolkit can help keep large amounts of service learning information organized for staff to reference during the development and implementation of their project/course. Resources for the development of a toolkit can be garnered from trusted organizations such as the Corporation for National and Community Service (2008), which addresses fundamental information about service learning as a teaching technique and special population considerations. One-hour lunch-and-learn opportunities, half-day or full-day workshops can be offered to staff to help faculty move through the process of initial idea to project development with a well-planned student assessment tool. One program enabled faculty to find a peer mentor to encourage collaboration of interests, support ideas, and celebrate successes (Bennett et al., 2016).

Often, the best service learning projects are ones that stem from a passion found within a specific faculty member or student. An active champion of a cause can provide critical practical information about a population or community partner that allows for the development of a meaningful project. Engaging community partners by developing community advisory boards or as active members of the project development and execution is more likely to result in a positive experience for all associated parties and the target population.

DEVELOPING ASSESSMENTS

Within service learning, there exists a variety of activities to enhance student experiences. It is, therefore, important that the service learning assessment be structured for optimal learning to occur. Three different tools used for assessing the service learning experience are reflection, portfolios, and written exams.

Reflection

The traditional method for service learning assessment is reflection, which has been an effective model used in community teaching experiences within the United States to allow students to better understand diverse populations, cultures, and health care disparities (Nickman, 1998; Piper, DeYoung, & Lamsam, 2000). The general effectiveness of reflection is based on the principle that learning does not necessarily occur as the result of experience itself, but rather as a result of reflection designed to achieve specific outcomes (Jacoby, 2015). In order to be effective, reflection principles should embody the four Cs—continuous, connected, challenging, and contextualized. *Continuous* reflection means that the work, readings, and critical evaluation occur before, during, and after the experience. It must also be *connected* to theory, the social determinants of health, and course objectives. It must *challenge* the student to think critically, continually ask questions, and look at situations in new ways to gain perspective. And finally, reflection must be *contextualized*. It should move the student from doing to thinking and should be meaningful in relation to his or her experience.

Portfolios

A portfolio is another method of assessment and is a collection of student handiwork that represents the student's achievements, growth, and products. Portfolios used for assessment purposes may also include a measurement on the impact of the portfolio itself upon student learning. (Carraccio & Englander, 2004; Plaza, Draugalis, Slack, Skrepnek, & Sauer, 2007). This is particularly important in the context of service learning. Outcomes, such as professionalism, are difficult to assess using traditional methods. As an assessment tool, portfolios help to guide future learning, provide reassurance, promote reflection, shape values, reinforce motivation, and inspire students to set higher standards for themselves (Zubizarreta, 2009).

Once the learning goal for the portfolio is identified, the "evidence" is collected to demonstrate progress toward the specified goal. Examples of potential pieces of evidence for a portfolio might include:

* Patient care plans/notes and letters
* Videotaped encounters
* Needs assessments/surveys
* Peer assessments

Students are encouraged to reflect on the evidence presented in the portfolio and include these reflections in their portfolio. Grading portfolios by rubric is common wherein the following questions are answered: (a) Did the portfolio meet the specified goal? (b) Did the evidence support the specified goal? (c) Were the four Cs of reflection met? (d) Was the format organized and the material punctual?

Written Exams

The didactic component of service learning is critical as credit is given for the learning. Required readings with quizzes and written exams allow for the assessment of knowledge gained in service learning. Examples of required readings include portions of *Healthy People 2020* for students who are participating in the promotion of wellness (Office of Disease Prevention and Health Promotion, 2016).

FUNDING FOR SERVICE LEARNING

Service learning project costs can vary from marginal fees for office-supply use to thousands of dollars in annual expenditures, depending on the size and longevity of the project. Many larger institutions have administrative offices to help with the financial support of smaller initiatives in the form of small internal grants. This type of grant tends to range in size from $500 to $1,500 and is solicited via a grant application process. Many institutions require that the service learning project reflect at least one area related to the mission and vision of the organization (Duncan, 2014; Office of Community Engagement, Virginia Commonwealth University, 2016; School of Medicine & Health Sciences, 2016).

Faculty wishing to incorporate service learning into their curriculum may not have the advantage of having an internal grant as seed money for their project. It may be advisable, therefore, to consider the community partner(s) involved in the proposed project and to develop relationships with community stakeholders who may be able to assist in the creation of a funding opportunity. It is important to remember that many effective service learning projects do not require monetary donations, but rather the cultivation of in-kind donations of time and resources for interested community partners. Developing relationships with an institution's business or development office can help determine whether in-kind donations may be eligible for a tax benefit.

CONCLUSIONS

Service learning is a powerful pedagogical tool that, if implemented properly, can positively influence the health professions student, the faculty and institution, as well as the community it serves. As service learning in health professions education has moved from a recommendation to an accreditation requirement in some disciplines, educators may find themselves overwhelmed by the challenge. Extensive planning and preparation must occur for successful execution of a service learning project. Equally important is the initiation and maintenance of ongoing community relationships. Yet, if educators can view learning as an experience that can meet a community need, the classroom will not only come alive but active learning will occur as well. Consideration of time commitments, course objectives, and desired outcomes will affect the type of service learning activity selected; whereas the choice of an appropriate method of assessment will enhance the student's experience. In addition, service learning programs offer opportunities for faculty scholarship. Thorough preparation for service learning projects and consistent faculty development before, during, and after a project are key elements of successful service learning programs. Finally, the funding needs for service learning projects vary greatly. Grant funding may partially or fully offset costs; and creative collaborations with community agencies can often provide the necessary resources.

REFERENCES

Anderson, J. B., & Pickeral, T. (1998). Challenges and strategies for success with service-learning in pre-service teacher education. *Service Learning, General*. Paper 17. Retrieved from http://digitalcommons.unomaha.edu/cgi/viewcontent.cgi?article=1021&context=slceslgen

Astin, A. W., Vogelgesang, L. J., Ikeda, E. K., & Yes, J. A. (2000). How service learning affects students. *Higher Education, 144*(3), 35–36. Retrieved from http://digitalcommons.unomaha.edu/slcehighered/144

Bennett, D., Sunderland, N., Barleet, B., & Power, A. (2016). Implementing and sustaining higher education service-learning initiatives: Revisiting Young et al.'s organizational tactics. *Journal of Experiential Education, 39*(2), 145–163.

Billig, S. H. (2000). The effects of service learning. *Service Learning, General*. Paper 42. Retrieved from http://digitalcommons.unomaha.edu/slceslgen/42

Busch, D. (2016). A brief history of service-learning. Retrieved from http://www.socialchange101.org/history-of-service-learning

Carraccio, C., & Englander, R. (2004). Evaluating competence using a portfolio: A literature review and web-based application to the ACGME competencies. *Teaching and Learning in Medicine, 16*, 381–387.

Civic Engagement and Service-Learning, University of Massachusetts Amherst. (2016). Service-learning: Building relationships with community organizations. Retrieved from http://cesl.umass.edu/SLBuildingRelationshipswithCommunityOrganizations

Colorado State University. (2016). Types of service-learning. Retrieved from http://tilt.colostate.edu/service/news/typesOfSL.cfm

Corporation for National and Community Service. (2008). Community service and service-learning in America's schools. Retrieved from https://www.nationalservice.gov/pdf/08_1112_lsa_prevalence.pdf

Dewey, J. (1938). *Experience and education*. New York, NY: Macmillan.

Duncan, L. (2014). Service Learning Grant—Office of Engagement—Purdue University. Community service/service learning grant program. Retrieved from https://slg.engagement.purdue.edu

Eyler, J., Giles Jr, D. E., Stenson, C. M., & Gray, C. J. (2001). *At a glance: What we know about the effects of service-learning on college students, faculty, institutions and communities, 1993–2000*. Nashville, TN: Vanderbilt University.

Frawley, R. G. (2013, June). *Developing a pilot program to embed service-learning in the curriculum of a Christian liberal arts college*. Regent University, Alexandria, VA. Retrieved from https://search.proquest.com/openview/36f9836ae19d13d7dcda5343e903a24b/1?pq-origsite=gscholar&cbl=18750&diss=y

Giles, D. E., Jr., & Eyler, J. (1994). The theoretical roots of service-learning in John Dewey: Toward a theory of service-learning. *Michigan Journal of Community Service Learning, 1*(1), 7.

Jacoby, B. (2015). *Service learning essentials questions answers and lessons learned.* San Francisco, CA: John Wiley.

Joyce, B. (2006). Introduction to competency-based residency education. Retrieved from http://www .acgme.org

LeCrom, C., Pelco, L., & Lassiter, J. (2016). Faculty feel it too: The emotions of teaching through service-learning. *Journal of Community Engagement and Higher Education, 8*(2), 41–56.

Nickman, N. A. (1998). Learning to care: Use of service-learning as an early professionalization experience. *American Journal of Pharmaceutical Education, 62*(4), 380–387.

Office of Community Engagement, Virginia Commonwealth University. (2016). Service-learning project small grants program. Retrieved from http://community.vcu.edu/faculty-support-/funding-/service -learning-project-small-grants-program

Office of Disease Prevention and Health Promotion. (2016). *Healthy People 2020.* Retrieved from https:// www.healthypeople.gov

Parsi, K., & List, J. (2008). Preparing medical students for the world: Service learning and global health justice. *The Medscape Journal of Medicine, 10*(11), 268.

Pelletier, S. G. (2016, September 27). Service-learning plays vital role in understanding social determinants of health. *AAMCNews.* Retrieved from https://news.aamc.org/medical-education/article/service -learning-vital-role-understanding

Piper, B., DeYoung, M., & Lamsam, G. (2000). Student perceptions of a service-learning experience. *American Journal of Pharmaceutical Education, 64*(2), 159–165.

Plaza, C. M., Draugalis, J. R., Slack, M. K., Skrepnek, G. H., & Sauer, K. A. (2007). Use of reflective portfolios in health sciences education. *American Journal of Pharmaceutical Education, 7*(2), 34.

Savanick, S. (2015). The Science Education Resource Center at Carleton College. What is service learning. Retrieved from http://serc.carleton.edu/introgeo/service/what.html

The School of Medicine & Health Sciences. (2016). Service to the community. Retrieved from http:// smhs.gwu.edu/academics/md-program/opportunities-students/service-community

Sørensen, K., Van den Broucke, S., Fullam, J., Doyle, G., Pelikan, J., Slonska, Z., & Brand, H. (2012). Health literacy and public health: A systematic review and integration of definitions and models. *BMC Public Health, 12*(1), 80.

Steinberg, K. S., Bringle, R. G., & Williams, M. J. (2010). Service-learning research primer. Retrieved from http://csl.iupui.edu/doc/service-learning-research-primer.pdf

Stewart, T., & Wubbena, Z. (2014). An overview of infusing service-learning in medical education. *International Journal of Medical Education, 5,* 147–156. doi:10.5116/ijme.53ae.c907

University of Central Arkansas. (2016). Types of service-learning. Retrieved from http://uca.edu/service learning/types

Zubizarreta, J. (2009). *The learning portfolio: Reflective practice for improving student learning* (2nd ed.). Bolton, MA: Anker.

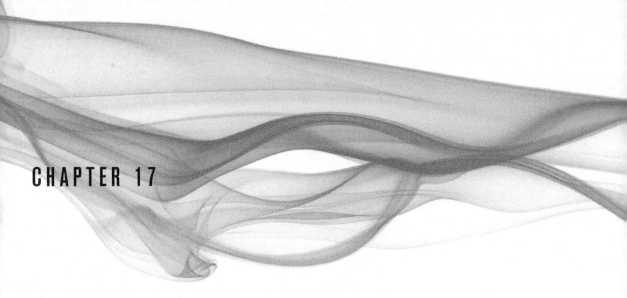

CHAPTER 17

Creating a Career Development Curriculum: Facilitating Transition to Professional Practice

Bonnie Jo Hanson and Matt Casey

CHAPTER OBJECTIVE

• Facilitate successful transitions from the student role to professional practice

---

In today's competitive marketplace, it is imperative that healthcare educators equip graduating students with negotiation skills. The art of negotiation is made up of a learned set of skills that should provide the student with the understanding that effective negotiations start with researching the market trends; focus on what value the applicant will add to the organization; consist of the applicant knowing what their deal-breakers are prior to entering into negotiations; are about learning to understand the "interests" of the parties concerned, not just their stated "positions"; and end with mutually agreeable terms.

—Madison Thompson, PA

In many health professions programs, the average age of applicants is declining (Hooker, Cawley, & Asprey, 2010). As a result, many students are now entering programs without significant prior work experience aside from any prerequired hours of direct patient care. This decline in prior work experience affects academic performance and personal characteristics necessary for career success (Scott, Patel, & Honda, 2016). Students often lack the skills needed to successfully transition from student to practicing clinician. In addition, as the health care system continues to encourage increased early specialization (despite the growing need for primary care providers), students begin to struggle with the process of career discovery while moving through their educational programs (Cassel & Reuben, 2011). Educators should provide learning opportunities for students to develop skills that will later translate into success as licensed providers (Haroun, 2016; Stiwne & Jungert, 2010). This chapter focuses on curricula that health care educators across the country are beginning to use to assist students with their transition to professional practice.

TEACHING STUDENTS HOW TO RECEIVE AND GIVE EFFECTIVE FEEDBACK

The ability to use effective feedback is an important transferable skill that benefits students in their professional lives. Many health care educators, including clinical preceptors, observe that some students' sense of entitlement affects their ability to receive and provide feedback effectively. Students who are not taught these skills will likely become professionals who lack the tools to provide meaningful peer reviews, to participate in morbidity and mortality conferences, and to conduct or respond well to annual evaluations (Anderson, 2012). It is thus imperative that health care educators incorporate feedback skills into the curriculum and ensure continuity of effective feedback throughout students' educations. However, feedback must be conceptualized as a supported sequential process rather than a series of unrelated events (Archer, 2010). Therefore, health care educators should reinforce effective feedback skills and role-model these behaviors during their encounters with students. Health professions programs also need to choose clinical preceptors who are good role models and should provide these preceptors with professional development opportunities that focus on giving and receiving feedback.

In addition, faculty members must work closely with students to help them understand that the objective of receiving feedback is to have new insights that stimulate reflection and growth. Students can be taught how to respond to difficult feedback by helping them replace behaviors that are reactive and/or defensive with behaviors that demonstrate interest in and acceptance of the information being offered. Exhibit 17.1 lists characteristics of effective feedback.

EXHIBIT 17.1 Characteristics of Effective Feedback

- Clear and specific
- Timely and immediate
- Carried out in private and with respect
- Focused on an observed behavior
- Solely about the individual receiving the feedback
- A tool that encourages self-reflection and evaluation
- Simplified and delivered slowly
- Focused on what can be changed by focusing on a specific action (e.g., what was said or done)
- Balanced
- Given frequently
- A method that recognizes that all learners can improve something
- Done using the first person in order to communicate perception rather than ultimate truth
- A way to create additional learning opportunities
- Includes an action plan as well as a plan for follow-up feedback

THE IMPORTANCE OF SELF-BRANDING TO FUTURE PROFESSIONALS

Health care consumers make important choices every day, including which brands of medicine to buy, where and from whom they seek medical treatment, and which insurance to purchase. Even though the terms *diversification* and *self-branding* are not typically associated with career planning and the management of aspiring health care professionals, the various employers, hiring managers, and recruiters are also consumers—of talented job candidates who meet their ideal criteria (the right skills, experience, interest, temperament, and personality).

The first goal of aspiring health care practitioners is to identify what their ideal employers are seeking. Potential candidates who do not yet meet the requisite requirements may need additional education, some amount of professional experience, or to acquire new skills. For those who meet those requirements, the next goal is to make their brand accessible to potential employers, who cannot hire people they do not know and cannot find (Bronstein & Cochran, 1995).

Curricula vitae (CVs) and cover letters are common branding tools, but another good way to make a student's brand accessible is to have a complete and current LinkedIn profile. Recent statistics show that 94% of recruiters use LinkedIn to vet candidates (Stadd, 2013), and LinkedIn users who keep their profiles current are 18 times more likely to be found in searches by members and recruiters (Fisher, 2016).

Finally, prospective professionals may need assistance in ensuring that their brand communicates who they are, and that they can communicate the unique value they can provide an employer and how they are distinct from other applicants.

The Value of Career Discovery

Career discovery is a lot like taking a patient history. Just as it is difficult to diagnose patients before understanding their background, current state, and symptoms, it is very challenging for individuals to identify and select the ideal job opportunity without first understanding pertinent information about themselves.

Not all positions are the same. Working in the emergency department of a large academic medical center is different from working in a rural, primary care clinic. For aspiring clinicians, evaluating their fit for a given role requires them to inventory and prioritize their skills (what can they do), interests (what they like to do), work styles (how they like to work, and how they like others to work with them), values and motivations (what is important to them), personal attributes (how they describe themselves), and goals (the achievements or outcomes they seek). It is how the unique combination of these elements measures up against different job profiles that determine whether one role is a better fit than another.

A variety of resources are available to those seeking to provide career discovery support for their students. Higher education institutions almost always have a dedicated career services department that focuses exclusively on the career needs of students and alumni. Often it provides access to and interpretation of specific assessments designed to help students learn more about themselves. Popular examples include the Myers–Briggs Type Indicator, Strong Interest Inventory, StrengthsFinder 2.0, and SkillScan Career Drivers, but there are many others. Career services departments also offer one-on-one coaching and consulting that provide individually focused counsel, advice, and resources. Career coaches in the community may be able to offer students seminars or individual attention to assist them in their transition from student to health care professional. In addition, professional bodies, such as the Association of American Medical Colleges (AAMC), American Nurses Association (ANA), and the American Academy of Physician Assistants (AAPA), offer links to career resources.

CURRICULUM VITAE DEVELOPMENT

The CV has long been the expected, standardized, documented, and detailed inventory of a person's academic and professional experience. CVs should also be recognized as a marketing document, and their purpose is to help health care professionals secure an interview for a job or academic opportunity. CVs can help students differentiate themselves from their competitors in a number of areas. Research has shown that recruiters and hiring managers spend between 6 and 10 seconds reading a job applicant's CV (Evans, 2012). A great CV, then, should have a clean, professional format and should be intuitive and easy to read. Making key information—including contact details, job titles and dates, and relevant academic credentials—most accessible is essential.

A well-differentiated CV is also contextual and informative. Single-sentence descriptions of organizations and outcome-specific bulleted phrases and/or sentences are excellent ways to convey specifically the importance and relevance of a candidate's professionalism, leadership, and volunteer work. Finally, there is no specific length requirement for a CV; experience and relevance should dictate its length. Students who have learned to include only pertinent information while documenting their clinical work with patients will likely have the most success in drafting a CV that includes only the relevant information employers seek. This is yet another example of a transferable skill.

WRITING COVER LETTERS

Although a CV is a document designed to convey skills, experiences, and accomplishments, a cover letter is a document designed to contextualize the content of a CV and explain why this particular candidate is the best one for this specific position. Writing this letter is an opportunity for students to create a concise, interesting, individualized message that outlines who they are, what value they have and can create, why they are uniquely qualified for the position, and how they can be differentiated from other candidates.

Cover letters have no one preferred style, length, or format—no one-size-fits-all standard. However, it is important to identify any industry- or organization-specific guidelines from which to begin. The most important feature of any cover letter is that it is customized for each specific career opportunity. In today's job market, it is not uncommon for a single open position to attract hundreds of applicants. When applying among a sea of equally talented and accomplished job hunters, a student's well-written, targeted cover letter may very well land that student in a hiring manager's "yes" pile.

JOB-SEARCH STRATEGIES

It is important that students understand their career possibilities and target roles by answering such questions as "What type of organization do I want to work for?" "What quality of life do I want?" and "What options are available to me that I have not yet considered?" Asking students these questions will help them identify positions that are best connected to who they are and what they want. Once students have identified the type of role they want to pursue, the next step is to craft a job-search plan.

It is estimated that 80% of the available positions in the marketplace are not advertised at sites, such as Indeed or Monster.com (Nishi, 2013), which means that most people are competing for the same 20% of positions if they rely solely on job boards. Clearly, those odds do not favor student job seekers. Good options for locating potential jobs include organization websites, industry-specific job boards, association job pages, LinkedIn, job fairs, alumni job boards, and career services departments at educational institutions. The armed forces offer scholarships and financial assistance programs for current and aspiring health care professionals. Employers and hiring managers continue to promote job opportunities across social media platforms, including Facebook, Twitter, Instagram, and YouTube.

INTERVIEW PREPARATION AND FOLLOW-UP

The ability to understand a question, formulate a precise answer, and speak in an interesting, relevant, and professional manner is an essential part of interviewing. However, there is much more to the interviewing process than just answering questions. It is paramount that students understand the type of interview they are preparing for. There are phone screenings, one-on-one interviews, panel interviews, case interviews, and experiential interviews; each requires a degree of customized preparation and delivery (Schaefer, 2014).

How candidates present themselves—an essential element of personal branding—is often as important as how they showcase what they know. Professionally appropriate attire presents a sense of credibility, seriousness, and interest in a role before a word is even spoken. Shaking hands, making eye contact, and mirroring behavior are other examples of nonverbal communication that convey confidence and professionalism and influence interviewers' perceptions of a job candidate (Schaefer, 2014).

Like many of the topic areas discussed in this chapter, interviewing is very much a skill that can be taught and improved. Identifying possible interview questions is an excellent way to prepare students for a career conversation. Instructors, professional colleagues, and career-specific websites are possible resources for gathering information on interviewing. Mock interviews are effective ways to educate students who are unfamiliar with the interviewing process and to prepare potential job candidates for actual interviews.

A job candidate's work is not complete once the interview is over. Hiring personnel who review applicants' CVs and their interview notes to assist in decision making indicate impressive follow-up by a candidate can tip the scales in the candidate's favor (Martin, 2014). After each interview, it is customary (and highly recommended) that interviewees send to each person they met a customized and conversation-specific "thank you" message. In the past, the letter was to be handwritten and mailed, but emailed messages of appreciation are now considered appropriate.

Students should be made aware that organizations differ in how they internally handle the interviewing and hiring processes. Some organizations are clear about their hiring process and specific about their decision and response timelines, whereas others are not. For those that are not, interviewees should follow up with the organization about the status of their job candidacy in 1 to 2 weeks. Job applicants should always be professional in their correspondence with companies, because even if a candidate is not hired at this time, organizations might yet reach out regarding future job opportunities.

NEGOTIATION CONCERNING JOB OFFERS

The negotiation is the time for employers and candidates to flesh out the details of a formal job offer with terms that are mutually agreeable and beneficial. Before entering into this conversation, job candidates must be prepared with respect to certain fundamental elements: marketplace trends, expectations, and opportunities that include (but are not limited to) national and local salary expectations, and benefit options and packages offered by comparable organizations and in the community outside of the organization. Applicants should also revisit their career discovery inventory and compare how the offer aligns with their values, needs, expectations, and goals. Areas in which there is some lack of alignment are potential topics for negotiation.

Candidates should not make decisions immediately after an offer is presented. They should be comfortable telling the hiring manager or recruiter that they need time to review and prepare for a follow-up conversation. Job candidates should never be the first to disclose their salary requirements to the employer. Instead, employers should reveal to the candidate their predetermined offer so the candidate can assess whether that is an area in which to negotiate. In some states, such as Massachusetts, it is now illegal for employers to ask candidates about their current or prior salary. Note as well that a job offer is more than a salary, so it is critical to understand the entire job package before making any decisions. Job-package components might include compensation (bonus plans, deferred compensation programs), transportation allotments, relocation reimbursement and support services, leave policies, and flexible work schedules. The negotiation is complete when both parties arrive at and sign an agreement.

CHECKLIST FOR THE TRANSITION FROM HEALTH CARE STUDENT TO LICENSED CLINICIAN

As students approach graduation, many become overwhelmed with licensing, credentialing, and preparing for their boards. Health care educators play a pivotal role in easing these anxieties by providing an outline of the many transitional steps from student to employed provider. In addition, members of licensing and certification boards and question-and-answer panels involving recent alumni may be able to share pearls of wisdom concerning the process.

The tasks involved can include the following:

- Instruction on test-taking strategies for preparing for the boards
- Creation of a filing system for storing copies of transcripts, patient encounter logs from supervised clinical experiences, procedure logs for privileging, CV iterations, letters of recommendation, licensure documentation, national practice certificate, Drug Enforcement Administration (DEA) certificate, state prescribing authorization certificate, advanced cardiovascular life support (ACLS)/basic life support (BLS) certificate, immunization records, state laws and regulations, hospital credentialing packet, ongoing professional education certificates, conference syllabi, awards, contracts, malpractice certificates, records of expenses and reimbursements, and so forth
- An introduction to state laws/regulations (ongoing professional education requirements that may differ from the national certification organization requirements) and to the process for obtaining licensure
- Information on how to register for the National Provider Identifier (NPI) and for state-specific organizations such as the MassPat program
- Information on how to obtain the federal DEA and state prescription authorization certificates
- Information on what to expect regarding hospital credentialing and privileging
- Information required to understand malpractice and insurance coverage
- Information on what to expect regarding the maintenance of all licenses/certificates
- An introduction to opportunities for new clinicians to become involved in state and national organizations, as well as future leadership opportunities

If time is limited, programs may want to develop a checklist (such as "New PA Checklists," which is offered to AAPA members at this website (www.aapa.org) for their students. Such checklists should provide students who are approaching graduation a proposed order for the tasks to complete as they take their first steps toward transitioning to licensed health care providers, as well as some links to the websites of various professional organizations.

THE NATURE OF CAREER DEVELOPMENT

Work, like life, is not static. Over the course of a career, an individual's personal and professional skills, values, styles, and goals can change. Matters that influenced a job choice in someone's 20s might be very different from those that matter in one's 40s.

Career development is not something done just once. It is a holistic, repeatable, ongoing process of assessment, evaluation, implementation, and measurement to ensure that professionals are making informed choices over time. Career development is not a solitary endeavor; it requires engagement, different perspectives, and feedback from others. It involves recognizing and acting on opportunities when they arise, and knowing why choices were made.

Students should learn to take advantage of the bounty of tools, professional development options, and organizational resources available to them. Before students graduate, health care educators may consider introducing them to a variety of future leadership roles, including participation in health care organizations; research projects and quality-improvement initiatives; and positions in the fields of policy development, education, and business management. Encouraging young clinicians to invest in strategic career development can help them achieve careers that are shaped by purposeful intention and based on sound choices.

CONCLUSIONS

Teaching students medical knowledge and clinical skills is an obvious component of the formal health care curriculum. However, the health care educator's job should not stop there. Providing students with opportunities to learn skills that will help them successfully transition from students to licensed professionals is an imperative part of ensuring that the future of our profession is a bright one. As Gerald Duffy, a Northeastern University Physician Assistant Program alum (class of 2016), reflects, "There are many concepts and skills that require teaching and understanding to help for a smooth transition from student to practitioner. Career development is an essential component in propelling a student beyond the classroom and into the work environment" (personal communication, September 29, 2016).

As the competition for professional health care positions rises, prospective employers can have difficulty differentiating among applicants. Programs that invest in helping students learn how to communicate how they are unique are certain to see a rise in the percentage of their students obtaining coveted positions. Health professions educators can assist their students by integrating a career development curriculum into their programs.

REFERENCES

Anderson, P. A. M. (2012). Giving feedback on clinical skills: Are we starving our young? *Journal of Graduate Medical Education, 4*(2), 154–158. doi:10.4300/JGME-D-11-000295.1

Archer, J. C. (2010). State of the science in health professional education: Effective feedback. *Medical Education, 44*, 101–108.

Bronstein, E., & Cochran, N. (1995). Preceptor Reference Manual: Academic Year 2013–2014. Hanover, NH: Geisel School of Medicine at Dartmouth Department of Family and Community Medicine Office of On Doctoring.

Cassel, C. K., & Reuben, D. B. (2011). Specialization, subspecialization, and subsubspecialization in internal medicine. *New England Journal of Medicine, 364*, 1169–1173. doi:10.1056/NEJMsb1012647

Evans, W. (2012). Keeping an eye on recruiter behavior. Retrieved from http://cdn.theladders.net/static/images/basicSite/pdfs/TheLadders-EyeTracking-StudyC2.pdf

Fisher, C. (2016, August 3). 5 steps to improve your LinkedIn profile in minutes [Web log message]. Retrieved from https://blog.linkedin.com/2016/08/03/5-steps-to-improve-your-linkedin-profile-in-minutes-

Haroun, L. (2016). *Career development for health professionals: Success in school and on the job.* St. Louis, MO: Elsevier.

Hooker, R. S., Cawley, J. F., & Asprey, D. P. (2010). *Physician assistants: Policy and practice.* Philadelphia, PA: F. A. Davis.

Martin, E. (2014, October 22). How to follow up after a job interview. *Business Insider.* Retrieved from http://www.businessinsider.com/how-to-follow-up-after-a-job-interview-2014-10

Nishi, D. (2013, March 24). Take your search for a job offline. *The Wall Street Journal.* Retrieved from http://on.wsj.com/1QJXuaq

Schaefer, P. (2014). Expert advice: 9 tips to nail an in-person interview. Retrieved from https://www.nerdwallet.com/blog/loans/student-loans/expert-advice-ace-inperson-interview

Scott, R., Patel, D., & Honda, T. (2016, October). *Admissions variables: Predictors of PA student success?* Oral presentation at the Physician Assistant Education Association Annual Conference. Minneapolis, MN.

Stadd, A. (2013, September 10). 55% of recruiters turn to Twitter, compared to Facebook's 65% and LinkedIn's 94%. *Adweek.* Retrieved from http://www.adweek.com/socialtimes/recruiters-twitter/490440?red=at

Stiwne, E. E., & Jungert, T. (2010). Engineering students' experiences of transition from study to work. *Journal of Education and Work, 23*(5), 417–437.

PART IV

Assessment and Evaluation of Learning Outcomes

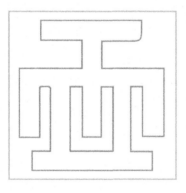

HWE MU DUA
"Measuring stick"

Symbol of examination and quality control

This symbol stresses the need to strive for the best quality, whether in production of goods or in human endeavors.

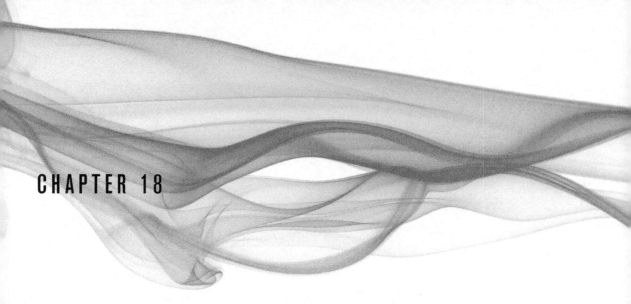

CHAPTER 18

Diverse Learner Assessment Strategies

Marie Meckel, Nadia Cobb, Aviwe Mgobozi, Evelien E. Cellissen,
Kristen Burrows, Theresa J. Riethle, and Htin Zaw Soe

CHAPTER OBJECTIVES

- Design assessments that fit diverse learning styles
- Compare qualitative and quantitative strategies for evaluating students' knowledge, attitudes, and skills, including writing assignments, standardized tests, and clinical evaluation

---

The hardest conviction to get into the mind of a beginner is that the education upon which he is engaged is not a college course, not a medical course, but a life course, for which the work of a few years under teachers is but a preparation.

—*William Osler*

Assessment of health professions students covers many domains and is deeply complex. Assessing students' knowledge, attitudes, and behavior progressively through didactic and clinical aspects of their training requires an understanding of evaluative tools, as well as how and when to use them (Schwartz, 2011). The educator must know how the qualitative and quantitative results correlate with the varied stages of learning, as well as with the end goal of graduating a competent fit-for-purpose provider who will not only provide the best care possible, serve the health care needs of communities, but also pass his or her examinations. Epstein and Hundert (2002) defined *competence in medicine* as "the habitual and judicious use of communication, knowledge, technical skills, clinical reasoning, emotions, values, and reflection in daily practice for the benefit of the individuals and communities being served" (p. 226). With the rise of competency-based medical education, learner assessment in the health professions continues to evolve. The shift to competency-based health professions education requires (a) identifying the desired outcomes, (b) clearly defining levels (e.g., milestones) of expected competencies, (c) determining an assessment rubric/framework for the competencies, and (d) using an evaluation process to determine whether trainees represent the outcome that is desired when they graduate (Academic Medicine Blog, 2015; Englander, Cameron, Addams, Bull, & Jacobs, 2015a,b; Englander et al., 2013). We see examples of competency-based education frameworks developed and subsequent assessment models implemented in medical education programs worldwide. The Canadian Physician Competency Framework (CanMEDS) has been adapted in many places globally and implemented in medical and health professions education (Frank, Snell, & Sherbino, 2015).

This chapter provides an overview of the principles of learning, as well as describes some of the common assessment tools currently used in health professions education. The tools are described through their use, domain, strengths, and challenges. New directions in assessment emerging from the evolution of person-centered health professions education are discussed, and global examples that present new options for assessment are included.

PRINCIPLES OF LEARNING

Learning is an individual process affected by multiple layers of intrinsic and extrinsic factors. These include students' learning styles (visual, auditory, kinesthetic), motivation (choice, challenge, control, collaboration, construct meaning, consequences), relationship with teachers (dependent students with expert teachers, interested students with motivating teachers, involved students with facilitating teachers, and self-directed students with delegating teachers), and personality-based preferences impacted by situational aspects (students as activists, pragmatists, theorists, or reflectors; Grow, 1991; Honey & Mumford, 2006; Khanal, Shah, & Koirala 2014; Turner & Paris, 1995). Bloom's taxonomy describes learning as occurring in three domains: knowledge (cognitive domain), skills (psychomotor domain), and attitudes (affective domain). These are hierarchal and demonstrate a developmental process. The cognitive domain begins with the lower order thinking skill of remembering and progresses through understanding, applying, analyzing, evaluating, and creating. Anderson and Krathwohl (2001) expanded Bloom's original affective domain to begin with the lower order action of receiving and to progress through responding, valuing, organizing, with characterizing at the highest order. Burch (1970s) expanded Bloom's psychomotor domain into the Conscious Competence Learning Model. The model centers on the journey from unconscious incompetence to unconscious competence. The learner starts with a lack of awareness of a skill (unconscious incompetence) and then moves through the following stages: realization of the need for the skill but failing to acquire it (conscious incompetence), acquiring the skill through practice (conscious competence), and then mastery of the skill to the point of no longer needing to think about how to do it (unconscious competence).

A useful conceptual tool for applying assessment to the stages of learning is Miller's prism (Figure 18.1), which has been adapted from Miller's original (1990) pyramid and is often used to describe assessment in medical education. Miller's prism suggests that as stages of learning become more complex, the ways in which the learner demonstrates skills (permitting observation and assessment) become congruently complex. The model integrates the aspects of attitudes, skills, and knowledge as contributors to how/whether a learner progresses to the next stage of competence.

Before considering specific assessment approaches to apply to student learning, it is important to understand the conceptual model of learning persistence. Studies have identified persistence as a critical aspect in determining academic success in minority as well as nonminority learners. Swail (2003) developed a model of student persistence and achievement demonstrating the inextricable relationships between them. Cognitive factors (academic rigor, quality of learning, critical thinking ability, study skills, time management), institutional factors (financial aid,

It is only in the "does" triangle that the doctor truly performs.

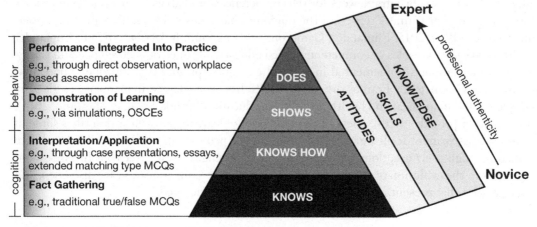

Based on work by Miller GE, The Assessment of Clinical Skills/Competence/Performance;
Acad. Med. 1990; 65(9): 63–67. Adapted by Drs. R. Mehay & R. Burns, UK (Jan 2009).

FIGURE 18.1 Miller's prism.

MCQs, multiple-choice questions; OSCEs, objective structured clinical examinations.

Source: Reprinted from Wass, Van der Vleuten, Schatzer, and Jones (2001).

student services, academic services, curriculum/instruction, recruitment/admissions), and social factors (socioeconomic issues, religious background, attitude toward learning, social coping skills, communication skills, cultural values, expectations, family/peer influence) are forces acting on all learners. The equilibrium between and among these factors and the reciprocity of various combinations shape the learning process. Stability and instability of these forces shape individual students, impacting their persistence and, thus, their academic performance (Figure 18.2). Swail's model (2003) can be used as a conceptual framework for the educator as well as the learner to better understand and meet the individual students where they are, and to provide resources to increase their persistence and achievement.

Assessment processes used in health professions education are multidimensional and curricular/instructional methodologies strive to have students gain the skills to be successful equitably.

ASSESSMENT

A first step for any health professions educator is to determine whether assessment of students is to be assessment *of* learning or assessment *for* learning. Assessment *for* learning is formative in nature. It is often used as a progressive guide for the learner, one in which reflection, feedback, shaping, and reassurance are key. Feedback that is constructive, timely, and detailed takes faculty commitment and resources. The outcome of formative assessment can help increase the learner's intrinsic motivation as well as his or her confidence and professional identity. Assessment *of* learning is summative in nature, seeking to evaluate benchmarks and assess mastery of material (Ferris & O'Flynn, 2015). Both types of assessment are important. Assessment *for* learning must necessarily come first if students are to be given a fair opportunity to develop progressively into independently practicing health care providers. Assessment *of* learning is necessary for educators to be able to fulfill their obligation to patients and society, that is, to certify that students are competent to take the next steps toward becoming independently practicing providers.

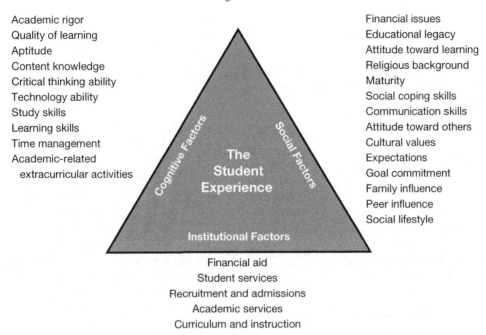

Academic rigor
Quality of learning
Aptitude
Content knowledge
Critical thinking ability
Technology ability
Study skills
Learning skills
Time management
Academic-related
   extracurricular activities

Financial issues
Educational legacy
Attitude toward learning
Religious background
Maturity
Social coping skills
Communication skills
Attitude toward others
Cultural values
Expectations
Goal commitment
Family influence
Peer influence
Social lifestyle

Cognitive Factors

Social Factors

The Student Experience

Institutional Factors

Financial aid
Student services
Recruitment and admissions
Academic services
Curriculum and instruction

FIGURE 18.2 Forces impacting student persistence and achievement.
Source: Adapted from Swail's Geometric Model (Swail, 2003).

Various assessment approaches available to educators are shown in Table 18.1. This table provides a description of assessment methods, domains that may be assessed with these methods (e.g., knowledge, attitudes, skills, and so forth), and types of assessments that can be accomplished with the methods (e.g., formative or summative assessment and other specific uses). The table also suggests the limitations and strengths of each method.

The portfolio has been used in health professions education programs as a way to gain a longitudinal, broader view of the learner's abilities, which include reflection, attitudes, as well as professionalism, in addition to the more traditional methodologies (Haldane, 2014). The portfolio is believed to show a more holistic view of the learner, demonstrating a progression in competencies in a way that enables individual strengths as well as weaknesses to be assessed. In this light, portfolios have been useful in both the formative and summative aspects of assessment. Challenges have arisen in the use of portfolios, including the intense mentor/faculty investment they require, the lack of standardization within and across disciplines/institutions, learners' variable comfort levels with the reflective aspects of portfolios as they know they are being evaluated, as well as the integration of portfolios into the educational process (Driessen, Van Tartwijk, Van Der Vleuten, & Wass, 2007).

Collaborative testing is another example of an assessment tool that has been used both in the United States and Canada. In Canada, collaborative testing has been used for more than 20 years, but it was not until 2014 that the University of British Columbia Department of Oceanic and Atmospheric Sciences actually studied its impact on learners (Gilley & Clarkston, 2014). This assessment tool has been implemented in clinical education programs as well, and an example of this can be seen at Bay Path University Physician Assistant Program in the United States. In this program, collaborative testing is done in the following manner. Physician assistant (PA) students are divided into groups of four and meet immediately after completing their individual exams. They are not allowed to interact or discuss the exam with each other until they meet as a group. One student in the group is assigned the role of moderator. This role rotates through the group to avoid dominant students from taking over the group. Students then go through the

TABLE 18.1 Methods of Assessment

Method	Domain	Type of Use	Limitations	Strengths
Written exercises				
Multiple-choice questions in either single best answer or extended matching format	Knowledge, ability to solve problems	Summative assessments within courses or clerkships; national in-service, licensing, and certification examinations	Difficult to write, especially in certain content areas; can result in cueing; can seem artificial and removed from real situations	Can assess many content areas in relatively little time, have high reliability, can be graded by computer
Key feature and script concordance questions	Clinical reasoning, problem-solving ability, ability to apply knowledge	National licensing and certification examinations	Not yet proved to transfer to real-life situations that require clinical reasoning	Assess clinical problem-solving ability, avoid cueing, can be graded by computer
Short-answer questions	Ability to interpret diagnostic tests, problem-solving ability, clinical reasoning skills	Summative and formative assessments in courses and clerkships	Reliability dependent on training of graders	Avoid cueing; assess interpretation and problem-solving ability
Structured essays	Synthesis of information, interpretation of medical literature	Preclinical courses; limited use in clerkships	Time-consuming to grade, must work to establish interrater reliability, long testing time required to encompass a variety of domains	Avoid cueing, using higher order cognitive process
Assessment by supervising clinicians				
Global ratings with comments at the end of rotation	Clinical skills, communication, teamwork, presentation, skills, organization, work habits	Global summative and sometimes formative assessments in clinical rotations	Often based on secondhand reports and case presentations rather than direct observation; subjective	User of multiple independent raters can overcome some variability due to subjectivity
Structured direct observation with checklists for ratings (e.g., mini-clinical evaluation exercise or video review)	Communication skills, clinical skills	Limited use in clerkships and residencies, a few board certification examinations	Selective rather than habitual behaviors observed, relatively time-consuming	Feedback provided by credible experts
Oral examinations	Knowledge, clinical reasoning	Limited use in clerkships and comprehensive medical school assessments, some board certification examinations	Subjective, gender and race bias have been reported; time-consuming; requires training of examiners; summative assessments need two or more examiners	Feedback provided by credible experts

(*continued*)

TABLE 18.1 Methods of Assessment (*continued*)

Method	Domain	Type of Use	Limitations	Strengths
Clinical simulations				
Standardized patients and objective structured clinical examinations	Some clinical skills, interpersonal behavior, communication skills	Formative and summative assessments in courses, clerkships, medical schools, national licensure examinations Board certification in Canada	Timing and setting may seem artificial, require suspension of disbelief; checklists may penalize examinees who use shortcuts; expensive	Tailored to educational goals; reliable, consistent case presentation and ratings; can be observed by faculty or standardized patients; realistic
Incognito standardized patients	Actual patient habits	Primarily used in research; some courses, clerkships, and residencies use them for formative feedback	Requires prior consent; logistically challenging, expensive	Very realistic; most accurate way of assessing clinician's behavior
High-technology simulations	Procedural skills, teamwork, simulated clinical dilemmas	Formative and some summative assessment	Timing and setting may seem artificial, require suspension of disbelief; checklists may penalize examinees who use shortcuts; expensive	Tailored to educational goals; can be observed by faculty; often realistic and credible
Multisource ("360-degree") assessments				
Peer assessments	Professional demeanor, work habits, interpersonal behavior, teamwork	Formative feedback in courses and comprehensive medical school assessments; formative assessment for board recertification	Confidentiality, anonymity, and trainee buy-in essential	Ratings encompass habitual behaviors; credible source; correlates with future academic and clinical performance
Patient assessments	Ability to gain patients' trust; patient satisfaction, communication skills	Formative and summative; board recertification; used by insurers to determine bonuses	Provide global impressions rather than analysis of specific behaviors; ratings generally high with little variability	Credible source of assessment
Self-assessments	Knowledge, skills, attitudes, beliefs, behaviors	Formative	Do not accurately describe actual behavior unless training and feedback provided	Foster reflection and development of learning plans
*Portfolios	All aspects of competence; especially appropriate for practice-based learning and improvement and systems-based practice	Formative and summative uses across curriculum and within clerkships and residency programs	Learner selects best case material; time-consuming to prepare and review	Display projects for review; foster reflection and development of learning plans

(*continued*)

TABLE 18.1 Methods of Assessment (*continued*)

Method	Domain	Type of Use	Limitations	Strengths
Milestones	All aspects of competence: medical knowledge, patient care, interpersonal skills/communication, professionalism, practice-based learning and improvement, systems-based practice	Formative and summative uses across curriculum and within clerkships and residency programs	Challenging to determine how detailed milestones should be; creating a very detailed tool becomes unwieldy for those performing the assessment	Outcome-based approach, integrated assessment that is multifaceted based on the progressive and incremental aspects of the learner
*EPAs (Association of American Medical Colleges, 2015)	All aspects of competence: medical knowledge, patient care, interpersonal skills/communication, professionalism, practice-based learning and improvement, systems-based practice	Formative and summative uses across curriculum and within clerkships and residency programs	Defining the activity; determining what/how aspects define ability to perform autonomously; who decides, how documented?	Address multiple competencies and skills at once—enabling assessment of entrusted activity with decreasing supervision to level of autonomy; these can be used in the Milestone model
*Collaborative assessments (Falchikov, 2013)	Knowledge, clinical reasoning, problem solving	Mostly formative, some summative uses	Building team trust and group dynamics may take some time; effectiveness depends on commitment of all team members (to show up for all team meeting and to remain engaged in the process)	Use of teams for learning enhances student learning, promotes group learning and collaboration, and increases motivation to learn; provides immediate feedback to learning; increases retention of knowledge
*OPAs (ten Cate, 2013)	Learners' knowledge, skills	Formative and summative uses across curriculum and within clerkships and residency programs	Determining which OPAs are truly useful without creating endless activities that slow and confuse the assessment process	Small units that are part of EPAs, milestones; more easily measured; help validate milestone/EPA mapping because they contain multiple OPAs
Social accountability (National Academies of Sciences, Engineering, and Medicine, 2016a; World Health Organization, 2013)	All competencies, social determinants of health, sustainable development goals	Formative and summative uses across curriculum and within clerkships and residency programs	Determining meaningful links between didactic and experiential learning and what and how to measure	Transformational in nature, reflective, meaningful connections and understanding of health rather than medicine

EPA, entrustable professional activities; OPA, observable practice activities.

*Methods with asterisks (*) are given further narrative explanation on pages 190 and 193.

Source: Adapted from Epstein (2007).

questions and, as a group, decide on the answer they believe is correct. Students are required to come to a general consensus before moving to the next question. For questions they are unsure of as a group, students look up answers individually; if they cannot find appropriate answers, they put aside those questions to discuss with an educator. Students then get feedback and guidance on the questions they have identified as unknowns. The group receives a group grade based on their answers. If the group's test score is more than 90%, then each student gets 2 extra points on the individual exam. Educators claim that the methodology gives students immediate feedback on their learning and, more important, it helps them develop skills in group dynamics and a comfort level in asking questions of each other. Studies done on collaborative testing demonstrated that this type of assessment tool enhances student learning, promotes group learning and collaboration, and increases motivation to learn (Gilley & Clarkston, 2014). Other studies done on collaborative testing demonstrated an in increased retention of course content in summative final exam (Sandahl, 2010). In general, the use of collaborative testing has had a positive impact on learners.

In 2014, the AAMC's guidelines used 13 core entrustable professional activities (EPAs) as a framework for describing necessary competencies of graduating medical students as they entered medical residency programs. The AAMC 2015 update of the core EPAs are defined as "a unit of professional practice that can be entrusted to a sufficiently competent learner or professional" (ten Cate et al., 2015, p. 983). Others have viewed the EPAs providing a method for identifying the professional competencies that require learners to progress through multiple domains to attain the highest level of Miller's prism (Mulder et al., 2010). Developing EPAs requires careful consideration of the activity's description; which knowledge, skills, and attitudes are required for the activity; what information is needed to assess progress; timeline of expected unsupervised practice; as well as the final formal determination (how many times performed, who decides, how documented). Currently, the EPAs are being piloted at 10 medical schools convened by the AAMC.

Observable practice activities (OPAs) are specifically defined elements within EPAs and milestone achievements. An example of an OPA would be demonstrate accurate medical reconciliation on a patient's chart in hospital. The EPA corresponding milestone achievement could be "management of patient medications." They represent daily activities that must be observed in order to advance professionally (ten Cate, 2013). An example of an OPA is the demonstrable ability for learners to communicate with patients in a manner that patients understand, that is, the practice of patient-centered communication (Teherani & Chen, 2014).

Over and above the adoption of any one assessment method or set of methods, Walubo and colleagues (2003) developed a tool to help guide educators to find the best assessment tools for their educational programs' needs. Each type of assessment tool (multiple-choice questions [MCQs], objective structured clinical examinations [OSCEs], short-answer questions, patient clinical examination, and oral exam) is given a score based on multiple factors. These factors include performance of the skill that is being measured (knowledge and facts recall, problem solving, communication, and practical skills), cost (human hours, materials, and cost of examiners), suitability (venue, resources, and time of exam preparation), and safety from cheating (risk of communication between candidates and probability of leakage). The scoring system allows programs and educators to determine which assessment tools may best address the factors most important to the program. For instance, if educators believe that student cheating is a major problem in their program, the scoring system will help them identify the assessment tools that are most resistant to students' ability to cheat.

The evolution of assessment options enables educators, institutions, and health professional training programs to consider learners in a different light than in the past, when MCQs provided the most prevalent (sometimes, the only) option from which to choose. Assessment processes have become much more holistic, with evidence that assessment often has secondary outcomes, such as improved team work, enhancement of learners' ability to self-assess, enriched context-specific scenarios, and reinforced retention of knowledge and skills. All students can benefit, no longer disadvantaging students from nontraditional educational paths, as well as from socioeconomic educational disadvantage.

GLOBAL EXAMPLES OF ASSESSMENT METHODOLOGIES

Diverse exemplars of learner assessment strategies can be seen from around the world. Here, we examine approaches to learner assessment in South Africa, Canada, the Netherlands, and Myanmar.

South Africa

South Africa has some of the most challenging health care issues in the world. For example, high rates of HIV and tuberculosis (World Health Organization, 2016) are complicated with the maldistribution of a health workforce within the rural areas (Shisana et al., 2009; Wilson et al., 2009). Rural recruitment and retention have been a challenge (Lehmann et al., 2008). In the late 1990s, the country introduced major reforms into its medical education to address these issues. Medical educators not only changed their recruitment and retention strategies, they also adopted new teaching tools to better suit rural underserved regions. Likewise, assessment tools were changed to better accommodate the new modes of learning. As a result, Walter Sisulu Medical School has had the following outcomes: 73% of graduates are practicing in the rural areas of the Eastern Cape and Kwa-Zulu Natal, 78% work in the public sector (full- and part-time), and 60% are in general practice (National Academies of Sciences, Engineering, and Medicine, 2016a).

Students recruited from rural underserved areas in many cases speak English as a second language and have an educational background that has not prepared them for the rigors of medical studies. A requirement was established in which students needed to demonstrate proficiency in English since medical textbooks are in English and not in indigenous languages. However, lectures in English and assessments that rely heavily on written language skills are often challenging for these students. To help address this issue, incoming students are tested for English-language skills and, if found to be weak, assistance is offered to improve these skills. Furthermore, it was decided that alternative educational and assessment tools should be employed to more fairly and effectively meet student learning needs. Thus, the program relied heavily on problem-based learning sessions to teach the different areas of medicine, and case write-ups and OSCEs were heavily used as assessment tools. These changes were implemented to accommodate the variety of learning styles to allow the program to better achieve its goal of being more inclusive. Much of the learning is based in communities similar to those from which students are recruited and to which they hope to return as health care providers. Attrition rates have dropped dramatically with the use of these new teaching and assessment tools, which are believed to have enhanced academic performance (Iputo et al., 2005). This case demonstrates how a country altered its medical and health professions training process, including assessment tools, to accommodate diverse learning styles and to include learners from disadvantaged educational backgrounds, with the ultimate outcome of increasing access to quality health care in the areas of high need.

Canada

In Canada, the McMaster University Physician Assistant Education Program utilizes assessment tools that encourage and reinforce the development of skills considered to be important for future practicing health professionals. Beginning as early as the admissions process, applicants are assessed on attitudinal and behavioral capacities by asking them to respond verbally to and thoughtfully evaluate medical ethical issues, such as doctor-assisted suicide. In coursework and clinical skills training, problem-based learning sessions incorporate the use of rubrics that assess students' abilities to address personal knowledge deficits and to work collaboratively with team members.

The Netherlands

In the Netherlands, the Dutch PA midwifery program at Rotterdam University bases its assessment on the CanMEDS competency categories, which include medical expert, communicator, collaborator, health advocate, leader, scholar, and professional (Frank & Danoff, 2007). Students build a portfolio based on all the aspects of the assessments. These portfolios are reviewed by clinical mentors over the course of the students' medical school careers. Portfolio reviews are both formative and summative in nature. Halfway through the program, students have a formative portfolio assessment of their development up to that point in time. Students who do not demonstrate developmentally appropriate progress toward master-level proficiency undergo an oral assessment conducted by two independent assessors. At the end of the program, a summative assessment is performed, again using the portfolio as the basis of this review. An exemplar of assessment rubric is available in the online supplemental materials.

Myanmar

In Myanmar's University of Community Health, Magway, the primary health professions program is the bachelor of community health (BCommH) degree course (4 years). In the first, second, and third years, students are assessed with three class tests for each subject as formative assessments throughout the academic year before final examinations. These class tests include classwork and final examinations. In the final examination, students have to sit for written (theory) and practical/viva examinations for each subject as summative assessments. Distributions of score marks in final examinations for each subject are written (50%), classwork (30%), and practical/viva (20%). A passing mark is 50% and, if a student fails in final examinations of the first year to third year, he or she has to resit for supplementary examinations 6 weeks later. In the fourth and final year, the Community Health classes are assessed by the same rubric as used in the first 3 years. For medicine and surgery, in addition to written (50%) and classwork (30%), students have to undergo bedside examinations with patients and viva in respective affiliated township hospitals, which accounts for 20% of total marks in final examinations. If they fail in final examinations, they have to resit for supplementary examinations 6 months later. After passing final examinations of the final year, they have to undergo Community Medicine Field Training for 2 months.

CONCLUSIONS

When contemplating assessment, there are many angles to explore. Why do we assess our learners (for formative or summative purposes)? What are we trying to assess (medical knowledge, skills, attitudes, behaviors, clinical reasoning, problem-solving ability, ability to apply knowledge, ability to gain patients' trust and satisfaction, social accountability, and so forth)? Once these questions are answered, one then asks, "Who should assess the students (faculty, supervisor, peer, self, multisource)?" and "What assessment methods are most appropriate (quantitative, qualitative, written, oral, individual student-based or team-based, and so forth)?" Seldom is it the case that one method or one type of evaluator will provide all the data needed to assess a learner in any single competency area. The general rule of thumb is that multiple methods and multiple evaluators will yield the best data to determine the learner's competency.

REFERENCES

Academic Medicine Blog. (2015). Retrieved from http://academicmedicineblog.org/understanding-com petency-based-medical-education/

Anderson, L. W., Krathwohl, D. R., & Bloom, B. S. (2001). *A taxonomy for learning, teaching, and assessing: A revision of Bloom's taxonomy of educational objectives.* Boston, MA: Allyn & Bacon.

Anderson, L. W., Krathwohl, D. R., Airasian, P., Cruikshank, K., Mayer, R., Pintrich, P., . . . Wittrock, M. (2001). *A taxonomy for learning, teaching and assessing: A revision of Bloom's taxonomy.* New York, NY: Longman.

Driessen, E., Van Tartwijk, J., Van Der Vleuten, C., & Wass, V. (2007). Portfolios in medical education: Why do they meet with mixed success? A systematic review. *Medical Education, 41*(12), 1224–1233.

Englander, R., Aschenbrener, C. A., & Call, S. A. (2014). Core entrustable professional activities for entering residency. *Association of American Medical Colleges.*

Englander, R., Cameron, T., Addams, A., Bull, J., & Jacobs, J. (2015a). Understanding competency-based medical education. Retrieved from http://academicmedicineblog.org/understanding-competency -based-medical-education

Englander R., Cameron T., Addams A., Bull J., & Jacobs J. (2015b). Developing a framework for competency assessment: Entrustable professional activities (EPAs), AM rounds. Retrieved from http://academic medicineblog.org/developing-a-framework-for-competency-assessment-entrustable-professional -activities-epas

Englander, R., Cameron, T., Ballard, A. J., Dodge, J., Bull, J., & Aschenbrener, C. A. (2013). Toward a common taxonomy of competency domains for the health professions and competencies for physicians. *Academic Medicine, 88*(8), 1088–1094.

Epstein, R. M. (2007). Assessment in medical education. *New England Journal of Medicine, 356*(4), 387–396.

Epstein, R. M., & Hundert, E. M. (2002). Defining and assessing professional competence. *Journal of the American Medical Association, 287*(2), 226–235.

Falchikov, N. (2013). *Improving assessment through student involvement: Practical solutions for aiding learning in higher and further education.* New York, NY: Routledge.

Ferris, H., & O'Flynn, D. (2015). Assessment in medical education: What are we trying to achieve? *International Journal of Higher Education, 4*(2), 139–144.

Frank, J. R., & Danoff, D. (2007). The CanMEDS initiative: Implementing an outcomes-based framework of physician competencies. *Medical Teacher, 29*(7), 642–647.

Frank, J. R., Snell, L., & Sherbino, J., (Eds.). (2015). *CanMEDS 2015 physician competency framework.* Ottawa, ON: Royal College of Physicians and Surgeons of Canada.

Gilley, B. H., & Clarkston, B. (2014). Collaborative testing: Evidence of learning in a controlled in-class study of undergraduate students. *Journal of College Science Teaching, 43*(3), 83–91.

Grow, G. O. (1991). Teaching learners to be self-directed. *Adult Education Quarterly, 41*(3), 125–149.

Haldane, T. (2014). "Portfolios" as a method of assessment in medical education. *Gastroenterology and Hepatology From Bed to Bench, 7*(2), 89.

Honey, P., & Mumford, A. (2006). *Learning styles questionnaire: 80-item version.* Maidenhead, UK: Peter Honey Publications.

Iputo, J. E., & Kwizera, E. (2005). Problem-based learning improves the academic performance of medical students in South Africa. *Medical education, 39*(4), 388–393.

Khanal, L., Shah, S., & Koirala, S. (2014). Exploration of preferred learning styles in medical education using VARK modal. *Russian Open Medical Journal, 3*(3), 305–312.

Lehmann, U., Dieleman, M., & Martineau, T. (2008). Staffing remote rural areas in middle- and low-income countries: A literature review of attraction and retention. *BMC Health Services Research, 8*(1), 19–28.

Miller, G. E. (1990). The assessment of clinical skills/competence/performance. *Academic medicine, 65*(9), S63–S67.

Mulder, H., ten Cate, O. T., Daalder, R., & Berkvens, J. (2010). Building a competency-based workplace curriculum around entrustable professional activities: the case of physician assistant training. *Medical Teacher, 32*(10), e453–e459.

National Academies of Sciences, Engineering, and Medicine. (2016a). *Global forum on innovation in health professional education.* Washington, DC: National Academies Press. Retrieved from http:// nationalacademies.org/hmd/Activities/Global/InnovationHealthProfEducation/2016-OCT-6 .aspx

National Academies of Sciences, Engineering, and Medicine. (2016b). *A framework for educating health professionals to address the social determinants of health*. Washington, DC: National Academies Press.

Sandahl, S. S. (2010). Collaborative testing as a learning strategy in nursing education. *Nursing Education Perspectives, 31*(3), 142–147.

Schwartz, A. (2011). Assessment in graduate medical education: A primer for pediatric program directors. Chapel Hill, NC: American Board of Pediatrics.

Shisana, O., Rehle, T., Simbayi, L., Zuma, K., & Jooste, S. (2009). *South African national HIV prevalence incidence behaviour and communication survey 2008: A turning tide among teenagers?* Cape Town, South Africa: HSRC Press.

Swail, W. S. (2003). *Retaining minority students in higher education: A framework for success* (ASHE-ERIC Higher Education Report). San Francisco, CA: Jossey-Bass.

Teherani, A., & Chen, H. C. (2014). The next steps in competency-based medical education: Milestones, entrustable professional activities and observable practice activities. *Journal of General Internal Medicine, 29*(8), 1090–1092.

ten Cate, O. (2013) Nuts and bolts of entrustable professional activities. *Journal of Graduate Medical Education, 5*(1), 157–158.

ten Cate, O., Chen, H. C., Hoff, R. G., Peters, H., Bok, H., & van der Schaaf, M. (2015). Curriculum development for the workplace using entrustable professional activities (EPAs): AMEE guide no. 99. *Medical Teacher, 37*(11), 983–1002.

Turner, J., & Paris, S. G. (1995). How literacy tasks influence children's motivation for literacy. *Reading Teacher, 48*(8), 662–673.

Walubo, A., Burch, V., Parmar, P., Raidoo, D., Cassimjee, M., Onia, R., & Ofei, F. (2003). A model for selecting assessment methods for evaluating medical students in African medical schools. *Academic Medicine, 78*(9), 899–906.

Wass, V., Van der Vleuten, C., Shatzer, J., & Jones, R. (2001). Assessment of clinical competence. *Lancet, 357*, 945–949.

Wilson, N. W., Couper, I. D., De Vries, E., Reid, S., Fish, T., & Marais, B. J. (2009). Inequitable distribution of healthcare professionals to rural and remote areas. *Rural and Remote Health, 9*(1060).

World Health Organization. (2013). *Health in the post-2015 development agenda: Need for a social determinants of health approach* [Joint Statement of the UN Platform on Social Determinants of Health]. Geneva, Switzerland: Author.

World Health Organization. (2016). TB/HIV fact sheet. Retrieved from http://www.who.int/tb/challenges/hiv/factsheets/en

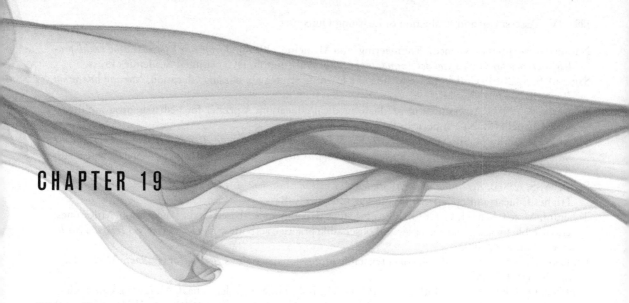

CHAPTER 19

Professionalism

April Gardner, Natalie Walkup, and Carolina Wishner

CHAPTER OBJECTIVE

- Integrate professionalism into the curriculum, including strategies for role development, assessment, and remediation of professionalism

---

The function of education is to teach one to think intensively and to think critically. Intelligence plus character—that is the goal of true education.

—*Martin Luther King, Jr.*

Teaching professionalism to future health care providers is an important task that often is inadequately covered in the formal health professions curriculum. Various studies suggest that unprofessional behaviors during training predict unprofessional behaviors in clinical practice and can lead to disciplinary sanctions from a state medical board (Papadakis, Hodgson, Teherani, & Kohatsu, 2004; Papadakis et al., 2005; Reed et al., 2008). Students report deficits in mentoring about professionalism and feelings of isolation during their education experience (Murr, Miller, & Papadakis, 2002). According to the current literature, students should be taught professionalism in both the didactic and clinical phases of their education to maximize learning experiences (Roth & Zlatic, 2009; Stern, 1998). In addition, educators need to develop expertise to engage students in learning professionalism (Shrank, Reed, & Jernstedt, 2004). There is also need for consensus about the definition of professionalism and to standardize assessment tools for measuring and monitoring professional behaviors.

DEFINING PROFESSIONALISM

No uniform definition of professionalism currently exists across the health professions. In 1995, the American Board of Internal Medicine (ABIM) developed a consensus description of professionalism for its specialty. The ABIM definition of professionalism includes six elements: altruism; accountability to patients, society, and the profession; excellence in exceeding expectations and committing to lifelong learning; duty to patients and professional organizations; volunteering, honor, and integrity in personal and professional behaviors; and respect for patients, families, and colleagues (ABIM, 1995).

Similarly, the American Association of Colleges of Pharmacy (Hill, 2000) has also developed guidelines for professional behaviors. It established 10 desired traits for professionals: knowledge and skills of a profession, commitment to self-improvement of skills and knowledge, service orientation, pride in the profession, covenantal relationship with the client, creativity and innovation, conscience and trustworthiness, accountability for his or her work, ethically sound decision making, and leadership (Popovich et al., 2011). AACP further defined professionalism as demonstrating the 10 traits of a professional, whereas *professional socialization* or *professionalization* is defined as developing professionalism in an individual by instilling the attitudes, values, and behaviors of the profession (Hill, 2000). The American Academy of Pediatrics (AAP) identified eight components of professionalism for it subspecialty: honesty/integrity, reliability/responsibility, respect for others, compassion/empathy, self-improvement, self-awareness/knowledge of limits, communication/collaboration, and altruism/advocacy (Klein et al., 2003). Using definitions and behaviors described in "Nursing: A Social Policy Statement" (American Nurses Association [ANA], 1980), the ANA *Code of Ethics for Nurses with Interpretive Statements* (ANA, 1985), and recommendations and policies from the ANA, Miller (1988) created a model for professionalism in nursing that includes behaviors such as scholarship, participation in professional organizations, autonomy, lifelong learning, and community service. Other generally acknowledged attributes for professionalism include self-reflection, awareness of one's own beliefs and culture, and respect for cultural differences.

FACTORS THAT INFLUENCE STUDENT PROFESSIONALISM

Chronic fatigue, sleep deprivation, stress, overwork and burnout, lack of confidence, lack of self-esteem, lack of experience, difficult patients, unprofessional attitudes and behaviors from educators, and unstructured or unsupervised clinical rotations were identified as factors that can negatively influence a student's attitudes toward professionalism (Schwartz, Kotwicki, & McDonald, 2009). In addition, the introduction of the Internet as a medical resource tool as well as a social media outlet brings professional challenges for students. In a small study of 56 medical student respondents reporting on Facebook use, 19% accepted friend requests from people they did not know well; 52% reported posting embarrassing pictures of themselves; and 54% reported seeing unprofessional behaviors of colleagues such as excessive alcohol use, being inappropriately unclothed, and discussions of clinical experiences with patients (Garner & O'Sullivan, 2010). Similar observations have been reported in other professions (Fang, Mishna, Zhang, Van Wert, & Bogo, 2014; Neville, 2016; Prescott, Wilson, & Becket, 2012). In a 2009 survey of U.S. medical schools deans, 60% of respondents (n = 47/78) reported unprofessional online conduct by medical students (Chretien, Greysen, Chretien, & Kind, 2009). Violations of professionalism included relaying unprofessional messages through email, social media, or a website; sexually suggestive materials, including pictures; requesting patients as Facebook friends; photographs, video, and descriptions of alcohol or substance abuse; blatant lapses in patient confidentiality; and negative comments about faculty, courses, rotations, or peers (Chretien, Greysen, Chretien, & Kind, 2009).

Stress among students can lead to unprofessional behaviors such as cynicism and academic dishonesty in addition to lower academic achievement, substance abuse, and suicide. Major causes of distress include separation from family and friends, increased academic rigor and concern for grade performance, a high-performing cohort, challenging exams, interpersonal conflicts with peers or faculty, separation from colleagues during the clinical experience, depression, burnout, patient death, student abuse, student debt, and personal or family changes in health status (Aradilla-Herrero, Tomás-Sábado, & Gómez-Benito, 2014; Dyrbye, Thomas, & Shanafelt, 2005).

ESTABLISHING PROFESSIONALISM IN A HEALTH PROFESSIONS CURRICULUM

It is important to establish a culture of professionalism, which includes faculty development in addition to student development. To be effective, professionalism must be established at matriculation, continue through the didactic curriculum, and fully extend through clinical rotations (Rivera & Correa, 2009). Students do not learn professionalism by chance, but by formal and active engagement (Gaiser, 2009). The role of the educator is to provide many learning experiences and tools to foster growth in attitudes and behaviors (Langendyk, Hegazi, Cowin, Johnson, & Wilson, 2015; Passi, Doug, Peile, Thistlethwaite, & Johnson, 2010). Professional competence should be considered using a milestone-based approach. Learners go on a journey of continued self-reflection and growth of professionalism. It is important to identify the professional attitudes and behaviors desired and then incorporate them into the curriculum. Some of the successful strategies include use of wikis, problem-based learning, faculty-led case scenarios (Lin, Lu, Chung, & Yang, 2010; Varga-Atkins, Dangerfield, & Brigden, 2010), use of reflective essays during clinical rotations (Rogers, Boehler, Roberts, & Johnson, 2012), small-group discussions of five to seven students, interactive lectures, case analyses, written exercises, role play (Rivera & Correa, 2009; Weisberg & Duffin, 1995), reflections on assigned reading, journal clubs, presentation of a prestigious annual award (Rivera & Correa, 2009), art and humanities (including poetry, drama, narrative, painting, sculpture, dance, etc.) and the humanities (Corri, 2003), CD-ROM modules (Boyle, Beardsley, Morgan, & Rodriguez de Bittner, 2007), and watching movies (Klemenc-Ketis & Kersnik, 2011).

Ceremony uses symbols, stories, feelings, and thoughts to connect people emotionally, intellectually, and physically to that which is spiritual and tradition (Neale, 2011). In medicine, the white-coat ceremony symbolizes entry into the profession and the transition from classroom learning to clinical practice (Rivera & Correa, 2009). In nursing, the pinning ceremony serves a similar purpose (Ball & McGahee, 2013; Cruz, Farr, Klakovich, & Esslinger, 2013). The University of Washington uses creative methods to develop professionalism with resident interns. Each new cohort of interns participates in a 5-day retreat with 11 sessions designed to help them manage ethical situations, assess and handle child abuse, advocate for children with special needs, and learn to work with dying patients. Each session is created to enhance learning and understanding of the eight components of professionalism identified by the AAP (honesty/ integrity, reliability/responsibility, respect for others, compassion/empathy, self-improvement, self-awareness/knowledge of limits, communication/collaboration, and altruism/advocacy). Small-group discussions, role-playing, and videotapes of difficult parent–physician discussions are used. Recent cases involving ethical issues are presented and time is allowed for residents to discuss the case. Communication and collaboration are taught through team-building skills. Residents must work together in small groups to solve a difficult situation, participate in a city-wide scavenger hunt, and prepare a meal for their small group, family, and faculty on a minimal budget (Klein et al., 2003). These ideas for a professional curriculum can be adapted to accommodate nearly any type of health professions program.

NEED FOR FACULTY DEVELOPMENT

Faculty development is often overlooked when incorporating professionalism into a curriculum. Faculty-development activities should aim at increasing knowledge and teaching skills around professionalism. Faculty should also be aware that sending subtle messages to their students about their own beliefs, both positive and negative, regarding health care culture can have a great impact on their students' professionalism. Gofton and Regehr (2006) call these subtle messages the *hidden curriculum*. They state, "We also transmit to the learner a vast array of behaviors, beliefs, and attitudes we never intended to share, nor even recognized we were imparting" (p. 20). Positive subtle messages are passed on when students hear providers congratulate a patient for maintaining achieving smoking cessation or making improvements on a goal. Providers endorse a healthy lifestyle when they indicate they are headed to the gym after their shift or are off to watch a child's soccer game. Conversely, providers convey negative messages when they complain about their schedules, colleagues, and patients. The hidden curriculum manifests in corridor conversations and comments we make to students about ourselves, our patients and their cultural or religious beliefs, other health care providers, health care reform, insurance companies, or malpractice insurance (Neutens, 2008).

Health professions educators have a responsibility to teach and model professional behaviors (Roth & Zlatic, 2009). Being a good role model is associated with listening, providing direct answers, showing respect, being trustworthy (Gaiser, 2009), creating a supportive learning environment (Passi et al., 2010), and upholding the defined values of professionalism (Shrank et al., 2004). Gaiser (2009) recommends a professionalism curriculum for faculty that includes reflective thinking and personal growth through transformational learning. Characteristics of reflective thinking include understanding that knowledge is partial and incomplete, that judgment and reasoning can be questioned, that patients are the center of a provider's considerations, that providers view themselves as a partner in the patient's care, and that the provider is able to consider personal practices and beliefs. Because transmitting the negative aspects of the hidden curriculum is unintended, assessments of professional behaviors are important. Shrank and colleagues (2004) suggest professionalism evaluations consist of student, colleague, and self-assessments in order to enhance the responsibility of the role model. Current literature suggests rewarding students and faculty with incentives for professional behavior (Rivera & Correa, 2009; Shrank et al., 2004) may add value in improving a culture of professionalism. Faculty incentives may include credit toward tenure and promotion or local or national awards for modeling professionalism.

ASSESSMENT

Assessing professionalism is challenging because professionalism is complex and evolves over time (Passi et al., 2010). Both formative and summative evaluations are important for the appropriate assessment of professionalism (Passi et al., 2010; Rivera & Correa, 2009). Assessment should begin early, be ongoing, be nurturing, and be based on clear and measurable objectives (Rivera & Correa, 2009). In the absence of a gold standard for valid and reliable assessment tools, multiple methods should be used for evaluating assessment and responses regarding student professionalism (Chisholm, Cobb, Duke, McDuffie, & Kennedy, 2006; Shrank et al., 2004).

Some of the strategies used to assess professionalism include educational portfolios, objective structured clinical examinations (OSCEs), use of patient simulation, peer evaluation, written evaluations, small-group discussions, oral presentations, written reports, self-evaluation reflective writings, oral exams, written exams, critical incident reports, global ratings, and checklists/rubrics. Professionalisms can also be assessed by formal evaluation sessions, direct observations, patient evaluation, and teamwork exercises. Other approaches include the Professionalism

Mini-Evaluation Exercise (P-MEX), attendance records, videotape analysis, interactive lectures, case analyses, journal clubs, and community service evaluation (Rivera & Correa, 2009). The 360-degree evaluation includes multiple assessments from multiple observers such as faculty, clinical preceptors, peers, physicians, physician assistants (PAs), nurse practitioners (NPs), and other medical staff (Passi et al., 2010; Reed et al., 2008; Rivera & Correa, 2009; Schwartz et al., 2009; Veloski, Fields, Boex, & Blank, 2005).

REMEDIATION AND CONSEQUENCES FOR UNPROFESSIONAL BEHAVIOR

Clear objectives for professional expectations should be developed and conveyed to students. Types of remediation and consequences for unprofessional conduct are important considerations and should be built into the professionalism curriculum prior to employing it. Remediation and consequences should be based on the offense. Strategies used in some programs include repeating a clinical rotation under a different preceptor, delivering a professionalism presentation to the matriculating class, participating in an intensive project with a preceptor committed to evaluating the project result and professional growth, stringent professionalism contract between the student and a faculty remediator, probation, and dismissal (Boyle et al., 2007). Other ideas for remediation include counseling the student, community service, nonpunitive support, documented hearings, and continued communication postremediation. Chapter 33 of this book discusses mechanisms of creating a culture of restorative justice and many of the strategies discussed in this chapter can also apply in dealing with professional challenges among students, faculty, and staff.

CONCLUSIONS

It is imperative that a culture of professionalism be built into both the didactic and clinical curriculum components of health professions education in order to develop professional students and future clinicians. A professionalism curriculum should be guided by clear objectives for professional expectations, competencies, and milestones. Health professions programs need to invest in an effective faculty–student mentorship, and should provide many learning experiences and tools to foster professional growth.

Professionalism is a process that takes time. It is important to build assessment into the curriculum to ensure that objectives are met. For individual students, assessment should begin early, be ongoing, be nurturing in quality, and be based on clear and measurable objectives. Focused remediation exercises and consequences for unprofessional conduct should be built into the professionalism curriculum prior to employing it. Consequences, such as suspension and dismissal, should be reserved for serious grievances and sequential failed remediation attempts.

REFERENCES

American Board of Internal Medicine. (1995). *Project professionalism*. Philadelphia, PA: Author. Retrieved from http://www.tau.ac.il/medicine/cme/pituach/030210/1.pdf

American Nurses Association. (1980). *Nursing: A social policy statement*. Kansas City, MO: Author.

American Nurses Association. (1985). Code for nurses: With interpretive statements. Kanses City, MO: Author.

Aradilla-Herrero, A., Tomás-Sábado, J., & Gómez-Benito, J. (2014). Associations between emotional intelligence, depression and suicide risk in nursing students. *Nurse Education Today, 34*(4), 520–525.

Ball, J., & McGahee, T. W. (2013). Dedication of hands to nursing: A ceremony of caring. *Journal of Nursing Education and Practice, 3*(10), 58.

Boyle, C. J., Beardsley, R. S., Morgan, J. A., & Rodriguez de Bittner, M. (2007). Professionalism: A determining factor in experiential learning. *American Journal of Pharmaceutical Education, 71*(2), 31.

Chisholm, M. A., Cobb, H., Duke, L., McDuffie, C., & Kennedy, W. K. (2006). Development of an instrument to measure professionalism. *American Journal of Pharmaceutical Education, 70*(4), 85.

Chretien, K. C., Greysen, S. R., Chretien, J., & Kind, T. (2009). Online posting of unprofessional content by medical students. *Journal of the American Medical Association, 302*(12), 1309–1315.

Corri, C. (2003). Medical humanities in nurse education. *Nursing Standard, 17*(33), 38–40.

Cruz, F. A. D., Farr, S., Klakovich, M. D., & Esslinger, P. (2013). Facilitating the career transition of second-career students into professional nursing. *Nursing Education Perspectives, 34*(1), 12–17.

Dyrbye, L. N., Thomas, M. R., & Shanafelt, T. D. (2005). Medical student distress: Causes, consequences, and proposed solutions. *Mayo Clinic Proceedings, 80*(12), 1613–1622. Retrieved from http://www.mayo clinicproceedings.org/article/S0025-6196(11)61057-4/fulltext

Fang, L., Mishna, F., Zhang, V. F., Van Wert, M., & Bogo, M. (2014). Social media and social work education: Understanding and dealing with the new digital world. *Social Work in Health Care, 53*(9), 800–814.

Gaiser, R. R. (2009). The teaching of professionalism during residency: Why it is failing and a suggestion to improve its success. *International Anesthesia Research Society, 108*(3), 948–954.

Garner, J., & O'Sullivan, H. (2010). Facebook and the professional behaviours of undergraduate medical students. *Clinical Teacher, 7*(2), 112–115. doi:10.1111/j.1743-498X.2010.00356.x

Gofton, W., & Regehr, G. (2006). What we don't know we are teaching unveiling the hidden curriculum. *Clinical Orthopaedics and Related Research, 449*, 20–27.

Hill, W. T. (2000). White paper on pharmacy student professionalism: What we as pharmacists believe our profession to be determines what it is. *Journal of the American Pharmaceutical Association, 40*(1), 96–102.

Klein, E. J., Jackson, J. C., Kratz, L., Marcuse, E. K., McPhillips, H. A., Shugerman, R. P., . . . Stapleton, F. B. (2003). Teaching professionalism to residents. *Academic Medicine, 78*(1), 26–34.

Klemenc-Ketis, Z., & Kersnik, J. (2011). Using movies to teach professionalism to medical students. *BMC Medical Education, 11*(60), 1–5. doi:10.1186/1472-6920-11-60

Langendyk, V., Hegazi, I., Cowin, L., Johnson, M., & Wilson, I. (2015). Imagining alternative professional identities: Reconfiguring professional boundaries between nursing students and medical students. *Academic Medicine, 90*(6), 732–737.

Lin, C. F., Lu, M. S., Chung, C. C., & Yang, C. M. (2010). A comparison of problem-based learning and conventional teaching in nursing ethics education. *Nursing Ethics, 17*(3), 373–382.

Miller, B. K. (1988). A model for professionalism in nursing. *Today's OR Nurse, 10*(9), 18.

Murr, A. H., Miller, C., & Papadakis, M. (2002). Mentorship through advisory colleges. *Academic Medicine, 77*(11), 1172–1173.

Neale, L. (2011). *The power of ceremony: Restoring the sacred in ourselves, our families, our communities*. Portland, OR. Eagle Spirit Press.

Neville, P. (2016). Clicking on professionalism? Thoughts on teaching students about social media and its impact on dental professionalism. *European Journal of Dental Education, 20*(1), 55–58.

Neutens, J. J. (2008). *The effective preceptor series: The hidden curriculum: What are you teaching?* [Brochure]. Crofton, MD: Association of Professors of Gynecology and Obstetrics.

Papadakis, M. A., Hodgson, C. S., Teherani, A., & Kohatsu, N. D. (2004). Unprofessional behavior in medical school is associated with subsequent disciplinary action by a state medical board. *Academic Medicine, 79*(3), 244–249.

Papadakis, M. A., Teherani, A., Banach, M. A., Knettler, T. R., Rattner, S. L., Stern, D. T., . . . Hodgson, C. S. (2005). Disciplinary action by medical boards and prior behavior in medical school. *New England Journal of Medicine, 353*(25), 2673–2682.

Passi, V., Doug, M., Peile, E., Thistlethwaite, J., & Johnson, N. (2010). Developing medical professionalism in future doctors: A systematic review. *International Journal of Medical Education, 1*, 19–29. doi:10,5116/ijme.4bda.ca2a

Popovich, N. G., Hammer, D. P., Hansen, D. J., Spies, A. R., Whalen, K. P., Beardsley, R., . . . Athay, J. L. (2011). Report of the AACP professionalism task force, May 2011. *American Journal of Pharmaceutical Education, 75*(10), S4.

Prescott, J., Wilson, S., & Becket, G. (2012). Students want more guidelines on Facebook and online professionalism. *Pharmaceutical Journal, 289*, 1–3. Retrieved from http://s3.amazonaws.com/academia .edu.documents/45905765/Pharmacy_students_want_more_guidelines_o20160524-28605-1501i6d.pdf? AWSAccessKeyId=AKIAIWOWYYGZ2Y53UL3A&Expires=1500868378&Signature=YoH75gLjlG fA33iS9XK1hQnf%2BGc%3D&response-content-disposition=inline%3B%20filename%3DPhar macy_students_want_more_guidelines_o.pdf

Reed, D. A., West, C. P., Mueller, P. S., Ficalora, R. D., Engstler, G. J., & Beckman, T. J. (2008). Behaviors of highly professional resident physicians. *Journal of the American Medical Association, 300*(11), 1326–1332.

Rivera, E., & Correa, R. (2009). Implementation of different initiatives to develop a culture of professionalism in the medical school. *Puerto Rico Health Sciences Journal, 8*(2), 135–139.

Rogers, D. A., Boehler, M. L., Roberts, N. K., & Johnson, V. (2012). Using the hidden curriculum to teach professionalism during the surgery clerkship. *Journal of Surgical Education, 69*(3), 423–427. doi:10.1016/j.jsurg.2011.09.008

Roth, M. T., & Zlatic, T. D. (2009). Development of student professionalism. *Pharmacotherapy, 29*(6), 749–756. doi:10.1592/phco.29.6.749

Schwartz, A. C., Kotwicki, R. J., & McDonald, W. M. (2009). Developing a modern standard to define and assess professionalism in trainees. *Academic Psychiatry, 33*(6), 442–450. doi:10.1176/appi.ap.33.6.442

Shrank, W. H., Reed, V. A., & Jernstedt, G. C. (2004). Fostering professionalism in medical education: A call for improved assessment and meaningful incentives. *Journal of General Internal Medicine, 19*(8), 887–892. doi:10.1111/j.1525-1497.2004.30635.x

Stern, D. T. (1998). Practicing what we preach? An analysis of the curriculum of values in medical education. *American Journal of Medicine, 104*, 569–575.

Varga-Atkins, T., Dangerfield, P., & Brigden, D. (2010). Developing professionalism through the use of wikis: A study with first-year undergraduate medical students. *Medical Teacher, 32*(10), 824–829. doi:10.3109/01421591003686245

Veloski, J. J., Fields, S. K., Boex, J. R., & Blank, L. L. (2005). Measuring professionalism: A review of studies with instruments reported in the literature between 1982 and 2002. *Academic Medicine, 80*(4), 366–370.

Weisberg, M., & Duffin, J. (1995). Evoking the moral imagination: Using stories to teach ethics and professionalism to nursing, medical, and law students. *Journal of Medical Humanities, 16*(4), 247–263.

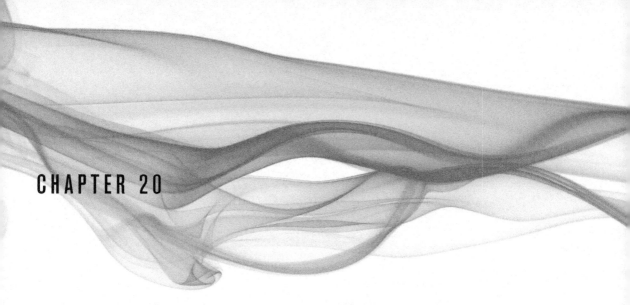

CHAPTER 20

Learner Assessment and Remediation

Jeanie McHugo

CHAPTER OBJECTIVES

- Identify students at risk
- Use best practices in the remediation process
- Design a successful remediation program

If a [student] can't learn the way we teach, maybe we should teach the way they learn.

—Ignacio "Nacho" Estrada

As discussed in preceding chapters, a multifaceted approach to learner assessment, including a wide array of methodologies, is critical to fully understanding the abilities of a student. Determining capability for clinical practice requires students to successfully complete the predetermined criteria defined by a professional body and interpreted by each educational institution. The ultimate goal for all involved is to ensure safety in medical practice. It is inevitable that a small proportion of students will struggle and perform poorly on various aspects of the learner assessment process. This is a concern for educators as student performance on program-related assessments often predicts subsequent performance on national certification board exams and clinical competence during medical practice thereafter. Retrospective studies of physicians disciplined by licensing boards have shown a prior history of academic performance difficulties during training (Cleland et al., 2013). Although this correlation has not been studied in other health professions, this pattern strengthens the case for early identification of underperformance.

From a broad perspective, federal experts are concerned about the current educational system and the acceptance of mediocrity (Maize et al., 2010, p. 1). Students are expected to perform as motivated adult learners who possess self-study skills to be successful in advanced degree programs. However, research suggests that students have not obtained the study and self-management skills within their earlier education to be successful in professional degree programs (Maize et al., 2010, p. 1). As stated by Winston, van der Vleuten, and Scherpbier (2010), education literature provides reasons why students struggle, which include problems with "time management; overreliance on passive learning; insufficient background and content knowledge; weakness in literacy, numeracy and study skills, test-taking strategies or critical thinking; and a general lack of the self-regulatory and metacognitive skills that are correlated with academic success" (p. 1039).

Accreditation standards require that health professions programs must have a published policy regarding grading, progression, remediation, and graduation requirements and provide documentation of identified deficiencies, remediation efforts, and outcomes (Accreditation Council for Pharmacy Education [ACPE], 2016; Accreditation Review Commission on Education for the Physician Assistant [ARCPA], 2016; Commission on Collegiate Nursing Education [CCNE], 2013; Liaison Committee on Medical Education [LCME], 2015). It is the role of the faculty member to help all learners reach their maximum potential; however, training and guidance on how to remediate struggling learners is severely lacking, and oftentimes, the remediation process is left to faculty availability and interest.

The approach to remediation needs to be individualized and targeted toward areas of weakness, with the goal of maximizing the potential of the learner (Guerrasio, 2016). Educators struggle to accurately and rapidly identify, diagnose, and remediate learners. There is uncertainty reported by faculty members regarding the efficacy of the remediation interventions, making outcome analysis difficult. Conclusions of several studies indicate the need for a rigorous approach to developing and evaluating remediation interventions (Cleland et al., 2013). A successful remediation process needs to fully challenge the student's concept of learning and must consider a blend of cognitive, behavioral, and affective factors (Winston et al., 2010, p. 1038).

LEARNING TO LEARN

An approach to prevention and a response to underperforming students is a focus on learning how one learns. For example, learners tend to spend too much time focusing on rote memorization, which will not facilitate critical thinking (Strout & Haidemenos, 2016). Taking the time earlier in the professional academic journey to study how one learns has the potential to prevent the cycle of underperformance characteristics of many struggling students. Frequently, struggling students have negative feelings and beliefs of low self-efficacy that directly influence their motivation to persist when learning becomes difficult. Students in this situation need to feel success early on in their struggles so that they feel a sense of control and confidence in their learning and subsequent academic performance. Furthermore, the change in focus of education, to include assessment of how each student learns, would enable a more accurate diagnosis of underperformance (Cleland et al., 2013). It is interesting to note that McGann and Thompson (2008) found that "students younger than 25 years of age often lacked effective learning strategies and were reluctant to access on-campus learning support" (p. 2).

According to Winston and colleagues (2010), an approach that focuses on active learning through collaboration, dialogue, self-direction, and reflection is found to be helpful. In the study, groups of six students met weekly throughout the semester to discuss study and reasoning skills, time management, strategies for integrating basic science material, as well as test taking and critical thinking. These students found the most useful aspect of the program was learning how to actively work with and organize lecture material; learning from test items and test-taking skills; and learning time management, general study skills, and critical thinking. Changes in ways to think and study allowed students the opportunity to recognize that their deficiencies lie in a combination of skills that led them to take a more active and involved approach in their learning.

They were able to "understand concepts as relationships, integrate the content of their various courses, and apply their knowledge in different contexts" (Winston et al., 2010, p. 1042). Furthermore, students identified the importance of attitude and motivation tied with their development as flexible, reflective learners in the learning process and were able to demonstrate increased accountability for their learning. Students identified the role of a teacher to be a combination of "rigorous expectations, facilitation skills, and honesty" (Winston et al., 2010, p. 1042) in pointing out deficits in study habits. Strategies for increasing active learning in the curriculum are covered in depth in Chapters 6, 7, and 8.

IMPORTANCE OF REMEDIATION

It is important to understand that deficiencies in learning often do not resolve without some aspect of intervention. Without intervention, underperforming learners eventually impact patient care, including patient satisfaction, patient safety, and overall quality of care. That said, it is our obligation to teach all of our learners, not only those who we feel are easier to teach, more enjoyable to teach, who are self-directed and can teach themselves, or with whom we have more in common. The best teachers are those who inspire achievement in all their students. They think not only about the individual student's problems but also about those problems in curriculum design that may be contributing factors to student deficiency (Bain, 2011).

There is a responsibility to self-monitor our professions—as educators, we are best qualified to assess the performance of our students and future clinicians. Preserving the integrity of our professions by preparing, evaluating, and providing remediation for our future colleagues is extremely important (Guerrasio, 2013).

PROGRESSION POLICIES, PREVENTIVE MEASURES, AND ACADEMIC RESOURCES

Clearly defined progression policies are intended to preserve the high academic standards dictated by the profession and thus the professional program. These policies define when a student cannot proceed in the curriculum and must remediate repeat portions of the curriculum and/ or be dismissed from the degree program. Academic progression policies vary among institutions and even among professional programs within the same institution. Because of the variability between didactic and clinically based learning experiences, policies can even vary among educational settings (Maize et al., 2010). According to McHugo (2017), a sample academic progression policy may read something like this:

Advancement through the program is based on the demonstration of the student's ability to master the content, skills, and professional behaviors consistent with the program's expectations and competencies. These expectations are delineated in the Policy and Procedure document, the Program Goals and Outcomes, and in course and lecture objectives. It is understood that a student must successfully complete all sequential coursework with a passing grade as defined previously prior to beginning the next curricular session. (pp. 20–21)

Policy contributors will have to determine how far to let student performance go before intervening with a remediation process. Discussion is needed at the faculty level to determine what is a passing score and whether there should be remediation offered after each poorly performed exam, after critical step exams, or after scoring low at the end of the entire course. If remediation is offered, then should it be a few days after or a few weeks after the failed exam and what will be a passing score? What happens in regard to clinical remediation and how is it similar to or different from didactic remediation? The remedy lies in the correct identification of the deficiency. These answers become complex as they may be different for an anatomy exam compared to a clinical medicine exam, clinical testing process, or clinical reasoning during patient involvement. Literature does not support best practice evidence to answer these questions and future research is needed in these areas.

Remediation Begins With Admissions

Preventing the need for remediation requires a review of the admission process. Theoretically, programs that intentionally seek to admit the most highly qualified students by identifying essential characteristics as accurate predictors of student success will have fewer underperforming students. These essential characteristics include both cognitive and noncognitive traits. Although grade point average (GPA) and graduate record exam (GRE) scores may be strong cognitive indicators of academic success, a holistic review also includes noncognitive qualities such as motivation, ethics, communication, responsibility, and professionalism. Most programs require a complex mix of both academic and nonacademic admission assessments to ensure selection of the most qualified candidates, thus minimizing the need for remediation (Maize et al., 2010, p. 2).

Addressing Academic Factors

Academic factors considered most important for retention and success in learning include personal study skills, study location and hours, class schedule comparative to personal focus level, and access to academic services. Limited time management skills, poor self-awareness, and inadequate social support are common barriers for students (Corrigan-Magaldi, Colalillo, & Molloy, 2014, p. 155). Although some of these aspects may not be changeable, information on how to efficiently use time and resources can be helpful. Academic success centers, library services, tutor resources, counseling, and disability support centers are essential resources for student referral and should be part of the remediation plan. These resources are typically covered by student fees and are often underutilized, as students may feel stigma associated with using them. Faculty members need to recommend and encourage struggling students to capitalize on provided resources. Directing students to the availability and use of academic support programs during new-student orientation can normalize and destigmatize their use.

IDENTIFICATION AND DIAGNOSIS

Successful remediation programs identify learning style strengths of participating students and employ a variety of active learning activities. This may include such things as web-based activities, summer restudy programs, performance reviews, practice with standardized patients, clinical observation and feedback, tutoring, and/or retesting (Corrigan-Magaldi et al., 2014; Hauer, Teherani, Irby, Kerr, & O'Sullivan, 2007; Maize et al., 2010). Assisting students to become more actively involved and motivated in their studies by implementing a variety of learning options allows for integration of experiential learning and technology. Faculty become the facilitators of the process as they mentor in promoting student success by providing an interactive, caring, and positive learning environment for students (Corrigan-Magaldi et al., 2014).

Because of the variability of potential deficits between students as well as the possibility of multiple deficits within a learner, it can be challenging for educators to identify underperforming learners and isolate an area of deficiency. Thus, an effective approach to remediation must include an assessment of the learner's competence, diagnosis of the deficiency, and development of an individualized learning plan that incorporates deliberate practice, feedback, reflection, and ultimately focused reassessment (Guerrasio, Garrity, & Aagaard, 2014, p. 352).

A Structured Approach to Remedial Assessment

Guerrasio (2013) has identified the need for a semistructured intake interview with each struggling learner. Addressing competencies based on the work of the Accreditation Council for Graduate Medical Education (ACGME), learning areas explored with the student include medical knowledge, clinical skills, clinical reasoning and judgment, time management and organization, interpersonal skills, communication skills, professionalism, practice-based learning and improvement, and systems-based practice (Guerrasio, 2013, p. 19). Using an interview guide, students are active participants in the deficit identification process (Guerrasio et al., 2014). Students need to be asked to identify strengths and things they should have done differently to ensure active engagement in a reflective process about what went well and what did not go so well (Hauer et al., 2007). If the student is unable to reflect appropriately, then remediation toward self-awareness and self-motivation need to be included in the plan (Guerrasio, 2013, p. 23). Competencies addressed with this approach can be tailored to those specific to various health professions.

The interview process needs to be transparent, instilling trust in the process. Learners want to know who knows of their struggles and what has been shared. It is important to destigmatize the problem by sharing with the learner, using unidentifiable information, how many others have been through this process and how they have continued to be successful in their career goals. It is also important to reflect on one's own level of transference in working with the student as well. Bringing implicit bias into awareness and separating one's own feelings from the situation are imperative in determining whether responses or actions are intended for the purpose of improving student performance (Guerrasio, 2013).

Using a Team Approach to Remediation

Often, more than one faculty member is involved in a remediation plan. In fact, some institutions develop a "success team," which may consist of the learner, a remediation specialist, a faculty member from the program, a mental health professional, and the student affairs dean or program director (Guerrasio et al., 2014). The team approach helps to objectively identify mechanisms to maximize remedial processes to maintain consistency and benefit a growing number of struggling learners without overburdening one or two faculty members. Then, the team works together to implement a remediation plan to address the identified deficit (Bierer, Dannefer, & Tetzlaff, 2015). The involvement of the student in this process is essential. Following the intake discussion, the student works with the team to identify the targeted areas of improvement and takes an active lead role in suggesting effective learning activities suitable to the learning style to construct a remediation plan. This team works with the student to ensure the plan is appropriate for the deficit(s) and the outcomes are measurable and sets due dates for progress reports. Regular meetings and frequent communication with the team ensure continued progress of the remediation plan (Bierer et al., 2015).

THE LEARNING PRESCRIPTION

The team must fully explore the potential for deficits, which may include multiple areas, and identify remedial activities for each deficit. The learning prescription is a one- to two-page analysis of performance specifically describing areas of strength, major areas of improvement, and case-specific comments (Chang, Chou, & Hauer, 2008, p. 1118). Each remediation plan must include deliberate practice, timely and regular feedback, and an assessment portion allowing the learning to reflect on his or her performance. Recommendations for change in the future are discussed, and, if reassessments are necessary, it is important to seek out additional assistance from other departments that are unaware of the learner's remediation status and perform routine aspects of the course or clinical experience (Guerrasio et al., 2014; Hauer et al., 2007).

According to Guerrasio (2013), there are many resources that can be used to obtain information about the performance of a struggling learner. The following information summarizes the resources that will help narrow the differential diagnosis and identify specific deficits:

- **Direct observation:** Ability to collect history, perform a physical exam, and collect additional patient information; efficiency; task prioritization; responsiveness to colleagues and other health care team members; interactions; and ownership of patient care
- **Presentation/rounds:** Integration of information; representation of the problem; formulation of differential diagnosis, assessment, and plan; ability to summarize the case; and formulation of questions
- **Interview the learner:** Review reading materials; explore social stressors and mental health; substance use/abuse; and gain learner's perspective
- **Other sources:** Chart review; arrival/departure time; 360-degree evaluations; multiple-choice exams; clinical skills exams; and patient/procedures logs.

In addition, Guerrasio (2013) provides key notable problems associated with each competency, which are helpful in determining the deficit(s). These are summarized in Table 20.1.

Although the most common deficits are found in medical knowledge, clinical reasoning, and professionalism, many students have multiple deficits and remediation must be prioritized to those deficits that are most severe. Often when one deficit is remediated, the others improve, but care must be taken to monitor growth and progression of all identified deficits (Guerrasio, 2013). Elements of remediation programs overlap extensively to include cognitive and affective behaviors. Students often need to identify themselves as "repeaters" and deal with self-esteem when accepting responsibility for their underperformance. They need to become active, flexible, and reflective learners who understand the complex interplay between their learning and their environment (Winston et al., 2010).

FACULTY FRAMEWORK AND EVALUATOR ROLE

Setting a Framework for Remediation

One of the key findings in remediation literature is the lack of a theoretical foundation to many remedial interventions. Faculty assigned to assist troubled learners feel unsure about how to develop an effective plan and adequately assess related outcomes without creating "more of the same" (Audetat, Laurin, & Dory, 2013, p. 230). Kalet, Guerrasio, and Chou (2016) have identified "twelve tips for best practices" (p. 787). These best practices are broadly categorized as (a) program vision and structure, (b) faculty roles and development, and (c) accountability and outcomes. They are summarized in Table 20.2.

Clearly define the role of the facilitator to provide learner feedback, review specific expectations, provide examples, prioritize deficits, and notify academic leaders when a student is falling behind help to clarify structure and framework for all involved. Warning signs for urgent student deficit identification include an inability to care for patients safely, acting dangerously toward self or others, or creating an impediment toward the learning of others (Guerrasio, 2013). The remediation facilitator must promote success in the learner by providing a supportive environment, exhibiting high expectations of growth, and respecting and challenging the learner with a mentorship connection (McGann & Thompson, 2008). Mentorship for at-risk students is known to foster motivation and chances for academic improvement (Robinson & Niemer, 2010). Students are appreciative of faculty availability, productive and honest feedback, a customized remediation plan, extra teaching and learning activities, and the recognition of their improvements. This process takes increased time on the part of the faculty facilitator, especially in learner deficits of clinical reasoning, communication, and mental well-being. Administrative officers

TABLE 20.1 Key Learner Deficits Associated With Core Competencies

Competency	Key Learner Characteristics or Deficits
Medical knowledge	• Unable to answer knowledge-based, fact-based questions • Lack of evidence of preparation/reading • Poor written exam scores
Clinical skills	• Physical exams may lack key elements or are performed incorrectly • Inaccurate information is obtained • Poor procedural skills • Unable to answer questions related to the exam or procedure

Clinical reasoning and judgment	• Learner has adequate knowledge and exam scores but:
	  • Is unable to focus the history and/or physical
	  • Orders too many tests
	  • Has difficulty prioritizing the differential diagnosis
	  • Includes extraneous information documentation

Time management and organization	• Unpreparedness • Unorganized appearance • Disorganized thought process in notes and case presentations • Multiple late and/or incomplete tasks
Interpersonal skills	• Difficulty functioning on a team • Many interpersonal conflicts • Transfer of blame • Inflexibility in compromise • Difficulty reading social cues and awkward peer interactions
Communication skills	• Poorly articulated oral presentations • Difficulty answering questions, but scores well on exams • Unable to convey differences in the level of urgency and severity • Poor communication in patient charts • Need to recontact patients to elicit more information
Professionalism	• Poor relationships with patients • Lack of respect • Use of technical verbiage with patients • Inappropriate dress or comments • Lack of punctuality • Dishonesty, laziness, or unethical actions
Practice-based learning and improvement	• Lack of self-directed learning • Does not set personal learning and patient care goals • Absence of quality-improvement methods • Defensive when receiving feedback • Does not seek help when needed or understand his or her own limitations
Systems-based practice	• Does not value interprofessional input • Neglects health care resources or cost/risk benefit analysis • Does not advocate for patients • Neglects transitions of care
Mental well-being	• Varies widely • Commonly includes inconsistent academic performance

Source: Adapted from Guerrasio (2013).

TABLE 20.2 Best Practices for Developing a Remediation Program

Category	Actions
Program vision and structure	1. Emphasize that remediation is a component of medical professionalism. 2. Adopt a programmatic approach. 3. Clearly articulate a framework for competence based on consensus. 4. Embrace a mastery learning approach that avoids arbitrary cutoffs. 5. Emphasize reflective practices associated with professional identity development and metacognitive competence.
Faculty roles and development	6. Structure remediation as an individual coaching relationship. 7. Separate remediation coaching from summative judgment roles. 8. Choose and develop appropriate faculty for remediation programs. 9. Develop and utilize a team of interdisciplinary experts. 10. Establish a community of practice for remediation coaching and allied experts.
Accountability and outcomes	11. Set clear expectations for success for all parties in a defined time frame. 12. Document remediation process and outcomes.

Source: Adapted from Kalet et al. (2016).

need to consider release of other responsibilities for faculty or alternative ways to assist in remediation of underperforming learners. This might include small-group remediation, which would also provide a means of peer-to-peer support or involving the clinical preceptor if the deficit is directly related to the clinical experience (Guerrasio et al., 2014; Hauer et al., 2007).

REMEDIATION STRATEGIES

Once the deficit has been identified, the team (with input from the student) develops a remediation plan. Remediation strategies may be more effective if sessions are viewed as learning opportunities to bridge the deficiencies to practice. This approach leverages the student's motivation for success, especially when there is a clear plan to guide the student toward future practice (Evans & Harder, 2013, p. 149). Components of the strategies are matched with each deficit and might include counseling, extra time, mentorship, one-on-one discussions, increased observation and feedback, role-modeling, special clinical experience, professional assessment, leave of absence, repeating of a course, clinical examination scenarios or simulation, and/or financial assistance (Szumacher et al., 2007, p. 729). Retesting is also a commonly used remediation strategy. There are many pros and cons to this strategy. Retesting allows students to reach their full potential and master the material. However, there is the risk that some students will "work the system" on the first exam, not realizing that in the real world there are not always second chances (O'Connell & Palfryman, 2015). The latter scenario can be curtailed by setting the maximum achievable score for the retest at the minimum passing score. According to McHugo (2017), an example of a general remediation policy may look something like this:

Every effort shall be made to give each student ample opportunity to demonstrate competency in each area of the program. If necessary, a process of remediation as a privilege earned by a student through active participation in the educational program as demonstrated by regular attendance, individual initiative, and utilization of resources available may be offered. Decisions regarding remediation will be determined on an individual basis after considering all pertinent circumstances, review of academic record, and consultation with the course instructor and faculty advisor. A regular performance-review process is designed to help faculty identify and assist students who may experience academic or professional difficulty. The process is proactive, with the goal of identifying at-risk students as early as possible. (p. 21)

For *all courses*, the process generally consists of the following:

1. **Identification:** The student is expected to be proactive and notify the course instructor if there are knowledge deficits. The course instructor works closely with the faculty advisor to identify the at-risk student through frequent faculty reports, exam grades, and advisory sessions.
2. **Evaluation and assessment:** Identified students will be referred to their faculty advisors for assessment of root causes. Referrals to campus assistance programs may be instituted (e.g., Student Success Center, Student Health, Disability Services for Students, or other resources).
3. **Plan development and implementation:** The faculty advisor, the student, and any other involved parties will design a remediation plan. Clear expectations will be documented and a contract for remediation developed. The department chair will then review the contract with the faculty advisor and student, placing the contract in the student's academic file. Depending on the plan for remediation, a timeline will be initiated for review of the student's progress. The faculty advisor and student will receive a copy of the contract and begin remediation.
4. **Plan evaluation:** Depending on the remediation needed, an evaluation instrument may be prepared to assess the student's progress. The course instructor and the faculty advisor may collaborate to design an appropriate tool to assess the progress. Evidence of compliance of mastery of a remediated knowledge deficit will be placed in the student's academic file with the contract.

Policies and procedures may also need to clearly identify remediation processes acceptable to the individual program. If retesting is allowed as a remediation strategy, will the exam have all new questions, a mix of previous questions and new questions, or only previous questions? Will the maximum grade achievable be 80%, 75%, or 70%? How will the math be calculated to determine the grade? A ratio formula? Will there be a review or some aspect of formative education prior to retesting? How much time will be allowed between notification of retesting and exam administration? These are all things to consider when discussing retesting as a remediation option. Ideally, these parameters are set prior to the situation within the program; however, they may need to be flexible to the needs of the student and the related scenario.

Guerrasio (2013) recommends that each deficit be aligned with a remediation strategy. After meeting with the remediation team to identify skill gaps and deficits and determining how the learner learns best, focused strategies can be employed. Table 20.3 illustrates an exemplar of possible remediation strategies based on identified deficit.

DETERMINING SUCCESS

McDowell (2008) points out the need for students to develop self-responsibility in their academic preparation; to be persistent and willing; to use a variety of resources to enhance their learning; and to follow the important practice of self-care. Much of remediation success is about self-mastery of nonacademic factors such as test anxiety, self-esteem, degree of fatigue, student-role strain, and balance of family and work obligations. Self-mastery is certainly part of educational success, along with satisfactory completion of remediating the identified deficit. Reassessment must be completed by a blind and neutral party so as to provide an objective view

TABLE 20.3 Sample Remediation Strategies Based on Identified Deficit

Deficit	Sample Remediation Strategies
Medical knowledge	• Change from disease-based reading to symptom-based reading • Link patient cases to reading • Create a list of items to look up

Clinical skills	• Assign readings or videos on physical exam skills or procedures
	• Digitally record students' performance of deficit skills and:
	  • Have student self-critique
	  • Give feedback
	  • Demonstrate missed elements

Clinical reasoning and judgment	• Review cases with the learner, and have learner:
	  • Develop differential diagnosis based on most likely, least likely, and emergent criteria
	  • Identify relevant history questions and physical exam elements
	  • Review diagnostic and treatment options

Time management and organization	• Teach a data-organization system • Have learners keep a log of daily activities (minute to minute) • Discuss activity log and help students identify and prioritize tasks to be completed
Interpersonal skills	• Address conflicts directly and privately with specific examples • Ask learner to provide model alternatives of positive interaction in conflict • Record simulated clinical interactions, have student view digital recording to foster self-reflection • Consider mental health evaluation
Communication	• Ask learner to identify how communication can facilitate or hinder patient care • Practice oral presentations emphasizing strong clinical reasoning • Role-play specific communicative skill sets • Have student summarize complex cases • Review clinical performance
Professionalism	• Review relevance of professionalism and consequences of being perceived as unprofessional • Review specific examples of learners' unprofessional behavior, emphasize high level of accountability and importance of self-reflection • Set clear expectations for professional behavior
Practice-based learning and improvement	• Have learner explore and write about benefits of lifelong learning • Discuss implementation of new knowledge to enhance patient care • Have learner complete quality-improvement project and reflect on the importance of continuous quality improvement
Systems-based practice	• Explore benefits of interprofessional input and team collaboration • Have learner seek health care resources to improve patient care • Have learner practice patient advocacy
Mental well-being	• Discuss concerns for students and their reflections • Provide supportive environment and activities that promote teamwork, stress reduction, and skills to overcome deficits • Consider evaluation for learning disabilities, psychiatric diagnosis, and substance use

Source: Adapted from Guerrasio (2013).

of the student's progress . . . or lack thereof. For some learners, success means being able to practice clinical medicine safely, whereas for others, it may mean changing career paths (Guerrasio et al., 2014, p. 357). Throughout this process, reflective journaling that outlines the experience and adapts the learning plan and career goals is a helpful tool that helps students develop strategies that will support goals of success, either within the physician assistant (PA) career or a new career path (Evans & Harder, 2013, p. 150).

GIVING MEANINGFUL FEEDBACK

Providing effective and meaningful feedback requires consideration of its content, location, timing, and technique used to deliver it. Setting clearly defined expectations for learners upfront is essential. Stated goals and objectives for each experience and added personal expectations based on teaching and learning styles will help set the stage for the remediation process. Feedback needs to be based on information rather than on judgment and limited to two or three areas of improvement. Careful choice of location along with optimal timing should be considered when providing clearly summarized feedback (Guerrasio, 2013, pp. 146–147). Some remediation specialists find success in a sandwich model: the learner is given positive, then negative, and then positive feedback. Others use the ask/tell/ask model, in which the interaction begins with the learner reflecting on his or her performance, after which the facilitator provides reinforcing and corrective feedback, and the session ends with the learner expressing his or her understanding of the feedback and summarizing the learning plan. Struggling learners strongly benefit from immediate directive feedback, which provides a framework for future learning activities. It is important to follow up with an email or memo summarizing the discussion and the plan to move forward. This also provides legal documentation for potential future needs (Guerrasio, 2013).

STARTING FROM THE GROUND UP

A successful remediation program must contain the following: a method to identify the struggling learner, a remediation team to identify the deficit and develop a plan, faculty development on remediation best practices and accessing academic services for struggling learners, measurable outcomes to determine success, financial resources and/or acceptance of release time within workflow, institutional support, and established policies and procedures (Kalet & Chou, 2014). Effective remediation programs are centralized, routinely evaluated, and have clearly defined goals and objectives. Many programs will develop threshold measures in determining need for and success of remediation practices. How you develop and determine the success of your program will need to be clearly defined in the planning phases of remediation plan development (Guerrasio, 2013, p. 155).

CONCLUSIONS

The challenge of struggling learners exists in all health professions programs. It is the role of the faculty member to help all learners reach their maximum potential, and therefore health professions programs must have remediation policies and procedure to remediate struggling learners. Each institution must determine its own remediation philosophy, goals, and processes as well as the expected outcomes needed to determine success. Remediation processes must be individualized. Without effective remediation, struggling learners are at risk of repeated failures and may be lost to the profession or graduate without the required competency to confidently and safely take care of patients.

REFERENCES

Accreditation Council for Pharmacy Education. (2016). Accreditation standards and key elements for the professional program in pharmacy leading to the doctor of pharmacy degree. Retrieved from https://www.acpe-accredit.org/pdf/Standards2016FINAL.pdf

Accreditation Review Commission on Education for the Physician Assistant. (2016). *Accreditation standards for physician assistant education* (4th ed.). Johns Creek, GA: Author. Retrieved from http://www.arc-pa.org/wp-content/uploads/2016/10/Standards-4th-Ed-March-2016.pdf

Audetat, M., Laurin, S., & Dory, V. (2013). Remediation for struggling learners: Putting an end to "more of the same." *Medical Education, 47*, 230–231.

Bain, K. (2011). *What the best college teachers do.* Cambridge, MA: Harvard University Press.

Bierer, S. B., Dannefer, E. F., & Tetzlaff, J. E. (2015). Time to loosen the apron strings: Cohort-based evaluation of a learner-driven remediation model at one medical school. *Journal of General Internal Medicine, 30*(9), 1339–1343.

Chang, A., Chou, C. L., & Hauer, K. E. (2008). Clinical skills remedial training for medical students. *Medical Education, 42*, 1118–1119.

Cleland, J., Leggett, H., Sandars, J., Costa, M. J., Patel, R., & Moffat, M. (2013). The remediation challenge: Theoretical and methodological insights from a systematic review. *Medical Education, 47*, 242–251.

Commission on Collegiate Nursing Education. (2013). Standards for accreditation of baccalaureate and graduate nursing programs. Retrieved from http://www.aacn.nche.edu/ccne-accreditation/Standards-Amended-2013.pdf

Corrigan-Magaldi, M., Colalillo, G., & Molloy, J. (2014). Faculty-facilitated remediation: A model to transform at-risk students. *Nurse Educator, 39*(9), 155–156.

Evans, C. J., & Harder, N. (2013). A formative approach to student remediation. *Nurse Educator, 38*(4), 147–151.

Guerrasio, J. (2013). *Remediation of the struggling medical learner.* Irwin, PA: Association for Hospital Medical Education.

Guerrasio, J. (2016). The crucial need for remediation. Retrieved from http://paeonline.org/need-for-remediation

Guerrasio, J., Garrity, M. J., & Aagaard, E. M. (2014). Learner deficits and academic outcomes of medical students, residents, fellows, and attending physicians referred to a remediation program, 2006–2012. *Academic Medicine, 89*(2), 352–358.

Hauer, K. E., Teherani, A., Irby, D. M., Kerr, K. M., & O'Sullivan, P. S. (2008). Approaches to medical student remediation after a comprehensive clinical skills examination. *Medical Education, 42*, 104–112.

Kalet, A., & Chou, C. L. (2014). *Remediation in medical education.* New York, NY: Springer Science+Business Media.

Kalet, A., Guerrasio, J., & Chou, C. L. (2016). Twelve tips for developing and maintaining a remediation program in medical education. *Medical Teacher, 38*(8), 787–792.

Liaison Committee on Medical Education. (2015). Functions and structure of a medical school: Standards for accreditation of medical education programs leading to the MD degree. Retrieved from http://lcme.org/publications/#Standards

Maize, D. F., Fuller, S. H., Hritcko, P. M., Matsumoto, R. R., Soltis, D. A., Taheri, R. R., & Duncan, W. (2010). A review of remediation programs in pharmacy and other health professions. *American Journal of Pharmaceutical Education, 74*(2), 1–9.

McDowell, B. M. (2008). KATTS: A framework for maximizing NCLEX-RN performance. *Educational Innovations, 47*(4), 183–186.

McGann, E., & Thompson, J. M. (2008). Factors related to academic success in at-risk senior nursing students. *International Journal of Nursing Education Scholarship, 5*(1), 1–15.

McHugo, J. (2017). *Student policies and procedures.* Grand Forks, ND: University of North Dakota Department of PA Studies.

O'Connell, C. B., & Palfryman, L. (2015, November). *Resting: Helpful remediation or academic crutch?* Paper presented at the PAEA Annual Education Forum, Washington, DC.

Robinson, E., & Niemer, L. (2010). A peer mentor tutor program for academic success in nursing. *Nursing Education Research, 31*(5), 286–289.

Strout, K., & Haidemenos, K. (2016). Eight remediation strategies to improve test performance. *Learning Curve, 46*(4), 21–22.

Szumacher, E., Catton, P., Jones, G. A., Bradley, R., Kwan, J., Cherryman, F., Palmer, C., & Nyhof-Young, J. (2007). Helping learners in difficulty: The incidence and effectiveness of remedial programmes of the medical radiation sciences programme at University of Toronto and the Michener Institute for Applied Sciences, Toronto, Ontario, Canada. *Annals of the Academy of Medicine, Singapore, 36*(9), 725–734.

Winston, K. A., van der Vleuten, C., & Scherpbier, A. A. (2010). At- risk medical students: Implications of students' voice for the theory and practice of remediation. *Medical Education, 44*, 1038–1047.

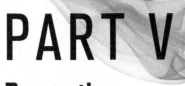

PART V
Promoting Diversity, Equity, and Inclusion

FUNTUNFUNEFU-DENKYEMFUNEFU
"Siamese crocodiles"

Symbol of democracy and unity

The Siamese crocodiles share one stomach, yet they fight over food. This popular symbol is a reminder that infighting and tribalism are harmful to all who engage in it.

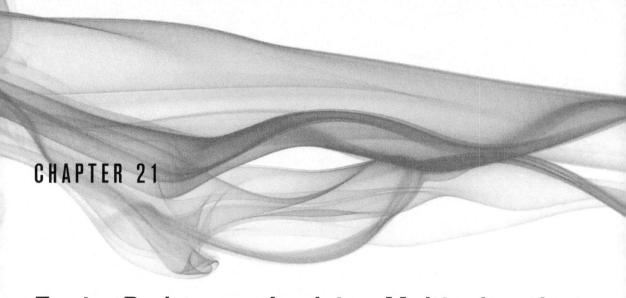

CHAPTER 21

Equity Pedagogy: Applying Multicultural Education in Health Professions Learning Environments

Kupiri Ackerman-Barger, David Acosta, Debra Bakerjian, Jann Murray-García, and Hendry Ton

---

CHAPTER OBJECTIVE

- Design and implement teaching strategies and learning environments that facilitate acquisition of knowledge and skills by students from diverse racial, ethnic, and cultural groups

---

However important they are, good intentions and awareness are not enough to bring about the changes needed in educational programs and procedures to prevent academic inequities among diverse students. Goodwill must be accompanied by pedagogical knowledge and skills as well as the courage to dismantle the status quo.

—Geneva Gay

EQUITY AND DIVERSITY AS DRIVERS FOR EXCELLENCE IN HEALTH PROFESSIONS

Academic health professions have begun to understand and embrace concepts such as equity and diversity. The word *equity* refers to a fair distribution of resources based on need. The term *education equity* acknowledges our history of legalized school segregation and the heritage of those

---

EXHIBIT 21.1 The Evolution of Diversity in Academic Health Professions

---

Diversity 1.0—Social Justice
Diversity 2.0—Cultural Competence
Diversity 3.0—Human Innovation

---

laws and taxation practices that have left some school districts without the funding they need to adequately prepare students (no matter their capability) for higher education. Because of education inequities, when students from underrepresented backgrounds and underserved communities seek health professions education, they often have a variety of learning needs that, thus far, health professions educators have been underprepared to meet. Although faculty may find it easier to "treat every student the same," this is not a realistic approach to education and can lead to missed learning opportunities for students and/or inadequate preparation of students for the role of health care provider.

The term *health equity* suggests that health care resources should be distributed based on the needs of individuals, families, and communities. In an equitable society, a community that has been historically underserved would have more service efforts directed toward it. One way to promote policies and resource allocation that promotes health equity is to ensure workforce diversity where representatives from underrepresented and underserved communities can advocate for and contribute to innovative solutions for the equitable distribution of health care resources.

Marc Nivet (2011) uses an IBM (International Business Machines) metaphor to describe how the term *diversity* has evolved in academic health professions over time (Exhibit 21.1). Initially, with Diversity 1.0, we thought of diversity mostly in terms of social justice, focusing on the legal and social barriers to the access of quality patient care. In the next phase, Diversity 2.0, we approached diversity from a cultural competence perspective, recognizing that with cultural awareness, skills, and knowledge, it may be possible to provide better care to a broader range of people. In the latest iteration of diversity, Diversity 3.0, we have begun to recognize that in addition to promoting social justice and cultural competence, there is also greater potential for human innovation when learning and working in environments that include a diversity of thinkers. Diverse learning and working groups provide a more robust environment for problem solving; thinking outside the box; and understanding individuals, families, and communities from a broader perspective.

Human innovation is needed so solve long-standing health disparities and structural problems within the health care system. In a health care system that has a pernicious history of perpetuating health disparities, it is imperative that we create a health professions workforce that understands what structural inequity means in a pluralistic society. Furthermore, the health professions workforce must be armed with the knowledge and tools needed to make significant changes in the health care system. Many of these skills can be fostered in learning environments that represent a diversity of perspectives. The purpose of this chapter is to present five distinct programs that use a multicultural education framework to promote education equity with a focus on underrepresented minority (URM) students and to enhance student learning related to equity and diversity.

MULTICULTURAL EDUCATION IN HEALTH PROFESSIONS

James Banks, an established scholar on multicultural education, says, multicultural education "is concerned with creating educational environments in which students from a variety of microcultural groups such as race/ethnicity, gender, social class, regional groups, and people with disabilities experience educational equality" (Banks, 2016, p. 80). Taxonomies are learning models that classify learning domains and promote a holistic approach to teaching and learning. Banks created such as taxonomy called the five dimensions of multicultural education:

1. Content integration
2. Knowledge construction
3. Equity pedagogy
4. Prejudice reduction
5. Empowering school culture and social structure

We explore these dimensions within the context of health professions education.

Content integration addresses the extent to which instructors use examples and content from a wide variety of cultures and groups to illustrate key concepts, principles, generalizations, and theories in a subject area or discipline. The National League for Nursing (NLN, 2016) supported this notion when it advocated that nursing education should embrace curricula that include culturally appropriate health care of diverse populations with attention to health disparities. In health professions, there is a multitude of opportunities to diversify the social groups, communities, and neighborhoods discussed in the curricula. Furthermore, we have unique leverage to illuminate the experiences and specific health care needs of invisible populations such as transgendered people, migrant workers, and victims of sex trafficking.

Knowledge construction encourages students to think about for whom, by whom, and about whom knowledge has been created and taught. It helps students understand the values, frameworks, and cultural assumptions that are implicit in what is taught. It considers how what we know and believe to be true has been influenced by people of certain dominant social groups, and how the information might be different if it were coming from different perspectives. Further, students are asked to avoid seeking singular answers (Mr. Jones is obese because of his lifestyle choices), but understand multiplicity (poverty, geographical location, access to food, chronic stress, and lack of community resources have contributed to Mr. Jones's obesity).

Equity pedagogy acknowledges that students from different backgrounds may learn in different ways. It, therefore, should inspire teachers to develop their curriculum and refine their teaching approaches to maximize the success of all students. In an article by Banks and Banks (1995), the authors focus on equity pedagogy as an essential component of multicultural education. In describing equity pedagogy, they emphasize that instructional approaches do not simply include techniques and methods, but need to include *context*. Banks (2016) stated that equity pedagogy exists when instructors modify and enhance their teaching to facilitate the academic achievement of diverse groups of students.

There are two key premises that are essential in equity pedagogy. First, individuals learn and assimilate information differently from one another. Learning preferences may be based on personality, culture, cognitive processes, and/or life experience. Understanding this dynamic may be especially salient when teaching URMs who are attending primarily White campuses. Second, material needs to be relevant and meaningful. In equity pedagogy, there is an active, purposeful movement away from a unimodal style, such as the use of lecture and PowerPoint as a primary teaching strategy. That is not to say that lecture and PowerPoint have no place in teaching, rather that when this style is the sole methodology used only a narrow group of learners benefit. Using an equity pedagogy approach would incorporate multiple teaching–learning strategies into a unit of teaching, thereby increasing opportunities for learners to grasp, integrate, and synthesize learning material.

Prejudice reduction asks all instructors to use teaching approaches that promote positive attitudes toward people from social groups different from their own. Banks (2016) suggests that this dimension addresses the attitudes and views of students and focuses on strategies that help students develop more democratic attitudes and values. One way to promote prejudice reduction is to create safe learning and discussion environments where participants who belong to

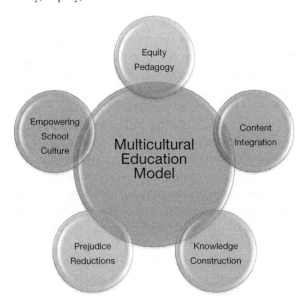

FIGURE 21.1 Five dimensions of multicultural education.
Source: Reprinted with permission from Banks (2016).

underrepresented groups can be honest about their experiences of racism, discrimination, and marginalization. During the process of typical classroom discourse, students would have the space to share positive exemplars of their social groups that counter negative stereotypes. Conversely, in a safe learning environment, students would also be able to confront personal biases so their views can be expanded.

Empowering school culture and social structure addresses the department or school as a whole. It means that schools create equal opportunities for success for all students by creating an overall positive learning community. In this dimension, schools would take steps to ensure the diversity of students, faculty, staff, and leaders. The total school environment is structured to promote inclusion and respect. The NLN (2016) recommended the cocreation of a "positive collaborative organizational culture that integrates the value of diversity and inclusivity into the functions of the nursing education program and academic institution" (p. 9). Addressing concepts, such as racism and structural exclusion, is essential to transforming a school environment (Banks, 2016; NLN, 2016). Some strategies include writing a strong mission statement; recruiting and retaining faculty, staff, leaders, and students from diverse backgrounds; holistic admission processes; establishing and monitoring metrics and benchmarks for diversity (Figure 21.1).

Multicultural Approaches to Teaching Health Professions Education

What follows are four exemplars of how health professions educators at a single university have created learning experiences for nursing and medical students. The overarching goal of these programs is to ensure URM students attain the knowledge and skills they need to be successful health professions clinicians, as well as to enhance student learning related to the concepts of diversity, equity, and inclusion. Each exemplar is followed by a table outlining how the principles of that learning activity are in alignment with the five dimensions of multicultural education.

INTEGRATED CASE-BASED LEARNING

Case-based learning (CBL) is a pedagogical method that is frequently used in education. There is no consensus on how to define CBL and there are a wide variety of ways that CBL is employed in the classroom (Thistlethwaite et al., 2012). The Harvard Business School was one of the first institutions to adopt CBL and has a long history of using this method in the classroom, but their focus has primarily been on business cases (Jonasson & Hernandez-Serrano, 2002). Subsequently, CBL has been increasingly used in health care education to make complex medical and nursing issues more applicable to patients and health conditions that students understand (Choi & Lee, 2009).

The nurse practitioner (NP) and physician assistant (PA) programs at our university have developed a novel model called Integrative Case-Based Learning, designed to incorporate social determinants of health into medical cases used in our clinical graduate programs. The integrative approach seeks to emphasize the context of a problem without sacrificing the clinical problem itself. We use a variety of methods, including automatic response systems and technology, to present the materials. Students are given pertinent information about a case focused on the key health issue and are challenged not only to think about the appropriate medical issue but also to explore the social determinants of the condition (poverty, education, socioeconomic status, regional variations, and cultural and linguistic needs of patients). Students typically work in teams to find resolutions to the realistic and challenging problems in the cases. This process has helped students link medical, social, and geographical issues that impact patient health.

Exemplar: Meet Jim

The goal of this case is to get the students to think more broadly about the patient's condition based on the minimal information they are given about the patient and then to lead them through a series of questions to help them focus on the issues. This case works well as an overview to why issues, such as the patient's context and social determinants of health, are important. The students are given a piece of information that is then followed by a discussion or with use of an audience-response system.

This case involves "Jim," a 35-year-old African American patient who presents to the primary care clinic to establish care with a complaint of fever, cough, and shortness of breath for the past 9 days. He provides a "history of present illness" of having gone to a local urgent care clinic 7 days ago, with similar symptoms, where he was prescribed a "Z-pack" and nothing else. His symptoms have not improved since that time.

At this point, students are asked, "Before you know anything about Jim, what do you think could be going on with him? What kinds of questions do you want to ask him?" Students are then prompted to think what else could be contributing to Jim's condition with each piece of information that is revealed.

Students are then introduced to Jim's family—he has a wife who is a preschool teacher and two children, ages 2 and 4 years. Students are told that Jim lives in the middle of an orchard in a company-owned home, where he and his family live rent free as part of his wages. He is a supervisor who oversees local laborers who work on several different orchards and fields in the area.

We then learn about Jim's community by showing students a Google Earth map of where he lives, 25 miles outside of Bakersfield, California. Within a 20-minute drive from his house there are no health care offices except the urgent care center and there are no hospitals; there is a pharmacy that is only open Monday through Friday, from 9 a.m. to 5:30 p.m.

Students discuss what each of these pieces of information mean and how it helps them really think about what might be going on with Jim. By this time, students generally identify asthma, upper respiratory infectious diseases, and pesticide exposure as possibilities.

TABLE 21.1　Applied Dimensions of Multicultural Education: Integrated Case-Based Learning

Critical Elements	Dimensions of Multicultural Education
Students are given key health information and asked to explore the social determinants of health using realistic, fully developed patient and family scenarios in nine different geographical regions in Northern California.	Content integration
Students explore a variety of cultures and environments in relation to specific health conditions and how those cultures and environments can impact health outcomes.	Knowledge construction
Integrative case-based learning and small-group learning allow students to explore the real challenges of access to high-quality health care.	Equity pedagogy
An integrative approach asks students to recognize a diversity of patients within the context of their circumstances. Students develop an empathetic approach to care through better understanding of each patient's situation.	Prejudice reduction

The next piece of the puzzle is that students learn that Jim lives in Kern County; they then are told to look up public health information on Kern County. They find out that Kern County has the highest incidence of heart disease in the state, the worst air quality in the nation, and that it is a medically underserved area. They find out that there are significant health disparities in the incidence of asthma based on race and ethnicity and that African Americans are more frequently treated in the emergency department (ED) for their asthma and are hospitalized at two to three times the rate compared with other races.

Students then are shown life expectancy along a 150-mile stretch of Highway 99, a main highway that traverses the central valley of California; there is discussion of how life expectancy differs by zip code by as much as a decade. And that, in fact, Sacramento's major medical center is located across the street from a zip code where the residents have a life expectancy 3.5 years less than their neighbors and where residents are three times more likely to go the ED for asthma, diabetes, and hypertension; and 50% more likely to have heart disease. This case provides the opportunity for rich discussion of the multiple factors that impact illness, such as geographical location, racial and ethnicity disparities, transportation, the impact of family and jobs, and lack of access to primary care and prevention services. Faculty can make this as short or as long as needed based on the objectives of the case. We have been able to have rich discussions taking anywhere from 15 minutes to 60 minutes.

Table 21.1 outlines how the critical elements of integrated CBL are in alignment with and exemplify the five dimensions of multicultural education.

TEAM PEACE IN HEALTH SERIES

Using an interprofessional education approach, a group of health professions students (medical, nursing, and PA) in their first year participate in cultural competence learning through the Teamwork for Professionalism, Ethics, and Cultural Enrichment (Team PEACE) Culture in Health Series. This series of five seminars given over a 9-month period combines principles of group development with cultural competence to engage nursing and medical students in small-group learning. There are four principal topics: becoming a culturally diverse learning community, narrative health care practice, social determinants of health, and unconscious bias. The final session is a large-group discussion called Conversation Café.

The Becoming a Culturally Diverse Learning Community seminar helps students establish a sense of community. As a strategy to build community and embrace difference, the first activity is a diversity potluck meal in which students share the personal and cultural significance of a dish they have chosen to share in a small group. In this session, basic cultural competence terminology and principles of community are discussed. Through individual and group reflection, students develop an appreciation for cultural inclusiveness and are able to see themselves as part of a greater campus and health care community.

In the Narrative Practice seminar, students learn about the important role of narratives in health care. Narrative practice in health care involves the sharing of stories as a way to find meaning in the health care experience. The sharing of narratives can improve sense of purpose and meaning, empathy, and reflection and enhances one's ability to understand the perspectives of another. Learners share a personal story of an illness with one another, practicing active listening and empathy. Using *Worlds Apart: A Four-Part Series on Cross-Cultural Health Care* by Fanlight Productions, students view and discuss a vignette of an African American man who relates his experience awaiting kidney transplant (Stanford Center for Biomedical Ethics, Grainger-Monsen, & Haslett, 2004). Students compare his experience with their own personal stories, and discuss the kinds of health care disparities people face. Students describe the evidence for and impact of health disparities as well the role of narrative practice in furthering a provider's understanding of the causes, impact, and potential solutions for health disparities.

In the Social Determinants of Health seminar, students grapple with the notion that the most powerful influences on health exist outside of health care. They discuss the sociopolitical and environmental factors that contribute to the economic and health struggles of patients, families, and communities. Local community-based strategies, including efforts by health care providers to support communities, are explored. Students leave the session with the ability to articulate why health care providers need to understand health at a community level and the impact health care providers can have as community advocates.

The Unconscious Bias seminar stresses the examination of one's own biases. Students learn about the hardwiring of unconscious bias and the role it has on human survival. They take implicit associations tests individually. Then, as a group, they reflect on the ways unconscious bias can become problematic within the role of health care providers and patient outcomes, with a particular focus on the lesbian, gay, bisexual, transgender and queer (LGBTQ) community as they view the film *GenSilent*. Finally, learners discuss strategies to recognize and manage unconscious bias.

The Team PEACE Culture in Health Series concludes with a large-group session using the Conversation Café format. The focus of a Conversation Café is to create an inviting climate where everyone is inspired to speak and listen and where diverse perspectives may emerge (Conversation Café, n.d.). The health professions students rotate among stations of four individuals to discuss strategies for implementing cultural humility and inclusiveness in their lives as developing health care providers. Table 21.2 outlines how the critical elements of Team PEACE are in alignment with and exemplify the dimensions of multicultural education.

BOOK CLUBS

The Interprofessional Book Club invites staff, clinicians, students, administrators, and faculty to gather during the lunch hour (lunch is served free of cost) over multiple book club sessions. An inclusive atmosphere is created when book club participants are told that they are voluntarily entering what is meant to be an emotionally safe and confidential space to practice

TABLE 21.2 Applied Dimensions of Multicultural Education: Team PEACE

Critical Elements	Dimensions of Multicultural Education
While analyzing the social determinant of health, students are able to conceive of broader systems that contextualize health diagnoses, interventions, and health outcomes.	Content integration
Examination of communities that are underserved in health care helps students understand how focus and resources have been allocated to certain groups to the exclusion of other groups. This is particularly identified when students watch the film *GenSilent* and learn about the intersection of aging and the LGBTQ community.	Knowledge construction
Students develop an appreciation for cultural inclusiveness and interprofessional collaboration and are able to see themselves as part of a greater campus and health care community.	Equity pedagogy
Exploring unconscious bias allows students to understand the nature of prejudice, explore their own biases, and have opportunities to expand their notions about others.	Prejudice reduction
The format of the Conversation Café creates a climate in which voices can be heard and students can collectively determine what they can do as students and as health care providers to create a culture of health equity.	Empowering school culture

LGBTQ, lesbian, gay, bisexual, transgender, queer.

cross-cultural dialogue and critical self-reflection. The facilitator should clarify this by saying, "Our dialogue is not meant to troll for proof of one another's racism, sexism, homophobia, and so on, but we *expect* such missteps in what can be an awkward and clunky discussion." The goal is to create an environment where previously silenced perspectives can be brought out of individuals often not recognized as experts or teachers within the academic environment. These individuals might include more relatively diverse groups of staff members than is typically found in a classroom, possessing less formal education or fewer degrees, or even underrepresented students whose usual posture is to receive from and not to give to an instructor. In this carefully facilitative, ongoing learning opportunity, there is an explicit goal of learning to care for and connect with other learners who share equal status as they embark into the uncertain and vulnerable territory of learning about the human condition.

The books are chosen to include historical or cultural facts and perspectives of interest to all cultural groups. For example, *The Warmth of Other Suns* by Isabel Wilkerson is a nonfiction masterpiece that interweaves stories of the Great Migration of African Americans from America's South. Attendees came to appreciate that the Great Migration exponentially dwarfed the Dust Bowl and Gold Rush migrations, though, as one White student pointed out, he had never heard of it. Participants begin to wonder about how and what they have learned previously in American educational institutions such as ours and to find that it is incomplete and has not necessarily prepared them to value and honor the stories of patients or colleagues. It is the role of the facilitator to relate the discussion back to the process of health care delivery and health professions education. These kinds of conversations have the potential to catalyze lifelong learning and a curiosity for a rich diversity of stories hidden and as yet uncovered by attendees. Table 21.3 outlines how the critical elements of book clubs are in alignment with and exemplify the dimensions of multicultural education.

TABLE 21.3 Applied Dimensions of Multicultural Education: Book Clubs

Critical Elements	Dimensions of Multicultural Education
This format gives participants an opportunity to delve deeply into issues that directly or indirectly impact health care.	Content integration
Books, such as *The Warmth of Other Suns,* exemplify a critical piece of U.S. history that is not taught in schools, yet have impacted generations of people.	Knowledge construction
The facilitated book clubs provide a space to care about and connect with others who share equal status while learning about the human condition.	Equity pedagogy
The book clubs stimulate conversation that brings forth the stories and perspectives of those who are often unheard. They catalyze curiosity and the desire for lifelong learning about others.	Prejudice reduction
This inclusive event held by the school reaffirms the school's commitment to important social issues and the importance of dialogue among students, faculty, and staff.	Empowering school culture

COMMUNITY ENGAGEMENT MODELS

Call to Action: A Course in Health Activism for Minority Students

The Summer Medical and Dental Education Program (SMDEP) is a summer residential pipe-line program that is offered at 12 health science institutions across the United States and is spon-sored by the Robert Wood Johnson Foundation (2016). The program targets college freshman and sophomores who come from population groups that are underrepresented in medicine and/ or dentistry and that have an expressed interest in a career in medicine or dentistry. Although this program focuses on prehealth professions students, the concepts used in this program can be applied at any level of health professions curricula. The curriculum focuses on development of key scientific concepts, leadership, career development, learning skills, and health policy. Each academic institution is allowed to add other curricular elements that they feel would add value and uniqueness to their program. The SMDEP at the University of Washington focused a por-tion of the curriculum on health disparities and the social determinants of health in the course, Call to Action: A Course in Health Activism. The instructor of record for this course (one of the authors) used Bank's Framework of Multicultural Education (Banks, 2016) to build the con-cept model for the health disparities project that each of the students was required to develop. Table 21.4 describes the project instructions and references each of the elements used in Bank's framework. Table 21.4 outlines how the critical elements of a health disparities project are in alignment with and exemplify the dimensions of multicultural education.

Bank's framework proved to be instrumental not only in the development of the course cur-riculum, but also in the effectiveness of its delivery. In addition, this approach created a col-laborative, multicultural learning environment that provided equitable opportunities for every student on the team to learn about a community they collectively cared about. The project empowered the students to create innovative solutions to address the health inequities they wit-nessed firsthand. In turn, the communities the students worked with were engaged and felt that they contributed to the learning of the students.

TABLE 21.4 A Call to Action: Health Disparities Project

Project Instructions	Dimensions of Multicultural Education
Choose a health inequity that significantly impacts one of the local communities.	Content integration
Work in teams of four to eight students (students were assigned to groups to ensure team diversity).	Prejudice reduction and inclusive learning environments
Interview community members to understand their perspective of the health inequity issue chosen.	Content integration and knowledge construction
Perform a literature search and construct two to three data points (at a minimum) that are evidence-based that validate your intended message.	Content integration
Create the best platform collectively to disseminate your message (your findings) to impact change.	Equity pedagogy

Community-Based Participatory Curriculum Development: A Tool for Teaching Health Professional Learners About Minority Health and Health Disparities

Reducing health care disparities among disenfranchised populations remains a major challenge in the United States, and those affected are integral to helping researchers and health care providers achieve a better understanding of their causes and potential solutions. Community-based participatory research (CBPR) has provided a process for obtaining input by partnering community members with academic researchers to jointly define issues needing study. The principles of CBPR (Zubaida, Grunbaum, Gray, Franks, & Simoes, 2007) were adopted, translated, and modified to develop a new curriculum tool for medical educators—the Community-Based Participatory Curriculum Development (CBPCD) tool (Acosta, 2013)—specifically designed to partner community members with medical educators at academic medical institutions to jointly define issues related to health disparities to teach and better prepare our future health care workforce. The critical elements of this CBPCD approach include:

1. Recognition that the community has important expertise
2. Partnering of community members with medical educators
3. Community members participate in every aspect of curriculum development
   a. Identify and define health concerns of the community
   b. Design meaningful learning objectives
   c. Delivery of educational material
4. Ensure a mutual sharing of knowledge, skills, resources, and power
5. Empower the community to inform and direct change in behavior, attitudes, knowledge, and skills of future health care workforce

Table 21.5 outlines how the critical elements of integrated CBL are in alignment with and exemplify the dimensions of multicultural education.

The CBPCD tool was used to develop three separate health care disparities courses at one of the major medical schools in the Pacific Northwest by one of the authors for three population groups: Hispanics, LGBTQ, and African American. This approach allowed the medical education team to engage the local community and was a part of directly and receive meaningful

TABLE 21.5 Applied Dimensions of Multicultural Education: Community-Based Participatory Curriculum Development

Critical Elements	Dimensions of Multicultural Education
Recognition that the community has important expertise	Knowledge construction
Partnering of community members with medical educators	Prejudice reduction
Community members participate in every aspect of curriculum development	Content integration, knowledge construction, prejudice reduction, equity pedagogy
Ensure a mutual sharing of knowledge, skills, resources, and power	Content integration, knowledge construction, prejudice reduction, equity pedagogy
Empower the community to inform and direct change in behavior, attitudes, knowledge, and skills of the future health care workforce	Equity pedagogy, empowering school culture

recommendations on curriculum content that matters (based on their personal experiences with medical students, residents, and faculty). The results from our annual graduate exit survey 5 years after launching the courses revealed that there was a significant improvement in students' perceptions of the instruction regarding health care disparities. Surveys of fourth-year medical students demonstrated that 86.1% felt their instruction in health care disparities was appropriate and 6.3% felt their instruction was inadequate, as compared to scores of 79% and 18.5%, respectively, in the fourth-year medical student cohort surveyed prior to the implementation of this curriculum. Medical students who participated in this curriculum cited that this approach provided them with a unique opportunity to hear testimony and witness the direct impact of health inequities on the community members affected, which enriched their learning (Acosta, 2013). The principles used in the CBPCD are in alignment with each element of Bank's Framework of Multicultural Education (Banks, 2016), and the tool can be used to demonstrate the effectiveness of this framework.

CONCLUSIONS

This chapter describes four innovative programs that have been implemented in health professions schools using the underpinnings of multicultural education. Each of these examples is distinctly different in its structure and processes and addresses different learning styles. There is no single educational approach to teaching for equity and diversity, rather a variety of strategies and methodologies are used. Health professions educators are encouraged to develop a broad teaching skill set and to seek out innovative teaching–learning approaches that meet the needs of their students within the context of their learning environment. In this chapter, we offer strategies for inspiration as well as for use and adaptation.

REFERENCES

Acosta, D. A. (2013). Using a community-based participatory (CBP) approach to teaching medical students about minority health and health disparities: The CBP Curriculum Development Tool. *Hawaii Journal of Medicine and Public Health*, 72(8, Suppl. 3), 11.

Banks, C. A., & Banks, J. A. (1995). Equity pedagogy: An essential component of multicultural education. *Theory Into Practice, 34*(3), 152–158.

Banks, J. A. (2016). *Cultural diversity and education: Foundations, curriculum, and teaching* (6th ed.). New York, NY: Routledge.

Choi, I., & Lee, K. (2009). Designing and implementing a case-based learning environment for enhancing ill-structured problem solving: Classroom management problems for prospective teachers. *Educational Technology Research and Development, 57*(1), 99–129.

Conversation Café. (n.d.). Conversations that matter! Retrieved from http://www.conversationcafe.org

Gay, G. (2010). *Culturally responsive teaching: Theory, research, and practice* (2nd ed.). New York, NY: Teachers College Press.

Jonassen, D. H., & Hernandez-Serrano, J. (2002). Case-based reasoning and instructional design: Using stories to support problem solving. *Educational Technology Research and Development, 50*(2), 65–77.

National League for Nursing. (2016, February). Achieving diversity and meaningful inclusion in nursing education. *NLN Vision Series*. Retrieved from http://www.nond.org/resources/NLN-vision-statement-achieving-diversity.pdf

Nivet, M. (2011). Diversity 3.0: A necessary systems upgrade. *Academic Medicine, 86*(12), 1487–1489.

Robert Wood Johnson Foundation. (2016). Summer medical and dental education program. Retrieved from http://smdep.org/about

Stanford Center for Biomedical Ethics (Producer), Grainger-Monsen, M. (Director), & Haslett, J. (Director) (2004). *Worlds Apart: A Four-Part Series on Cross-Cultural Health Care* [Motion picture]. United States: Fanlight Productions, Inc. (Available from Fanlight Productions, Inc., http://www.fanlight.com/catalog/films/912_wa.php)

Thistlethwaite, J. E., Davies, D., Ekeocha, S., Kidd, J. M., MacDougall, C., Matthews, P., . . . & Clay, D. (2012). The effectiveness of case-based learning in health professional education. A BEME systematic review: BEME Guide No. 23. *Medical Teacher, 34*(6), e421–e444.

Wilkerson, I. (2010). *The warmth of other suns: The epic story of America's great migration*. New York, NY: Random House.

Zubaida, F., Grunbaum, J. A., Gray, B. S., Franks, A., & Simoes, E. (2007). Community-based participatory research: Necessary next steps. *Preventing Chronic Disease, 4*(3), 1–5.

ADDITIONAL RESOURCES

American Association of Colleges of Nursing. (2014). Enhancing diversity in the workforce. Retrieved from http://www.aacn.nche.edu/media-relations/fact-sheets/enhancing-diversity

American Association of Medical Colleges. (2010). Roadmap to diversity: Integrating holistic review practices into medical school admission process. Retrieved from www.aamc.org/morediversity

Cohen, J. J., Gabriel, B. A., & Terrell, C. (2002). The case for diversity in the healthcare workforce. *Health Affairs, 21*(5), 90–102.

Institute of Medicine. (2002). Unequal treatment: What healthcare providers need to know about racial and ethnic disparities in health care. Retrieved from http://www.nationalacademies.org/hmd/~/media/Files/Report%20Files/2003/Unequal-Treatment-Confronting-Racial-and-Ethnic-Disparities-in-Health-Care/Disparitieshcproviders8pgFINAL.pdf

Fink, L. D. (2013). *Creating significant learning experiences: An integrated approach to designing college courses*. San Francisco, CA: Jossey-Bass.

Lang, J. M. (2016). Making small changes in teaching: Giving them a say. Retrieved from http://chronicle.com/article/Small-Changes-in-Teaching-/235918

Maddux, S., & Applebaum, J. (Producers), & Maddux, S. (Director). (2010). *GenSilent* [Motion Picture]. United States: Interrobang Productions.

Mehl-Madrona, L. (2007). *Narrative medicine*, Rochester, VT: Bear and Company.

Page, S. (2007). Making the difference: Applying a logic of diversity. *Academy of Management Perspective, 21*(4), 6–20.

Phillips, J. M., & Malone, B. (2014). Increasing racial/ethnic diversity in nursing to reduce health disparities and achieve health equity. *Public Health Reports, 129*(Suppl. 2), 45–50.

Saha, S. (2014). Taking diversity seriously: The merits of increasing minority representation in medicine. *Journal of the American Medical Association, 174*(2), 291–292.

Sullivan Commission. (2004). *Missing persons: Minorities in the health professions. A report from the Sullivan Commission on diversity in the healthcare workforce* [Monograph].

U.S. Department of Health and Human Services and Health Resources and Services Administration Bureau of Health Workforce. (2006). *The rationale for diversity in the health professions: A review of the evidence.* Washington, DC: U.S. Government Printing Office. Retrieved from http://bhpr.hrsa.gov/healthworkforce/reports/diversityreviewevidence.pdf

U.S. Department of Health and Human Services and Health Resources and Services Administration Bureau of Health Workforce. (2015). Sex, race, and ethnic diversity of U.S. health occupations (2010–2012). Retrieved from http://bhpr.hrsa.gov/healthworkforce/supplydemand/usworkforce/diversityushealthoccupations.pdf

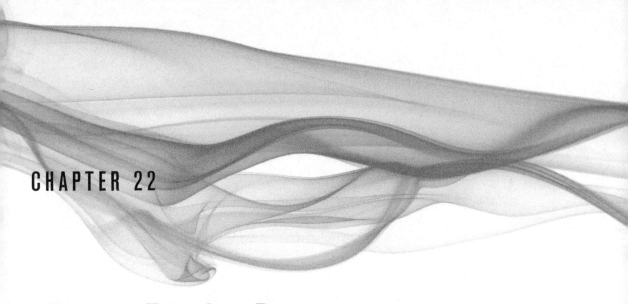

CHAPTER 22

Minority Faculty: Recruitment, Retention, and Advancement

Karen Mulitalo, Kupiri Ackerman-Barger, Darin T. Ryujin, and Maha B. Lund

CHAPTER OBJECTIVES

- Outline strategies to use to recruit and retain minority faculty
- Discuss strategies for minority faculty success in the academic environment
- Create successful mentoring programs, networking, and resources specific for minority groups

Almost always, the creative dedicated minority has made the world better.

—*Martin Luther King, Jr.*

Diversity is central to achieving academic excellence within health professions schools. Diverse viewpoints create a robust learning environment for scholars to explore and develop knowledge. A diverse faculty is essential to diversity efforts because it contributes to the recruitment and retention of a diverse student body; provides support, role-modeling, and mentoring for students from underrepresented backgrounds; contributes to robust curricula and new forms of pedagogy; and can provide insights into the planning of resource allocation, institutional policy, and research that is equitable and representative. However, gaping disparities exist in the number of minorities entering and being promoted within health professions schools (Hagan, Campbell, & Gaither, 2016; Rodríguez, Campbell, & Mouratidis, 2014; Salvucci & Lawless, 2016). This chapter reviews reasons for minority faculty attrition in health professions education, current best practices in minority faculty recruitment and retention strategies, and a section on minority faculty mentoring to assure that minority faculty can successfully meet the unique challenges they may face in meeting expectations for promotion and tenure.

ATTRITION OF MINORITY FACULTY IN HEALTH PROFESSIONS EDUCATION

Increasing and maintaining a diverse faculty presence on most campuses, especially predominantly White institutions, has been difficult at best. The National Center for Education Statistics (2016) reported that only 11% of full-time faculty in higher education were African American/Black, Hispanic/Latino, and Native American, defined here as *underrepresented minority* (URM) faculty. This disparity exists for health professions faculty as well. The Association of American Medical Colleges (AAMC; 2012) report that URM faculty constitute only 8.8% of all medical school faculty. The American Academy of Physician Assistants (2013) reported that 9.7% of physician assistant (PA) faculty were URM. According to the American Association of Colleges of Nursing (AACN; 2015), 12.3% of full-time nursing school faculty come from minority backgrounds. However, these data on nursing faculty did not disaggregate minority categories that define URM. URM faculty is similarly underrepresented in pharmacy schools (Hagan et al., 2016).

Attrition among minority faculty, in general, is a problem. Faculty attrition among minority faculty in health professions education is especially concerning. There are a variety of reasons minority faculty leave academic settings. The literature provides considerable evidence that experiences of marginalization, racism, and sexism play a significant role in faculty attrition. More specific, minority faculty are more likely than their nonminority counterparts to experience isolation, tokenism, devaluation of scholarship, and a lack of recognition for contributions to the academy (Diggs, Garrison-Wade, Estrada, & Galindo, 2009; Rockquemore & Laszloffy, 2008; Salvucci & Lawless, 2016; Smith, 2015). Minority faculty are often expected to go above and beyond other faculty by mentoring and advising minority students, teaching topics related to diversity (whether related to their area of expertise or not), and representing diversity on initiatives and in committees. This phenomenon is often called the *diversity tax* or the *diversity burden*. Furthermore, there tends to be a lack of minority mentors to help minority faculty navigate these obstacles (Rodríguez et al., 2014). Additional reasons for attrition include low salaries (Cropsey et al., 2008; Salvucci & Lawless, 2016) and lack of opportunity for promotion (AAMC, 2012; Salvucci & Lawless, 2016). These attrition issues can be addressed with intentional recruitment and retention efforts that focus on institutional inclusion and support.

STRATEGIES FOR MINORITY FACULTY RECRUITMENT AND RETENTION

Cutting-Edge Advertising and Outreach

Recruitment should be continuous and proactive rather than periodic or reactive to faculty attrition (Parson, 2016). With the explosion of social media over the last decade, organizations are compelled to conduct ongoing public relations and marketing assessments to stay abreast of marketing trends and popular job-posting sites. Organizations are well served to identify affinity groups and to create a network of individuals who can provide contact information for potential candidates from underrepresented groups. Up-to-date local and national marketing information should be readily available to hiring units.

In addition to advertising, health professions schools should engage in ongoing outreach. Outreach can include attending professional organizations' conferences, reaching out to health professions graduate programs, and incentivizing careers as health professions academics. Furthermore, institutions should look toward long-term outreach by increasing the diversity of their own student bodies and grooming graduate students for the role of health professions educator. Page, Castillo-Page, and Wright (2011) found that schools that have larger numbers of minority students tend to have more minority faculty. This may be because many of those students became faculty at the same institution. Therefore, pipeline programs may be an important means to increase diverse faculty. Yet, without compositional diversity in the classroom, this natural "pipeline" may not occur. Thus, the importance of fostering a diverse student body remains critical.

Strong Mission Statements and an Inclusive Campus Climate

Health professions schools need strong, inclusive mission statements that are part of the fabric of the institution. However, a mission statement is only useful when the day-to-day expectations of behavior are congruent with the mission statement and members of the school community hold each other accountable for the mission. There should be robust policies that promote inclusivity, the principles of community, and uphold a hate-free work environment. Leadership must be vigilant about addressing discriminatory behaviors and workplace bullying and have strong clear enforcement mechanisms to ensure that all people know they are respected and valued at the organization. Exhibit 22.1 provides examples of institution-wide strategies for training and support for institutional culture change.

Schools should post their strategic plan, clearly stating an institutional commitment to supporting students, faculty, and staff from underrepresented backgrounds and the steps the institution plans to take to honor this commitment. It is through mission statements followed by impactful diversity efforts that a university demonstrates its commitment to stakeholders and communities. One of the best ways for schools to demonstrate their vow to diversity to potential faculty hires is through strategic and in-depth campus visits during which candidates can hear from students and faculty who can speak to how the institution lives its mission and commitment to diversity on a daily basis. Furthermore, schools should be prepared to provide examples of scholarship related to diversity and work with underserved communities.

The value of inclusion cannot be understated. Inclusion is the mechanism that makes diversity work. It is through inclusion that members of the academic community feel respected, valued, and appreciated for the many aspects of their individual identity and intellectual capabilities. A climate of inclusion is not always the default in universities where individualism, competition, and elitism are embedded as a hidden curriculum. Therefore, explicit efforts should be taken by leadership and the campus as a whole to create inclusive environments. This process has to be modeled and emphasized by academic leaders. However, every individual at the university plays a part in the inclusive environment. When we smile, say hello, invite, and engage in meaningful conversations and interactions with individuals or social groups different from

---

EXHIBIT 22.1 Institutional Strategies That Support a Culture of Diversity and Inclusion

- Consistent training on implicit bias at all levels
- Minority affairs webpage, email, or monthly newsletter that provides updates on campus-wide diversity and inclusion initiatives and activities
- Communication about key minority faculty data to institutional leadership and key stakeholders
- Expansion of leadership positions at department, school, and institutional levels with special training of search committee members
- Increase grant support for research of underserved communities and minority workforce-related issues
- Increase funds for staffing of diversity-related activities
- Formation of diversity committees at department level to review policy and address issues of equity within each department

our own, we live inclusion. When prospective hires visit our campus, frequent and clear evidence of inclusion can be very appealing, especially for faculty who are looking to escape "chilly" work environments. The experience of inclusion should not end upon hire. Organizing breakfast clubs or lunch buddies is a way for new faculty to develop a professional network and to discover potential collaboration opportunities.

Diverse and Well-Trained Search Committees

Unconscious bias refers to the stereotypic associations or preconceived notions an individual may have about particular social groups. It is argued that this process relates to an innate tendency for our brains to categorize and organize information. However, these biases are often based on assumptions about others that are not accurate. Moody (2012) describes cognitive errors that can occur during the hiring process. These include positive and negative stereotyping, elitism, first impressions, good fit/bad fit, shifting standards, and provincialism. Research has indicated that during the hiring process unconscious bias and cognitive errors are more likely to negatively affect women and under-represented racial and ethnic groups (Corrice, 2009).

In order to mitigate unconscious bias in the hiring process, there are several steps that can be taken. The composition of the search committee should be constructed to be as diverse as possible, including women and people of color. These individuals can be faculty, staff, or students. They can also be members external to the department or school. All individuals who serve on a search committee should be required to participate in diversity and unconscious bias training. This training should emphasize the value of diversity and the role it plays in academic excellence and service to the community. Exploring how our unconscious bias can manifest, even when these biases are not in alignment with our personal values, is another essential element of search committee training. Cultural humility can serve as a framework to help individuals grapple with unpacking unconscious bias. Because working on unconscious bias is lifelong work, faculty should be expected to refresh or renew their skills.

Consider creating a toolkit for the recruitment and retention of minority faculty. This is an institution-specific guideline that aligns with the mission of the school and could be easily accessed by department chairs and search committees. The toolkit would include strategies for writing job descriptions that are both broad enough to appeal to a variety of applicants, but clear enough to give search committees specific criteria by which to evaluate candidates objectively. The toolkit would guide search committee members on how to screen applicants using concrete evidence rather than "gut feelings" or opinions. This would also be a place to describe how to use gender-neutral and culturally appropriate language during construction of interview questions as well as dos and don'ts during the interviewing and selection process.

Another best practice for ensuring that diversity and inclusion are central to the hiring process is the use of diversity advocates. An example of this practice in action is found at the University of California, Berkeley, which has adopted the role of faculty equity advisors. These are individuals who are appointed by the department chair or dean, receive in-depth training, and are tasked with ensuring that diversity and equity are considered in all aspects of the academic mission and departmental functions. One of the roles of the faculty equity advisor is to provide advice to chairs or search committees that ensure inclusive search practices are used in recruiting faculty. The role of diversity advocates can also be applied by having a committee for faculty diversity. University of California, Davis, created a committee, Underrepresented Groups in Medical and Biological Sciences, whose charge is to implement best practices for recruiting, retaining, and promoting minority faculty. This committee makes recommendations to the Office for Equity, Diversity, and Inclusion; Academic Personnel and health system leaders. Furthermore, this committee organizes networking events and workshops designed to recognize the accomplishments of minority faculty and to provide group mentoring.

Competitive Hiring Packages and Promotion Opportunities

Recruitment and retention efforts must also address equable salaries and opportunity for growth and promotion within the organization. Careful negotiation of competitive compensation packages need to occur. Universities should consider special hires for spouses/significant others, family-friendly policies (including childcare), and housing resources. There is evidence that women and minorities are not as well compensated or as frequently promoted as White men; and once faculty members discover these disparities in their school, there is often a sense of betrayal that can result in turnover (AAMC, 2012; Cropsey et al., 2008; Salvucci & Lawless, 2016). Routine and transparent annual salary equity reviews can demonstrate the university's commitment to valuing the contributions of each of its faculty members.

Robust faculty development programs related to merit and promotion expectations within the university should occur. Because minority faculty may have additional obstacles to navigate in the academy, a program with targeted workshops, resources, and mentors can be developed that address the unique needs of minority faculty.

In summary, despite the current and usual difficulty of recruiting and hiring faculty members of color, constructing and implementing different and intentional policies and practices centered around the recruitment and hiring of minority faculty can improve this process (Exhibit 22.2). Furthermore, the hiring of minority faculty should not be optional, but is considered essential for health professions programs to improve the overall education of students and to also improve the health professions workforce and, subsequently, the health of all individuals (Smith, 2011).

STRATEGIES FOR MINORITY FACULTY TO SUCCEED IN THE ACADEMIC ENVIRONMENT

Minority faculty face a wide range of challenges in the academic environment. These may include isolation, stress, and lack of support, bias, and colleagues' perception that they may be less qualified (Turner, Gonzalez, & Wood, 2008). Establishing strong mentoring relationships with senior faculty or peers who have experience on how the academic environment works is critical to the success of minority faculty. Harte and colleagues (2011) summarized a number of strategies for success, such as the formation of faculty collaboratives, which have been used successfully in various institutions. In addition, there are a number of national resources that are dedicated to helping minority faculty succeed. For instance, the National Center for Faculty Development and Diversity (NCFDD) offers programs on increasing research productivity, time management, and work–life balance. Other organizations that are dedicated to the success of minority faculty include the Robert Wood Johnson Foundation Harold Amos Medical Faculty Development Program (www.amfdp.org), Latina Researchers Network (www.latinaresearchers .com), Annie E. Casey Foundation Leaders in Equitable Evaluation and Diversity (LEEAD) Program (www.aecf.org/work/research-and-policy/research-and-evaluation/leaders-in-equitable -evaluation-and-diversity-lead), and the American Association of Hispanics in Higher Education (AAHHE) Multidisciplinary Faculty Fellows Program (www.aahhe.org/Programs/FacFellows ProgramDescription.aspx).

EXHIBIT 22.2 Practices to Increase Recruitment and Retention of Minority Faculty Candidates

---

1. Cutting-edge advertisement and outreach
2. Strong mission statement and an inclusive campus climate
3. Diverse and well-trained search committees
4. Competitive hiring packages

Active involvement in discipline-specific professional organizations is also essential. These organizations are (a) AAMC, (b) Physician Assistant Education Association (PAEA), (c) AACN, (d) National Organization of Nurse Practitioner Faculties (NONPF), (e) American Association of Colleges of Pharmacy (AACP), and (f) American Council of Academic Physical Therapy (ACAPT). Involvement in these associations provides opportunities for networking, sponsorship, mentorship, learning about promotion and tenure processes, and opportunities for scholarship such as presenting posters, coauthorship of articles, and peer reviews.

EXPANDING THE SCOPE OF SCHOLARSHIP

The percentage of minority faculty at academic medical centers remains disproportionately small despite many efforts to increase both student and faculty diversity over the past several decades (Rodríguez et al., 2014). As mentioned previously, this can lead to a diversity tax, or diversity burden. These additional responsibilities related to institutional diversity efforts are often not valued as scholarship or counted toward the promotion and tenure process, despite the institution's stated values and mission concerning diversity and inclusion. This can leave minority faculty with less time to spend on activities that nonminority faculty are encouraged to pursue to achieve promotion (Pololi, Cooper, & Carr, 2010).

Some institutions are revisiting their promotion and tenure guidelines and expanding the definition of scholarship (see Chapter 25). Coupled with effective mentoring, many of the outreach, community engagement, student mentoring, and clinical pursuits of minority faculty can be channeled into scholarly projects or research that furthers the minority faculty's academic career. Addressing the issues of diversity tax directly in the context of a mentoring relationship can help to guide choices and career paths and prevent diversion of minority faculty from true research or career interests.

EXTERNAL MINORITY LEADERSHIP PROGRAMS

There are increasing opportunities for leadership development for minority faculty in health professions education. These programs offer a setting for faculty to network, discuss issues faced by minority faculty in an open, safe space, and hear from successful minority leaders and faculty where there may be few opportunities to do so in their home institutions. Funded institutional support in terms of faculty release time and tuition fees help to increase participation. Such support can be negotiated as part of an employment package or during the annual review of one's teaching and workload. Faculty that successfully demonstrate leadership skills in academic settings can serve as a leadership pipeline for future positions and are role models and mentors for minority students and upcoming minority faculty. Minority faculty leadership training workshops are offered by several national organizations (Exhibit 22.3).

EXHIBIT 22.3 Minority Faculty Leadership Workshops

- AAMC Minority Faculty Development Seminar (www.aamc.org/initiatives/diversity/portfolios/260940/minorityfacultycareerdevelopmentseminar.html)
- Minority Nurse Leadership Institute at Rutgers School of Nursing (www.nursing.rutgers.edu/mnli/index.html)
- PAEA Minority Leadership Workshop (www.paeaonline.org/my-experience-at-the-leadership-101-developing-minority-faculty-leaders-pando-workshop)
- Johnson & Johnson/AACN Minority Nurse Faculty Scholars Program (www.aacn.nche.edu/students/scholarships/minority)

AACN, American Association of Colleges of Nursing; AAMC, Association of American Medical Colleges; PAEA, Physician Assistant Education Association.

MINORITY FACULTY MENTORING AND SPONSORSHIP

It is known in the health professions education field that diversity in the institution is considered important; however, it continues to be a difficult goal to achieve (Hamann, 2015). Mentoring and sponsorship may be a means to improve the persistence, advancement, and retention of diverse faculty. Blackwell (1989) describes mentoring as a process in which a faculty member of higher rank and special achievements instructs, counsels, guides, and facilitates the intellectual or career development of an individual identified as a mentee. The mentoring of a junior faculty member consists of instruction, promoting the acquisition of knowledge, providing psychological support, socialization into the culture and environment, modeling professionalism and building self-confidence, and navigation through the tumultuous higher education domain (Blackwell, 1989).

Mentorship is important for all, but for minority faculty it has arguably been considered the most dominant factor for career success (Turner et al., 2008). Specifically, diverse faculty disclose that building social capital, creating relationships with those individuals who have power and prestige, and developing uniquely independent scholarship and an active-participatory approach are ideal mentoring characteristics (Zambrana et al., 2015). Political guidance was principally critical to diverse faculty career success by improving knowledge regarding institutional norms and how to navigate the system, thus increasing social capital. This in turn may reduce the relinquishment of autonomy centered on scholarship and other academic pursuits that may otherwise occur as a form of assimilation if political guidance were absent.

A formal mentoring program is necessary for effective mentoring to occur. Despite the benefits of mentoring for diverse faculty, there are numerous barriers that may make mentoring nonexistent or inadequate for diverse faculty. There is clear lack of systematic formal mentoring of early-stage minority faculty (Moody, 2012). Reasons for the absence of a formal mentoring program typically include an institutional or systemic belief that informal or minimal mentoring is sufficient because the organization is successful, mentoring is not needed, or that mentoring prevents spontaneity. Likewise, formal mentoring is also avoided because departments and programs are concerned about the lack of faculty time and/or that a single mentor for the entire program is adequate for mentoring to occur. Training programs or seminars considered satisfactory for developing junior faculty, although helpful, are not sufficient for faculty mentoring. Informal mentoring may include only career advice; infrequent meetings; and an assumption that deans, chairs, and provosts are capable of mentoring junior faculty of color. Along these lines, it can be assumed that informal mentoring lacks quality control and improvement, which should be a component in a formal mentoring program.

Additional barriers to formal mentoring include difficulties with cross-cultural relationships, which may be prominent in health professions education because of the deficiency of diverse faculty in most health professions programs (Hamann, 2015). Minority faculty therefore may encounter more social and institutional isolation (Zambrana et al., 2015). Because diverse faculty often find themselves the only diverse faculty in their institution, there is heightened contrast between them and the majority faculty, which isolates the diverse faculty. Furthermore, the isolated faculty may also have to debunk stereotype threat or serve as a representative for the group to which they belong. Being the only minority faculty can bring a visibility that may bring unwanted, harmful attention, and a concurrent invisibility that is oppressive. Moreover, "othering" by faculty who feel comfortable only with their own in-groups disrupts collegiality. Finally, minority faculty often feel intense performance pressure (Moody, 2012). Power differentials may play a significant role in the development of relationships, especially between White mentors and mentees of color and male mentors and female mentees (Cowin, Cohen, Ciechanowski, & Orozco, 2011). Nevertheless, successful cross-cultural mentoring can occur between a White mentor and a diverse mentee; however, certain conditions need to occur. Diverse faculty seek to identify true allies who understand and are also sensitive to cultural differences. In addition, mentors who belong to the dominant group must avoid trying to duplicate their own career paths, scholarship, and personal constructs in mentees of color. Moreover, the development of mutual respect is of critical importance for the development of cross-cultural relationships. Overall, mentors who recognize differences in cross-cultural communication styles and power differentials, and who demonstrate sincere concern about the well-being and identity of the mentee, are more likely to have successful mentor–mentee relationships (Turner & Gonzalez, 2015). Cross-racial mentors have characteristics of multicultural sensitivity, self-reflection regarding privilege, and the understanding that many faculty of color are interested in research centered on race, ethnicity, diversity, and social justice topics (Stanley & Lincoln, 2009). Cross-racial mentorship goes beyond the concept assigned. It is critical that strong positive relationships are created and maintained despite the risk of discomfort that occurs when differences arise. Moreover, it is also imperative that the mentee not feel that he or she is being mentored because of his or her nondominant status or because of a deficiency in scholarship (Stanley & Lincoln, 2009).

CONCLUSIONS

Programs to increase the recruitment and retention of diverse faculty should have intentional, employable methods to break the aforementioned barriers. Specifically, institutional policies and norms must reflect a culture of equity and inclusion. Formal mentoring techniques and themes should be employed, with acknowledgment of explicit topics that concern diverse faculty. Education of faculty mentors regarding URM-specific experiences, networks outside the institution for URM faculty, and forming specific policies and practices regarding the mentoring of URM faculty are essential to promoting minority faculty success. Improving social capital through advisement regarding the political climate and how to navigate it is also critical. These considerations should be part of institutional culture and structure. As it is often said, "a lot of different flowers make a bouquet"; diversity is central to achieving academic excellence within health professions schools, and minority faculty need to not only be recruited and retained, but also to be supported to succeed.

REFERENCES

American Association of Colleges of Nursing. (2015). Enhancing diversity in the workforce. Retrieved from http://www.aacn.nche.edu/media-relations/fact-sheets/enhancing-diversity

American Academy of Physician Assistants. (2013). 2013 AAPA annual survey report. Retrieved from https://www.aapa.org/wp-content/uploads/2016/12/Annual_Server_Data_Tables-S.pdf

Association of American Medical Colleges. (2012). *Diversity in medical education: Facts & figures 2012*. Washington, DC: Author. Retrieved from https://members.aamc.org/eweb/upload/Diversity%20in%20Medical%20Education%20Facts%20and%20Figures%202012.pdf

Blackwell, J. E. (1989). Mentoring: An action strategy for increasing minority faculty. *Academe, 75*(5), 8–14.

Corrice, A. (2009). Unconscious bias in faculty and leadership recruitment: A literature review. *AAMC Analysis in Brief, 9*(2), 1–2.

Cowin, K. M., Cohen, L. M., Ciechanowski, K. M., & Orozco, R. A. (2011). Portraits of mentor-junior faculty relationships: From power dynamics to collaboration. *Journal of Education, 192*(1), 30–47.

Cropsey, K. L., Masho, S. W., Shiang, R., Sikka, V., Kornstein, S. G., & Hampton, C. L. (2008). Why do faculty leave? Reasons for attrition of women and minority faculty from a medical school: Four-year results. *Journal of Women's Health, 17*(7), 1111–1118. doi:10.1089/jwh.2007.0582

Diggs, G. A., Garrison-Wade, F., Estrada, D., & Galindo, R. (2009) Smiling faces and colored spaces: The experiences of faculty of color pursuing tenure in the academy. *Urban Review, 41*, 312–333.

Hagan, A. M., Campbell, H. E., & Gaither, C. A. (2016). The racial and ethnic representation of faculty in US pharmacy schools and colleges. *American Journal of Pharmaceutical Education, 80*(6), 108.

Hamann, R. A. (2015). *Comparison report: State of diversity among pa faculty and matriculants.* Washington, DC: Physician Assistant Education Association. Retrieved from http://paeaonline.org/research/comparison-report-state-of-diversity-among-pa-faculty-and-matriculants

Harte, H. A., Gilbert, J. L., Chai, H. H., Soled, S. W., Ofori-Attah, K., & Gunn, K. (2011). Perspectives on facilitating minority faculty success in higher education. *Kentucky Journal of Excellence in College Teaching and Learning, 7*(1), 5.

Moody, J. (2012). *Faculty diversity: Removing barriers.* New York, NY: Routledge.

National Center for Education Statistics. (2016). *Fast facts: Race/ethnicity of college faculty.* Washington, DC: U.S. Department of Education. Retrieved from https://nces.ed.gov/fastfacts/display.asp?id=61

Page, K. R., Castillo-Page, L., & Wright, S. M. (2011). Faculty diversity programs in U.S. medical schools and characteristics associated with higher faculty diversity. *Academic Medicine, 86*(10), 1221–1228.

Parson, P. (2016). Recruitment and retention at the intersections. In B. Barnett & P. Felton (Eds.), *Intersectionality in action: A guide for faculty and campus leaders for creating inclusive classrooms and institutions* (pp. 15–24). Sterling, VA: Stylus.

Pololi, L., Cooper, L. A., & Carr, P. (2010). Race, disadvantage and faculty experiences in academic medicine. *Journal of General Internal Medicine, 25*(12), 1363–1369.

Rodríguez, J. E., Campbell, K. M., & Mouratidis, R. W. (2014). Where are the rest of us? Improving representation of minority faculty in academic medicine. *Southern Medical Journal, 107*(12), 739–744. doi:10.14423/SMJ.0000000000000204

Rockquemore, K., & Laszloffy, T. A. (2008). *The black academic's guide to winning tenure—Without losing your soul* (p. 261). Boulder, CO: Lynne Rienner.

Salvucci, C., & Lawless, C. A. (2016). Nursing faculty diversity: Barriers and perceptions on recruitment, hiring and retention. *Journal of Cultural Diversity, 23*(2), 65–75.

Smith, D. G. (2015). *Diversity's promise for higher education: Making it work* (2nd ed.). Baltimore, MD: John Hopkins University Press.

Smith, D. G. (2011). Identifying talent, disrupting the usual. In L. M. Stulberg & S. L. Weinbberg (Eds.), *Diversity in American higher education* (pp. 142–152). New York, NY: Routledge.

Stanley, C. A., & Lincoln, Y. S. (2005). Cross-race faculty mentoring. *Change, 37*(2), 44–50.

Turner, C. S. V., & Gonzalez, J. C. (2015). What does the literature tell us about mentoring across race/ethnicity and gender? In C. S. V. Turner & J. C. Gonzalez (Eds.), *Modeling mentoring across race/ethnicity and gender* (pp. 1–41). Sterling, VA: Stylus.

Turner, C. S. V., Gonzalez, J. C., & Wood, J. L. (2008). Faculty of color in academe: What 20 years of literature tells us. *Journal of Diversity in Higher Education, 1*(3), 139–168.

Zambrana, R. E., Ray, R., Espino, M. M., Castro, C., Cohen, B. D., & Eliason, J. (2015). "Don't leave us behind": *The importance of mentoring for underrepresented minority faculty. American Educational Research Journal, 52*(1), 40–72.

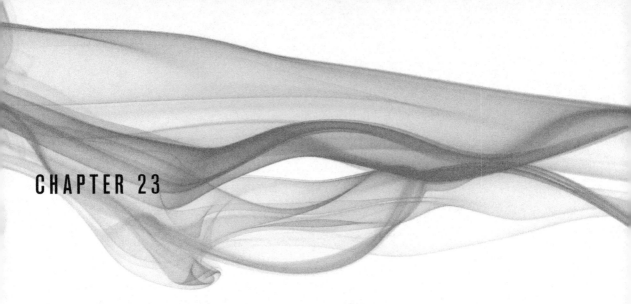

CHAPTER 23

Achieving Inclusive Excellence

Kenyon Railey, Jacqueline S. Barnett, and DeShana Collett

CHAPTER OBJECTIVES

- Explain key components of creating an organizational culture of equity, diversity, and inclusion
- Design measures of inclusive excellence in your program and classroom

---

We cannot seek achievement for ourselves and forget about progress and prosperity for our community. . . . Our ambitions must be broad enough to include the aspirations and needs of others, for their sakes and for our own.

—*Cesar Chavez*

The U.S. Census Bureau projects that the U.S. population will become "majority–minority" by the year 2044, and nearly one in five of the nation's total population is projected to be foreign born by 2060 (Colby & Ortman, 2014). This anticipated demographic shift, coupled with current judicial decisions and challenges related to ethnicity, gender identity, and sexual orientation, has heightened awareness of inequity in a variety of settings. Educational institutions, specifically those tasked with training medical providers, have seen a simultaneous increase in the recognition of health disparities among vulnerable populations.

This trend was largely influenced by the release of two sentinel reports, *Crossing the Quality Chasm* (Committee on Quality Health Care in America, Institute of Medicine, 2001) and *Unequal Treatment: Confronting Racial and Ethnic Disparities in Healthcare* (Committee on Understanding and Eliminating Racial and Ethnic Disparities in Health Care, Institute of Medicine, 2002). These documents were among the first to address the influence that bias, prejudice, and stereotyping have on differences in care, but they also highlighted the importance of increasing the proportion of underrepresented minorities (URMs) among health professionals. Since then, researchers have explored the implications of inequality and the roles that institutions of higher learning should play in mitigating them. Discussions about health equity are therefore intricately tied to discussions about diversity. Consequently, organizations are being asked to reexamine their institutional culture and diversity-related initiatives in the classroom and the clinic in order to promote education, improve health, and achieve social equity.

The Association of American Colleges and Universities (AAC&U) created the concept of inclusive excellence to help leaders understand the interplay between diversity and educational quality. This framework addresses the complex dimensions of organizational behavior, culture, and change that have served as barriers to inclusion, and it reinforces the concept that diversity is vital to institutional success. As defined by the AAC&U, *inclusive excellence* consists of four primary elements (Clayton-Pedersen, O'Neill, & McTighe Musil, n.d.):

1. A focus on intellectual and social development
2. Purposeful development and utilization of organizational resources to enhance learning
3. Attention to cultural differences that enhance the educational experience
4. A welcoming community that engages all of its members in learning

The work of the AAC&U highlights the need to integrate diversity and quality to place inclusion efforts at the core of institutional functioning while producing a product that is durable and beneficial to all within the organization. This chapter explores the current scope of diversity and inclusion within the health professions and medical education, and recommends strategies to achieve inclusive excellence in the classroom, across the organization, and beyond.

DIVERSITY VERSUS INCLUSION

It is crucial to understand that diversity and inclusion are not synonymous. In "Reinventing Diversity," Howard Ross defines *diversity* as an acceptance of difference, a lack of discrimination due to difference, and a presence of different kinds of people in organizations (Ross, 2011). This definition is both specific enough to address the many demographic differences related to race, ethnicity, gender, and sexuality, and flexible enough to be inclusive of other measures of diversity as our understanding of culture evolves. *Inclusion*, by contrast, is a "function of how involved people are in the structures of their organization" (Ross, 2011, p. 38). Ultimately, inclusion requires an engagement with diversity and the creation of a climate that promotes a sense of belonging, respect, and value for every member of the community. In the simplest terms, diversity is invitation, inclusion is involvement.

Within the academic medical sphere, demographic diversity remains a problem for students and faculty from traditionally underrepresented groups. It remains apparent that even if institutions were to achieve parity between population and provider demographics, a deficit would remain in the number of nonmajority individuals being promoted and holding key positions of influence. Efforts to establish inclusion therefore require organizations to address exclusionary policies and practices that compromise a sense of belonging while simultaneously celebrating the coexistence of individuals from different backgrounds.

BENEFITS OF DIVERSITY

As economies and people become more connected, organizations that best attract and retain diverse members will have a competitive advantage (Williams, Berger, & McClendon, 2005). Page utilizes the concepts of heuristics (i.e., tools to find solutions) and perspectives (i.e., how people see problems) to explore how diverse teams consistently outperform homogenous ones. He suggests that "diversity trumps ability," and that for certain tasks, diversity leads to greater innovation (Page, 2007). Given the complexity of our current health care situation, achieving diversity in classrooms, clinics, and teaching hospitals sets the stage for medical organizations to address societal needs.

The evidence suggests that a diverse student population promotes the cultural, civic, and intellectual learning of all trainees, broadens perspectives on race, and improves students' learning experience (U.S. Department of Health and Human Services and Health Resources and Services Administration Bureau of Health Workforce, 2006). Trainees also experience positive long-term effects on personal growth, purpose in life, and increased volunteer behaviors when educated in diverse settings (Locks, Hurtado, Bowman, & Oseguera, 2008). In 2008, investigators surveyed more than 20,000 graduating medical students to assess whether student body diversity was associated with educational benefits. The authors concluded that white students attending more racially diverse medical schools rated themselves as better prepared than students at less diverse schools to care for racial and ethnic minority patients, and had stronger attitudes about inadequate access to health care (Saha, Guiton, Wimmers, & Wilkerson, 2008). Ethnic and racial diversity is therefore an important cornerstone of enhanced learning environments for all.

For faculty members, diversity provides opportunities for role-modeling, contributes to a learning environment in which minority students feel included instead of marginalized, and helps in the recruitment and retention of future underrepresented students (Metz, 2013). In addition, it has been suggested that minority faculty recruits are attracted to a workplace where they perceive a presence of similar "faces" and backgrounds (Smith, 2012).

Improving the pipeline of URMs therefore not only improves the educational environment, but also holds a promise of positive consequences for traditionally underserved areas. A diverse workforce is associated with improvements in patient access and public health for underserved populations, patient satisfaction, and quality care (U.S. Department of Health and Human Services and Health Resources and Services Administration Bureau of Health Workforce, 2006). Medical providers from underrepresented racial and ethnic backgrounds are more likely to practice primary care than are their White counterparts. Furthermore, these individuals are also more likely to practice in medically underserved areas. These findings were validated in a study that examined physician assistant (PA) practice patterns and demonstrated that PAs from underrepresented groups are more likely to work in underserved areas, and that a higher proportion of non-White versus White PAs chose to work in primary care settings (Coplan, Cawley, & Stoehr, 2013).

It is important to add that diversifying the provider workforce with respect to race, ethnicity, and gender is important, but it will not sufficiently address projected deficits in access and quality as health care is reformed. Inclusion with respect to who manages patients is an important consideration with implications for the pipeline for students and access for patients. The PA profession, which emerged out of a need to increase primary care providers in underserved areas (LeLacheur, Barnett, & Straker, 2015), as well as the proliferation of other advanced practice providers such as nurse practitioners (NPs), has increased the number of potential professionals at the point of patient care. In certain states, many PAs and NPs are providing care in rural and medically underserved areas (Mulitalo & Straker, 2007; Pomeranz, Bailey, & Bradley-Guidry, 2014).

With today's changing demographics, it is expected that future health professions students will be increasingly differentiated by race, ethnicity, age, sexual identity, social class, culture, and so on. It will be vital for health educators to have the knowledge, skills, and attitudes to use (not ignore) difference to enrich the curricula and promote a culturally competent learning environment. As hospitals and clinics continue to explore more team-based delivery models, health professionals urgently need to work together in teams and move beyond traditional, physician-driven models of care.

BARRIERS TO INCLUSION

One of the current challenges to diversity and inclusion relates to how organizations view diversity. Over the past two decades, efforts to address diversity generally have involved strategies that create immediate changes, often as a reaction to a particular event or problem. Success has too often been determined by activities, defined by fewer complaints, and characterized by "making halfhearted commitment to increasing diversity in the future" (Ross, 2011, p. 32). Unfortunately, this pattern has created cynicism and contributed to prevailing and persistent negative views of affirmative action, leading many to continue misinterpreting the data on whom affirmative action programs benefit most. Prevailing misperceptions that diversity entails "unqualified" individuals taking the "spots" of "better" individuals have persisted. By themselves, diversity programs and activities rarely lead to change at levels deep enough to ultimately transform climate; thus, a key barrier to address is overcoming activity-focused initiatives and the resulting negative perceptions of diversity and inclusion work (Ross, 2011).

Even when diversity programs exist, their lack of integration presents a further challenge in academic medical centers. Projects and programs that run parallel to core processes, where many diversity efforts have remained, are insufficient to "move the needle." In 2011, Marc Nivet, the chief diversity officer of the Association of American Medical Colleges (AAMC), published a landmark article recommending a transformation of how diversity and inclusion are viewed in achieving a more equitable health system (Nivet, 2011). He concluded that diversity and inclusion are solutions, not problems, and he ultimately recommended that institutions work to integrate these tenets within their core policies. In an update to the 2011 article, he advocated an emphasis on how "all community members experience the institution's culture" (Nivet, 2015, p. 1592). This is not to say that organizations should discontinue initiatives that address historically unfinished business as it relates to race, social class, and gender; rather, diversity programs must continue in these areas while simultaneously engaging new concerns about disability, gender identity, immigration, and religion, among others (Smith, 2012). These programs contribute to inclusive excellence by addressing campus climate, but efforts must be integrated into core instructional and institutional processes.

One cannot discuss contributors to a lack of inclusion without also discussing the systematic barriers related to race, ethnicity, and gender that remain within society broadly, and in medicine specifically. Many of the diversity issues facing institutions are related to power and equity concerning groups for whom access and inclusion are lacking (Smith, 2011). The persistent lack of URMs in the health workforce may be a symptom of the nation's "long and unresolved struggle to come to terms with the uncomfortable and often divisive issue of race and racism" (Grumbach & Mendoza, 2008, p. 421), which is deeply rooted in American history. The marginalization of racial and ethnic minorities is arguably the root cause of the disparities experienced in today's health care system, and such marginalization may be the major barrier to the creation of inclusive climates.

SPECIFIC STRATEGIES TO DIVERSITY AND INCLUSIVE EXCELLENCE

The AAC&U's concept of inclusive excellence reimagines traditional ways of thinking about institutional function. The AAC&U recommends that organizations think beyond traditional pipeline- and demographic-focused diversity initiatives. Given that subgroups themselves are multifaceted, true institutional transformation and excellence are rooted in recognizing the value of multiple individuals within organizations. An inclusive community holds everyone responsible for creating a culture of belonging, and it implements strategic systemic change to build a capacity for diversity. This section addresses a few strategies for building diverse organizations and addressing exclusionary processes that have been barriers to inclusive excellence.

Make Inclusion Central to the Mission

Making inclusion central to an organization's mission has bearing on the experience of faculty and students alike. Just as textbooks, small groups, and lectures have a direct effect on the educational process, so, too, does the institution's learning environment—"the institution's ethos, teachers, modeling, policies, and processes" (Murray-García & García, 2008, p. 646).

Most academic health centers share the tripartite goal of teaching, research, and patient care. To better serve populations and achieve excellence in the original tripartite goals, diversity and inclusion are now considered necessary to achieve strategic imperatives and academic excellence. Smith (2011) has suggested that leaders within academic health centers consider building the capacity for diversity in a manner similar to that used for building the capacity for technology. As the Internet and computer-based skills and knowledge grew, the viability of various organizations in and out of health education was linked to technological capability. Institutions invested in human and financial capital to build a technological framework that promotes educational excellence. Initially, implementing technology was a struggle because it challenged the status quo (Smith, 2012). Over time, however, technology became a dynamic yet simultaneously stable entity. Learning about the effects of race, ethnicity, gender, and sexual orientation on health, diversity, and inclusion on the core of an organization will increase our capacity for adaptation and advancement in much the same way technology has.

Improve Access and Success for Underrepresented Students

Evidence suggests that the use of traditional measures of aptitude and ability (i.e., grade point average [GPA], standardized testing scores, and so on) to predict success have led to restrictive admission decisions that often benefit White students (Bleich, MacWilliams, & Schmidt, 2015; Hassouneh & Lutz, 2013). To build inclusive organizations, institutions should consider other metrics to identify successful applicants, especially given that standardized tests, such as the medical college admission test (MCAT), do not seem to correlate with clinic performance (Gohara et al., 2011). In addition, URMs admitted to medical schools with lower MCAT scores are as likely to graduate and pass licensing boards as nonminority students (Davidson & Lewis, 1997). One study evaluating the use of graduate record examination (GRE) scores in PA admissions concluded that only 40% of programs were using scores in accordance with guidelines, and that current data on the predictive value of the GRE is incongruent (Hocking & Piepenbrock, 2010). Organizations should consider interview processes that consider other attributes of success and alternate measures of intelligence. Such metrics as resiliency, resourcefulness, engagement with diversity, and inclusion should be considered (Clayton-Pedersen et al., n.d.).

To promote success, institutions should provide a diverse learning environment by attending to the recruitment, retention, and achievement of all students while simultaneously enhancing curricular instruction, assessment, mentorship, and overall campus climate.

Improve Access and Success for Underrepresented Faculty

A shortage of URM faculty in medicine and health professions training programs persists. Efforts to recruit and retain URM faculty must address historical policies of exclusionary practices and a culture that promoted elitism and systemic discrimination, both of which caused URM faculty to feel devalued and marginalized (Whittaker, Montgomery, & Martinez Acosta, 2015). To improve the retention and success of URMs, Whittaker and colleagues (2015) suggest that institutions should implement steps to (a) assess the institutional climate; (b) establish faculty mentoring and retention programs; (c) promote equity in faculty workload, grant and research support, and academic rank, promotion, and tenure; (d) ensure balanced faculty governance and promotion and tenure structures; and (e) educate and engage leaders to be agents of change. Language used in recruiting materials should be welcoming and inclusive to encourage women and URMs to apply, and unbiased selection and promotion criteria should be established in advance to reduce the likelihood that some groups benefit over others.

Promote Education and Scholarship in Cultural Competency

In the early development of inclusive excellence, education is vital. Although the exact methods of training and overall effectiveness of inclusive excellence remain in debate and are beyond the scope of this chapter, it is clear that improving learners' and employees' cultural humility will enhance the educational environment by raising awareness and aiding the development of shared perceptions. Health professionals should be educated in diverse environments in which they can better understand the impact of an individual's needs, values, and preferences on interpersonal relationships and patient care (Nivet, 2011).

Even though behavioral change can occur through education, training alone will not change organizational culture unless a critical mass of individuals participates. Poorly designed and "one-off" initiatives (those without follow-up or reinforcement) can contribute to additional stereotypes and alienation (Holvino, Ferdman, & Merrill-Sands, 2004). Cultural competency integration over time has been shown to improve cultural awareness. Beck, Scheel, De Oliveira, and Hopp (2013) demonstrated that education throughout the preclinical year of a PA training program improved scores on cultural awareness surveys given at multiple times during the didactic year. A study conducted during the clinical year of a PA program yielded similar results. Using a qualitative analysis of a course that included self-reflection, oral presentations, and cultural awareness discussion groups, investigators concluded that integration throughout the clinical phase improved cultural competency (Bahrke, De Oliveira, Scheel, Beck, & Hopp, 2014).

Not only should institutions provide trainings, workshops, and other opportunities to improve exposure and instruction, they should also simultaneously pursue opportunities to perform educational research in these areas. Given a lack of consensus concerning the best means of evaluating the many methods for assessing cultural competency, new tools for assessing progress and effectiveness should be developed and validated.

Incorporate Multicultural Education Strategies and Equity Pedagogy

If education and scholarship in cultural competency are to succeed, educators must create initiatives that are based on multicultural education strategies. Multicultural education involves providing knowledge about such key concepts as immigration, racism, sexism, cultural assimilation, stereotypes, prejudice, and institutional racism (Banks & Banks, 1995). Multicultural education emerged in the United States during the profound social change of the 1960s and 1970s, when minority groups demanded inclusion in the curricula of schools, colleges, and universities. Today, it continues to evolve as population demographics shift, and it remains rooted in the transformation of education as a force for promoting equity and the ideals of a just and pluralistic society (Hanley, n.d.). To help students explore feelings and facilitate linkages, educators need to incorporate these concepts into the learning milieu (Banks & Banks, 1995).

James A. Banks developed and conceptualized multicultural education along five dimensions: (a) content integration, (b) knowledge construction, (c) prejudice reduction, (d) equity pedagogy, and (e) empowering school culture and social structure (Banks, 1994, 2013; Banks & Banks, 1995). Chapter 21 includes details of Banks's dimensions of multicultural education. Understanding the concept of equity pedagogy is important because it can help educators make reforms and create meaningful learning experiences.

Equity pedagogy involves teaching students more than just the medical facts about a particular disease or illness; it involves directing learners to pay attention to assumptions, biases, and societal determinants related to that same illness. Learning becomes more meaningful because it also includes a consideration of the experiences and attitudes of others. A skilled educator in equity pedagogy can help students learn about the effects of illness on a patient's functional ability, employment, and family dynamics. A curriculum that integrates the concepts of multiculturalism with equity pedagogy can help students gain and retain the knowledge and skills they need to act thoughtfully regarding patient care.

Discuss Unconscious Bias, Microaggressions, and Stereotype Threat

To create a climate in which constituents thrive rather than merely survive, institutions working toward inclusive excellence must discuss and address the effects of bias, prejudice, and stereotypes on the learning environment. Academic medical centers must dedicate resources and training to the ways unconscious bias compromises inclusion efforts at multiple levels. Current and future clinicians must understand the effects of unconscious bias on health inequity in the United States. In addition, administrators must understand that implicit associations at the recruitment and retention levels and unconscious biases contribute to microaggressions, which compromise efforts to achieve inclusive excellence among learners, faculty, and staff.

Racial microaggressions were first defined in the 1970s by Chester Pierce as "brief and commonplace daily verbal, behavioral, or environmental indignities, whether intentional or unintentional, that communicate hostile, derogatory, or negative racial slights and insults toward people of color" (Sue et al., 2007, p. 271). Microaggressions can be environmental as well as result from human encounters. Although the perpetrators of microaggressions are often unaware, these indignities have real implications for peer and patient relationships in academic medicine. Institutions should therefore provide members with examples of microaggressions to raise awareness and promote opportunities for reflection on the effects of race and racism in the workplace. It is important to note that microaggressions can also relate to gender, sexual orientation, and disability, producing equally detrimental effects on women, lesbian, gay, bisexual, transgender, and queer (LGBTQ) individuals, and individuals with disabilities. All microaggressions must be managed if institutions are to establish the climates of belonging required for achieving inclusive excellence.

A stereotype threat occurs when negative remarks on the characteristics of a group of people trigger "physiological and psychological processes that have detrimental consequences for behavior" (Burgess, Warren, Phelan, Dovidio, & van Ryn, 2010, p. S169). In medical education, such threats have real-time implications for trainee performance.

Create Communities of Support

In a qualitative analysis that examined minority faculty members' experience with discrimination in academic medicine, faculty described the need for adequate support to succeed, including noninstitutional support from sources such as family, clergy, and community (Carr, Palepu, Szalacha, Caswell, & Inui, 2007). This type of support is crucial for health professions learners as well. Affinity groups, such as the Student National Medical Association (SNMA), Latino Medical Student Association (LMSA), Asian Pacific American Medical Student Association (APAMSA), and local and national LGBTQ professional and student associations, positively affect student environments within institutions and communities. Supportive educational communities foster a campus culture in which diversity is essential to intellectual and social development. These organizations naturally sustain and promote mentorship at the peer and faculty levels. Furthermore, these groups often coordinate social events, hold discussion groups, create celebrations of heritage, and initiate educational events that improve the cultural awareness of the broader academic community.

Create Organizational Transparency

To improve transparency and ultimately accountability, organizations should monitor and report their hiring practices and hold regular reviews of their mentoring and promotion processes. They should simultaneously conduct an assessment that includes a systematic review and evaluation of the current state of diversity and inclusivity within their organization. Collecting and sharing demographic information based on various institutionally directed imperatives are crucial to stakeholder accountability. Transparency concerning these data can help leaders establish accountability metrics that are intentional and visible. Both qualitative and quantitative data provide a broader, more in-depth understanding of the current state of an organization's diversity and inclusivity, and sharing this information facilitates an assessment of the data's impact.

A variety of strategies—including facilitating structured dialogue among URM and non-URM groups, teaching effective feedback methods to faculty, increasing exposure to role models who exhibit counterstereotype behaviors (Burgess et al., 2010), and others (see Table 23.1)—can contribute to the cultivation of a sense of belonging for all.

MEASURING INCLUSION

Research into change and organizational transformation has shown that monitoring progress is absolutely essential (Smith, 2012). Developing a framework for the organization's process of data collection and assessment is an important first step. The framework should consist of comprehensive performance measures directly tied to the institution's mission, goals, strategies, and outcomes. The culture and climate baseline assessment should be conducted before the implementation of any strategies or action plans. Another assessment should then be performed to monitor progress, especially as it relates to organizational learning. This information will ultimately allow teaching hospitals to make data-driven conclusions that support previously implemented initiatives.

An example of a baseline assessment tool is the Diversity Engagement Survey (DES), which was created in partnership by the AAMC, the University of Massachusetts Medical School, and DataStar. The DES is a diagnostic and benchmarking tool that contains 22 items. From 2011 to 2012, researchers piloted the survey and administered it to 13,694 respondents at 14 academic medical centers; they concluded that the DES was a reliable and valid instrument for assessing engagement around inclusion (Person et al., 2015). Metrics should be multifaceted to cover a wide range of areas throughout the organization. Refer again to Table 23.1 for some metrics organizations can use to establish benchmarks that adhere to the mission of promoting inclusive excellence.

CONCLUSIONS

Projected shifts in our nation's demographics highlight the current imbalance between the percentage of racial and ethnic minorities in the general population and their representation in the health professions. These changing demographics suggest that educational and medical institutions must undergo major shifts if they are to respond to the diverse array of future patient, personnel, and provider needs.

TABLE 23.1 Strategies for Achieving Inclusive Excellence

Mission	Objective	Strategies	Measures/Benchmarks
Improve access and success: URM students	▪ Increase matriculation and graduation of URM students ▪ Implement admission processes that consider resourcefulness, resiliency, leadership, altruism, and diversity/inclusion engagement in line with the institution's mission	▪ Consider holistic admission processes and nontraditional measures of candidate assessment and evaluation ▪ Discuss measures beyond GPAs and standardized testing in admissions criteria ▪ Provide longitudinal cultural humility training ▪ Perform an annual review of recruitment and retention data ▪ Identify areas of improvement ▪ Review financial aid/scholarship programs ▪ Review pipeline programs ▪ Increase networking/mentoring efforts ▪ Perform student exit surveys/interview	▪ Numbers/percentages of URM applications and matriculation ▪ Numbers/percentages of URM students regarding retention and attrition ▪ Length of time until graduation ▪ Board/certification exam passage rates

Improve access and success: URM faculty	▪ Recruit and retain
	▪ Ensure balanced promotion and tenure structures
		▪ Employ intentional recruitment efforts
		▪ Provide cultural humility/implicit bias training for all search committees
		▪ Institute competitive salaries
		▪ Identify barriers for academic success
		▪ Cluster hiring efforts
		▪ Perform faculty exit surveys/interview
			▪ Numbers/percentages of URM faculty:
			  ▪ Recruited, hired, promoted
			  ▪ Retained and separated
			  ▪ Serving in leadership positions (dean, chairs, and others)
			  ▪ Received research support/funding
			  ▪ Reported job equity, job satisfaction, presence of inclusive climate

Promote education and scholarship in cultural competency	▪ Improve diversity and cultural awareness throughout formal and informal components of curriculum ▪ Enhance patient care ▪ Reduce health care disparities	▪ Review curricular and noncurricular components for integration of culturally relevant material ▪ Perform regular ongoing curricular mapping for diversity and inclusion content ▪ Integrate cultural competency in a longitudinal fashion, not in isolated lectures ▪ Review methods/time frame for evaluating the curriculum and learning objectives to ensure that diversity and inclusivity are appropriately assessed ▪ Review the effectiveness of current programming, activities, and trainings, and establish valid pre/post assessment measures ▪ Examine course content delivery methodology and teaching styles for appropriateness for all students ▪ Perform ongoing training sessions for faculty ▪ Review content that may perpetuate stereotypes and may include forms of microaggressions or implicit bias ▪ Perform educational research in cultural competency	▪ Analyze course/instructor evaluations ▪ Analyze qualitative learner feedback on courses ▪ Review publication frequency

(continued)

TABLE 23.1 Strategies for Achieving Inclusive Excellence (*continued*)

Mission	Objective	Strategies	Measures/Benchmarks
Incorporate multicultural education strategies and equity pedagogy	▪ Deliver course content in a culturally appropriate manner ▪ Improve attitudes, knowledge, and skills regarding culturally appropriate care	▪ Explore and define racism, sexism, privilege, and social determinants of health ▪ Use self-reflection exercises ▪ Provide data beyond scientific facts on patients and populations ▪ Enhance social history taking skills ▪ Explore the meaning of illness for patients ▪ Explore impact of disease on patient's functional ability, employment, and family dynamics	▪ Analyze patient satisfaction data ▪ Analyze standardized patient experiences ▪ Analyze qualitative learner feedback on courses
Discuss unconscious bias, microaggressions, and stereotype threat	▪ Improve awareness of specific attitudes and behaviors that contribute to marginalization ▪ Create identity-safe environments	▪ Have members take implicit association tests ▪ Identify specific examples of microaggressions ▪ Discuss race and racism within a historical context but also within health care settings ▪ Review concepts related to privilege ▪ Respond to microaggressions and develop methods to address in learner and workplace settings ▪ Discuss and acknowledge microaggressions related to gender, sexual orientation, and disability ▪ Promote self-affirmation activities ▪ Increase exposure and visibility of positive role models that counter stereotype threat ▪ Provide alternative external explanations for anxieties and distractions that do not validate the stereotype ▪ Conduct structured dialogues among URM and non-URM groups ▪ Teach effective feedback methods	▪ Collect qualitative data on member experiences ▪ Review mistreatment reports and bias incidence data (sexual, racial, harassment, sexual assault, bias reporting, and so on) ▪ Compile minority representation numbers
Create communities of support	▪ Provide essential intellectual and social support of all students, faculty, staff, and campus community members	▪ Establish organizational structural support for inclusive excellence ▪ Establish climate survey ▪ Establish a bias incidence response team (BIRT) ▪ Develop workshops and diversity forums that promote community interaction	▪ Assess campus-wide climate survey data annually, trend data ▪ Review bias incidence data (sexual, racial, harassment, sexual assault, bias reporting, and so forth)
Create organizational transparency	▪ Enhance accountability ▪ Promote equity among constituents	▪ Review policies, procedures, and program handbooks, including strategic plans, mission, and vision statements related to equity, diversity, and inclusivity ▪ Institute diversity and unconscious bias training ▪ Review marketing materials, website, and social media to determine whether they are consistent with the mission and goals of the institution ▪ Review and create professional development activities related to diversity and inclusivity ▪ Conduct faculty exit surveys/interview	▪ Establish and review performance evaluations and diversity metrics for deans and administrators ▪ Establish accountability metrics for colleges and incentives for meeting benchmarks ▪ Ensure that reporting on accomplishments and challenges in meeting institutional diversity benchmarks are visible ▪ Establish a diversity dashboard with metrics, and publish it on the institution's website ▪ Conduct and review faculty exit interview data

GPAs, grade point averages; URM, underrepresented minority.

To address dilemmas related to disparities in academic success, the absence of comprehensive guidelines that incorporate diversity at its core, and an overall lack of coordination of diversity efforts, the AAC&U created the concept of inclusive excellence. It provides an excellent framework for academic medical centers that seek to improve educational climate, health care quality, and health disparities.

To truly achieve inclusive excellence and lessen the impact of bias and exclusionary practices, educational and medical institutions should align their personnel, policies, politics, and procedures. They should also support these efforts not only through the formation of actual bodies, offices, and centers dedicated to the task, but also through the financial backing that such efforts require to achieve long-lasting effects. Working and learning in environments of inclusive excellence will affect future recruitment and retention and will ultimately attract outstanding and talented members who are fully engaged while working to improve teaching, learning, and service in an increasingly diverse world.

REFERENCES

Banks, C. A. M., & Banks, J. A. (1995). Equity pedagogy: An essential component of multicultural education. *Theory Into Practice, 34*(3), 152–158.

Banks, J. A. (1994). *An introduction to multicultural education*. Needham Heights, MA: Allyn & Bacon. Retrieved from http://eric.ed.gov/?id=ED372129

Banks, J. A. (2013). *An introduction to multicultural education* (5th ed.). Boston, MA: Pearson.

Bahrke, B., De Oliveira, K., Scheel, M. H., Beck, B., & Hopp, J. (2014). Longitudinal integration of cultural components into a physician assistant program's clinical year may improve cultural competency. *Journal of Physician Assistant Education, 25*(1), 33–37.

Beck, B., Scheel, M. H., De Oliveira, K., & Hopp, J. (2013). Integrating cultural competency throughout a first-year physician assistant curriculum steadily improves cultural awareness. *Journal of Physician Assistant Education, 24*(2), 28–31.

Bleich, M. R., MacWilliams, B. R., & Schmidt, B. J. (2015). Advancing diversity through inclusive excellence in nursing education. *Journal of Professional Nursing: Official Journal of the American Association of Colleges of Nursing, 31*(2), 89–94. doi:10.1016/j.profnurs.2014.09.003

Burgess, D., Warren, J., Phelan, S., Dovidio, J., & van Ryn, M. (2010). Stereotype threat and health disparities: What medical educators and future physicians need to know. *Journal of General Internal Medicine, 25*(Suppl. 2), S169–S177. doi:10.1007/s11606-009-1221-4

Carr, P. L., Palepu, A., Szalacha, L., Caswell, C., & Inui, T. (2007). "Flying below the radar": A qualitative study of minority experience and management of discrimination in academic medicine. *Medical Education, 41*(6), 601–609. doi:10.1111/j.1365-2923.2007.02771.x

Clayton-Pedersen, A., O'Neill, N., & McTighe Musil, C. (n.d.). Making excellence inclusive: A framework for embedding diversity and inclusion into colleges and universities' academic excellence mission. Retrieved from https://www.uwp.edu/explore/offices/diversityinclusion/upload/Making-Inclusive-Excellence.pdf

Colby, S. L., & Ortman, J. M. (2014). *Projections of the size and composition of the U.S. population: 2014 to 2060* (Report No. P25-1143). Washington, DC: U.S. Census Bureau. Retrieved from http://www.census.gov/library/publications/2015/demo/p25-1143.html

Committee on Quality of Health Care in America, Institute of Medicine. (2001). *Crossing the quality chasm: A new health system for the 21st century*. Washington, DC: National Academies Press. Retrieved from https://www.nap.edu/catalog/10027/crossing-the-quality-chasm-a-new-health-system-for-the

Committee on Understanding and Eliminating Racial and Ethnic Disparities in Health Care, Institute of Medicine. (2002). *Unequal treatment: Confronting racial and ethnic disparities in health care*. Washington, DC: National Academies Press. Retrieved from http://www.iom.edu/Reports/2002/Unequal-Treatment-Confronting-Racial-and-Ethnic-Disparities-in-Health-Care.aspx

Coplan, B., Cawley, J., & Stoehr, J. (2013). Physician assistants in primary care: Trends and characteristics. *Annals of Family Medicine, 11*(1), 75–79. doi:10.1370/afm.1432

Davidson, R. C., & Lewis, E. L. (1997). Affirmative action and other special consideration admissions at the University of California, Davis, School of Medicine. *Journal of the American Medical Association, 278*(14), 1153–1158.

Gohara, S., Shapiro, J. I., Jacob, A. N., Khuder, S. A., Gandy, R. A., Metting, P. J., & Kleshinski, J. (2011). Joining the conversation: Predictors of success on the United States Medical Licensing Examinations (USMLE). *Learning Assistance Review*, *16*(1), 11–20.

Grumbach, K., & Mendoza, R. (2008). Disparities in human resources: Addressing the lack of diversity in the health professions. *Health Affairs (Project Hope)*, *27*(2), 413–422. doi:10.1377/hlthaff.27.2.413

Hanley, M. (n.d.). The scope of multicultural education. Retrieved from http://education.jhu.edu/PD/newhorizons/strategies/topics/multicultural-education/the-scope-of-multicultural-education

Hassouneh, D., & Lutz, K. F. (2013). Having influence: Faculty of color having influence in schools of nursing. *Nursing Outlook*, *61*(3), 153–163. doi:10.1016/j.outlook.2012.10.002

Hocking, J. A, & Piepenbrock, K. (2010). Predictive ability of the graduate record examination and its usage across physician assistant programs. *Journal of Physician Assistant Education*, *21*(4), 18–22.

Holvino, E. H., Ferdman, B. M., & Merrill-Sands, D. (2004). Creating and sustaining diversity and inclusion in organizations: Strategies and approaches. In M. S. Stockdale & F. J. Crosby (Eds.), *The psychology and management of workplace diversity* (pp. 245–276). Malden, MA: Blackwell.

LeLacheur, S., Barnett, J., & Straker, H. (2015). Race, ethnicity, and the physician assistant profession. *Journal of the American Academy of Physician Assistants*, *28*(10), 41–45. doi:10.1097/01.JAA.000047 1609.54160.44

Locks, A. M., Hurtado, S., Bowman, N. A., & Oseguera, L. (2008) Extending notions of campus climate and diversity to students' transition to college. *Review of Higher Education*, *31*(3), 257–285. doi:10.1353/rhe.2008.0011

Metz, A. M. (2013). Racial and ethnic underrepresentation in medicine: Lessons from the past and a vision of the future. *Teaching and Learning in Medicine*, *25*(Suppl. 1), S33–S38. doi:10.1080/10401334.2013.84 2908

Mulitalo, K. E., & Straker, H. (2007). Diversity in physician assistant education. *Journal of Physician Assistant Education*, *18*(3), 46–51.

Murray-García, J. L., & García, J. A. (2008). The institutional context of multicultural education: What is your institutional curriculum? *Academic Medicine*, *83*(7), 646–652. doi:10.1097/ACM.0b013e3181782ed6

Nivet, M. A. (2011). Commentary: Diversity 3.0: A necessary systems upgrade. *Academic Medicine*, *86*(12), 1487–1489. doi:10.1097/ACM.0b013e3182351f79

Nivet, M. A. (2015). A diversity 3.0 update: Are we moving the needle enough? *Academic Medicine*, *90*(12), 1591–1593. doi:10.1097/ACM.0000000000000950

Page, S. E. (2007). Making the difference: Applying a logic of diversity. *Academy of Management Perspectives*, *21*(4), 6–20. doi:10.5465/AMP.2007.27895335

Person, S. D., Jordan C. G., Allison, J. J., Fink Ogawa, L. M., Castillo-Page, L. C., Conrad, S., Nivet, M. A., & Plummer, D. L. (2015). Measuring diversity and inclusion in academic medicine: The diversity engagement survey. *Academic Medicine*, *90*(12), 1675–1683. doi:10.1097/ACM.0000000000000921

Pomeranz, H., Bailey, J. R., & Bradley-Guidry, C. (2014). Primary care and diversity in the physician assistant profession. *Journal of Physician Assistant Education*, *25*(4), 47–51.

Ross, H. J. (2011). *Reinventing diversity: Transforming organizational community to strengthen people, purpose, and performance*. Lanham, MD: Rowman & Littlefield.

Saha, S., Guiton, G., Wimmers, P. F., & Wilkerson, L. (2008). Student body racial and ethnic composition and diversity related outcomes in U.S. medical schools. *Journal of the American Medical Association*, *300*(10), 1135–1145. doi:10.1001/jama.300.10.1135

Smith, D. G. (2011). *Diversity's promise for higher education: Making it work*. Baltimore, MD: Johns Hopkins University Press.

Smith, D. G. (2012). Building institutional capacity for diversity and inclusion in academic medicine. *Academic Medicine: Journal of the Association of American Medical Colleges*, *87*(11), 1511–1515. doi:10.1097/ACM.0b013e31826d30d5

Sue, D. W., Capodilupo, C. M., Torino, G. C., Bucceri, J. M., Holder, A. M., Nadal, K. L., & Esquilin, M. (2007). Racial microaggressions in everyday life: Implications for clinical practice. *American Psychologist*, *62*(4), 271–286. doi:10.1037/0003-066X.62.4.271

U.S. Department of Health and Human Services and Health Resources and Services Administration Bureau of Health Workforce. (2006). *The rationale for diversity in the health professions: A review of the evidence*. Washington, DC: U.S. Government Printing Office. Retrieved from http://docplayer.net/255577-The-rationale-for-diversity-in-the-health-professions-a-review-of-the-evidence.html

Whittaker, J. A., Montgomery, B. L., & Martinez Acosta, V. G. (2015). Retention of underrepresented minority faculty: Strategic initiatives for institutional value proposition based on perspectives from a range of academic institutions. *Journal of Undergraduate Neuroscience Education: JUNE: A Publication of FUN, Faculty for Undergraduate Neuroscience, 13*(3), A136–A145.

Williams, D. A., Berger, J. B., & McClendon, S. A. (2005). Toward a model of inclusive excellence and change in post-secondary institutions. Retrieved from https://www.aacu.org/sites/default/files/files/mei/williams_et_al.pdf

PART VI
Promoting Leadership and Scholarship

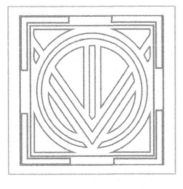

NEA OPE SE OBEDI HENE
"He who wants to be king."

Symbol of service and leadership

Comes from the expression, "Nea ope se obedi hene daakye no, firi ase sue som ansa" meaning, "He who wants to be king in the future must first learn to serve."

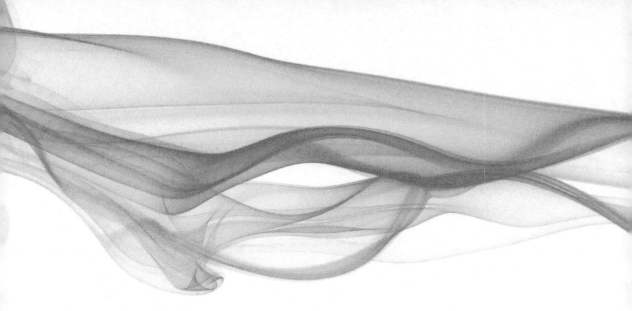

CHAPTER 24
Effective Ways to Promote Scholarship: The Academic Scholarship Portfolio

Douglas Brock and Susan Symington

CHAPTER OBJECTIVE

- Establish an academic scholarship portfolio that addresses the four legs of health professions scholarship: clinical work, teaching, service, and research

---

You have to learn the rules of the game. And then you have to play better than anyone else.

—*Albert Einstein*

DEFINING SCHOLARSHIP

It is often useful to begin a chapter with an established definition of the topic under discussion. A definition of the academic scholarship portfolio can establish a reader's expectations, create common ground for discussion, and provide a nod to the authors' own perspectives on the topic. Unfortunately, even a cursory review of the health sciences educational literature demonstrates considerable difference of opinion on the definitions of scholarship, academic portfolios, and the relationship between scholarly activities and the creation of an academic portfolio. Thus, we needed to make some decisions and acknowledge some accompanying limitations. As medical, physician assistant (PA), and interprofessional educators, working in a large academic health care center, we confess a bias. However, most of the principles underlying scholarship are widely applicable across varying types of training institutions, disciplines, and faculty roles. The broader

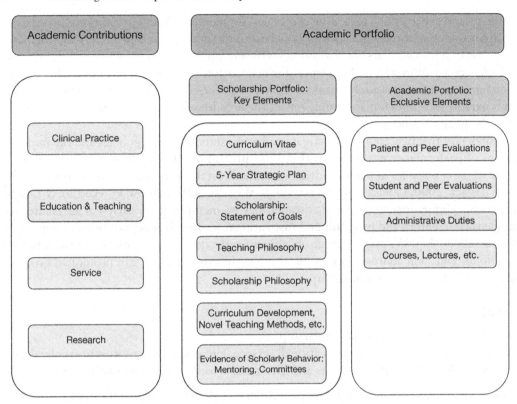

FIGURE 24.1 The academic and the scholarship portfolio.

academic portfolio contains a range of materials, of which only some belong to the scholarship portfolio (Figure 24.1). Our focus is on the scholarship components of an academic portfolio (Seldin & Miller, 2009). This chapter is not intended to address the many important aspects of an academic career that typically do not constitute scholarship (e.g., student and peer evaluations, supervisor assessments). Rather, it compiles some of the most commonly described and useful portfolio elements applicable to health sciences educators, and provides recommendations for documenting scholarship.

We define scholarship applying conceptual models first advocated by Boyer (1990) and widely adopted and advocated by others (American Association of Colleges of Nursing [AACN], 1999; Peterson & Stevens, 2013). Broad surveys of granting agencies, scholarly press directors, and journal educators reveal key themes underlying scholarship. Scholarly work has clear goals, requires adequate preparation and the use of appropriate methods, may achieve outstanding results, and may be effectively communicated and reflective (Glassick, Huber, & Maeroff, 1997). A scholarship portfolio documents scholarly achievements, but also includes personal goals and philosophies that guide academic progression. The portfolio shows evidence of active engagement in a scholarly community as both contributor and participant. Planning and building a scholarship portfolio helps guide early career faculty in tracking their professional achievements, communicating these achievements to others, establishing a career trajectory, and defining a personal niche in their discipline. The scholarship portfolio also provides critical evidence to support academic appointments and promotions.

Navigating Academia

Early-career health sciences faculty often enter their new roles with little preparation or experience navigating the often confusing and contradictory nature of the academic world, and its requirements and expectations regarding career development. Different institutions, programs, and disciplines present divergent views for how best to integrate clinical practice, teaching, service, and research into scholarship. Sometimes, conventional academic practice takes a narrow view of what constitutes acceptable venues for acquisition and dissemination of scholarship (e.g., conducting original research that is published in a peer-reviewed scientific journal). However, this narrow view does not accurately reflect the breadth of what constitutes modern scholarship in the health sciences.

It is important that new faculty investigate and understand both the policies and the implicit definitions of performance evaluation within their institution. The challenges can be significant, but are necessary for academic advancement and establishing one's self as an academic scholar (Glassick, 2000; Goldszmidt, Zibrowski, & Weston, 2008; Zibrowski, Weston, & Goldszmidt, 2008). Unfortunately, it can also sometimes be incumbent on early-career faculty to encourage their mentors and program and institutional leaders to accept of broader approach to defining scholarship. We present three objectives for the development and use of the scholarship portfolio, and then address options by which early-career faculty can promote a broader definition of what constitutes scholarship.

Objectives

1.   Describe common elements of scholarship
2.   Describe how to link clinical, educational, service, and research activities to scholarship
3.   Describe a portfolio that documents and illustrates broadly defined scholarly achievement

Some of this chapter expands on Seldin and Miller's work to better integrate clinical practice, teaching, organizational and community-focused service, and research as contributors to scholarship (Seldin, 1998a, 1998b; Seldin & Miller, 2009). Faculty roles, positions, and opportunities will differ; many faculty will not have clinical roles, whereas others may principally teach and never take part in formal research investigations. However, in all cases, our central argument is that much of the work of early career faculty can be interpreted and disseminated as scholarship—whether through clinical practice, teaching students, developing curriculum, professional leadership activities, unit service activities, or participating in the conduct of formal scientific investigations. The next four sections describe the scholarly contributions associated with clinical practice, education, service, and research.

THE FOUR LEGS OF SCHOLARSHIP

Clinical Work

There are benefits and challenges associated with remaining active in clinical practice while also working in academia (Christmas, Durso, Kravet, & Wright, 2010). A rich and current base of clinical practice experience and knowledge helps maintain clinical relevance in the health professions classroom and is a vital component of successful teaching. Students appreciate the clinical pearls, case studies, and ongoing advice available from seasoned health care providers. Faculty educators, who practice clinically, can also provide shadowing opportunities for students and help support precepting opportunities for other faculty.

Clinical expertise and clinical teaching can enhance opportunities for publication and editing for refereed clinical or practice-based journals. These same journals also commonly seek expert peer reviewers—a means for new faculty to gain an introduction to publication. Most clinical and practice-focused journals also provide opportunities for clinically practicing educators to publish case studies, brief reports, and clinical discussion articles. These types of publications often demand less formal scientific rigor, focusing more on the personal and professional insights of the contributor.

Successful scholarship is more than a product; it is also acting and collaborating in ways that support the work of others. Clinical practice can provide ongoing engagement and potential collaborative efforts on scholarly work in clinical settings. Success in creating clinical scholarship is often dependent on establishing a niche through recognized expertise in an area of clinical practice. Engaging in professional activities at local, state, regional, national, and international levels, and in developing and providing continuing health care education, offers further avenues to network and meet providers, scholars, and potential collaborators.

Education and Teaching

Today's educators, across all disciplines, actively seek to understand the relationship between education, their profession, and interprofessional work (Huber & Morreale, 2002). Tracking one's teaching methods and the associated learning that occurs is no longer simply an exercise in self-monitoring, but a body of work worth disseminating. Portfolios can help enable the capture of teaching as scholarship (Reece, Pearce, Melillo, & Beaudry, 2001; Seldin, 1998a, 1998b; Tofade, Abate, & Fu, 2014).

A Scholarship of Teaching and Learning

Boyer (1990) redefined scholarship to include the scholarship of teaching and learning (SoTL). Glassick (2000) and Beckman and Cook (2007) later strengthened the perspective that teaching can be scholarship. Boyer described scholarship activities to include each of the following (Boyer, 1990):

- **Scholarship of discovery:** A commitment to the development of knowledge, moving beyond the reporting of outcomes to include dissemination of processes and passion that benefit one's institution and program as well as the broader academic community
- **Scholarship of integration:** Activities that connect, integrate, and reinterpret existing knowledge to expand, broaden, and deepen its scope; in the health sciences, interprofessional education collaborations integrate insights gained across disciplines, to improve education for all
- **Scholarship of application and engagement:** Activities that apply existing knowledge and skills to solve problems within one's own institution but also "connecting the rich resources of the university to our most pressing social, civic and ethical problems, to our children, to our schools, to our teachers and to our cities (Boyer, 1996, pp. 19–20)

Further refining the work of Boyer (1990, 1996), Shulman (1999) and Hutchings and Schulman (1999) identified the critical aspects for the successful translation of teaching to scholarship. Excellent teaching becomes scholarly as sound assessment tools and evidence-gathering procedures are employed to systematically collect and report educational activities. Philosophies common to traditional research are used. A teacher first develops a question, founded in his or her teaching, and makes inquires of the recent and relevant literature and scholarly works in the field to ascertain the relevance of the question. These inquiries include both the topic of study (e.g., anatomy) and the current teaching methods (e.g., the flipped classroom). Teaching moves further toward scholarship when work is peer reviewed. Teaching scholarship should constitute "community property." Successful translation is then judged by the extent the work is publically disseminated, responded to, and built upon by other teachers and investigators.

MedEdPORTAL provides one good venue for publishing and disseminating educational scholarship (Reynolds & Candler, 2008; Shankar, 2014). Developed by the Association of American Medical Colleges (AAMC), MedEdPORTAL provides a prestigious peer-reviewed publishing site. The portal is open to submissions from all health sciences disciplines. Submissions need to be full stand-alone learning modules, with learning objectives and outcomes, of value to and available for free to educators. In addition, MedEdPORTAL's i-Collaborative provides a non-peer-reviewed venue to share works in progress. Curriculum developers can obtain feedback and engage other educators around topics of common themes. The interested reader is also encouraged to explore MedEdWorld (2016) and Multimedia Educational Resource for Learning and Online Teaching (2016). These resources each provide valuable opportunities for educators to publish and disseminate work.

It can be a challenge for educators to find the time and to reconcile scheduling conflicts so as to be able to engage in scholarship development (Schrager & Sadowski, 2016). Schrager and Sadowski (2016) provide an excellent summary to assist busy academics in achieving success in scholarship. One of their most important recommendations for academics is "making everything count twice" (p. 11). In Table 24.1, we provide a modified table, analogous to the work by Schrager and Sadowski, to illustrate common examples of scholarship taken from everyday academic responsibilities.

Service

Most institutions require some form of service to support promotions and appointment processes. The majority of universities consider service to include participation in program, departmental, institutional, local, and national organizational activities. Opportunities can include

TABLE 24.1 "Making Everything Count Twice," Translating Everyday Work to Scholarship*

Context	Scholarship Opportunity
Clinical: Interesting patients?	Develop case studies, present in local and national venues, publish brief reports.
Education: Challenging students? Exemplary mentors? Teaching moments?	Develop case studies, present in local and national venues, publish brief reports.
Education: Developing new curriculum?	Is the curriculum novel? Consider publishing in a journal specific to health care education.
Education: Lectures as scholarship?	Academic environments offer many opportunities to share information in a scholarly manner. Is the work publishable or suitable for national meetings? Can your lecture be presented as in grand rounds? Can you present your materials to students outside your specific discipline? Can your work be turned into continuing education (e.g., CME, CNE) for practitioners?
Education: Innovative teaching methods?	Innovative teaching methods can be published in journals focused on both health care education and education in general.
	Increased use of social media in teaching can be recognized as scholarship (Sherbino et al., 2015).
Service: Institutional and program committee work?	Is the committee work innovative in approaching problems? Novel solutions, even those from a single institution, can be presented in local and national venues, even published if the committee tracks change and demonstrates impact of its work and decisions.

CME, continuing medical education; CNE, continuing nursing education.

*The authors acknowledge Sarina Schrager and Elizabeth Sadowski for developing this work. We have modified their work to more broadly reflect health care educators.

Source: Adapted from Schrager and Sadowski (2016). Reproduced with permission. Copyright *Journal of Graduate Medical Education.*

admissions, administrative roles, committee work, and membership on professional boards. Administrative roles are commonly counted as organizational service, as they can involve a significant amount of time away from typical faculty responsibilities. Advising students and mentoring, including serving on thesis, doctoral, and project committees, is often considered institutional service, or it is considered a teaching function.

Volunteering time or expertise, clinical or otherwise, to service organizations and participating in or organizing a service learning project with students can each constitute evidence of scholarly engagement (e.g., providing health screenings). This work can be translated into scholarship as either products (e.g., publications) resulting from service, or as a demonstration of integration in a community (e.g., health care personnel serving the homeless). It is important to find out what activities constitute service at your institution, and to record service activities in one's curriculum vitae (CV) and portfolio.

Editorial opportunities may arise, not only in relation to clinical practice, but they may also extend to service, teaching and education, and other areas of content expertise. These include opportunities for the review and evaluation of work submitted for publication, conference presentations, continuing education, research grant applications, and moderating professional education meetings. Although these may not always constitute a tangible scholarship product, they demonstrate a faculty member's status as a respected member of a scholarly community.

Service Learning

Service learning is an educational strategy and learning experience that integrates community service with instruction and self-reflection to strengthen learning, teach civic responsibility, and strengthen communities. Service learning has links to cultural competency (Albritton & Wagner, 2002), increased community involvement (Jones, Blinkhorn, Schumann, & Reddy, 2014), and empathy (Brazeau, Schroeder, Rovi, & Boyd, 2011). See Chapter 16 for a further discussion of service learning. Finding and developing links between education and community needs can constitute strong scholarship. For example, working with a local church on a service learning project may provide evidence of community involvement that also supports an institutional mission ("Building Trust Between the Homeless," 2016). Describing this work with regard to the existing literature, carefully collecting and interpreting evaluation data from project activities, and then disseminating conclusions locally or more broadly can constitute scholarship.

Research

Institutional appointments and promotions often require that educators conduct independent research, building a line or lines of research that characterize their career. Although it is beyond the scope of this chapter to describe the full range of research activities commonly recognized as constituting scholarly activities, some definitions are useful to consider. The Code of Federal Regulations (45 CFR 46.102(d)) defines *research involving human subjects* as: "a systematic investigation, including research development, testing and evaluation, designed to develop or contribute to generalizable knowledge" (U.S. Department of Health and Human Services, 2009). The National Academy of Sciences describes research as work to "extend human knowledge of the physical, biological, or social world beyond what is already known" (National Academies Press, 1995, p. 3). Other research methods of inquiry common in the social and behavior sciences emphasize different means of interpretation, are often not driven by a distinct question, but instead are more exploratory, often even seeking findings to emerge from naturalistic observations rather than from prescribed scientific method-based designs. Figure 24.2 provides an expanded view of traditional scientific method-based research, to broadly illustrate processes more common to scholarship based on education, clinical work, and service. In summary, most

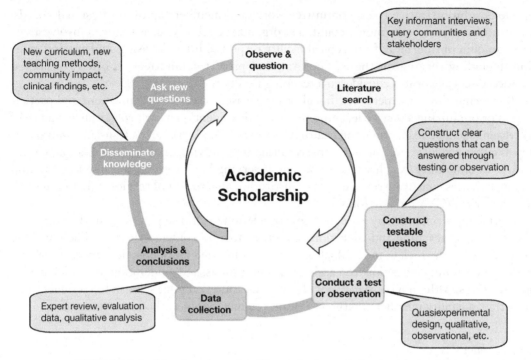

FIGURE 24.2 Adapting the scientific method to academic scholarship.

approaches to research include observations that nurture questions, investigations that further knowledge, each involving the collection, assessment, and reporting of data. For those interested in readable and general descriptions of both the more quantitative (e.g., scientific method) and qualitative approaches (e.g., observational) to research, we encourage exploring the works of John Creswell (2013, 2014).

THE SCHOLARSHIP PORTFOLIO

We have described an academic portfolio consisting of both scholarship elements and more purely academic elements. It is also useful to think of these scholarship elements as pieces of a cohesive portfolio. A scholarship portfolio tracks and records scholarly activity, but also includes detailed descriptions of a scholar's goals, paths to achieving these goals, a teaching philosophy, and its author's self-defined success (e.g., a 5-year plan) and an awareness for potential challenges to achieve success. The portfolio provides a tool for self-reflection on one's career, aspirations, and achievement (Pinsky & Fryer-Edwards, 2004; Zobairi, Nieman, & Cheng, 2008). Components of this portfolio can also serve as an introduction, informing prospective colleagues, appointment and promotion committees, and potential employers about the individual. Different audiences vary in their interest and need to see different selections from the portfolio. Think of a portfolio as a collection of useful elements rarely presented in their entirely, but instead filtered for specific purposes. When applying for an academic position, the CV is essential. But a teaching philosophy, an organized statement of goals, and the story of how your original educational aspirations led you to your current position can be equally important.

A well-developed scholarship portfolio allows you to provide consistent, accurate, and self-reflective information across a multitude of academic needs. Cristancho and Varpio (2016) provide 12 tips for guiding new medical educators in developing their career. These recommendations are valuable across all health care disciplines. In Exhibit 24.1, we have summarized the key findings, and have modified the tips to be applicable to the broader health sciences education

---

EXHIBIT 24.1 Twelve Career Tips for Early-Career Health Care Educators*

---

1. Articulate your area(s) of interest
2. Define what success is to you
3. Create a 5-year strategic plan
4. Develop strong communication skills
5. Cultivate relationships with mentors
6. Be a good mentee
7. Build a network of peers
8. Craft multiple elevator speeches
9. Be a team player
10. Build resilience as your armor
11. Understand health care education is a field not a discipline
12. Embrace your identity as part of health care education

---

*The authors acknowledge Sayra Cristoancho and Lara Varpio for developing these criteria for medical educators. The criteria have been slightly modified to reflect health care educators more broadly.

Source: Christancho and Vapiro (2016).

community. Exhibit 24.1 provides a good introduction on how to think like an experienced academic, to increase the likelihood of success and help limit the hurdles encountered in academia.

Scholarship Portfolio Components

Each element of a scholarship portfolio must make a strong and accurate impression. The portfolio must be appropriately formatted and its materials carefully proofed. Its introductory materials set a tone and must concisely convey the essence of your work and your aspirations. Once you have clearly established your goals, your portfolio focuses on building and reinforcing these early statements. Next, we discuss the most basic elements of a scholarship portfolio.

Professional Goal Statement

Even a novice academic needs to establish both short- and long-term goals (e.g., a 5-year plan) to guide his or her career. Many of these goals will be intrinsic, such as ensuring that one's work instills pride and confidence. Some are more extrinsic goals that describe the mark of the academic's work on the world. Most goals have both intrinsic and extrinsic elements. A goal statement can fit your individual preferences. Some are only a few sentences declaring your direction and aspirations. Others consist of an evolving list of subgoals or a single expanding narrative. The document is fluid and personal, providing a compass when conflicting responsibilities threaten to overrun your goals. Keep the statement simple. Do not set unachievable or inherently unrealistic goals. Align your goals with your position or the position you aspire to attain. State or have implicit time estimates for achieving goals. These are your goals; there is no need to provide a justification or establish their foundation.

Curriculum Vitae

In much of the work world, the résumé serves the purpose of describing, usually in 1 or 2 pages, the attributes, education, and skills an applicant brings to a particular position. It is a focused record, designed for quick appraisal. The CV, on the other hand, records all educational and professional experiences and accomplishments that define the academic scholar's career, at length and without editorial comment. This vital component of the portfolio asks for a highly detailed, "just-the-facts" description of the academic's life. Its focus on accurate and complete reporting makes it the most commonly evaluated component of the scholarship portfolio. However, the CV is limited, lacking sufficient color and depth to fully describe one's goals and philosophies; the author's career trajectory can only be partially inferred from it.

When incorporating educational work into a CV and scholarship portfolio, it is important to understand and reflect your institution's requirements and mission. In many cases, there will be institutional standards for the contents and layout of the CV. Requirements can vary widely by discipline and institution. However, in most cases, the CV details one's educational preparation, clinical and administrative experience, teaching experience, scholarly activity, and service contributions. The CV provides the reference material for appointment and promotion decisions, grant submissions, and academic hiring decisions. Table 24.2 illustrates one common layout for a CV, with examples taken from other common formats. See online supplement for an example of a CV.

Teaching Philosophy Statement

Academic programs often ask faculty to describe their teaching philosophy for purposes of appointment, review, and promotion. For many educators, this constitutes the first time they have considered a philosophy of education; certainly, they hold beliefs about education, but

TABLE 24.2 Common Elements of the Curriculum Vitae

Personal data	Place of birth, citizenship
Education	Undergraduate and graduate, indicate dates
Postgraduate training	Internships, fellowships, residencies
Faculty appointments	Place and dates
Clinical appointments	Place and dates
Honors and awards	Program specific, local, national, teaching, publications
Licensure/certification	Boards, licenses, states, and dates
Professional organizations	Membership and offices held
Teaching responsibilities	Courses, lectures, mentoring, role in educational committees
Editorial responsibilities	Editorial boards, editorial review
Special responsibilities	National: Professional organizational committees, study sections, training grant committees
	Local: Institutional and program committees, workgroups, hospital committees
Research funding	Title, funder, funding amount, principal investigator, active/pending, completed, submitted
Bibliography	Refereed journal articles, book chapters, books and videos, other publications, manuscripts submitted for review, abstracts
Innovations	Patents, software, curriculum development

perhaps not a philosophy. Although a teaching philosophy is a common requirement for promotion, it should be considered less of an obligation and more an opportunity for reflection and self-assessment.

Different recommendations for developing a teaching philosophy reveal some common threads (Medina & Draugalis, 2013; Owens, Miller, & Grise-Owens, 2014; Schonwetter, Sokal, Friesen, & Taylor, 2013). First, start building your teaching philosophy as *early* as possible in your career. The associated tasks will not become easier; nor will your memory of your accomplishments improve with time. Developing a teaching philosophy is a personal exercise in *self-reflection*. Both new and experienced academics have goals they hope to attain, experiences that support their beliefs, and have envisioned paths to achieving success. Writing a teaching philosophy helps solidify your beliefs. However, as your teaching *matures* and your experiences accumulate, you will find your beliefs about education change markedly. A teaching philosophy should therefore be a *dynamic* document, responsive to growth and change. Make the teaching philosophy statement truly your own. Limit your use of references or quotes from established theories of education. Instead, *in your own voice*, limiting the use of jargon and seeking to communicate to a broad audience, write what you honestly feel and believe. Be *concise*, as these documents commonly are less than a page or two in length. Focus on illuminating how your teaching achieves the mission of your institution, the innovations you have incorporated that improve student learning, your accommodations to different learning styles, and collaborative relationship with students.

Scholarship Philosophy Statement

A scholarship philosophy is also sometimes required in academic appointments and promotions. Like the teaching philosophy, the scholarship philosophy documents one's research and scholarship interests in a manner that links individual goals to proposed and already implemented activities necessary to achieve success. Early-career faculty may want to structure their statement in alignment with institutional criteria for advancement. However, the scholarship statement also benefits its author to a greater extent if success is defined through careful self-reflection. This is also a dynamic document that evolves across time. The statement should be understandable to a broad audience. Again, be concise, avoid jargon, and focus on describing the links among interests, goals, activities, and successes.

A Proper Scholarship Portfolio

A CV serves as a ledger and reference. A professional goal statement sets your stage. Teaching and scholarship statements connect the dots, telling the story. The scholarship portfolio combines these important elements and can add more, such as video records, collections of your presentations and publications, and curriculum descriptions.

Ultimately, the scholarship portfolio should be *purposeful*. A scholarship portfolio that does not fill a need or needs should not be created. The portfolio must be sufficiently *flexible* to serve multiple purposes across your career. It should be sufficiently *inclusive* to list all relevant aspects of your service, academic, and clinical work. Scholarship portfolios benefit from a *modular* format. Keep the components of the scholarship portfolio separate, not integrated as a whole. Your portfolio should serve as a tool for *self-reflection*, allowing you to review and guide your scholarly activities. Your portfolio must be *sustainable*; its scope must be manageable to ensure you will continuously monitor and update your materials. Designate a block of time each month to add to and modify your evolving portfolio.

Online electronic portfolios have gained momentum, providing novel means to capture and display student work and the scholarship of faculty (Butler, 2006; Hoekstra & Crocker, 2015; Kelly & Lewenson, 2010). Familiar social media (e.g., Facebook, YouTube) and web-based tools (e.g., Google Docs) provide faculty with alternative mediums to easily share and showcase scholarly work, create graphically rich displays, and provide hyperlinks for dynamic interconnectivity between different elements of a portfolio.

CONCLUSIONS

A successful academic life needs to balance many demands, often including practice, teaching and educational activities, service, and research into a focused and intentional career trajectory. A well-composed scholarship portfolio documents all outcomes and activities in teaching, clinical practice, professional/community service, and scholarly outcomes. A scholarship portfolio selects, expands upon, and integrates these components to describe your scholarly activities and achievement into the creation of new works and active engagement in the scholarship community. The trajectory connects aspirations to actions, actions to outcomes, and outcomes to impact, telling a story that is unique to the individual. The path is not always clear or without hurdles, but through self-reflection, collaboration, and an openness to the academic experience, you will achieve success.

REFERENCES

American Association of Colleges of Nursing. (1999). Defining scholarship for the discipline of nursing. (1999). Retrieved from http://www.aacn.nche.edu/publications/position/defining-scholarship

Albritton, T. A., & Wagner, P. J. (2002). Linking cultural competency and community service: A partnership between students, faculty, and the community. *Academic Medicine, 77*(7), 738–739.

Beckman, T. J., & Cook, D. A. (2007). Developing scholarly projects in education: A primer for medical teachers. *Medical Teacher, 29*(2), 210–218.

Boyer, E. (1990). *Scholarship reconsidered: Priorities of the professoriate.* Princeton, NJ: Carnegie Foundation for the Advancement of Teaching.

Boyer, E. (1996). The scholarship of engagement. *Journal of Public Outreach, 1*(1), 11–20.

Brazeau, C. M., Schroeder, R., Rovi, S., & Boyd, L. (2011). Relationship between medical student service and empathy. *Academic Medicine, 86*(Suppl. 10), S42–S45.

Building trust between the homeless & the medical community. (2016). Retrieved from https://depts .washington.edu/medex/magazine/building-trust-between-the-homeless-the-medical-community

Butler, P. (2006). A review of the literature on portfolios and electronic portfolios. Retrieved from http:// www.eportfoliopractice.qut.edu.au/docs/Butler%20-%20Review%20of%20lit%20on%20ePortfolio%20 research%20-%20NZOct%202006.pdf

Christmas, C., Durso, S. C., Kravet, S. J., & Wright, S. M. (2010). Advantages and challenges of working as a clinician in an academic department of medicine: Academic clinicians' perspectives. *Journal of Graduate Medical Education, 2*(3), 478–484.

Creswell, J. W. (2013). *Qualitative inquiry and research design: Choosing among five approaches* (3rd ed.). Los Angeles, CA: Sage.

Creswell, J. W. (2014). *Research design: Quantitative, qualitative, and mixed method approaches* (4th ed.). Los Angeles, CA: Sage.

Cristancho, S., & Varpio, L. (2016). Twelve tips for early career medical educators. *Medical Teacher, 38*(4), 358–363.

Huber, M. T., & Morreale, S. P. (Eds.). (2002). *Disciplinary styles in the scholarship of teaching and learning: Exploring common ground.* Sterling, VA: Stylus.

Glassick, C. E. (2000). Boyer's expanded definitions of scholarship, the standards for assessing scholarship, and the elusiveness of the scholarship of teaching. *Academic Medicine, 75*(9), 877–880.

Glassick, C. E., Huber, M. T., & Maeroff, F. I. (1997). *Scholarship assessed.* San Francisco, CA: Jossey-Bass.

Goldszmidt, M. A., Zibrowski, E. M., & Weston, W. W. (2008). Education scholarship: It's not just a question of "degree." *Medical Teacher, 30*(1), 34–39.

Hoekstra, A., & Crocker, J. (2015). Design, implementation, and evaluation of an ePortfolio approach to support faculty development in vocational education. *Studies in Educational Evaluation, 46,* 61–73.

Hutchings, P., & Schulman, L. (1999). The scholarship of teaching: New elaborations, new developments. *Change, 31*(5), 10–15.

Jones, K., Blinkhorn, L. M., Schumann, S. A., & Reddy, S. T. (2014). Promoting sustainable community service in the 4th year of medical school: A longitudinal service-learning elective. *Teaching and Learning in Medicine, 26*(3), 296–303.

Kelly, M., & Lewenson, S. B. (2010). Making time: Moving the faculty dossier to an electronic format. *Journal of Professional Nursing, 26*(2), 90–98.

Medina, M. S., & Draugalis, J. R. (2013). Writing a teaching philosophy: An evidence-based approach. *American Journal of Health-System Pharmacy, 70*(3), 191–193.

MedEdWorld. (2016). A global medical education community. Retrieved from http://www.mededworld.org/Home.aspx

Multimedia Educational Resource for Learning and Online Teaching. (2016). Retrieved from https://www.merlot.org/merlot/index.htm

National Academies Press. (1995). *On being a scientist: Responsible conduct in research* (2nd ed.). Washington, DC: Author.

Owens, L. W., Miller, J. J., & Grise-Owens, E. (2014). Activating a teaching philosophy in social work education: Articulation, implementation, and evaluation. *Journal of Teaching in Social Work, 34*, 332–345.

Peterson, K., & Stevens, J. (2013). Integrating the scholarship of practice into the nurse academician portfolio. *Journal of Nursing Education and Practice, 3*(11), 84–92.

Pinsky, L. E., & Fryer-Edwards, K. (2004). Diving for PERLS: Working and performance portfolios for evaluation and reflection on learning. *Journal of General Internal Medicine, 19*(5, Pt. 2), 582–587.

Reece, S. M., Pearce, C. W., Melillo, K. D., & Beaudry, M. (2001). The faculty portfolio: Documenting the scholarship of teaching. *Journal of Professional Nursing, 17*(4), 180–186.

Reynolds, R. J., & Candler, C. S. (2008). MedEdPORTAL: Educational scholarship for teaching. *Journal of Continuing Education in the Health Professionals, 28*(2), 91–94.

Schonwetter, D. J., Sokal, L., Friesen, M., & Taylor, K. L. (2013). Teaching philosophies reconsidered: A conceptual model for the development and evaluation of teaching philosophy statements. *International Journal for Academic Development, 7*(1), 83–87.

Schrager, S., & Sadowski, E. (2016). Getting more done: Strategies to increase scholarly productivity. *Journal of Graduate Medical Educators, 8*(1), 10–13.

Seldin, P. (1998a). *Successful use of teaching portfolios* (2nd ed.). Hoboken, NJ: John Wiley & Sons.

Seldin, P. (1998b). *The teaching portfolio: A practical guide to improved performance and promotion/tenure decisions* (2nd ed.). Hoboken, NJ: John Wiley & Sons.

Seldin, P., & Miller, J. (2009). *The academic portfolio: A practical guide to documenting teaching, research and service.* San Francisco, CA: Jossey-Bass.

Shankar, P. R. (2014). MedEdPORTAL: A resource for health educators. *Clinical Teaching, 11*(4), 315–316.

Sherbino, J., Arora, V. M., Van Melle, E., Rogers, R., Frank, J. R., & Holmboe, E. S. (2015). Criteria for social media-based scholarship in health professions education. *Postgraduate Medical Journal, 91*(1080), 551–555.

Shulman, L. (1999). The scholarship of teaching. *Change, 31*(5), 11.

Tofade, T., Abate, M., & Fu, Y. (2014). Perceptions of a continuing professional development portfolio model to enhance the scholarship of teaching and learning. *Journal of Pharmacy Practice, 27*(2), 131–137.

U.S. Department of Health and Human Services. (2009). Code of Federal Regulations, Title 45 Part 46. (2009). Retrieved from https://www.hhs.gov/ohrp/regulations-and-policy/regulations/45-cfr-46/#46.102

Zibrowski, E. M., Weston, W. W., & Goldszmidt, M. A. (2008). "I don't have time": Issues of fragmentation, prioritisation and motivation for education scholarship among medical faculty. *Medical Education, 42*(9), 872–878.

Zobairi, S. E., Nieman, L. Z., & Cheng, L. (2008). Knowledge and use of academic portfolios among primary care departments in U.S. medical schools. *Teaching and Learning in Medicine, 20*(2), 127–130.

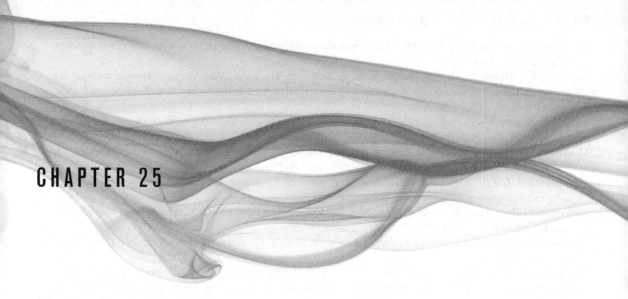

CHAPTER 25

Scholarship Reconsidered for Health Professions Educators

Karl Terryberry and Gerald Kayingo

CHAPTER OBJECTIVE

- Apply the elements of professional writing and creating an inclusive view of scholarship: discovery, integration, application, and teaching, including the Boyer Model

---

[T]he work of a professoriate might be thought as having four separate, yet overlapping functions. These are the scholarship of discovery; the scholarship of integration; the scholarship of application; and the scholarship of teaching.

—Ernest L Boyer

Scholarship and professional writing drive the dissemination of evidence collected during practice. Health care is advanced when clinicians practice with investigative minds, and when they observe their actions and search for relationships between treatment and outcomes. Such inquisitive clinicians can then report their findings, which might in turn stimulate more advanced, controlled studies. To present their findings to other practitioners, clinicians must produce manuscripts that meet standards of professionalism.

The first part of this chapter provides general principles of professional writing that health professions educators should reinforce, practice, and promote. The second part defines scholarship as it applies to health professions educators, and how they can contribute to the development of knowledge in their field.

ESSENTIAL ELEMENTS OF PROFESSIONAL WRITING

Unity of Message

One fundamental, but often overlooked, element of professional writing is unity of message. Manuscripts should have a singular purpose that is maintained throughout. A potential trap for writers in health professions is to assume that once the piece's purpose is stated, readers will not lose sight of it. However, because authors often unintentionally impose cognitive demands on readers, they may be offering readers different ways to think about the details being presented. For example, when reporting methods of data collection, writers may assume that the information provided clearly reflects the article's purpose because the data are meaningful to them. However, readers often fail to interpret the data in the same way.

Writers need to remind readers about the piece's purpose and clearly connect the data, charts, and graphs to their intended meaning. Constantly reinforcing the message helps readers stay on task. One way to ensure unity of message is to find parts of the manuscript that seem to reach conclusions, and then offer clarifying statements to reorient readers to the intended message.

Coherence, Information Management, and Sentence Development

Any writer's goal is to retain the interest of the reader, but choppy and disconnected ideas disrupt the coherence of a document. To establish control over the presentation of ideas, writers often move from one idea to another by embedding certain transitional elements in sentences, such as introductory words, phrase, and clauses. Such subordinate elements serve to identify what is important in the sentence and what is not.

Coding what is important in writing is supported by research on cognition. Our brains tend to retain information if it is presented in certain forms (such as actions and images) and if it is located in certain positions within sentences. For example, in a long passage, our brains recognize the importance of information at the beginning, lose focus in the middle, and retain the greatest amount of information from the end (Savin & Perchonock, 1965). Writers who understand the cognitive principles associated with processing information can meet their readers' needs by positioning information in alignment with cognitive expectations.

Not only are the *locations* of sentence elements important to readers, the elements themselves convey levels of importance. For example, the independent clause, which contains the subject and verb, is the most powerful part of a sentence. It draws an image and conveys an action that readers can retain. In contrast, dependent clauses—so named because they depend on the independent clause—are inherently subordinate; readers recognize that the information in dependent clauses relates to the independent clause. Finally, nonessential elements, which are located within commas and read like afterthoughts, are the weakest parts of a sentence. Readers expect that any information in them is relevant but not the focus of the sentence's intended meaning. Therefore, the rules of punctuation are important: punctuation controls these elements by separating the important information from the supportive elements.

English employs four different types of sentences to produce different types of meanings. A simple sentence, which is composed of one independent clause, is one idea that is often supported by phrases. Writers use this type of sentence the most to present their important points. A compound sentence contains two independent clauses in conjunction with each other, which enables writers to develop two important points or show the relationship between two important ideas. A complex sentence contains one independent clause and one or more dependent clauses that present some information that is subordinate to the main point in the independent clause. This sentence type is especially useful in discussing cause-and-effect relationships. Finally, in a compound–complex sentence, the subordinate clauses provide some relevant details that are associated with two equally important independent clauses. Sentences of this type are usually longer than the others, so writers need to be aware of the cognitive demands they put on their readers' brains. Too much information, especially if not well controlled by punctuation, can create confusion or overwhelm readers (Lester & Beason, 2012).

Grammatical Correctness

In writing, nothing is more recognizable—or often, more damaging—than grammar errors. Many health professions educators can identify good writing and poor writing, but often they do not know why it is good or bad. Because most people remember some of the rules of writing from elementary school, they tend to associate grammatical errors with elementary-level thinking. Thus, even if the message is clear and cogent, mistakes in grammar and in the conventions of professional writing often suggest a lack of preparedness and professionalism, whether fair or not. Grammar errors cannot be tolerated because they can damage our authority as writers (Terryberry, 2005).

Professional writers generally agree that some mistakes are more damaging than others. Primary mistakes, such as a lack of subject–verb agreement, sentence fragments, comma splices, and run-on sentences, are considered the most egregious of grammatical errors because they indicate that the author cannot perform the most basic writing tasks. These errors can be easily identified and corrected. Subject–verb agreement means that a singular noun (e.g., "patient") requires a singular verb ("has"), whereas a plural noun ("patients") requires a plural verb ("have"). Subject–verb disagreement can be identified using a simple sentence-analysis strategy in which the writer breaks every sentence into its independent clauses, dependent clauses, and phrases, and then associates each subject with the correct form of its verb. This process, called *sentence diagramming*, is not taught much anymore, but it allows writers to eliminate many mistakes before they show up in print (Terryberry, 2005).

Sentence diagramming can also be applied to the primary errors associated with incomplete thoughts. These errors are damaging because communicating in complete sentences is a basic skill in formal writing. Comma splices, sentence fragments, and run-on (fused) sentences are often products of informality, not educational unpreparedness. Although conversational (informal) forms of language are fine in emails or texts to our friends, they are not acceptable in formal manuscripts or presentations. When writing professionally, we need to play by and practice the rules of formality so that they become habit (Terryberry, 2005).

Secondary mistakes, such as nonparallel structure, dangling modifiers, or pronoun–noun disagreement, often result from a lack of attention to detail (Terryberry, 2005). These errors can occur when authors are so concerned with the message that they lose sight of the forms in which the ideas are presented. Putting a proofreading and editing strategy in place can find and correct these secondary errors.

Language Standards for Professionals

Every day we choose different words or phrases to express our ideas in different contexts. With our friends, we easily employ slang and even words that do not exist. When we meet new people, we may use more formal language until we become more familiar with them. We may even adopt a higher level of language and presentation when we speak with our superiors. Even then, these forms of language are not identical to the forms of language we employ in professional writing. Unfortunately, many writers fail to recognize that conversational forms of language are not typically acceptable in a professional context.

Many students wish they could "write like they speak" or simply transcribe their thinking onto the page, but such a conversational style does not convey professionalism. In popular, conversational language, we often use words ambiguously or in new ways to convey new meanings. In professional writing, however, our goal should be to reach the more formal end of the language spectrum in which words are used for purposes that are specific and agreed upon in the field. Using language that everyone can understand and recognize for its exact meaning helps to ensure that our message is not lost.

Every writer needs to develop a strategy to meet readers' expectations of language. Research has shown that certain forms of language presented in consistent ways can result in a clearer message. The human brain processes information from language by recognizing patterns. When writers know those patterns and use them in their writing, then the cognitive processing of information becomes easier for readers.

Verb-based strategies are the easiest for readers to understand and incorporate. Among the most useful strategies are the following:

1. Use verbs, not nouns, to convey action.
2. Use strong verbs instead of weak verbs that camouflage meaning.
3. Recognize proper applications of the passive and active voices.
4. Eliminate vague expressions that contain indefinite pronouns.
5. Replace static verbs with action-oriented verbs.

Problem 1: Writers sometimes use nouns to represent the action in a sentence instead of using verbs.

The verb is the strongest part of speech because readers are more likely to retain ideas presented through action. Experienced, professional writers craft their sentences around verbs, which, when used effectively, help readers visualize the action of a sentence.

Reading specialists and psychologists tell us that readers remember an action or hold the image of an object performing that action in their minds more readily than when visualizing a static object (Terryberry, 2005). When we converse, we tend to focus on nouns because they are easily identifiable, quickly recalled, and at the forefront of the limited vocabulary we use during conversations. As a result, the sentences we create around nouns are not tightly constructed, nor are they crafted into powerful ideas presented through carefully chosen words. Instead, our spoken sentences are filled with excess words that help us communicate about the nouns we choose from our limited, conversational vocabulary. Ultimately, the wordiness of speech gives us time to think and finish our thoughts while we are talking. For these reasons, professional writers should not write the way they speak. Instead, mature writers rewrite, edit, and revise their sentences until they perform their intended function: to communicate clearly, effectively, and more formally.

Attempting to write effective, verb-based sentences can be difficult in a first draft. Implement this verb-based strategy after the document has been edited for coherence and unity. Once the document is clearly organized and follows a rational line of thinking, writers can use this verb-based strategy to sharpen sentences and to communicate the intended message with precision and accuracy.

Writers who use nouns formed from words that express the action of the sentence bring their readers close to the message but often fail to communicate that message precisely. By using nouns to express action, they miss the opportunity to use powerful verbs, and they create sentences whose excessive words cloud the intended meaning.

Example: The CEO gave the indication that he would step down if the board asked him to do so.

In this sentence, the CEO did not really *give* anyone anything. Instead, the CEO *indicated* his future actions.

Revision 1: The CEO indicated that he would step down if the board asked him to do so.

Although the main subject and verb combination is strong, the remainder of the sentence is filled with the weak verb phrases *step down* and *asked him to do so*. Because the CEO is not literally stepping, this sentence uses conversational language instead of precise language that creates specific meanings. Also, *asked him to do so* is wordy, and *do so* is a vague construction. Consider the following revisions:

> *Revision 2: The CEO indicated that he would resign if the board asked him to.*
> *Revision 3: The CEO indicated that he would resign if the board requested it.*

Problem 2: Writers sometimes use weak, meaningless verbs when they are unsure of their intended meaning. Use strong verbs instead.

We have seen that if we write as we speak, we rely on the limited vocabulary available to us during conversation. As a result, we use only a limited number of words that come quickly to mind, and thus we choose language that is close to our intended meaning, not the sentence's intended meaning. This often involves using weak verbs—verbs that offer vague meanings—and we often attempt to supplement their vague meanings by adding adverbs, which are words that modify or explain verbs. We do this because weak verbs and adverbs come to mind more quickly than do strong verbs that elicit a more precise meaning.

When we write down our thoughts, we have time to scrutinize the words we have used, and to choose verbs that express our ideas more forcefully. So instead of writing that someone "looked over the text," we should write "reviewed the text," because "reviewed" conveys an action that is more specific than a simple matter of looking. In this case, we used a single accurate word instead of a couple that are more vague.

Problem 3: Writers use the passive voice when action is necessary.

It is important to know when to use the passive and active voices. Sentences in the active voice have a clear "a doer did a certain action to something" structure, whereas those in the passive voice have a "something received a certain action from a doer."

> *Example of active voice: Lightning struck the tree.*
> *Example of passive voice: The tree was struck by lightning.*

The active voice is typically used more often; it is a stronger writing tool because it is direct and emphasizes the doer over the receiver of the action. The passive voice is a weaker writing tool because it emphasizes the receiver of the action, not the doer. Moreover, the verb used in the passive voice typically includes a form of "to be" (*is, are, was, were, be,* or *been*), which creates a static (less active) relationship between the doer and the receiver. Active (dynamic) verbs aid our ability to encode information and create a mental image of action that is retained by the reader. Strong writers limit the use of "to be" verbs in their professional documents because they want to create stimulating sentences that show action.

In the sentences about the tree and lightning, the passive voice literally creates a static relationship between the two nouns. The helping verb *was* indicates that the tree simply existed, and that something was done to it. The tree is not the doer, but it *is* the subject of the sentence, and readers typically expect the subject of a sentence to be the doer of the action. When the subject is not the doer of the action, the word order of the sentence has been changed, and readers' expectations are subverted. Thus, the relationship of words in the passive voice is more convoluted; it does not allow readers to figure out which noun is the doer, and which is the receiver, according to the positions of the words alone.

In the sentence in the active voice, *lightning* is the subject and therefore the doer, and the sentence uses a powerful verb in *struck*. The reader can now more easily visualize the action being performed.

Note that in some cases, the passive voice is preferred or even necessary:

- To express an action when the doer is unknown. (Example: "The pool had been emptied before we arrived.")
- To express an action when the writer does not want to disclose the doer. ("Mistakes were made and documents were shredded.")
- To emphasize the receiver instead of the doer. ("Group A was assigned to be the control group.")

This last case is the one that is most applicable to scientific writing. In many cases, the writer is also the researcher and wishes to avoid writing "I performed . . ." "I then studied . . .," and "I then proposed. . . ." The scientific community has accepted this use of passive voice because it moves the focus of the study away from the scientist and onto the activities and results of the study itself.

Problem 4: Writers fill their papers with indefinite pronouns that have no meaning.

Avoid using *it* and *there* as subjects. Consider the following examples:

Example 1: <u>There is</u> no prior knowledge required for this job other than a general understanding of accounting principles.
Example 2: <u>It has been</u> indicated by our analysis that the new policies will cost millions.

In these sentences, *it* and *there* appear to be the subjects of the sentences. If we want to create a clear "a doer did a certain action to something" structure, then we start sentences with the doers of the action. However, in these sentences, *it* and *there* are not the doers of action, but instead are pronouns, which take the place of nouns. But we cannot know what word or words *it* and *there* replace in these examples. Actually, in these sentences those words are meaningless and do not communicate the point clearly; in addition, note that these sentences are in the passive voice. Let us consider revising them:

Example 1: There is no prior knowledge required for this job other than a general understanding of accounting principles. (To what does "there" refer?)
Revision: This job requires only a general understanding of accounting principles.
Example 2: It has been indicated by our analysis that the new policies will cost millions. (To what does "it" refer?)
Revision: Our analysis indicates that the new policies will cost millions.

Problem 5: Writers tend to use static verbs too often.

Recall that "to be" verbs (*is, are, was, were, be,* and *been*) tend to make sentences boring because they create a static relationship between the subjects and the verbs; in those instances, the subjects are not really acting at all. Just as in Problem 4, using "to be" verbs in this way often encourages the use of indefinite pronouns and leads writers into the passive voice. Thus, it is good practice to limit the use of "to be" verbs to instances in which the subjects are in fact in a state of being, when they are not acting in any way. So, whenever sentences contain "to be" verbs, check to see whether the subject is in a state of being; if it is not, revise it so that it contains action-oriented verbs.

SCHOLARSHIP FOR HEALTH PROFESSIONS EDUCATORS

Promotion, Tenure, and the Meaning of Scholarship in the Profession

Many health professions educators have historically worked under clinical faculty tracks, focusing mostly on clinical practice and teaching with less emphasis on scholarly activity. For these reasons, many clinical faculty have had fewer opportunities to apply for tenure or even promotion (Levinson & Rubenstein, 2000). In many academic centers, faculty promotion requires evidence of some form of scholarship. It is also essential for the health professions educator to participate in the full range of academic life: serving on committees, collaborating with faculty from other disciplines, taking on administrative tasks or mentoring new faculty, developing new courses, reshaping existing courses, mentoring student research projects, and advising students—and the list goes on.

As central as these tasks are to every academic's professional life, they do not necessarily translate into promotion and tenure because of failure to turn these activities into the scholarship that counts. Scholarship is the primary component of an academic's job, and recent research seems to suggest that faculty members are slowly accepting this expansion of roles (Garino, 2014; Miller & Dehn, 2014; Ritsema & Cawley, 2013; Starck, 1996). In addition to disseminating new knowledge, health professions educators need to broaden the definition of *scholarship*.

Ernest Boyer's work has changed the perspective on what scholarship means to many academics (Boyer, 1990). In the past, academia valued a linear approach to the development of knowledge: Scholarship was the investigative form of research that led to publications, which disseminated that information to other professionals and then to students in the classroom. Boyer argues, however, that investigative research such as original research in a biology laboratory, is only one component of developing knowledge. Results from these experiments need to be applied, and that application may generate more research questions.

By connecting more theoretical research findings to practice, and then allowing practice to develop more theories and thus more research, the development of knowledge becomes less linear and more circular. According to Boyer, new knowledge stimulates scholarship not only in the forms of publications and presentations, but also in practice and teaching. Consequently, Boyer sees scholarship as four interconnected functions: *discovery* (traditional research), *integration* (synthesis of knowledge), *application* (moving theory into practice or service), and *teaching* (encouraging others to learn and investigate further). In their book *Scholarship Assessed*, Glassick, Huber, Maeroff, and Boyer (1997) recommend that to give these four types of scholarship activities the same weight they all deserve, they all must be held at the same standards of scholarly performance.

Effective service and teaching have great potential of generating novel research questions and should be counted as scholarship. In the area of service, for example, a faculty member who has observed the health habits of the population in a specific neighborhood might help to staff a clinic there that both provides care to the population and helps evaluate whether certain clinical approaches are applicable in a real-world setting. This information could be used in curriculum design to tailor remediation for the struggling students. In addition, data gathered to assess teaching effectiveness can be used to develop best practices and thus can be transformed into scholarship. Other examples include mentoring outcomes of new faculty members by experienced faculty and oral presentations at conferences.

Although teaching and service are becoming recognizable forms of scholarship (Glassick et al., 1997; Hutchings & Shulman, 1999), published research is still the strongest and most formal contribution to the field's scholarly dialogues. Publishing in peer-reviewed journals is often viewed as the most objective, quantifiable measure for evaluating faculty for promotion and tenure. How then do clinicians and health educators improve their publication record given their limited time and resources?

We must first realize our limitations, recognize and overcome the barriers, and aim to produce research that is reasonable for our circumstances. Achieving these goals is possible by understanding the three main type of research: *quantitative*, *qualitative*, and *interventional*.

Quantitative Research

The quantitative forms of research—descriptive, correlational, quasiexperimental, and experimental—have varying degrees of strength and reliability. The stronger types of quantitative studies use controls and measures to increase reliability. Descriptive and correlational forms of research are designed to describe or explore correlations and relationships; they lack experimental controls and do not measure outcomes. Quasiexperimental studies determine cause-and-effect relationships between variables, but the levels of control are weak because, for example, the populations may not be randomized. Experimental studies are highly controlled studies in which typically a single variable is manipulated to determine causality. A type of experimental research called a *randomized controlled trial* provides the strongest form of evidence; it is typically conducted in institutions where research is a primary focus. As Boyer claims, not all contributions to knowledge in the health professions derive from experimental research (discovery) because its results are theoretical and must be generalized to the populations being served (integration).

Qualitative Research

Qualitative research explores the subjective nature of health care in that it helps explain the perspectives, beliefs, or feelings of patients. Although these types of studies include no controls, they offer ways to understand the social aspects of health care that often drive patients' behaviors and responses to practitioners. Two examples of qualitative research are studies that examine the "lived experiences" of groups (the most common form of student research) and studies that seek to analyze the belief systems of cultural groups.

Interventional Research

Interventional research (another form of integration scholarship) includes any type of study that assesses whether a treatment actually produces the desired effects in patients. Such a study might investigate whether a given treatment protocol produces certain specific treatment goals in a set of patients, whether those goals are set by established standards or by patients' needs.

Planning Your Research Study

Choosing the right type of research among studies that are diverse in scope and purpose can be a daunting process. Consultation with experienced faculty and researchers for their guidance in planning research is recommended. In addition, many universities have research centers or departments that provide education, mentoring, and career development in the area of research. Online resources are also available. One such example is "Research to Publication" (www.rtop.bmj.com), a partnership between the University of San Francisco and the BMJ Publishing Group. The website listed offers online modules on research design and writing for publication and is a comprehensive resource on research design, research ethics, manuscript writing, manuscript submission, and the peer-review process.

The Contributions of Health Professions Educators to Scholarship

The scholarship of clinicians and health professions educators makes essential contributions to the scholarly dialogues of the field. The high-quality research conducted in pure research institutions likely does not exist unless clinicians and health professions educators provide a reasonable body of evidence that suggests the need for such research. Working clinicians are on the front lines of health care, so they are best equipped to observe trends that appear in practice and to report them in case studies, which then become the foundation for further investigations. If clinicians do not publish their observations and findings, their knowledge may be lost.

In some work environments, the trends and consistencies of practice may be further investigated in cohort studies, which compare a given population with similar populations to see whether the given population has or has not changed relative to the other populations over time. Such studies can lay the foundation for future research about factors affecting this group by making their findings available to those who can conduct more rigorous studies.

Another contribution to the field that requires no clinical facilities or patients is systematic reviews, in which authors (reviewers) critically evaluate the body of research in a given field. These reviews compile studies in a given area of health care to evaluate the strength of the research so that practice can be more precisely directed. When a body of research begins to point in one direction, reviewers process that information and publish it so that teachers can prepare students with knowledge that is current and supported by research.

Grant procurement can also be considered scholarship. Just as conferences and poster sessions are preliminary stages to publication, getting grants is a preliminary stage of research. For health professions educators, community grants, internal funding support, or grants from professional organizations can help defray costs and also legitimize the research being conducted. Most grant-giving agencies require evidence that the goals of the proposal are reached, and the best evidence of that achievement is a published article.

CONCLUSIONS

Scholarship and professional writing are important components in the career of a health professions educator. They are the foundations of evidence-based practice. Today's health educators need to be fully aware of the various forms of scholarship, which include research, integration, application of scholarship, and teaching. It is also important to be familiar with the three main types of research: quantitative, qualitative, and interventional so as to choose a method that best fits one's circumstances. Mentorship, forming research groups, and seeking faculty development workshops are some of the commonly used strategies to improve scholarship. Good writers are made, not born. Like effective leadership or excelling at a sport, writing needs to be practiced early and often.

REFERENCES

Boyer, E. L. (1990). *Scholarship reconsidered: Priorities of the professoriate*. Princeton, NJ: Carnegie Foundation for the Advancement of Teaching.

Garino, A. (2014). Set the world on fire: Sparking research interest in physician assistants. *Journal of Physician Assistant Education, 25*(3), 21–25.

Glassick, C. E., Huber, M. T., Maeroff, G. I., & Boyer, E. L. (1997). *Scholarship assessed*. San Francisco, CA: Jossey-Bass.

Hutchings, P., & Shulman, L. S. (1999). The scholarship of teaching: New elaborations, new developments. *Change: The Magazine of Higher Learning, 31*(5), 10–15.

Lester, M., & Beason, L. (2012). *The McGraw-Hill handbook of English grammar and usage* (2nd ed.). New York, NY: McGraw-Hill.

Levinson, W., & Rubenstein, A. (2000). Integrating clinician-educators into academic medical centers: Challenges and potential solutions. *Academic Medicine, 75*(9), 906–912.

Miller, A. A., & Dehn, R. (2014). Physician assistant research culture: Another view. *Journal of Physician Assistant Education, 25*(3), 7–8.

Ritsema, T. S., & Cawley, J. S. (2013). Building a research culture in physician assistant education. *The Journal of Physician Assistant Education, 25*(2), 11–14.

Savin, H. B., & Perchonock, E. (1965). Grammatical structure and the immediate recall of English sentences. *Journal of Verbal Learning and Verbal Behavior, 4*(5), 348–353.

Starck, P. L. (1996). Boyer's multidimensional nature of scholarship: A new framework for schools of nursing. *Journal of Professional Nursing, 12*(5), 268–276.

Terryberry, K. J. (2005). *Writing for the health professions*. Clifton, NY: Cengage Learning.

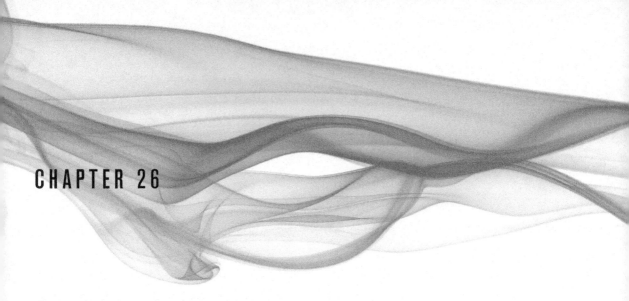

CHAPTER 26

Promoting Academic and Student Leadership

Reamer L. Bushardt, Teri L. Capshaw, and Sonia J. Crandall

CHAPTER OBJECTIVES

- Describe leadership styles and theories, tools, and skills to navigate leadership roles
- Discuss communication and conflict management
- Formulate a plan for leading change and role modeling for students

---

Without courage, we cannot practice any other virtue with consistency. We can't be kind, true, merciful, generous, or honest.

—*Maya Angelou*

More than 15 years ago, in "Educational Outcomes and Leadership to Meet the Needs of Modern Health Care" Spencer and Jordon (2001 p. ii44) described the need to evolve health care education and to create better alignment with the needs of a changing clinical practice environment. Vision in such an environment requires educational leadership that can "digest, assimilate, and provide evidence for the various demands and requirements and to synthesize and express the 'digest' in terms of a set of measurable and achievable outcomes fit for the purpose. The second leadership role is to facilitate change and realise the vision" (p. ii44). We exist in era in which health care and health care education must be reinvented to create value and improve patient experience; capable, creative leaders are critically needed within training programs and the practice environment to guide innovation and this necessary reinvention.

Through models like the National Institute for Health and Care Excellence, the United Kingdom has been on the front line for many years in exploring ways to maximize value and cost-effectiveness in health care (Nuffield Trust and Institute for Fiscal Studies, 2013). As health care in the United States increases its focus on improving health care access, cost, quality, efficiency, and patient experience, the guidance from Spencer and Jordon (2001) is timely and significant. To achieve the goals set out by contemporary health policies shaped around value, coupled with a general need to lower overall health care costs, tremendous efforts are needed not only to redesign current health care delivery systems, but also to evolve existing educational models to better prepare the current and future health care workforce for a team-based, value-based practice environment. It is necessary to enrich leadership training and professional development for students and faculty across medicine, nursing, and the health sciences. Leadership skills and abilities should prepare faculty to adapt and sustain health professions education in a rapidly changing and uncertain world. Traditional models for leadership development are likely inadequate if consideration of generational differences within today's health care workforce and new paradigms for care delivery, such as interprofessional collaborative practice, patient empowerment and increased utilization of health information technologies, and greater scopes of practice for myriad health care professionals. Traditional models often lack a board functional orientation, tools to increase self-awareness, and guidance for career management, which new leaders require for long-term success in today's health care market.

In this chapter, we explore these six key areas related to leadership for new and established faculty and health care professional students: the theoretical basis of leadership, fundamentals of leadership in health care education and clinical practice, a model for faculty and student leadership development, leadership assessment, women and leadership, and future trends in leadership development. Whether in the classroom or at the patient's bedside, leadership will be critical to accelerate innovation within education and practice and to align it with considerable changes in U.S. health care policy. Let us build an understanding and practical plan for leadership capacity building across these six key areas.

THE THEORETICAL BASIS OF LEADERSHIP

Leadership is most often defined by traits, qualities, and behaviors. Common examples of the myriad characteristics a leader might possess are a clear personal vision; a sense of purpose; being knowledgeable, strong, courageous, tenacious, powerful, resourceful, and resilient; as well as being a good communicator. Values and personal integrity are integral to this role. Good leaders exhibit many styles and they possess a diverse array of qualities. There is no single recipe for good leadership. Although a foolproof formula for effective leadership remains elusive, research suggests leadership requires aptitude (Drucker, 1986). John W. Gardner challenged the concept of leadership existing within a single designated individual and situation. Gardner (1990, p. 30) postulated that "leadership is the accomplishment of group purpose, which is furthered not only by effective leaders but also by innovators, entrepreneurs, and thinkers; by the availability of resources; by questions of value and social cohesion." In any group, there are different roles that individuals occupy, and one of the roles is that of leader. "Leaders cannot be thought of apart from the historic context in which they arise, the setting in which they function. . . . They are integral parts of the system, subject to the forces that affect the system" (Jossey-Bass, 2007, p. 17).

Leadership has been studied extensively for many years and an examination of popular theories can be helpful in providing context for and insight into effective models of leadership development.

Contingency Theory and Situational Leadership

Fred Fiedler was the first management theorist to assert that leadership effectiveness is contingent upon situation. In his book *A Theory of Leadership Effectiveness* Fiedler (1967) described situational factors in interaction with leader traits and behavior that influence leadership effectiveness. The theory suggests there is no single ideal leadership behavior. Both task-oriented and relationship-oriented leaders can equally be successful if their style fits the given situation. Wheatley (1994) endorses situational leadership, or how a specific situation should affect the approach of a leader. She believes leaders should be empowered to make intelligent decisions based on how they comprehend a given situation, versus through a simple understanding of policy or procedure. Wheatley (1994, p. 144) states, "leadership is always dependent on the context, but the context is established by the relationships we value."

The Vroom–Yetton Model of Leadership is a contingency theory that suggests leaders should vary the extent to which they allow followers to participate in decisions based on certain factors and the context of the situation (Vroom & Yetton, 1973). The model uses a decision tree to assess the nature of the task, the extent to which followers can be expected to disagree over the best solution, and the extent to which followers will accept decisions they do not support (Parker, 1999).

Servant Leadership

Robert Greenleaf, in his 1970 essay, "The Servant as Leader," explored the idea of the philosophy of servant leadership. A servant leader is community minded, focusing on the growth and well-being of people and community. Power is shared, the needs of others are made subservient to those of the leader, and the leader focuses on helping others develop and succeed. Servant leadership has often been described as a common phenomenon among health care professionals and student leaders within health care education programs.

Transactional and Transformational Leadership, Ethical Leadership, and Authentic Leadership

J. M. Burns, in the late 1970s, developed a theory to explain the differences among behaviors of political leaders using the terms *transactional* and *transformational leadership* (Burns, 1978). B. M. Bass modified Burns's theory to propose that transformational leadership augmented the effects of transactional leadership on the efforts, satisfaction, and effectiveness of followers (Bass, 2008). Transactional leaders reward effort and strive to ensure subordinates' behaviors conform to expectations. As a result, this type of leader tends to concentrate on compromise, intrigue, and control (Bass, 1993).

Transformational leadership is a form of moral leadership. Transformational leaders inspire their followers to look beyond self-interest and work together toward a collective goal (Burns, 1978). Transformational leadership converges with the more contemporary construct of ethical leadership in a focus on personal characteristics and integrity. Brown and Trevino (2006, p. 597) state, "Ethical and transformational leaders care about others, act consistently with their moral principles (i.e., integrity), consider the ethical consequences of their decisions, and are ethical role models for others". In ethical leadership, traits of a moral leader include integrity, honesty, and trustworthiness.

Bill George (2003) is credited with creating the model of authentic leadership. In his seminal work, *Authentic Leadership: Rediscovering the Secrets to Creating Lasting Value*, George demonstrated, through illustrative examples from corporate leaders, that authentic leaders in mission-driven companies create greater shareholder value than financially driven firms. Authentic leaders are sincere in striving to serve others by empowering the people they work with to make a difference. The model proposes five qualities that authentic leaders possess: pursuing purpose with passion, practicing solid values, leading with the heart, establishing enduring relationships, and demonstrating self-discipline. Traits of an authentic leader include self-awareness, openness, transparency, and consistency. An authentic leader is motivated by positive end values and concern for others, as opposed to self-interest. The construct of authentic leadership has also been well described in nursing, associating this leadership model with the creation of healthier work environments (Shirey, 2006).

Four Frames for Leadership

Lee G. Bolman and Terrence E. Deal developed four orientations or "frames" that characterize the way leaders think about issues and problems: a structural frame, human resource frame, political frame, and symbolic frame (Bolman & Deal, 1991). The structural frame stresses goals and efficiency. A structural leader values analysis and data, while keeping eyes on the bottom line and setting clear directions. Structural leaders use new policies, rules, or restructuring to try to solve organizational problems (Bolman & Deal, 1991).

The human resource frame emphasizes human needs. Human resource leaders value relationships and feelings; they lead through facilitation and empowerment. Bolman and Deal's (1991) political frame sees organizations as areas of continuing conflict and competition among various interests for scarce resources. Political leaders are advocates and negotiators, who spend their time networking, negotiating, building a power base, and forming coalitions. The fourth frame, the symbolic one, "sees a chaotic world in which meaning and predictability are social creations and facts are interpretative rather than objective" (Bolman & Deal, 1991, p. 512). A symbolic leader tries to instill a sense of enthusiasm and commitment, while paying attention to myth, ritual, ceremony, and stories.

Charismatic Leadership

Jay A. Conger and Rabindra N. Kanungo advanced the study of leadership in organization by developing a behavioral theory of charismatic leadership. Conger and Kanungo's (1987) model builds on the concept that charisma is an attributional phenomenon. Charisma is viewed both "as a set of dispositional attributions by followers and as a set of leaders' manifest behaviors. The two are linked in the sense that the leaders' behaviors form the basis of followers' attributions" (Conger & Kanungo, 1987, p. 645).

They identified several behavioral components of charisma that include opposition to the status quo; an idealized vision; and unconventional, transformative, and strong articulation of future vision. "A leader becomes charismatic when he/she succeeds in changing his/her followers' attitudes in accept the advocated vision," according to Conger and Kanungo (1987, p. 640).

The Five Practices of Exemplary Leadership

Researchers James Kouzes and Barry Posner identified five fundamental practices that enable leaders to get extraordinary results, published in their landmark book, *The Leadership Challenge: How to Make Extraordinary Things Happen in Organizations*. Kouzes and Posner conceptualize leadership as "the art of mobilizing others to want to struggle for shared aspirations" (Kouzes & Posner, 2012, p. 30). Their research demonstrated that leadership is teachable and that ordinary people who guide others along trailblazing paths follow similar journeys. They synthesized their findings into five fundamental practices (Table 26.1).

A Model for Faculty and Student Leadership Development Based on Competencies, Character, Commitment, and Empowerment

The most successful health care professionals integrate both art and science into the care of patients and families. Leadership is fundamental to patient care, including routine activities such as building rapport with patients, motivating patients to adopt healthy behaviors, collaborating

TABLE 26.1 Five Practices of Exemplary Leadership

1. Model the way	Exemplary leaders establish standards of excellence and they practice what they preach, aligning words and deeds.
2. Inspire a shared vision	Leaders are passionate about making a difference and they engage others in creating a shared vision.
3. Challenge the process	Leaders forge new trails; they are not afraid to experiment and take risks on the path to success.
4. Enable others to act	Exemplary leaders foster collaboration and involve others in decision making and goal setting.
5. Encourage the heart	Leaders realize that work is hard, so they share the limelight and celebrate others' accomplishments.

effectively with members of an interprofessional team, and advocating for resources to support our teams and the communities they serve. Health care providers have a unique and inherent obligation to grow and develop continuously as professionals. Further, faculty must facilitate within their students the formation of a professional identity as a core component of all health professions education. Tenets of professionalism should be seamlessly integrated within the leadership development for anyone who cares for patients and families. Regulatory bodies for health care professionals routinely license and evaluate practice with attention on both clinical competence and professional conduct.

There is value in incorporating skills and competencies that emphasize empowerment and interprofessional collaborative practice. To prepare professionals for a complex practice environment filled with numerous challenges, these skills are critical. Maintaining high-quality interpersonal dynamics within a care team not only can improve the quality of the care delivered but also facilitate healing care environments for patients and families. In "Professionalism in Healthcare Professions," a report published by the Health and Care Professions Council (2014), a description of professionalism as a fluid construct had similarities with situational leadership:

> Professionalism . . . was not seen as a static well-defined concept, but rather was felt to be constructed in specific interactions . . . definitions of professionalism were fluid, changing dynamically with changing context . . . this contextual influence was perceived, both in terms of the clinical, patient-centred context, and of the organizational and interprofessional context. (p. 22)

We propose a model for leadership development, applicable to health care professional faculty and students, that is built on leadership character development within an empowerment framework. In their work "Developing Leadership Character," Gandz, Crossan, Seijts, Stephenson, and Mazutis (2010) ask three questions in assessing leaders at any level in an organization:

1. Do they have the competencies to be a leader?
2. Do they have the commitment to be a leader?
3. Do they have the character to be a good leader?

These authors previously described requisite knowledge, skills, understanding, and judgment that leaders need and categorized these into four competency areas: strategic, business, organizational, and people. These competencies share general intellect as a common underpinning

(Figure 26.1). The critical interplay between these leadership competencies with commitment and character, as described by these authors, we believe is highly relevant to health care professionals and students.

The character traits that support leadership, similar to the construct of professionalism within health care professions, can be hard to define, measure, assess, and develop. Consider the last person you were unable to work with successfully. What precipitated the breakdown? Consider the last two major failures of leadership within your institution. What were the underlying causes of the failure? Research suggests that character was involved as a central theme in the failures or the relationship breakdown. Character fundamentally shapes our behaviors. It profoundly influences how we engage with the world around us, what we notice, what we reinforce, what we value, what we choose to act on, how we make decisions, and who we engage in conversation. For the purposes of this model for leadership development, *character* is defined as a composite of personality traits, values, and virtues.

Whether developing leadership curricula for health professions education or constructing an individualized professional development plan for a faculty member, we recommend attention to leadership competencies across the four key areas previously described (e.g., strategic, business, organizational, and people), as well as attention to commitment and character development. Within each of these areas, educational activities and assessments should address knowledge, understanding, skills, and judgment. Admission processes used in health professions education frequently identify students who are aspirational, engaged, and altruistic; however, the rigor of training and impact of exposure to challenging clinical environments may warrant ongoing surveillance and reinforcement. Measures of empathy may be useful in surveillance of commitment and student response to training. For example, Nunes, Williams, Sa, and Stevenson (2011) examined empathy levels among undergraduate students in five different health sciences disciplines and found a decline in self-reported empathy scores began during the first year of training. The authors noted the decline may be caused in part by a "settling in" effect, with a change from idealism to realism, but they also postulated students may be exhibiting an adaptive response to new responsibilities and heavy workloads. The extent to which faculty

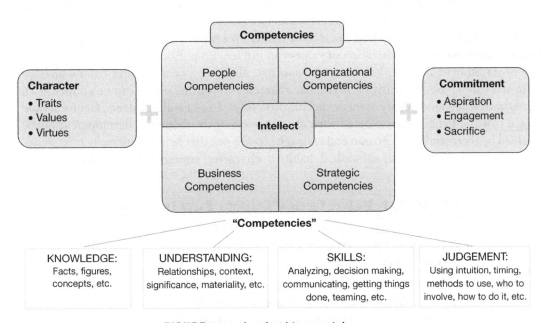

FIGURE 26.1 Leadership on trial.

Source: Gandz, Crossan, Seijts, and Stephenson (2010).

physicians are able to focus on the aspect of work that is most meaningful to them has a strong inverse relationship to their risk of burnout. Efforts to optimize career fit may promote physician satisfaction and help reduce attrition among academic faculty physicians. Similar attention to commitment should be directed to faculty members, who are often subject to numerous factors associated with burnout. Based on findings from Shanafelt and colleagues (2009), the extent to which individuals are able to focus on aspects of work that are most meaningful to them is inversely related to their risk of burnout. Steps taken to optimize career fit and individualize career development plans to the needs and interests of the faculty member may pay dividends on maximizing commitment. These authors recommend presenting faculty with a broad list of leadership skills, tasks, and competency areas, then soliciting their input to prioritize areas of perceived need and personal interest. This information can be used to produce a discrepancy analysis, which can inform an individualized professional development plan, as well as inform key target areas for development across the entire body of faculty assessed.

Character Development

Crossan and colleagues describe an approach to developing leadership character at the individual, group, and organizational levels, which these authors believe is applicable to health professions education. To focus on approach, health professions educators may adopt groupings of common virtues or define a set of values or virtues that are important to a particular profession or program. Peterson and Seligman (2004) identified six universal virtues that were common across a diverse sample of cultures, religions, and moral philosophies: wisdom, courage, humanity, justice, temperance, and transcendence. Col. (Ret.) Eric Kail (2011) defined six core facets of character-based leadership: courage, integrity, selflessness, empathy, collaboration, and reflection (Exhibit 26.1).

Alternatively, it may be practical to adopt the set of nine behaviors described by Swick (2000) in his normative definition of medical professionalism. Various national professional organizations, such as the American Academy of Physician Assistants, also publish core values for the profession they represent. It is important to remember that an individual's character is composed of both habitual qualities (also known as *character strengths*) as well as a motivational component (Figure 26.2). In the approach described by Crossan and colleagues, values are leveraged as motivational factors that may lead a person or constrain a person to prefer a specific end goal. As a result, a purposeful prioritization of values can influence a person in selecting a particular course of action over another. Values can be conceptualized as a central point from which we operate and can be used to cultivate particular character strengths, which can be aligned with goals of the health education program or specific profession. In assessing students, faculty should be aware that the behaviors associated with character strengths shape the development of the values held by their students. Crossan and colleagues point out that personality traits exist somewhere between the previously described habitual character strengths (or weaknesses) and

---

EXHIBIT 26.1 Six Core Facets of Character-Based Leadership

Courage: moral resilience and bravery under pressure
Integrity: how well your life reflects your values
Selflessness: placing the needs of the organization and followers above your own
Empathy: understanding others' perspectives, leveraging diversity
Collaboration: capacity for supporting peers as teammates; seeing the big picture
Reflection: translating performance into potential

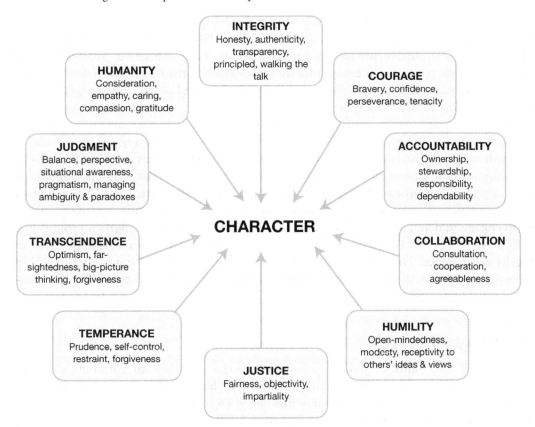

FIGURE 26.2 Developing leadership character.

Source: Crossan, Gandz, and Seijts (2012).

motivational values. For faculty and students, having baseline awareness of personality traits, or their natural tendencies, can be instrumental in constructing and managing a personal leadership development plan.

Crossan and colleagues constructed the Virtue-Based Orientation (VBO) Model, which places character development at the center of ethical decision making. Their model adds reflection as a mediator to the four-stage process, developed by James Rest (1984, p. 19), built on awareness, judgment, intent, and behavior. The VBO Model focuses on the outcomes of ethical decisions as offering learning opportunities for future ethical decision making, and by design it develops the character strengths of the person making the decisions. Such a process is not so different from paradigms for clinical decision making already used by numerous health professions education programs, which incorporate empiric evidence, provider experience, and patient preferences into decision making. In both models for evidence-based practice and the VBO Model, deliberate practice is a proven pathway for the acquisition of expert performance and can guide curricular development.

Character can be taught, and intentional curricular activities and mentoring can help prioritize values in such a way that decision making aligns with accepted standards for a particular profession or discipline. As Crossan and colleagues assert, "Deliberate teaching interventions such as role-plays, collaborative learning techniques, service learning opportunities, and self-reflection exercises in the classroom appear to affect character development through increased moral awareness and moral reasoning" (p. 290). Similarly, in clinical training environments, if subject to reflection, the patient and trainee experience can provide powerful opportunities to refine and strengthen character-based leadership and solidify ethical decision making. These authors recommend the "parallel chart" approach developed by Rita Charon of Columbia University, which blends narrative into patient care. To illustrate, Charon listens as patients tell their stories and then she writes down everything she remembers, in the order in which it was told. Charon offers that that this method does not take longer than traditional charting methods but produces notes that are far more telling. More important, she indicates that this approach has ripple effects: The narratively retrained eye sees three dimensions when it examines any patient. Students do not have to write about every patient they encounter, but writing about some of them can dramatically increase the attention they pay to all of them. This approach provides an opportunity for health professions students to develop character strengths and documents an experience they may choose to share with faculty or preceptors, which can serve as a useful tool to facilitate mentoring and professional development. Similarly, opportunities for groups of students to engage in dialogue that draws from clinical experiences can strengthen professional identity formation, ethical decision making, and appreciation for how individual character strengths shape values. Through faculty facilitation, this approach can be meaningful within interdisciplinary groups of students and can be used to help develop competencies for interprofessional collaborative practice.

LEADERSHIP ASSESSMENT

Leadership skills and abilities should be assessed to ascertain whether students and faculty are adequately prepared for the rapidly changing and uncertain health care environment. An assessment and feedback process is instrumental in measuring a leader's skill set, clarifying needs and goals, and setting a direction for future development. A 360-degree assessment tool—a method of collecting opinions about an individual's performance from a range of coworkers—is especially beneficial in providing a panoramic view of perceptions rather than just self-perception, which affords a complete picture. Notable other assessment tools include:

- Using benchmarks to assess leadership skills
- Campbell Leadership Index
- Cardinal Leadership Inventory
- Leadership Virtues Questionnaire
- Multifactor Leadership Questionnaire

WOMEN AND LEADERSHIP

This chapter would be incomplete without addressing women in leadership. This topic is important because parity has not been achieved between the percentage of women in the health professions and their representation in executive leadership within clinical and academic enterprises.

Dan Diamond (2014), former managing editor of *Daily Briefing*, the Advisory Board's leading newsletter for health care executives, notes that nearly 80% of hospital and clinic employees are women, but only 43% of health care executives are women, according to the 2014 Advisory Board Survey Solutions Employee Engagement Benchmark. The Association of American Medical Colleges' 2013 to 2014 publication on the state of women in academic medicine reports that 38% of all full-time faculty members are women. However, only 5% hold the rank of full professor, whereas 18% of the men hold that rank. "Women are continuing to make progress in obtaining administrative positions in the dean's office, yet the percentage of women in department-level [15%] and decanal positions [16%] remains low compared to men" (Lautenberger, Dander, Raezer, & Sloane, 2014, p. 11).

There are several features that may help explain why women are not better represented in health care leadership. McDonagh and Paris (2012, p. 24) describe these features as barriers that create "a labyrinth that women have to navigate to advance into leadership positions," such as women's perceived leadership and communication styles, unconscious bias and gender stereotype (Anderson et al., 2015), limited opportunity for formal leadership development and mentoring, an individual's level of confidence and competence and self-awareness, competing family needs and career demands, conscious choice not to pursue leadership, and intentionality (McDonagh & Paris, 2012).

There is increasing evidence that paying attention to specific elements is having a positive influence on women in leadership. For example, a study by Chang and colleagues (2016, p. 694) of participants of formal career development programs (CDPs) designed specifically for women in academic medicine found that "women faculty participating in CDPs were less likely to leave academic medicine than their men and women faculty peers." Other features being studied and confronted are the unconscious (implicit) bias and gender stereotypes that disadvantage women seeking leadership opportunities. Deliberate transformation is needed and proven strategies to ameliorate bias and stereotyping have been described (Carnes et al., 2015; Easterly & Ricard, 2011). The good news is that women are often seen as transformative and collaborative leaders, characteristics of which are highly correlated with leadership effectiveness (McDonagh & Paris, 2012).

CONCLUSIONS

As the health care environment becomes more complex, uncertain, and volatile, new models for leadership development will emerge. In recent years, there has been increased attention on accreditation standards related to interprofessional health care education, and health care delivery systems are investing in models that leverage interprofessional collaborative practice. As a result, more training for health care providers, faculty, and students will be needed that address team-based practice and greater capacity for more complex and adaptive thinking. Leadership and its associated risks will likely be shared more collaboratively in a health care market designed to deliver value-based care. This transfer will require new skills for those delegating authority and those receiving it; in some cases, those individuals will be patients and families.

Drawing from a project commissioned by the Center for Creative Leadership (2016) and the resultant "Future Trends in Leadership Development," we relate four trends anticipated to impact leadership development for health professions students and faculty in the future. The first anticipated trend is a greater focus on vertical development. An adaptive leader must be able to self-direct his or her own professional development and earn new skills and abilities through stages of development and lifelong learning. The second trend, related to the first, is the transfer to the individual of more ownership for professional development. Faculty and students alike are subject to significant quantities of training that they are not interested in or find little value in. Social psychology tells us that a person's motivation to grow and learn is highest when that person feels authority over his or her own development. Empowering patients to be more engaged in self-care is a commonly accepted goal in health care, and the same perspective can be adopted for leadership development among faculty and students. Institutions should provide a vision and desired outcomes, offer tools for self-assessment and development, and empower learners to self-direct relevant aspects of their own leadership development. The third expected trend is increased focus on collective, rather than individual, leadership. Leadership will evolve in many situations to a collective process that is spread among a community of stakeholders. The fourth trend is a necessary focus on innovation in leadership development methodologies. The health professions education and health care delivery environments are subject to rapid transformation to meet goals for value-based care and greater capacity for learning health care systems. As a result, the market will demand innovation in how we develop leaders to keep up with the accelerated pace of health care delivery redesign.

REFERENCES

Anderson, A., Ahmad, A., King, E., Lindsey, A., Fevre, R., Ragone, S., & Kim, S. (2015). The effectiveness of three strategies to reduce the influence of bias in evaluations of female leaders. *Journal of Applied Social Psychology, 45*, 522–539.

Audi, R. (2012). Virtue ethics as a resource in business. *Business Ethics Quarterly, 22*(2), 273–291.

Bass, B. M. (1993). Transformational leadership and team and organizational decision making. In B. Bass & B. Avolio (Eds.), *Improving organizational effectiveness through transformational leadership*. Thousand Oaks, CA: Sage.

Bass, B. M. (2008). *The Bass handbook of leadership: Theory, research, and managerial applications* (4th ed.). New York, NY: Free Press.

Bolman, L. G., & Deal, T. E. (1991). Leadership and management effectiveness: A multi-frame, multisector analysis. *Human Resource Management, 30*(4), 509–534.

Brown, M., & Trevino, L. (2006). Ethical leadership: A review and future directions. *Leadership Quarterly, 17*(4), 595–616.

Burns, J. (1978). *Leadership*. New York, NY: Harper & Row.

Carnes M., Devine, P., Manwell, L., Byars-Winston, A., Fine, E., Ford, C., . . . Sheridan, J. (2015). Effect of an intervention to break the gender bias habit for faculty at one institution: A cluster randomized, controlled trial. *Academic Medicine, 90*(2), 221–30.

Center for Creative Leadership. (2016). Assessments. Retrieved from http://www.ccl.org/leadership/assessments/index.aspx

Chang, S., Morahan, P. S., Magrane, D., Helitzer, D., Lee, H. Y., Newbill, S., . . . Cardinali, G. (2016). Retaining faculty in academic medicine: The impact of career development programs for women. *Journal of Women's Health, 25*(7), 687–696.

Charon, R. (2006). *Narrative medicine: Honoring the stories of illness*. New York, NY: Oxford University Press.

Conger, J. A., & Kanungo, R. N. (1987). Toward a behavioral theory of charismatic leadership in organizational settings. *Academy of Management, 12*(4), 637–647.

Crossan, M., Gandz, J., & Seijts, G. (2012). Developing leadership character. *Ivey Business Journal*. Retrieved from http://iveybusinessjournal.com/publication/developing-leadership-character

Crossan, M., Mazutis, D., Seijts, G., & Gandz, J. (2013). Developing leadership character in business programs. *Academy of Management Learning and Education, 12*(2), 285–305.

Diamond, D. (2014, August 26). Women make up 80% of health care workers—but just 40% of executives [Web log post]. Retrieved from https://www.advisory.com/daily-briefing/blog/2014/08/women-in-leadership

Drucker, P. F. (1986). *The practice of management*. New York, NY: Harper & Row.

Easterly, D., & Ricard, C. (2011). Conscious efforts to end unconscious bias: Why women leave academic research. *Journal of Research Administration, 42*(1), 61–73.

Fielder, F. E. (1967). *A theory of leadership effectiveness*. New York, NY: McGraw-Hill.

Gandz, J., Crossan, M., Seijts, G., & Stephenson, C. (2010). *Leadership on trial: A manifesto for leadership development*. London, Ontario, Canada: Ivey Publishing.

Gandz, J., Crossan, M., Seijts, G., Stephenson, C., & Mazutis, D. (2010). Leadership on trial: A manifesto for leadership development. Retrieved from http://www.ivey.uwo.ca/research/leadership/research/books-and-reports.html

Gardner, J. (1990). *On leadership*. New York, NY: Free Press.

George, B. (2003). *Authentic leadership: Rediscovering the secrets to creating lasting value*. San Francisco, CA: Jossey-Bass.

Health and Care Professions Council. (2014). Professionalism in healthcare professions. Retrieved from http://www.hpc-uk.org/assets/documents/10003771Professionalisminhealthcareprofessionals.pdf

Jossey-Bass. (2007). *The Jossey-Bass reader on educational leadership*. San Francisco, CA: Author.

Kail, E. (2011). Take the CTI. Retrieved from http://www.performanceprograms.com/self-assessments/leadership-effectiveness/cardinal-leadership-inventory-cli

Kouzes, J., & Posner, B. (2012). *The Leadership challenge: How to make extraordinary things happen in organizations* (5th ed.). San Francisco, CA: Jossey-Bass.

Lautenberger, D., Dandar, V., Raezer, C., & Sloane, R. (2014). *The state of women in academic medicine: The pipeline and pathways to leadership.* Washington, DC: Association on American Medical Colleges.

McDonagh, K., & Paris, N. (2012). The leadership labyrinth: Career advancement for women. *Frontiers of Health Service Management, 28*(4), 22–28.

Nuffield Trust and Institute for Fiscal Studies. (2013, May). Public payment and private provision: The changing landscape of health care in the 2000s. Retrieved from http://www.nuffieldtrust.org.uk/sites/ files/nuffield/publication/130522_publicpayment-and-privateprovision.pdf

Nunes, P., Williams, S., Sa, B., & Stevenson, K. (2011). A study of empathy decline in students from five health disciplines during their first year of training. *International Journal of Medical Education,* (2), 12–17. Retrieved from https://www.ijme.net/archive/2/empathy-decline-in-first-year-students.pdf

Parker, C. (1999). The impact of leaders' implicit theories of employee participation on test of the Vroom–Yetton Model. *Journal of Social Behavior and Personality, 4*(1), 45–61.

Peterson, C., & Seligman, M. (2004) *Character strengths and virtues: A handbook and classification.* New York, NY: Oxford University Press.

Shanafelt, T., West, C., Sloan, J., Novotny, P., Poland, G., Menaker, R., . . . Dyrbye, L. (2009). Career fit and burnout among academic faculty. *JAMA Internal Medicine.* Retrieved from http://medicine.uams .edu/files/2012/10/Career-Fit-and-Burnout.pdf

Shirey, M. (2006). Authentic leaders creating healthy work environments for nursing practice. *American Journal of Critical Care, 15*(3), 256–267. Retrieved from http://ajcc.aacnjournals.org/content/15/3/256 .abstract

Spencer, J., & Jordan, R. (2001). Educational outcomes and leadership to meet the needs of modern health care. *Quality in Health Care, 10*(Suppl. II), ii38–ii45.

Swick, H. (2000). Toward a normative definition of medical professionalism. *Academic Medicine, 75*(6), 612–616.

Vroom, V. H., & Yetton, P. W. (1973) *Leadership and decision-making.* London, UK: Feffer and Simons.

Wheatley, M. (1994). *Leadership and the new science.* San Francisco, CA: Berrett-Koehler.

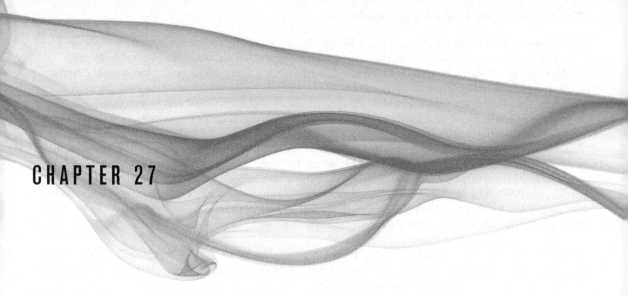

CHAPTER 27

Giving and Receiving Feedback
Craig Keenan

CHAPTER OBJECTIVE

• Discuss how to give effective feedback to students and colleagues

---

We all need people who will give us feedback. That's how we improve.

—*Bill Gates*

Feedback in health care education can be defined as the method by which teachers observe and describe their learners' activities, and feed information back to them to reinforce appropriate behaviors and correct mistakes. Feedback is perhaps the most powerful teaching tool that the health care educator has in his or her toolbox. Ideally, giving effective feedback to learners improves their clinical performance and fosters their continuous improvement as clinicians. Yet learners vary widely in their acceptance and application of feedback. Educators can learn skills that make learners more receptive to feedback.

Health care educators themselves must also be receptive to feedback about their teaching. Educators can develop their own skills at receiving feedback. By understanding the process of both giving and receiving feedback, health care educators can master the feedback process and truly enhance their teaching.

GIVING FEEDBACK

Feedback comes in three basic forms—appreciation, coaching, and evaluation—which are outlined in Table 27.1 (Stone & Heen, 2014). *Appreciation* is pure "positive" feedback that shows that you value the learner's contribution. It thanks and motivates the learner to repeat the behavior.

TABLE 27.1 Key Differences Among Appreciation, Coaching, and Evaluation

Feedback Type	Purpose	Teacher's Role	Timing	Content	Example
Appreciation	Connecting Reinforcing	Team member	Immediate	Acknowledgment Thanks	"Thank you for seeing that extra patient."
Coaching	Improving ("negative") Reinforcing ("positive")	Coach	Immediate	Information Description of behavior Development of improvement plan	"Your cardiac exam was incomplete. You should also assess the point of maximal impulse and jugular venous pressure."
Evaluation	Grading	Judge	Delayed	Judgment Grade	"You are not meeting expectations on your clinic efficiency. As a third-year resident, I expect you to be able to see six patients per clinic session."

Coaching is what is more classically viewed as feedback. Coaching feedback can be "positive," in which the teacher observes a proper behavior, and describes and praises it in order to reinforce it. The more impactful coaching feedback, however, is usually the constructive, or "negative" feedback, wherein the teacher describes a deficiency in behavior and provides specific feedback to improve knowledge and/or skills. Thus, coaching feedback ideally provides the learner with information that is both descriptive and formative.

Evaluation is a judgment or grading of a learner's performance. It typically occurs at the end of a clinical rotation or course, and incorporates multiple observations to provide a *summative* assessment of performance. Coaching and evaluation do have some overlap. In reality, effective coaching feedback requires real-time evaluation of the learner's behavior, as the teacher will need to "grade" the learner to determine what he or she is doing right or wrong, which then informs subsequent coaching. This on-the-fly evaluation is not summative. Ideally, more formal evaluation summarizes many coaching interactions that a teacher has had with a learner to make a final judgment. Of course, evaluation sessions may include coaching feedback on behaviors and suggestions for improvement. However, coaching given during evaluation sessions is often less impactful because it is delayed and does not refer to explicit, observed behaviors.

BARRIERS TO GIVING FEEDBACK

Although health educators and learners both agree that feedback is essential to improving, learners often report not receiving adequate feedback. There are many barriers to providing effective feedback (Exhibit 27.1). Health education often occurs in fast-paced clinical environments. This leads to minimal direct observation of learners' behaviors at the bedside with patients or colleagues. Teachers more often observe oral presentations or written chart notes, which only allow an inference on actual behaviors. This lack of direct observation greatly limits the amount of effective feedback that can be given. Even when direct observation does occur, it can be challenging to find time to provide feedback in these hectic environments, which can be exacerbated by having a large number of learners to supervise.

Some teachers avoid giving negative feedback for fear of being disliked by learners, or fear of damaging learners' self-esteem. Others fear retaliatory negative evaluations by learners, which

> **EXHIBIT 27.1** Barriers to Providing Effective Feedback

Inadequate observation of learners' activities and behaviors
Lack of time to give feedback
Excessive number of learners to give feedback to
Fear of retaliation (i.e., poor teaching evaluations)
Fear of being disliked by learners
Fear of damaging learners' self-esteem

can impact promotions or pay. With all of these barriers, it is easy for teachers to rationalize not providing feedback.

Health educators must remain aware of the potential consequences of not providing feedback. Without it, learners must interpret their performance based on vague external clues. They may feel that no feedback indicates that they are doing well. Relying on inappropriate cues, they can become overconfident in their rudimentary abilities, or unconfident in their strongest skills. Most important, patient care may suffer because learners' mistakes are overlooked or uncorrected. Once established, attitudes, behaviors, and skills can endure beyond the training period, affecting learners' ultimate practice. Thus, the failure to provide corrective feedback can seriously threaten a health professional's career by allowing incorrect behaviors to flourish while failing to reinforce good behaviors. Giving effective feedback is a critical teaching responsibility, and it is essential that educators overcome the barriers so as to develop competent professionals.

ESSENTIAL QUALITIES OF GIVING EFFECTIVE FEEDBACK

Everybody likes to receive appreciation and positive coaching feedback. Negative coaching feedback, no matter how enlightened the learner or how deftly delivered by the teacher, is always at its core a "criticism." As such, it usually will have an emotional impact on the learner, especially if it is unexpected. This can impact how well a learner receives and acts on feedback. Health educators must always keep this fact in mind as they deliver constructive feedback.

The effectiveness of feedback and learners' perceptions of its value can be enhanced by imbuing it with specific qualities (Delva et al., 2013; Lefroy, Watling, Teunissen, & Brand, 2015). Table 27.2 uses the FEARLESS mnemonic to summarize these essential qualities (Keenan, Swenson, & Henderson, 2016). If these qualities are combined with the essential conversational skills discussed later, the negative impact of feedback can often be minimized.

1. **Formative:** *Emphasize the formative intent of feedback.* Learners learn best when they consider their teachers an ally. On the first day of any class or rotation, educators should explicitly state that they will give feedback regularly and that its purpose is to improve the learner's performance and patient care, and to foster their personal and professional growth. Also, it is good practice to preface negative feedback by explicitly repeating these goals, which may help minimize negative emotional responses.
2. **Expected:** *Create a culture in which feedback is expected.* Educators must create an environment where self-assessment, feedback, and growth are emphasized. Such a culture will make feedback more prevalent and less threatening for all involved.

TABLE 27.2 FEARLESS: Qualities of Effective Feedback

Formative	Emphasize **formative** intent
Expected	Create a culture in which feedback is **expected**
Aligned	**Align** feedback with the learner's goals and expectations
Recent	Give feedback on **recent** behaviors
Less	Limit the amount of feedback: **Less** is more
Environment	Deliver feedback in a respectful, nonjudgmental, nonthreatening learning **environment**
Specific	Feedback should describe **specific**, observed, "first-hand" behaviors
Success	Develop an action plan for **success**

Effective health educators must make time at the outset of a rotation to discuss learners' goals, to encourage learners to ask for feedback, and to set learners' expectations to receive it. Many learners avoid seeking feedback for fear of exposing their deficiencies. Encouraging learners to proactively seek feedback reduces such fear and creates in them a learning frame of mind. Learners who ask for feedback often are more receptive when it is delivered. Studies in nonmedical fields have found that persons who ask for feedback more frequently have higher job performance and job satisfaction.

3. **Aligned:** *Align feedback with the learner's goals and expectations.* Ideally, this is done in two steps at the orientation session. First, the educator delineates performance expectations. Second, the educator should try to elicit learners' learning objectives for the course or rotation. The pair then will use this information to establish learning goals at the outset of the rotation, and to also guide educators' observations, teaching, learning, and feedback. Tailoring feedback to the individual increases the effectiveness of the feedback.

4. **Recent:** *Give feedback on **recent** behaviors.* Timely feedback is best: The most effective feedback occurs close to the observed behavior. Feedback that is late or unexpected, especially if negative, is nearly always met with a negative reaction. Educators must not have timeliness overrule common sense. Specifically, most negative feedback should be given in private. And after emotionally charged moments (e.g., right after an unsuccessful Code Blue), postponing the feedback until emotions calm down often allows the learner to be better prepared to have a feedback conversation.

5. **Less:** *Limit the amount of feedback: **Less** is more. Don't overwhelm learners with excessive feedback in one session.* Teachers should address the most important, changeable behaviors first. Usually two to three items of constructive feedback are the most that can be given in one setting, but sometimes only one item is reasonable if it is challenging (e.g., professionalism issues). When considering the amount of feedback to give, teachers must also try to balance positive and negative feedback, which can help improve receptivity and create a positive learning climate.

6. **Environment:** *Deliver feedback in a respectful, nonjudgmental, nonthreatening learning environment.* Feedback that occurs in a safe, convenient, comfortable place and time is more likely to be delivered and received well. Positive feedback can generally be given anywhere. Corrective feedback, however, is best given in private. Learners often feel humiliated when feedback is given in public, even when teachers view it as minor. This negative emotional reaction can contribute to rejection of the feedback.

7. **Specific:** *Feedback should describe specific, observed, "first-hand" behaviors.* When providing constructive feedback, it is essential to describe the exact behavior, discuss why it was wrong, and what it looks like when correct. By simply describing the erroneous behavior, teachers can avoid the trap of inferring the knowledge or motivations behind learners' behaviors. Such inferences are often incorrect, add a personal emphasis, and can make learners less receptive to the feedback. "You have arrived late to rounds the last 3 days" is better than "It seems that you do not like this rotation, because you have been late the last 3 days."

   Positive feedback is easier to deliver, but, too often, is just vague generalizing (e.g., "great job"). Positive feedback also needs specificity to tell learners exactly what to continue to do, such as: "You had a nice list of potential pathogens for the meningitis, and chose the antibiotics based on that—good work."

8. **Success:** *Develop an action plan for success.* The best feedback has the learner determine the action plan to get to the next level. For negative feedback, the educator and learner ideally discuss a plan for change that makes the behavior correct then next time. For instance, if a resident chooses an improper antibiotic for pneumonia, the teacher may ask the resident to read the guidelines and report back to the team on the pathogens and currently recommended antibiotic options based on them. For positive feedback, educators can add next steps to grow even further, such as: "For the future, you should read up on the differences in community-acquired versus hospital-acquired pneumonia and how that would change your antibiotic choice."

MODELS OF GIVING EFFECTIVE FEEDBACK

Most educators now feel that feedback is best delivered via a conversation with the learner in which self-reflection is a strong component. The three most commonly used feedback models are the feedback sandwich, Pendleton Model, and reflective feedback conversation.

The feedback sandwich is probably the most well-known method, and is the most rudimentary. It begins and ends with statements of positive feedback (the bread), with the constructive (negative) coaching feedback sandwiched between them (the meat). This method is less likely to elicit a negative response from the learner, but may dilute the important constructive feedback. Some educators start with positive feedback and end with negative feedback—the "open-faced feedback sandwich." Many learners are very familiar with this method, and tend to discount the positive, waiting for the "but" before the negative feedback. Conversely, learners who overestimate their skills focus on the positive statements and may fail to take in the negative feedback. This method is teacher centered, and lacks learners' self-assessments or conversations. It can be effective for small pieces of on-the-fly feedback.

Learners' self-reflections and self-assessments are key components of the coaching and feedback process and of practice-based learning, and improvement more generally (Branch & Paranjape, 2002). Having learners share their self-reflections is an important first step in the process of setting learning goals. Moreover, hearing learners' perspectives on their performances yields valuable information on the learners' levels of insight. Learners generally fall into one of three basic categories of self-assessment. One group assesses its own strengths and weaknesses with good accuracy. A second group, often high performers, tends to underestimate its skill level. These individuals tend to dismiss positive statements and fixate on the negative feedback. A third group comprise the "unskilled and unaware" (Kruger & Dunning, 1999). These learners tend to overestimate their skills and are the most difficult to improve. Hearing how learners assess their skills can help teachers better gauge whether the learners over- or underestimate their skills and, thereby, frame their feedback optimally.

The Pendleton Model and reflective feedback conversation both use self-assessment as the starting point for delivering feedback. The Pendleton Model uses a structured four-step approach. In step one, the learner is asked to state what was good about his or her performance. In step two, the teacher states areas of agreement and elaborates on other areas of good performance. In step three, the learner states what was poor or what could have been improved. In step four, the teacher states what he or she thinks could have been improved. The model is conversational, requires self-assessment, balances positive and negative feedback, and encourages a safe and supportive environment. This model relies heavily on learners' self-assessments and works well for learners who can accurately assess their skills. With learners who over- or underestimate their skills, the dialogue enables teachers to recalibrate the learners' inaccurate self-assessments. Having learners start with their own self-assessments also opens the dialogue and allows the teacher to highlight unrecognized resident strengths and performance issues. In the long term, residents who engage in this recalibration process could potentially improve their self-assessment skills, which are critical for physicians as lifelong learners.

Though similar to the Pendleton Model, the reflective feedback conversation model (Exhibit 27.2) adds the exploration of reasons for underperformance and adds an explicit step for developing improvement (Cantilon & Sargeant, 2006). An easy way to remember this model is ask–tell–ask–tell.

Although these actions describe key components of effective feedback, the relationship between the learner and the teacher is equally important. Teachers who give the feedback must be viewed by the learner as a credible source. They must be experts in the content, with appropriate clinical experience, and ideally should have directly observed the learner (Lefroy et al., 2015). As mentioned, feedback can be emotional and personal for learners. Given this, a trusting and supportive relationship with the teacher can improve learner's acceptance of feedback (Delva et al., 2013). Thus, organizing health training programs in which learners develop longitudinal, trusting relationships with supervisors can increase the credibility and acceptance of feedback by learners, enable teachers to set learning goals with their learners, and optimize opportunities for the teacher to provide feedback that furthers these goals over time.

RECEIVING FEEDBACK

Health educators will routinely get feedback on their own teaching or courses. They are just as susceptible to not hearing or acting on feedback as are their learners. Learning how to better receive feedback can help educators both receive and deliver it.

EXHIBIT 27.2 The Reflective Feedback Conversation

Step 1: Teacher asks the learner to share any concerns about his or her performance and what he or she would like to have done better (Ask).
Step 2: Learner describes concerns and areas for improvement.
Step 3: Teacher provides views on performance and offers support to learner. (Tell) Ideally includes discussion of positive and negative aspects of performance.
Step 4: Teacher asks learner to reflect on what might improve the performance. (Ask)
Step 5: Learner responds with ideas for improvement.
Step 6: Teacher elaborates on learner response, makes corrections, and checks for learner understanding. (Tell)

Stone and Heen (2014) discuss three common triggers that block the receipt of feedback. The first is called the *truth* trigger, in which the learner simply believes that the behavior described is not accurate, and thus disagrees with or fails to act on the feedback. The second is the *relationship* trigger, in which the wrong person is actually giving the feedback. This may include a person whom the learner does not respect or who did not actually observe the behavior in question. The third trigger is the *identity* trigger, in which getting negative feedback actually threatens a learner's self-identity. This is especially true in the health professions, where many learners are constant high achievers and have self-esteem that is strongly linked to perfect performance. Learners vary widely in their sensitivities and responses to negative feedback.

As "experts," health educators are also prone to all of these triggers when they receive feedback on their teaching and/or courses. Educators may dismiss the feedback, viewing the learners as novices without the knowledge or skills to understand or criticize the teaching (a combination of the truth and relationship triggers). Educators are also prone to the identity trigger, as their teaching abilities are often strongly linked to their self-esteem.

To combat the truth and relationship triggers, educators must recognize that any negative feedback is worthy of close consideration. Precisely because they do view the material with fresh eyes, students provide an important perspective. An honest appraisal of student feedback allows health professions educators to clarify and improve the student-centeredness of their teaching. They must recognize that learners are the ultimate judges of their teaching, so dismissing learners' concerns is not helpful. The goal should not be to argue about feedback's validity, but rather to understand it more fully by discussing it further with the learners, if possible. Educators might also enlist trusted education colleagues to discuss their impressions and provide separate feedback. This might include having highly rated educators come observe their teaching to get "unbiased" feedback. Only by fully discussing areas of feedback can teachers avoid blind spots of continued underperformance.

These techniques fall in line with the concept of developing a "growth mind-set." Carol Dweck (1999) studied children's responses to failure at progressively complex puzzles. As the puzzles got harder, some children got frustrated and gave up, viewing their inability to solve them as failures. These children were found to have a "fixed mind-set." Another group of children, however, did not give up as quickly and viewed the harder puzzles as making them better puzzle solvers overall—this group was labeled as having a "growth mind-set." Subsequent research has found that these mind-sets can be changed, and people can move from more fixed views ("failure is an indication of how bad I am") to growth views ("failure is a way for me to grow and get better").

The growth mind-set concept is easily applied to feedback. Describing suboptimal behavior so it can be changed to improve, doing a meaningful self-assessment to develop an action plan for improvement, seeking out feedback, or asking to understand feedback more carefully are all processes that could be considered as integral to a growth mind-set. Challenges are viewed as opportunities. Health educators who recognize this will continue to improve. They can emphasize to their learners that being a health professional requires constant self-directed improvement over an entire career. They will be able to role model for their learners a positive way to respond to constructive feedback. Educators will also be able to instill the importance of a growth mind-set in their learners for their own lifelong learning.

CONCLUSIONS

Feedback is the health educator's most powerful teaching tool. Giving effective feedback means overcoming barriers, understanding the key qualities of effective feedback, mastering the reflective feedback conversation, and helping learners develop a growth mind-set.

REFERENCES

Branch, W. T., & Paranjape, A. (2002). Feedback and reflection: Teaching methods for clinical settings. *Academic Medicine, 77*, 1185–1188.

Cantilon, P., & Sargeant, J. (2006). Teaching rounds: Giving feedback in clinical settings. *British Medical Journal, 337*, 1292–1294.

Delva, D., Sargeant, J., Miller, S., Holland, J., Alexiadis, B. P., Leblanc, C., Lightfoot, K., . . . Mann, K. (2013). Encouraging residents to seek feedback. *Medical Teacher, 35*, e1625–e1631. doi:10.3109/01421 59X.2013.806791

Dweck, C. S. (1999). *Self-theories: Their role in motivation, personality, and development*. Philadelphia, PA: Psychology Press.

Keenan, C., Swenson, S., & Henderson, M. (2016). Feedback in residency training. In F. Williams & D. A. Wininger (Eds.), *A textbook for internal medicine education programs* (12th ed.). Alexandria, VA: Alliance for Academic Internal Medicine.

Kruger, J., & Dunning, D. (1999). Unskilled and unaware of it: How difficulties in recognizing one's own incompetence lead to inflated self-assessments. *Journal of Personality and Social Psychology, 77*, 1121–1134.

Lefroy, J., Watling, C., Teunissen, P. W., & Brand, P. (2015). Guidelines: The do's, don'ts and don't knows of feedback for clinical education. *Perspectives on Medical Education, 4*, 284–299.

Stone, D., & Heen, S. (2014). *Thanks for the feedback: The science and art of receiving feedback well*. New York, NY: Viking Penguin.

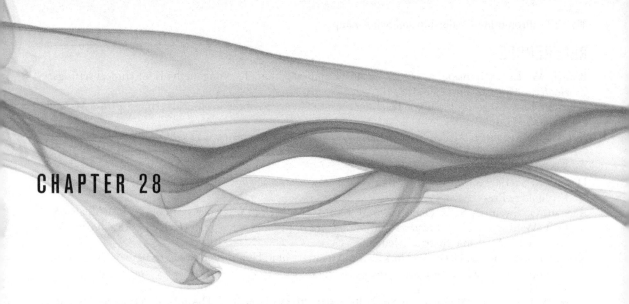

CHAPTER 28

Successful Mentoring: Socialization of Faculty and Students

Ruth Ballweg

CHAPTER OBJECTIVES

- Examine the nature of mentoring
- Explain why both mentoring and being mentored enhance faculty and student development in the health professions

---

A teacher affects eternity. No one can tell where his influence stops.

—*Henry Adams*

THE NATURE OF MENTORING

Mentoring in health professions education is relatively underdeveloped compared to the corporate world, where mentoring activities were formally introduced in the 1970s (Frei, Stamm, & Buddeberg-Fisher, 2010). The ways companies use mentoring processes to increase their competitive edge, develop and retain employees, and build "brand loyalty" are instructive. Corporate mentoring consists of informal, individual relationships, as well as formal mentoring projects operated as part of human resources departments. Corporations and institutions that place a high priority on mentoring typically include training for mentors and mentees, "matching processes," recommended mentoring strategies, evaluation processes, and sometimes even extra compensation (Rowley, 1999). In health professions education, mentoring may be more informal, although some academic settings include mentoring as a regular academic duty and therefore a criterion for recognition and promotion (Beckel & Brown, 2005).

A quick online search of mentoring websites reveals a wide range of mentoring software products, including mentoring guides for specific generations, mentoring "matching services" (somewhat similar to online dating sites), and even online mentoring sites. The topics covered include concerns such as frustration, career advancement, boredom, efficiency, obstacles, workload, and even treating others thoughtfully.

Mentoring provides many benefits. Mentees obviously benefit from improvement in their professional positions. However, mentoring has two other prime beneficiaries: (a) the mentors, who, as role models of "lifelong learning," learn from their mentees and receive the satisfaction of investing in the future and (b) the organization, which retains employees in a work environment in which turnover is costly (Wilson & Elman, 1990).

Mentoring, which differs from coaching and counseling, is a cost-free career promotion strategy based on a personal relationship in a professional context (Frei et al., 2010). Mentors can also be confused with tutors, teacher/educators, or supervisors, all of whom may perform formal assessments and/or evaluations as part of their interactions with students or employees. A mentor is an active partner in an ongoing relationship which helps a mentee to reach personal professional goals (Frei et al., 2010).

HISTORY OF HEALTH PROFESSIONS MENTORING

Health professionals may incorrectly think that mentoring is not important because we spend so much time with patients, we are educated and trained in communications skills, and we pride ourselves on being problem solvers and critical thinkers. However, this viewpoint can isolate us from our leaders, colleagues, and students; it also eliminates opportunities for input and feedback.

Historically, only doctors were seen as the leaders of the health care system. The accompanying view was that processes to develop leaders—such as mentoring—just were not necessary in the emerging health professions. The doctors would "take care" of everything. Of course, this was a simplistic, unrealistic, and even shortsighted view. As nurses moved into leadership positions throughout health care, they had pride in their hard-won status and were not always supportive of leadership growth in the new professions that developed and expanded in the 1960s, 1970s, and 1980s.

In the current climate of interprofessional emphasis in health professions education, each professional group fiercely maintains its own culture; little sharing occurs between disciplines. Thus, as we recognize and teach about the possibilities of interprofessional practice (IP), interprofessional leadership development—including the development of IP mentoring relationships—should be a high priority on our list of strategies for successful project implementation.

A common theme in the professional development literature across all health professions is that the absence of mentoring can be detrimental to professional growth and disruptive to educational programs. Janne Dunham-Taylor has written in the nursing literature about the importance of mentoring: "In the midst of a nursing faculty shortage, recruitment and retention of new faculty are of utmost importance if the country is to educate and graduate a sufficient number of nurses to meet care demands. The pressure of horizontal hostility combined with lack of support, guidance and knowledge about the education system makes novice nurse faculty members vulnerable to burnout and early resignations" (Dunham-Taylor, Lynn, Moore, McDaniel, & Walker, 2009, p. 337). Dr. Phyllis Carr and colleagues identified the absence of mentoring as the most important factor hindering career progress in academic medicine (Carr et al., 2003). They reported that 98% of participants identified the lack of mentoring as either the first (42%) or second (56%) most important factor hindering progress in academic medicine.

The "content" of mentoring also varies among professions. Terms that describe nursing mentoring include *socialization, collaboration, operations, validation/education, expectations, transformation, reputation, documentation, generation,* and *perfection* (Dunham-Taylor et al., 2009). To describe the content and activities of mentoring in medicine—with regard to academic surgeons specifically—Dr. F. Souba created an acronym from the word *mentor:* **m**otivate, **e**mpower/encourage, **n**urture self-confidence, **t**each by example, **o**ffer wise counsel, and **r**aise the performance bar (Souba, 1999). Other health professions have their own recommended list of mentoring duties, some of which come from agreed-upon "competencies" for their professions. It is hoped that the mentoring activities for all professions will soon include such issues and concerns as advocacy, equity, and patient-centered care.

TYPES OF MENTORING

Mentoring relationships include one-on-one mentoring, group mentoring, team mentoring, peer mentoring, and even e-mentoring. Ideally, new mentoring relationships involve face-to-face discussions; more well-established mentoring relationships may take place by phone or by using digital tools such as Skype and FaceTime.

Participants have given formal (as opposed to more informal) mentoring programs' mixed reviews on the issues of structure, documentation, and evaluation. Some mentoring programs may pair up mentors and mentees, thereby eliminating the need to "find" a mentor. Mentoring programs may also offer helpful—and sometimes required—training sessions for mentors and mentees.

Peer mentoring is an often-overlooked type of mentoring that may reap the greatest benefits over time. Colleagues with similar roles but in different communities or regions can provide valuable suggestions, reality checks, and support. Peer mentors report career-long relationships with their mentees as the mentees' careers develop. Shared knowledge of daily/weekly schedules can help maximize the peers' availability for conversations via phone or teleconferencing.

FINDING A MENTOR

Health professions educators who have not been matched with a mentor should constantly "be on the lookout" for potential mentors. Mentors can be recommended by colleagues, identified and/or cultivated through contacts at meetings or on shared projects, or sought during participation in professional organizations. Educators' experiences as mentees may encourage them to become mentors and find new mentees. Successful educators and leaders often describe mentoring as a "way of life" in their careers.

Based on the needs, expectations, and availability of mentors or mentees, mentoring timelines may be short or long—several months, a year, or even off and on throughout a long career. Despite differing opinions from other experts, a review of literature by Dr. Phyllis Carr suggests that making same gender or same race-race matches is relatively unimportant (Carr et al., 2003). They do, however, point out the importance of maintaining clear boundaries in cross-gender mentoring relationships.

MENTOR CHARACTERISTICS

Many publications and websites list helpful characteristics of a mentor. An overall requirement is that mentors "know the territory"—are up to date and aware of current methods, materials, and procedures (Haack, 2006). Other important characteristics include consistent ongoing availability and reliability, commitment to the mentee's professional and personal development, and the ability to maintain confidentiality in the relationship (Frei et al., 2010).

Skill sets for effective mentors include being nonjudgmental, demonstrating lifelong learning, and being transparent about their own experiences in seeking better answers and more effective solutions in their own careers (Frei et al., 2010; Rowley, 1999). Mentoring skills are especially important when rapid changes in the health care system require hope and optimism with respect to effective problem solving and innovation.

The time commitment involved in being a mentor is a serious consideration. Structured mentoring programs typically require 4 hours per month in regularly scheduled sessions (Management Mentors, 2015). "Mentoring . . . is anchored in the knowledge that mentoring can be a challenging endeavor requiring significant investments of time and energy" (Rowley, 1999, p. 20).

THE MENTEE ROLE

Being a mentee is hard work, too. Mentees agree to bring to their mentors their candid concerns about daily challenges and successes, as well as their perceptions about professional and personal development. Mentees agree to receive feedback, criticism, and even praise as they work through the issues they have identified. In an environment in which time is precious, gossip, moaning, and "dramatics" are not appropriate. Mentees also agree to maintain the confidentiality of mentoring conversations—especially given that mentors may share examples of their own personal challenges.

Mentees should not completely emulate their mentors; their challenge is to become themselves. Mentors do not enter into mentoring relationships because they want their mentees to "be just like them."

COMMONALITIES OF MENTORS AND MENTEES

Recognizing the shared "habits" of mentors and mentees can help identify mentors and mentees who are likely to provide optimum mentoring experiences. The following list of characteristics provides some helpful insight into the mentoring experience (Management Mentors, 2015):

1. Active listening
2. Dedication to success
3. Dedication to others' success
4. Curiosity
5. Engagement with one's surroundings
6. Willingness to step outside of comfort zones
7. Practice of the three Rs: responsible, respectful, and ready

In the words of Gwen Ifill, the well-known PBS commentator and role model, "your responsibility isn't just to climb the ladder of success, even more importantly your responsibility is to bring up others behind you" ("Tribute to Gwen Ifill," 2016).

EXPLORING SOME MENTORING SITUATIONS

Situation 1

You have taken a new job. Previously you worked in a private institution; now you are in an academic health center at a large public institution. You are leaving a job as "vice chair" to become the "chair" of a department. You know you have a lot to learn. When and how will you let people know that you are looking for one or more mentors who can help you learn the culture and to function most effectively within this environment? What sort of person(s) will you be looking for? What type of help/perspective are you seeking? What are your next steps?

Also, many of the people you have mentored at your "old job" are concerned that you will no longer be available to them. How will you manage this situation, and what will you tell them?

And finally, there is the matter of your interest in someday mentoring people within your new environment, although obviously this is not an immediate goal as you settle into your new job. What types of people will you "be on the lookout" for, and how might you identify them as you integrate yourself into a new culture?

Situation 2

Some of the most valuable advice/support comes from "peer mentoring." Discussing reality-based shared experiences, conflicts, and successes provides long-lasting and satisfying rewards. Consider how you might identify and develop peer-mentoring relationships across your career—including identifying potential peer mentors and then defining and organizing your relationship and interactions over time. What are your expectations of how this might work for you?

Situation 3

A compelling feature of health professions education is that our students quickly become our peers. Consider how you might provide mentoring to program graduates and other practicing clinicians in your community and profession. What do you have to offer? What types of issues would you choose to avoid? How might you organize these relationships to include regular meetings by phone, in person, or at conferences, as needed?

Situation 4

You have heard from several colleagues that they have had some bad experiences with mentors, which makes them reluctant to enter into this type of relationship again. Several of these negative experiences involved breaches in confidentiality: The mentors revealed confidential or sensitive information that had been part of their mentoring discussions. In another situation, the mentor had suddenly dropped the mentee over political differences relating to a contentious election. What other types of issues or conflicts might come up during the mentoring process, and how might you avoid them?

Situation 5

Your department has signed on to a successfully funded interprofessional grant, and you have been named to the steering committee. Given what you have now learned about mentoring, you bring the topics of joint IP leadership development and mentoring into the conversation. What steps for moving this forward could be taken? Who should be involved? Might there be a way to involve students in this process?

CONCLUSIONS

Health care is a rewarding career that also presents specific challenges. Being a health professions educator adds extra challenges. Some of these include difficult conversations with students or faculty, managing up and managing down, and balancing the three legs of academia: teaching, scholarship, and service. For one to succeed and enjoy the rewards of this career, it is important to seek mentoring at all stages. The mentoring process provides benefits for both the mentee and the mentor and the mentoring relationship may be informal or structured as a regular academic duty. Successful educators and leaders often describe mentoring as a "way of life" in their careers. Key characteristics of successful mentor–mentee relationships include consistent commitment and accountability, confidentiality, clear communication and boundaries, as well as respecting individual differences.

REFERENCES

Beckel, J., & Brown, A. (2005). Generation X: Implications for faculty recruitment and development in academic health centers. *Academic Medicine, 80*(3), 205–210.

Carr, P., Jackson, V., Palepu, A., Szaleche L, Casewell, C., & Inui, T. (2003). Having the right chemistry: A qualitative study of mentoring. *Academic Medicine, 67*(3), 328–324.

Dunham-Taylor, J., Lynn, C., Moore, P., McDaniel, S., & Walker, J. (2009). What goes around comes around: Improving faculty retention through more effective mentoring. *Journal of Professional Nursing, 24*(6), 337–346.

Frei, E., Stamm, M., & Buddeberg-Fisher, B. (2010). Mentoring programs for medical students—A review of PubMed literature 2000–2008. *BioMed Central Medical Education, 10*, 32.

Haack, P. (2006). Mentoring and professional development programs: Possibilities and pitfalls. *Music Educators Journal, 92*(4), 60–84.

Management Mentors. (2015). Corporate mentoring tips: 7 habits of highly successful mentors & mentorees. Retrieved from http://www.management-mentors.com/resources/june-2010-mentor-mentoree-habits

Rowley, J. (1999). The good mentor: Supporting new teachers. *Educational Leadership, 56*(8), 20–22.

Souba, W. (1999). Mentoring young academic surgeons, our most precious asset. *Journal of Surgical Research, 82*, 113–120.

"Tribute to Gwen Ifill." (2016). What Gwen Ifill taught us. *PBS Evening News*. Retrieved from http://www.pbs.org/newshour/bb/gwen-ifill-taught-us

Wilson, J., & Elman, N. (1990). Organizational benefits of mentoring. *Academy of Management Executives, 4*(4), 88–94.

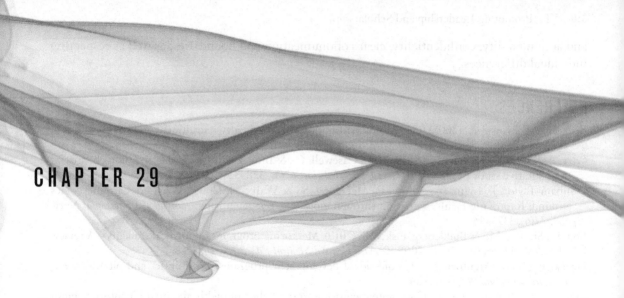

CHAPTER 29

Creating a Faculty and Student Mentoring Program

Michael Estrada and Laura Estrada

CHAPTER OBJECTIVE

- Create an effective mentoring culture, including characteristics of a good mentor, strategies for engaging emerging leaders, developing power, enhancing intrinsic motivation, and creating meaningful leadership experiences

---

The delicate balance of mentoring someone is not creating them in your own image, but giving them the opportunity to create themselves.

—Steven Spielberg

The rapid growth of the physician assistant (PA) profession and educational programs ("Physician Assistants," 2016) has created the need for mentors of faculty and students. Currently there are no standards for mentoring of PAs when they are students, clinicians, or academic faculty. However, an abundance of literature related to nursing and medical mentorship exists. Furthermore, the mentoring relationship has been defined, roles and characteristics of a mentor and a mentee have been identified, and critical components necessary for a successful mentorship have been described. Once a mentoring relationship has been established, some events that may transpire can lead to an unsuccessful mentorship.

THE MENTORING RELATIONSHIP

A mentoring relationship can occur at any time; it is a reciprocal partnership of teaching and learning (Hnatiuk, 2013) that facilitates professional growth and development. Effective mentors recognize that the time invested in a mentoring relationship provides a high rate of return and increases the professional self-reliance of mentees, increasing their leadership and networking capability. Mentors are also beneficial in decreasing the challenges related to professional growth and transitions (Lynch, 2016) that can be found in underrepresented faculty and students such as minorities and women. The mentoring relationship is a lifelong journey that at times can be limited in which the mentee absorbs the mentor's knowledge and develops a robust set of skills. Through this lifelong journey the mentor serves as an "emotional and psychological support" for the mentee (Meinel, Dimitriadis, von der Borch, Stormann, & Niedermaier, 2011, p. 2). It is important for both mentors and mentees to acknowledge and understand that the relationship being nourished is intended to increase their self-awareness and growth development in their respective roles. The mentorship relationship should not be used as a competitive tool with others in their profession by either the mentee or the mentor. If competitive feelings occur within the mentoring relationship from either the mentee or the mentor, the consequences are detrimental. The mentor loses credibility as a role model because he or she no longer displays the characteristic of collegiality.

THE MENTORING PROGRAM

Creating a successful mentoring program begins with screening, training, and support of mentors and mentees, referred to as a *mentoring pair*. The identification of unique faculty and student qualities will help in matching the right mentor to a mentee so that the relationship created through mentoring provides the right guidance necessary for success, support, and closure ("Elements of Effective Practice for Mentoring," 2016). Successful mentoring socializes the neophyte faculty member and student into their respective roles as health care providers and industry leaders through thoughtful facilitation, assessment, and formation. Mentoring programs can also provide the academic institution with insight into obstacles and/or barriers encountered by students that need to be addressed to ensure the academic success of the student (Dimitriadis et al., 2012). Furthermore, the academic institution can use the results of the mentoring relationship when reviewing a faculty member's academic performance and productivity (Straus, Johnson, Marquez, & Feldmen, 2013).

Successful Mentoring: Definition and Characteristics

The term *mentor* has been widely used in multiple settings and has been primarily used by academic institutions or corporate entities to define a reciprocal relationship that focuses on experiences, achievement, and influence (Berk, Berg, Mortimer, Walton-Moss, & Yeo, 2005). A mentor refers to an individual who helps with the professional development of another person (Seisser & Brown, 2013), whereas the *mentee* is the beneficiary of that development. In many instances the mentor–mentee relationship is founded on trust, integrity, experience, and professional expertise.

Characteristics of a mentoring relationship vary depending on the relationship. Some relationships are "informal" and others are "formal." An example of an informal relationship is one that occurs with family, friends, and, in some instances, students and peers. The focus of an informal mentoring relationship is to provide support to the mentee and to help overcome barriers of social stigma and serve as a confidence builder. Formal mentoring is structured and organized and has a positive impact on the development of both social and professional skills (Pathways to College Network and National College Access Network, 2011). It is "tangible"

EXHIBIT 29.1   Elements of a Mentoring Relationship

Goal setting
Meetings
Shared contact information
Types of mentoring activities to be pursued
Assessment tool to consider efficacy of activities

---

advice and provides solutions that will help the mentee advance in a professional role, career, or academics. A formal mentorship is developed with intent and purpose with expected outcomes or goals that benefit both the mentor and the mentee. Faculty, for example, would enter into a formal mentoring relationship with a student or peer.

A formal mentoring relationship requires basic elements (Exhibit 29.1): goal setting, meetings, shared contact information, and the identification of the types of mentoring activities desired as well as a measurable assessment plan to document the progress of goals and outcomes.

Two additional critical elements needed for a successful mentor–mentee relationship are approachability and availability of both parties involved. Successful mentoring characteristics identified in a study through the Department of Medicine at the University of Toronto Faculty of Medicine and the University of California, San Francisco, School of Medicine, determined that reciprocity, mutual respect, clear expectations, personal connection, and shared values fostered successful mentoring relationships (Straus et al., 2013). Formal and informal mentoring has been associated with leadership development and in safeguarding the future of the profession (Bower, 2000). The wide variance and range of mentoring relationships and research in this area agree that positive attitude, strong self-esteem, and effective communication directly relate to the success and outcome of mentoring relationships (McCloughen, O'Brien, & Jackson, 2009).

The Right Match

Finding the right mentor can be a challenging but equally rewarding experience when the "right match" is found. Mentoring is an interpersonal relationship between two people; like most voluntary relationships it will not last unless both parties benefit from the relationship (Lee, Anzai, & Langlotz, 2006). A process for screening, selecting, and matching must be established and followed. This can be done informally at first to determine compatibility and "comfort" level of both the mentor and the mentee before entering into a formal relationship (Pathways to College Network and National College Access Network, 2011). Venues for informal meetings can include a prearranged luncheon or activity. Communication style, personality traits, and a clear understanding of self-awareness are part of a successful match. Being able to share one's self-journey and positive and negative experiences requires a deep understanding of self and how the journey has contributed to personal and professional career challenges and successes. This will serve as the foundation of the mentoring pair.

Selecting the right mentee takes thoughtful introspection regarding availability, commitment, and skill set. The mentee should have a clear understanding of why he or she chose to be mentored (American College of Healthcare Executives, 2014). Mentees should be flexible and willing to accept constructive criticism and committed to achieving the outcomes and goals established for the relationship. It is the responsibility of mentees to ensure that scheduled meetings and appointments with their mentors are kept. The development of a simple work plan that describes the background, preferences, and perceived strengths and areas of needed improvement of the mentee that include target goals and timelines will serve as a blueprint of the mentoring relationship (see the Mentorship Blueprint in the online supplement).

The Mentoring Pair

There has to be multiple areas of compatibility when matching the mentor with the mentee (mentoring pair), understanding that the relationship is multifaceted and complex (Kram, 1985). Social factors, academic experience, cultural background, work ethic, gender, and personality traits that can be identified on self-assessment surveys help discover talents and unique strengths. A self-assessment survey of both the mentor and the mentee should be done prior to initiating a potential mentor relationship. A self-assessment survey can help in identifying areas of commonality between the two.

It has been suggested in the literature that social and emotional factors contribute to student success (Pritchard & Wilson, 2016). In a mentoring relationship, although not always possible, the importance of finding social compatibility may have an impact on outcomes and goals. The need for a better understanding of cultural influences on leadership and professional practice (House et al., 1999) has reached its peak with the changing demographics of local and global populations. Cultural background is important to academic achievement and maintaining cultural attachments to ensure success (Willetto, 1999). It is important to explore the cultural differences of the mentoring pair as this may have an impact on the approach and style of mentoring. Consider how giving and getting advice might differ in certain cultures (American College of Healthcare Executives, 2014).

Mentoring is important for a career in academic medicine (Beech et al., 2013), particularly when minority populations experience unique challenges in workforce and professional development. Many new minority faculty members are unaware of the value of mentoring due to a lack of minority representation in the healthcare workforce and academic setting. Therefore new minority faculty members find it difficult to identify compatible and willing mentors. There is little research in the area of gender and mentoring. Several patterns emerge in gender socialization that affects coping, experiences, and opportunity. Matching gender compatibility successfully should prevent miscommunication that could be attributed to gender differences (Liang, Bogat, & Duffy, 2013).

The Design of a Mentoring Program

In reviewing the literature on mentoring, there are many models and tools to choose from when designing a mentoring program. Structured rubrics, outlines, and plans are examples of the types of designs that were easily found when searching online for sample models. It is the opinion of the authors that a mentoring program should be unique to the needs of the mentee and be simple, easily implemented, and measurable. The Triangular Model, or tier mentoring (Kosoko-Lasaki, Sonnino, & Voytko, 2006), in which new students are mentored by advanced students, advanced students are mentored by faculty members or senior researchers/fellows fulfills the features of simplicity, implementation, and measurability. This model can easily be modified to meet the needs of any academic program and can be used in the mentoring of both students and faculty members (Figures 29.1 and 29.2). The success of any model is based on the mentor's desire to educate, share, and become a role model for the mentee.

A formal mentorship program should also have a facilitator or director who can help with organization, pairing, and assessment of the program activities. At very least, informal mentorship relationships should have a mechanism of providing feedback and assessment through thoughtful reflection and critique. Goal setting is an important part of a successful mentoring program, but of equal importance is the assessment of whether goals are achieved and the mentoring relationship is a success. This will evaluate the effectiveness of the program, as well as identify any shortcomings (Kosoko-Lasaki et al., 2006). Periodic informal assessments can be

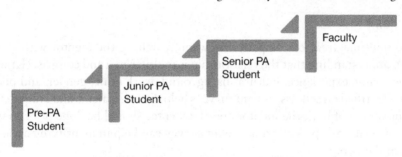

FIGURE 29.1 Modified tier student model.

PA, physician assistant.

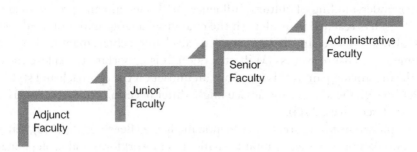

FIGURE 29.2 Modified tier faculty model.

done as needed, whereas formal assessments should be conducted at regular intervals: quarterly, biannually, and annually.

CONCLUSIONS

Mentoring is important to students and faculty for professional and personal growth and advancement. It is a process that provides socialization to a specific environment or profession that increases self-awareness and development. It is done through formal and informal relationships with a mentor who possesses desired qualities, skills, and experience in a chosen profession. The mentoring relationship is reciprocal and secures longevity of a profession by instilling the noncognitive characteristics necessary to be a professional. Faculty and students can seek out mentoring relationships in an effort to enhance career choices and promotion. Mentoring is a method that also provides opportunity to faculty and students to serve as role models to peers and colleagues.

REFERENCES

American College of Healthcare Executives. (2014). *ACHE mentor guide*. Chicago, IL: Author.

Beech, B., Calles-Escandon, J., Hairston, K., Langdon, S., Latham-Sadler, B., & Bell, R. (2013). Mentoring programs for underrepresented minority faculty in academic medical centers: A systematic review of the literature. *Academic Medicine: Journal of the Association of American Medical Colleges*, *88*(4), 541–549.

Berk, R. A., Berg, J., Mortimer, R., Walton-Moss, B., & Yeo, T. (2005). Measuring the effectiveness of faculty mentoring relationships. *Academic Medicine: Journal of the Association of American Medical Colleges*, *80*(1), 66–71.

Bower, F. (2000). *Nurses taking the lead: Personal qualities of effective mentorship*. Philadelphia, PA: W. B. Saunders.

Bureau of Labor Statistics, U.S. Department of Labor. (2015). *Occupational outlook handbook, 2016–2017 edition.* Retrieved from https://www.bls.gov/ooh/healthcare/physician-assistants.htm

Coles, A. (2011). *The role of mentoring in college access and success: Research to practice brief.* Washington, DC: Institute for Higher Education Policy.

Coles, A. (2011). *The role of mentoring in college access and success: Research to practice brief.* Washington, DC: Institute for Higher Education Policy.

Dimitriadis, K., von der Borch, P., Störmann, S., Meinel, F. G., Moder, S., Reincke, M., & Fischer, M. R. (2012). Characteristics of mentoring relationships formed by medical students and faculty. *Medical Education Online, 17.* doi:10.3402/meo.v17i0.17242

Elements of effective practice for mentoring. (2016, June 20). Retrieved from http://www.nationalmentoringresourcecenter.org/index.php/what-works-in-mentoring/elements-of-effective-practice-for-mentoring.html

Hnatiuk, C. (2012, March 30). Mentoring nurses towards success. *Minority Nurse, 5,* 42–45.

House, R. J., Hanges, P. J., Ruiz-Quintanilla, S. A., Dorfman, P. W., Dickson, M., & Gupta, V. (1999). Cultural influences on leadership and organizations. *Advances in Global Leadership, 1*(2), 171–233.

Kosoko-Lasaki, O., Sonnino, R., & Voytko, M. L. (2006). Mentoring for women and underrepresented. *Journal of the National Medical Association, 98*(9), 1449–1459.

Kram, K. E. (1985). *Mentoring at work: Developmental relationships in organizational life.* Glenview, IL: Scott Foresman.

Lee, J. M., Anzai, Y., & Langlotz, C. (2006). Mentoring the mentors: Aligning mentor and mentee expectations. *Academic Radiology, 13*(5), 556–561.

Liang, B., Bogat, G. A., & Duffy, N. (2013). Gender in mentoring relationships. In D. L. Dubois & M. J. Karcher (Eds.), *Handbook of youth mentoring* (pp. 159–173). Newbury Park, CA: Sage.

Lynch, S. (2016, August 24). Maximizing mentorship: Strategies for academic success. Retrieved from http://paeaonline.org/maximizing-mentorship-strategies-for-academic-success

Meinel, F. G., Dimitriadis, K., von der Borch, P., Störmann, S., & Niedermaier, S. (2011). More mentoring needed? A cross-sectional study of mentoring programs for medical students in Germany. *BMC Medical Education, 11,* 68. doi:10.1186/1472-6920-11-68

McCloughen, A., O'Brien, L., & Jackson, D. (2009). Esteemed connection: Creating a mentoring relationship for nurse leadership. *Nursing Inquiry, 16*(4), 326–336.

Pritchard, M. E., & Wilson, G. S. (2016). Using emotional and social factors to predict student success. *Journal of College Student Development, 44*(1), 18–28.

Seisser, M. A., & Brown, R. (2013, April 8). Mentoring programs: Essential for sustaining a culture of safety. Retrieved from http://www.psqh.com/news-and-analysis/?cat=0&keywords=mentoring+programs

Straus, S. E., Johnson, M. O., Marquez, C., & Feldmen, M. D. (2013). Characteristics of successful and failed mentoring relationships: A qualitative study across two academic health centers. *Academy of Medicine, 88*(1), 82–89.

Willetto, A. A. (1999). Navajo culture and family influences on academic success: Traditionalism is not a significant predictor of achievement among Navajo youth. *Journal of American Indian Education, 38*(2), 1–24.

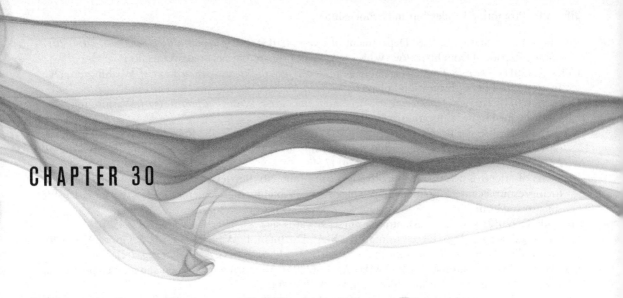

CHAPTER 30

Managing Up and Managing Down: Getting Along With Others

Ruth Ballweg

CHAPTER OBJECTIVE

- Formulate a strategy to successfully navigate the culture, structure, and function of academic educational settings

---

The art of effective listening is essential to clear communication, and clear communication is necessary to management success.

—*James Cash Penney*

TRANSITIONING TO ACADEMIA

Moving from clinical practice to health professions education—and then moving forward into academic leadership— requires cultural adjustment and new skill sets. In the clinical role, medical knowledge, effective communication/documentation skills, and "being a good team member" are necessary to maximize patient care. Clinical settings most often have well-defined roles and structures that are easily recognized and understood by individuals in clinical practice.

In contrast, the culture, structure, and function of academic educational settings vary markedly among institutions and educational programs—even those within the same discipline. "Onboarding" and "orientation" to academic settings are less structured than similar processes in clinical settings and new educators or leaders must take it upon themselves to learn "how it works" and "where they fit" with minimal support from others who also may not fully understand the academic environment of a specific institution and program.

Most clinicians moving into academia understand that they will have teaching and scholarly assignments, that they will work with and mentor students, and that they will have curriculum development responsibilities. There is little recognition, however, of the many administrative tasks that they will be required to take on, as well as committee work, having to write reports, conduct evaluations and data analyses, and integrating themselves into the larger community within the department, the school, and the institution. Without some understanding of these additional roles, some faculty members become embittered and move on. Here, as throughout the health care environment, prevention is the solution.

SETTING EXPECTATIONS AND UNDERSTANDING ROLES

In academic settings, the department chair, division chief, or program director has the responsibility for setting expectations for the work environment and how people will work together. New leaders at the department/divisions/program level often express surprise at the amount of time they spend "managing" people. This includes faculty, staff, students, and preceptors.

Seemingly small decisions, such as the structure of committees and teams, the frequency and structure of meetings, and even the entity's customs for social events such as celebrating individual birthdays and holidays, set the tone for how the group works together. Depending on the size and geographic distribution of the group, a leadership team may provide feedback and assist the designated leader in management and planning.

Academic settings are hierarchical by definition, which is why it is critical that faculty and staff members understand each other's ranks, roles, and rules within the institution. A helpful way to provide correct information about these processes is through an all-inclusive meeting that describes human resources (HR) processes for each group (e.g., staff, faculty, unionized personnel, etc.). HR representatives for the various groups can explain the process of hiring for each group and how this is carried out by differing administrative structures and processes.

One of the most common disagreements between faculty and staff members arises from very different expectations about "time management," including formal and planned time off for staff, as compared to flexible time off for faculty. The staff may think: "Those faculty should be here every day, just like they're required to be! Working at home doesn't count!") Similarly, the faculty—not understanding the more structured schedules of staff members— may assume that they can hand off last-minute staff assignments for producing tests or uploading course materials without understanding the staff's responsibility to support the work of multiple faculty members in a limited amount of time. Among faculty members there may be misunderstandings of institutional academic HR policies for hiring, promotion, and tenure. If all faculty and staff have at least a general knowledge of these issues and HR rules, the better the climate will be for collaboration, productivity, and mutual support.

On a larger scale, it is critical for academic leaders and faculty to have an understanding of where they and their department/division/program fall within the larger school and institution. In a large academic health center this may involve where they "fit" academically and clinically. For example, the program may be in a specific department within the school of medicine or nursing, whereas individual faculty members may each provide clinical care within entirely different clinical departments of the institution's health care delivery systems (hospitals and clinics). Similarly, because of the unique features of physician assistant (PA) and nurse practitioner (NP) education, these programs may be in a specific department of the school of medicine or nursing—with a reporting structure up to a chair—and the leader may also have appointments to higher level and more overarching executive committees of the school or hospital. It is important to differentiate where one's reporting functions are (the chair or dean of the school) and also where one's "advisory" functions fit (overarching executive/advisory committees). Ideally, it is important for leaders of NP and PA programs to have a relationship and direct access to the dean of "their school" without obtaining permission from the person to whom they directly report. This type of access is especially important for emergent political or policy issues about which the dean may need to be supportive when suddenly called upon to comment on issues relating to PA or NP practice.

Knowledge of the infrastructure—as well as "learning from experience"—gives academic leaders an understanding of who they can appropriately go to within the upper administration to ask for help on complex policy issues such as professional practice, human resources concerns, or legislative issues. Examples of these contacts include the university's or the school's legal staff, disability office, faculty governance officers (e.g., faculty senate), communications department, development office, or even the provost.

UNDERSTANDING "DIRECT REPORTS"

The HR "unit" of management in most academic, corporate, and governmental agencies is based on the principle of direct reports. A *direct report* is an employee who reports directly to someone else (Hedges, 2011). Direct reports also typically have their own direct reports who report to them. Business and administrative literature is thick with scholarly projects to define the ideal number of direct reports—typically ranging from six to eight individuals. This theory is called the *span of control*. Some experts recommend restructuring and reorganizing if the span of control in an organization greatly exceeds the six to eight range of direct reports (Topp & Desjardins, 2011). One of the most common reasons that leaders "burn out" is that they manage many more direct reports than is reasonable.

The assumption of direct reporting is that the "report" will freely and appropriately communicate and share information with the person to whom he or she reports. The manager agrees to listen, to "be present," and to participate in a conversation to move the work or products forward.

MANAGING UP

One major application of the direct report theory is the principle of "managing up." As many academic administrative leaders would say: "The perfect administrative entity under my leadership is one that causes few problems, has outstanding outcomes, and allows me to take credit for its successes. Making that happen is your responsibility!"

In the "managing up" process, the "boss" agrees to let the direct report initiate the communication between the two of them by providing draft agendas—and potential solutions—in advance of meetings as a "first pass" about how they will spend their time together. This agreement comes as the "boss" and the direct report get to know each other in their respective roles and consider how best to maximize their relationship to benefit the department, section, or program. In managing up, "reports" guarantee that they will never let their managers be surprised by a lack of accurate and timely information (Garone, 2008; McMullen, 2015).

Although this approach may at first seem inappropriate, it is common practice in corporate and academic environments. Managing up allows "reports" to state their needs in a concise and efficient manner. Managers may, of course, freely edit the proposed agenda by removing or adding topics for discussion depending on their own priorities and knowledge. The advantage is that they do not need to start every meeting "from scratch" in considering what the report wants to talk about and consider (Garone, 2008; Turk, 2007).

Typically, a managing-up agreement also includes an agreed-upon schedule for regular meetings, plans for communicating progress/follow-up, agreement on methods of communication (emails/memos/letters/phone calls), and even plans for emergencies.

MANAGING DOWN

Just as a leader may be a direct report to someone who ranks higher than him or her (a dean, a chair, a "chief"), leaders also work with individuals (faculty and staff) who directly report to them. Although the activities and outcomes in academia may be markedly different from corporate and governmental structures, the principles of managing down can still be applied to create an effective and productive culture and work environment. The leader sets the tone by being visible, accessible, and responsive. An "open door" policy and a daily strategy of "management by wandering around" flatten out hierarchy and promote collaboration and innovation (Garone, 2008).

Open communication is the key to these management strategies, including shared calendaring reports on external meetings and projects, and recognition/ praise for accomplishments and successes. In working with direct reports it is critical that the leader be seen as fair and consistent, nurturing but firm, and responsive to feedback about her or his own performance (Hedges, 2011).

Direct reports typically value clarity from the leader in the negotiation and assignment of expectations and timelines. Agreed-upon plans for reporting and follow-up are also key features of this management approach.

The same types of behavior that are expected in the "managing up" relationship apply here as well. The direct report is encouraged to bring ideas, solutions, and potential innovations to the leader. Similarly, the leader recognizes that not all projects go as planned and that each person has his or her own skill set as well as areas that require growth and development.

A word on "language" here: some leadership writers—although still supporting the principles of direct reporting, span of control, managing up, and managing down—suggest that more positive and inclusive words may be more appropriate in the current workplace. Possible replacement terms are *constituency management* and *span of influence and awareness*.

BUILDING FEEDBACK INTO THE WORK ENVIRONMENT

Both giving and receiving feedback are key components of success in working with others. A quick search of the Internet will provide many websites with tips for delivering feedback and for graciously receiving it. From a manager's/leader's point of view, creating an environment for feedback can make a big difference. It is most useful if feedback takes place regularly and routinely rather than in response to crises or errors. It is also helpful if it takes place in a carefully chosen location so that there is no perception of criticizing or belittling a person in front of his or her coworkers.

In providing feedback, it is a good idea to ask for permission—for example, "Would now be a good time for me to provide you with some feedback?" It is also important that the feedback has the intent of being "caring" rather than critical. Leaders and workers can sometimes lose track of the fact that feedback ideally is not just negative—and that positive comments and support are welcomed. In other words, it is helpful to balance negative feedback with praise. Details should always be supplied rather than stating nonspecific feelings or descriptions. Overall, feedback should be realistic, doable, and focus on the fix.

Receiving feedback is also an art. At first, it may be difficult not to take the criticism personally. It is a good idea to seek regular feedback and to welcome it as a strategy for personal growth and improvement. Although it is reasonable to ask for specifics and details to help you, it is important not to put the person on the defensive. Thank the person for his or her input, and plan for follow-up reporting or conversation if this will be helpful. See Chapter 27 for more information about giving and receiving feedback.

TOOLS TO FACILITATE GROUP INTERACTIONS

Successful corporate, academic, and administrative groups often use personality assessment tools to facilitate group work, support, and mutual understanding. Regardless of the tool (Myer Briggs, StrengthsFinder [Rath, 2013], Keirsey Personality Testing [Keirsey, 1998]) the purpose is to recognize, acknowledge, and value the differing personality strengths that individuals bring to the work environment. An overarching principle is that the "best teams" are made up of individuals with varying skill sets and personality types in contrast to groups made up of individuals with identical approaches to work and problem solving. These tools can be used for individual assessment; however, this work is maximized in group sessions facilitated by a trainer who can offer useful interactive sessions to demonstrate group strengths and optimum interactions.

EXEMPLARS

Exemplar A

The rapid growth of the health care systems—and health professions education—has led to new schools and programs and new leadership arrangements and "developing" structures as compared to "traditional" structures. The changes also include increased diversity of all types, the emergence of new leaders, and a growing list of expectations for academic leaders and clinicians. Although you have been a senior faculty member in your program, your responsibilities up until now have primarily been to teaching clinical practice and do research. You have recently applied for—and been chosen—as the division chief reporting to a new chair who is new to your institution. Neither of you have been in these leadership roles before. Consider how you might work together to develop your leadership skills, recognize your relative "rank" with respect to your working relationship, and build structures for working and communicating with each other in your new roles.

Exemplar B

In preparing for an upcoming accreditation site visit, an external consultant has advised the school it has incorrectly interpreted the requirement for a leader's supervision of faculty and staff to refer to direct-reporting relationships. As a result, the understanding was that you personally had over 20 direct reports to include all faculty and staff. This was challenging to manage and meant that you were not always able to devote your full attention to other administrative priorities.

As a result of the consultation, the school's administration has asked that all departments and programs redesign their administrative structures to reflect "span of control" principles. Consider how you might accomplish this, including the appropriate reassignment of supervisory and reporting functions.

Exemplar C

You are the leader of a well-established clinical training program that has moved along without any major changes for a number of years. There has been little turnover of faculty or staff and even when "new hires" were brought on, they were graduates of the program and well known to you and others. The culture of the program was "everyone works hard, knows what they're supposed to do . . . and does it." Because of some recent retirements and also administrative decisions to expand the program, you now have two new staff members and three new faculty members who come from "outside" of your institution . . . and your program. They recently met with you as a group to tell you that the culture is "old-fashioned" and that they do not know how to fit in. They say they are willing to work hard but they do not know how to work with you or the other long-standing faculty and staff. How will you approach this problem? Who will you go to for guidance? What will be your short- and long-term goals?

Exemplar D

An ongoing topic in your group's meeting is an interest in learning more about "personality strength tools" such as Myers Briggs and StrengthsFinder. In exploring this possibility you are pleased to find that your institution's administration offers access to a trainer facilitator who regularly works with on-campus groups on these topics. You schedule a time to meet with this person, who describes her or his work and asks you the following questions: "What is your goal with these training sessions?" "To whom will you offer these sessions?" "Faculty?" "Staff?" "Faculty and staff?" "Students?" The trainer also suggests that you consider not just "one-time sessions," but also that you come up with a 3- to 5-year plan for integrating these principles into your program at all levels. How do you respond to these questions? What are your next steps?

CONCLUSIONS

For the health professions educator to be successful, it is important to understand the roles and expectations of the various stakeholders such as the immediate supervisor, mentors, colleagues, staff, students, accrediting bodies, alumni, and the community. The educator needs to be aware of the reporting functions and also to understand the direct reports. Department chairs or program directors have the responsibility for setting expectations for the work environment and how people will work together. These processes are called managing up and managing down. In the managing-up process, the educator needs to clearly understand and prioritize his or her departmental chair's expectations, have regular communication, and, when necessary, provide potential solutions rather than presenting with problems all the time. The supervisor and the direct report should create opportunities to know each other in their respective roles and consider how best to maximize their relationship to benefit the department. In managing down, you are implementing and directing the work while mobilizing your staff to fulfill the department's priorities. Whether it is managing up or managing down, it is essential to communicate clearly, and provide specific, timely, and constructive feedback. In academia, the reality is that we are not only managing up or down, but we are always managing in all directions: up, down, and sideways.

REFERENCES

Garone, E. (2008, October 30). What it means to manage up. *The Wall Street Journal*. Retrieved from http://www.wsj.com/articles/SB1225119313313072047

Hedges, K. (2011, October 24). Five things never to say to your direct reports. *Forbes*. Retrieved from http://www.forbes.com/sites/work-in-progress/2011/10/24/five-things-to-never-say-to-your-direct-reports/#4b624e2727ee

Keirsey, D. (1998). *Please understand me II: Temperament, character, intelligence*. Del Mar, CA: Prometheus Nemesis Books.

McMullen, L. (2015, August 3). Six tips for managing up and what that even means: Helping your boss help you. *U.S. News & World Report*. Retrieved from http://money.usnews.com/money/careers/articles/2015/08/03/6-tips-for-managing-up-and-what-that-even-means

Rath, T. (2013). *StrengthsFinder*. Omaha, NE: Gallup Press.

Topp, K., & Desjardins, J. H. (2011). Span of control: Designing organizations for effectiveness. In J. Wolf, H. Hanson, & M. J. Mohr (Eds.), *Organization development in health care: High impact practices for a complex and changing environment*. Charlotte, NC: Information Age Publishing.

Turk, W. (2007, March–April). *The art of managing up*. Washington, DC: Department of Defense Acquisition, Technology and Logistics. Retrieved from http://uthscsa.edu/gme/documents/TheArtofManagingUp.pdf

ADDITIONAL RESOURCES

Briggs-Myers, I., & Meyers, P. (2010). *Gifts differing: Understanding personality type*. Boston, MA: Nicholas Brealey.

Goldsmith, M. (2007). *What got you here won't get you there*. New York, NY: Hachett Books.

Myers and Briggs Foundation. Resources for Myers Briggs training. Retrieved from http://www.myersbriggs.org/myers-and-briggs-foundation

Sheryl, S. (2013). *Lean in: Women, work and the will to succeed*. New York, NY: Knopf.

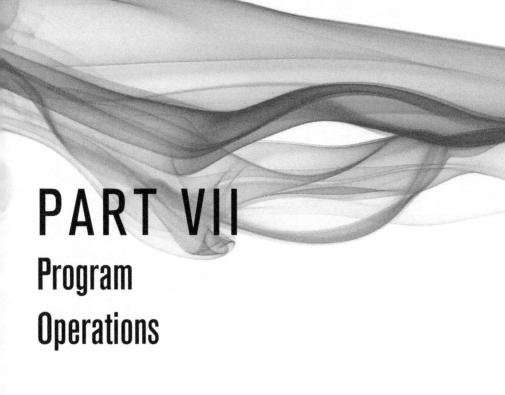

PART VII
Program
Operations

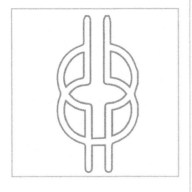

NYANSAPO
"Wisdom knot"

Symbol of wisdom, ingenuity, intelligence, and patience

An especially revered symbol of the Akan, this symbol conveys the idea that "a wise person has the capacity to choose the best means to attain a goal. Being wise implies broad knowledge, learning and experience, and the ability to apply such faculties to practical ends."

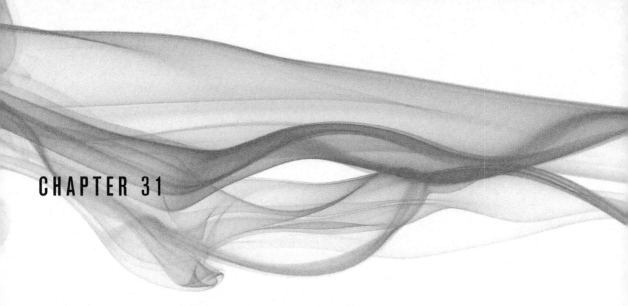

CHAPTER 31

Admissions Best Practices

Mariah Kindle and Douglas Brock

CHAPTER OBJECTIVES

- Develop transparent admission policies
- Review legal and compliance implications, applicants, common admission parameters, interview processes, and selection of candidates

---

[N]ot everything that can be counted counts, and not everything that counts can be counted.

—*William Bruce Cameron*

In the mid-1990s the World Health Organization (WHO) stated that universities and medical schools are "obligated to direct their education, research and service activities toward addressing the priority health concerns of the community, region, or nation they serve" (Roberts & Prideaux, 2010, p. 1054). In answering this call to action, colleges and universities began to develop more holistic admissions processes based on the published mission and goals of the institution. The overarching goal of holistic admissions processes is to generate a more diverse student body that will impact access to care in underserved communities. Underlying the holistic admissions process is the understanding that diversity in the classroom creates an opportunity to provide unique learning experiences for all students (Milem, 2003). Diversity is more than just race, ethnicity, and gender. The holistic admissions process also explores individual history, noncognitive attributes, clinical experiences, and socioeconomic and educational disadvantage.

Holistic admissions can be defined as the "university admissions strategy that assesses an applicant's unique experiences alongside traditional measures of academic achievement such as grades and test scores" (Urban Universities for Health, 2014, p. 2). The four tenets of holistic processes include: (a) broad-based selection criteria linked to the institution's and program's missions and goals; (b) a balance of applicant experience, personal attributes, and academic achievement; (c) individualized consideration to how each applicant might contribute to the learning environment and the profession; and (d) race and ethnicity, but only for decisions that are related to the published mission and goals associated with student diversity (Urban Universities for Health, 2014).

Holistic admissions policies begin with the mission and goals of the training program. Clearly defined vision and values statements will help support this process. It is important to clearly define how each of the four tenets relates to individual programs. Taking a "cookie-cutter" approach to building holistic admissions processes by copying another program's approach, does not lend itself to success. Programs must create their own application review policies, establish stakeholder agreements on selection variables to prioritize, determine the type of interview and who will be interviewed, and establish valid final selection criteria. Establishing or modifying holistic processes requires time and commitment from all stakeholders, but ultimately results in cohorts of academically strong, emotionally intelligent, mission-fit students. In the following sections, we lay out the essential elements of the admissions process (Figure 31.1).

OUTREACH

Health care training programs have witnessed rapid workforce growth with projected demands continuing through 2025. Expectations for a livable wage, high job satisfaction, and job availability have sparked a marked increase in the number of people applying to health science programs. Programs can receive hundreds of applications per available seat. Many of these applications are based solely on a program's public reputation, whereas other applicants will have responded solely to glowing media descriptions of a profession's desirability, often rooted

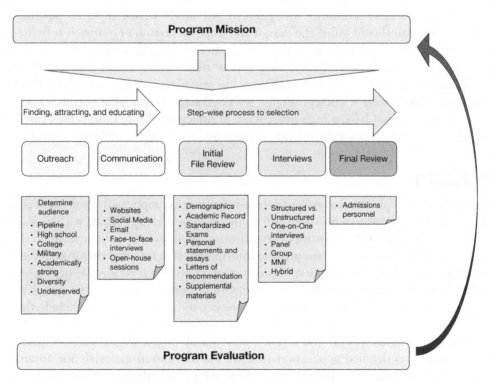

FIGURE 31.1 The holistic admissions process.
MMI, multiple mini-interview.

in financial and employment security. But are these applicants mission fit? As part of the holistic admissions process, programs develop and filter their applicant pools by creating outreach activities designed to attract applicants whose training goals align with the mission and goals of the program. Holistic outreach activities provide prospective applicants with the information to accurately self-assess their readiness, motivation, financial resources, and interest for training in a health science career.

Two distinct applicant pools dominate admissions: those ready to apply now, and those preparing to apply in the future. Each pool must receive information tailored to its specific needs and state of readiness. Applicants ready to apply now will likely be interested in the details of the application process, the mission-focused application review criteria, interview and selection processes, and details about how to make themselves competitive in the current cycle. Future applicants seek information on prerequisites, on how to strengthen their academic record, increase their knowledge of the health profession, and details about the program itself. Outreach events also attract those principally seeking only information. Having materials available to suit all attendees requires building comprehensive presentations and informational brochures, but also a willingness to adjust one's presentation on the fly to fit the audience. Even if an outreach event is specifically designed to attract one type of attendee, outreach materials should be sufficiently broad to ensure the most common questions and concerns of all are addressed.

Universities and colleges commonly hold large outreach events on campus, often targeting new freshman still trying to determine a major, or specific to soon-to-be graduates deciding on postbaccalaureate education programs. These on-campus activities are useful for reaching students already interested in health care education and students considering options that include the health sciences. Attendees at these events may not be aware of your program's mission. Targeted community advertising may increase awareness. These large events can increase diversity in the applicant pool, drawing prospective applicants who may not have believed a health care career could be within their reach. Broadening community-based outreach activities to include collaboration with local high schools and community colleges serves to build a strong applicant pipeline.

A program's mission should guide the design and implementation of outreach activities. If, for example, the program's mission seeks to increase diversity in the student body or prepare students to practice in underserved communities, research will be needed to identify which high schools and colleges have the greatest potential to provide mission-fit attendees. Working with schools that have strong science programs is a good start. Developing outreach activities specifically for schools that have a high percentage of underrepresented minorities can often target and inspire students toward health care careers otherwise considered to be out of reach.

COMMUNICATION

Communicating with applicants has never been easier or more complicated. Program websites, social media, and easy access to admissions offices by email provide applicants with a wealth of information. This information can prove overwhelming and is sometimes inconsistent. To aid preliminary decisions about a program, provide information that is comprehensive and understandable. Applicants often get their first impression of a university, college, or health science program based on the look, navigability, and information presented on a website. Website layout, ease of use, and clear and concise messaging are key to holding interest. Include the following when building or updating a website: (a) clearly state the mission, vision, values, and goals of the program; (b) provide specific and detailed prerequisite information, grade requirements and any exceptions; (c) detailed application timelines and required materials for admission; (d) financial aid, grant, and scholarship information; (e) a comprehensive "Frequently Asked Questions (FAQ)" page; (f) curriculum and student expectations; and (g) contact information for the program admissions office. Often, accrediting bodies require that specific information be readily available to applicants and when creating websites, programs must include the details as mandated. Building a website takes time, and routine updating and maintenance are necessary to remain compliant with accreditation requirements. Many institutions now have resources available, through a dedicated web development group or computer science students. In each case it is advised to have dedicated personnel or faculty to oversee website management. So, rather than go it alone, tap into the resources available through the institution. The benefits of a well-designed website will outweigh the challenges. Applicants will be better prepared, have fewer and more fully formed questions, and have a better understanding of the program's mission, goals, and expectations.

Social media can be both a friend and a foe to admissions personnel. Programs can use social media to reach a broad audience of prospective applicants, publish special interest stories about the activities of the program, advertise outreach activities and special events on campus, and more. However, social media sites must be monitored to ensure that published information is in the best interest of both the program and the applicant. Programs often have incomplete control of what can be displayed on social media sites. Postings may be made that are incorrect or inappropriate. Programs can ensure the quality of the materials they develop and promote online, can monitor user posts, and limit or increase the ability of the applicant to interact directly with a program's admissions personnel. It may be advisable to incorporate social media management into the job description of an admissions staff person's list of daily tasks. Prospective applicants will also find forums and blogs dedicated to the experiences of applicants applying to medical and nursing schools, physician assistant (PA) programs, pharmacy and dentistry schools, and so forth. Support for these forums range from well-monitored professional sources to more questionable sources that may provide incomplete or incorrect information.

Program websites and social media provide answers to many applicant questions, but there will be applicants who reach out directly to admissions personnel and academic advisors. Admissions personnel are familiar with never-ending queues of daily email, voice mail, and unannounced drop-ins. Many applicants request general information about the program that is clearly stated on the program's website. When a website is well designed, a respectful response providing clear information on how to access the information directly can be appropriate. It is not acceptable to simply point applicants back to the website to hunt for the answers—there is the potential to lose qualified applicants if giving them the email runaround. When possible, it is best to answer each question asked in a reply email.

Prioritizing email is essential to tackling the mountain of email programs receive. Sensitive email should be prioritized and responded to quickly. General questions can often be categorized into specific topics. Email templates can be developed to answer common questions, including program requirements, application deadlines, and outreach events. Many applicants ask questions that cannot be addressed by templates and are not available through an existing source. These questions are often personal or idiosyncratic in nature and must be responded to in an expedient and direct manner.

Admissions personnel have long lists of email pet peeves—emails from smartphones without salutations, rudely toned emails, entitled applicants, and the list goes on. The applicant does not realize admissions personnel may assess an applicant's readiness based not only on what the applicant says, but how he or she says it. If an applicant sends frequent emails that clearly show the information being provided is not being attended to, it could indicate the applicant has trouble following directions. If the email is rudely toned and questions the authority of admissions personnel, it may indicate professionalism concerns. However, most emails are professional with direct and sincere questions. In all cases, responses from admissions should be quick, respectful, and as complete as possible. Maintaining a complete record of all communications is strongly encouraged.

APPLICATION REVIEW

Admissions selection processes vary by program and by discipline. Prescribing a single strategy to serve all programs is not possible. However, all programs have expectations with common underlying dimensions. Some dimensions focus on academics, others speak to personal character, whereas others seek to understand motivation and readiness. Broadly, we expect an academic background that is sufficient to master training and personal qualities essential to clinical practice. We frame our discussion around cognitive and noncognitive applicant characteristics. Selection criteria for these characteristics can be defined by objective, quantitative evidence (e.g., grade point average [GPA]) or by more subjective, qualitative evidence (e.g., reference letters).

Holistic review processes aggregate applicant information from multiple sources employing a variety of methods. Logistic, resource, and cost constraints typically require reducing the full applicant pool to a manageable number of qualified applicants. This process, commonly called *file review*, constitutes inspection, evaluation, and selection of applicant files based on evidence assembled from demographics, academic records, standardized tests, clinical experience, personal statements, and letters of reference. This evidence can be described as cognitive (Exhibit 31.1) or noncognitive (Exhibit 31.2).

Cognitive Evidence

Academic Record

The academic record has long served as a principal, sometimes even the sole source of decision making in admissions. Academic records typically include a GPA—an overall average of all

---

EXHIBIT 31.1 File Review: Cognitive Evidence

Cognitive evidence is typically objective and quantitative, with numeric values that can be compared directly against a standard.

Academic Record: Demonstrates academic achievement

- GPA, adjusted for variation across schools
- GPA subscores: Last 90 credits, prerequisite credits, science versus nonscience, upper division course credits, and graduate credits
- Degrees, awards, licensure, and certification achieved
- Research and dissemination of work (e.g., publications and presentations)

Standardized Exams: Standardized exams typically provide national norms and evaluation recommendations

- Graduate Record Exam and subject exams
  - General scores: verbal, quantitative, and written analytical
  - Subject exams: biology, biochemistry and cell and molecular biology; biology; chemistry; literature in English; mathematics; physics; and psychology
- Medical College Admission Test
  - Sections: Chemical and Physical Foundations of Biological Systems; Biological and Biochemical Foundations of Living Systems; Critical Analysis and Reasoning; Psychological, Social and Biological Foundations of Behavior
- Millers Analogy Test
  - Assesses mental ability through analogies
- Test of English as a Foreign Language
- Assesses ability to use and understand English at the university level

---

GPA, grade point average.

grades recorded—and GPA subsets, which provide a more focused understanding of the applicant's performance. Common credit subsets include: "science and nonscience," "last 60 or last 90 hours," "graduate," and "prerequisite."

Institutional graduate programs and individual programs commonly require standardized tests that allow comparison of applicant scores with national norms. Common tests include the Graduate Record Examination (GRE), the Medical College Admission Test (MCAT), and the Miller Analogies Test (MAT). The GRE General Test—verbal, quantitative, and analytical writing scores—is required by the majority of American graduate-level programs. Seven optional GRE subject tests assess knowledge in specific domains (e.g., biology, biochemistry, and cell and molecular biology). The MCAT is principally used in the selection of medical students. The exam consists of four sections: chemical and physical foundations of biological systems; critical analysis and reasoning skills; biological and biochemical foundations of living systems; and psychological, social, and biological foundations of behavior. The MAT assesses mental ability through problems stated as analogies. International applicants, whose first language is not English, may be required to take the TOEFL or similar assessment of English competence.

Empirical studies show academic records constitute strong predictors of success in didactic training and for passing posttraining licensure exams better than interviews, personal statements, references, or tests of aptitude or situational judgment (Edwards, Friedman, & Pearce, 2013; Ferguson, James, & Madeley, 2002; Higgins et al., 2010; McManus et al., 2013; Patterson, Knight, et al., 2016; Salvatori, 2001; Schripsema, van Trigt, Borleffs, & Cohen-Schotanus, 2014; Sladek, Bond, Frost, & Prior, 2016; Utzman, Riddle, & Jewell, 2007a, 2007b). However, there is no consensus on how to best apply different components of the academic record in determining selection standards. Many programs focus on the science GPA as evidence for success in the health sciences disciplines. Other programs emphasize the last 60 or 90 credits as the most current demonstration of an applicant's academic acumen. When employing GPAs for selection purposes it is always important to adjust for differences resulting from variations in institutional grading standards (Didier, Kreiter, Buri, & Solow, 2006). Most programs examine multiple aggregate indicators; many also explore the applicant's full academic trajectory. Some applicants have poor early grades that cloud later more mature demonstrations of performance, an issue often underlying discrepancies between the last credits completed and the overall GPA. Success in higher level science coursework or a demonstration that the applicant's interest and aptitude for the sciences is consistent across his or her education, not strictly as a function of recently completed program prerequisites, can be useful. Some programs have success examining course withdrawals and failed courses as predictive of later difficulties. Even when the overall GPA is high, withdrawals from courses and failing scores, which are not explained in the applicant's personal statement, can indicate difficulties following through on academic commitments.

Academic records are less predictive of clinical skill and ability to apply health care knowledge to treat patients (Saguil et al., 2015; Silver & Hodgson, 1997). Still, the relationships between academic training and clinical success are complex and many questions remain (Jones, Simpkins, & Hocking, 2014).

Clinical Experience

The extent to which health science training programs require or value pretraining clinical experience and hours spent shadowing health care providers varies widely. Pretraining health care experience does not consistently predict academic performance, and indeed there may be an inverse relationship between pretraining clinical experience and performance in later training (Artino et al., 2012; El-Banna et al., 2015). The relationship between pretraining clinical experience and later clinical skill is also questionable (Hegmann & Iverson, 2016).

Noncognitive Evidence

Cognitive criteria provide a reasonable estimate of an applicant's ability to achieve academically, but poorly predict clinical skill or reveal the personal characteristics vital to providing ethical, empathetic, and professional care. Noncognitive evidence allows the opportunity to assess the alignment of an applicant's personal characteristics with a program's mission and goals. Unfortunately, during both file review and interviews, personal judgments are prone to explicit (prejudice and stereotyping) and implicit biases (subconscious decision making). To reduce bias, admissions processes must remove ambiguity from all decision-making processes, make decisions in emotionally neutral settings, and increase awareness of bias. Interviewers must be engaged, unpressured, and provide respectful feedback. Measuring noncognitive attributes in an unbiased and reliable fashion is challenging, but is required to ensure fairness (Albanese, Snow, Skochelak, Huggett, & Farrell, 2003a). Familiar noncognitive approaches include personality tests, interviews, reference letters, and personal essays or statements (Exhibit 31.2).

Analysis of this evidence allows the examination of complex constructs, including an applicant's personality traits (Conrad, 2006; Komarraju, Karau, Schmeck, & Avdic, 2011; Rothbart, Ahead, & Evans, 2000), values (Patterson, Prescott-Clements, et al., 2016), emotional intelligence (Chew, Md Zain, & Hassan, 2015; Chew, Zain, & Hassan, 2013), resilience (Carrothers, Gregory, & Gallagher, 2000; Gillespie, Chaboyer, & Wallis, 2009; Gillespie, Chaboyer, Wallis, & Grimbeek, 2007; McCann et al., 2013), maturity, motivation, professionalism, and communication skills. These variables have been associated with success in clinical practice and demonstrate an applicant's readiness for training. Many constitute personal attributes prioritized by health care programs (Jones et al., 2014).

Demographics

Common demographic characteristics evaluated in the admissions process include cultural identification, ethnicity and race, gender, age, and socioeconomic status. Life experiences, such as volunteer work, geographic upbringing (e.g., rural), military service, economic or educational disadvantage, and cross-cultural living, often weigh heavily in reviewers' decision making. The academic predictive power of demographics is highly debated. In some cases, the application of specific demographic criteria to selection processes can be unethical, illegal, or both (e.g., race, gender, color, ethnicity, or national origin). When using demographic measures, it is important that these are in line with the program and institutional mission statements, for example, rural colleges and programs that serve educationally underserved communities. All policies employing demographic criteria must also be compliant with the overarching policies of the institution. In addition, variations occur by state and federal statutes. Consequently, admissions personnel are cautioned to be intimately aware of institutional, program, state, and federal requirements.

Personality Variables

Admissions have a long history of incorporating personality testing, but supportive evidence is limited (Patterson, Knight, et al., 2016). Some specific traits, including conscientiousness, neuroticism, dominance, and empathy, have demonstrated predictive evidence (Chamberlain, Catano, & Cunningham, 2005; Chamorro-Premuzic & Farnham, 2003; Ferguson, Sanders, O'Hehir, & James, 2000; Griffin & Wilson, 2012; Hojat, Erdmann, & Gonnella, 2013; Lievens, Peeters, & Schollaert, 2008). One construct, emotional intelligence, has received considerable attention in health care training program admissions processes. Some findings are emerging that emotional intelligence may predict later performance, whereas other findings are less supportive (Carr, 2009; Carrothers et al., 2000; Chew et al., 2013; Chew et al., 2015; Lin, Kannappan, & Lau, 2013).

EXHIBIT 31.2 File Review: Noncognitive Evidence

Noncognitive evidence, often approached in a qualitative fashion, evaluates personal characteristics of applicants and often compares applicant qualities with a program's mission.

Demographics:

- Age, gender, ethnicity, race, citizenship, military veteran, other
- Schools attended
- Program's geographic catchment area, hometown
- Economic or educational disadvantage

Clinical experience:

- Hours of employment in clinical domains
- Degree of responsibility and independence
- Interprofessional team experience
- Provider type (e.g., registered nurse, pharmacy tech)
- Type of care or care setting (e.g., primary versus specialty care environment; hospital versus small clinic)

Clinical shadowing

- Hours of shadowing in separate clinical domains
- Providers shadowed (e.g., physician, nurse)
- Type of care or care setting (e.g., primary versus specialty care environment; hospital versus small clinic)

Service and volunteering

- Medical volunteer work or nonmedical community service
- Hours of service and volunteer work
- Service aligned with program mission
- Service not aligned with program mission

Reference letters

- Academic: professors, instructors
- Clinical: clinical colleagues, providers shadowed
- Personal: friends, family, clergy, and so on

Personal statements and essays

- Maturity, motivation, readiness, confidence
- Leadership, trustworthiness, honesty, altruism
- Cultural experiences
- Challenges faced and achievements
- Rationale for deficits in applicant's packet

Personal Statements and Reference Letters

Personal statements and references have been widely studied, but even early work questioned their value (Friedman, 1983). Professional references (DeZee et al., 2014) and personal references demonstrate little to no predictive value (Ferguson et al., 2002; Poole, Moriarty, Wearn, Wilkinson, & Weller, 2009). Reported limitations of reference letters include inflated estimates of applicant attributes, the impact of the reviewer's writing competence on file-review decisions, and concerns of confidentiality (Mason & Schroeder, 2014). Despite the lack of predictive evidence, personal statements and references are common to most admissions processes.

INTERVIEWS

Holistic selection processes commonly include interviews. Although quantitative data is common to file review, final decisions typically incorporate qualitative findings from interviews to ensure a holistic effort. Interviews provide an opportunity to delve deeply into the applicant's personal attributes and academic record, and draw direct comparisons between the applicant's and program's goals. However, the costs to both the program and the applicant can be high, and demands placed on interviewers can be excessive. We discuss five categories of interviews: one-on-one, group, panel, multiple mini-interviews (MMIs), and hybrid.

One-On-One Interviews

One-on-one interviews—whether in-person or via telephone or teleconference—are deeply enculturated into admissions processes. Reviewers elicit responses to specific questions, and can address a wide range of applicant qualities and values (Albanese et al., 2003a). Interviews allow admissions personnel to "get to know" the applicant, yet demonstrate relatively low reliability and poor predictive validity for academic performance, and at best moderate predictive validity for clinical skills (Basco, Gilbert, Chessman, & Blue, 2000; Basco, Lancaster, Gilbert, Carey, & Blue, 2008; Edwards et al., 2013; Patterson, Knight, et al., 2016; Prideaux et al., 2011; Wilkinson et al., 2008). Interviewers may overestimate their objectivity. Positive findings are achieved with more structured interview protocols (Levashina, Hartwell, Morgeson, & Campion, 2014) or innovations in the interviewing process (Donnon, Oddone-Paolucci, & Violato, 2009; Donnon & Paolucci, 2008; Kleshinski, Shriner, & Khuder, 2008). If using the one-on-one format, we recommend not heavily weighting interviewer judgments.

Panel and Group Interviews

Panel and group interviews are designed to allow multiple interviewers to simultaneously interview a single applicant (panel), or to allow one or more interviewers to simultaneously interview multiple applicants (group). These interviews, similar to one-on-one interviews, are limited in predictive validity (Iddekinge, Sager, Burn field, & Hefner, 2006) and provide only incremental support beyond more objective evidence (Dipboye, Gouger, Hayes, & Parker, 2001). They can be perceived as more threatening, especially to women and minority applicants (Albanese, Snow, Skochelak, Huggett, & Farrell, 2003b). In group interviews, question order can significantly impact the quality of interview ratings (Tran & Blackman, 2006). Group discussions following interviews may further reduce objectivity of group interviews (Palmer & Loveland, 2008).

Multiple Mini-Interviews

MMIs, are an "admissions the objective structured clinical examination (OSCE)" (Eva, Rosenfeld, Reiter, & Norman, 2004, p. 316) to improve on the reliability and predictive validity of traditional interview formats (Brownell, Lockyer, Collin, & Lemay, 2007; Dore et al., 2010; Grice, 2014; Husbands & Dowell, 2013; Knorr & Hissbach, 2014; Lemay, Lockyer, Collin, & Brownell, 2007; Patterson, Knight, et al., 2016; Patterson, Rowett, et al., 2016; Pau, Chen, Lee, Sow, & De Alwis, 2016; Pau et al., 2013; Sebok, Luu, & Klinger, 2014; Sladek et al., 2016; Thomas, Young, Mazer, Lubarsky, & Razack, 2015). Noncognitive attributes are assessed across multiple, focused, brief—typically 8- to 10-minute—standardized interview "stations." Stations can address personal attributes and values (e.g., professionalism and empathy) or program-specific goals or mission (e.g., interest in rural practice). Quantitative scoring protocols (e.g., Likert-type ratings) are completed by the interviewer. Although MMI ratings are less strongly associated with academic measures of success (Knorr & Hissbach, 2014; Pau et al., 2013, 2016), they demonstrate value in predicting later clinical skill (Knorr & Hissbach, 2014; Pau et al., 2013, 2016) and performance on clinically focused examinations (Eva, Reiter, Rosenfeld, & Norman, 2004; Reiter, Eva, Rosenfeld, & Norman, 2007). MMIs are reported by applicants as fair and believed to be more likely than traditional interviews to demonstrate an applicant's strengths (Razack et al., 2009). They may also be less prone to implicit bias (Jerant et al., 2015). It is useful to consider stations to represent situational judgment (e.g., responding to a hypothetical scenario); free form, in which interviewers focus on a specific skill, but do not follow a fixed structure; structured form, in which questions follow a scripted protocol; and behavioral interviews, in which applicants recall real-life experiences. Some evidence exists that self-reflection on one's own actual life events, versus the use of hypothetical scenarios, holds the strongest predictive value (Eva & Macala, 2014).

Hybrid Approaches

Some programs combine elements from traditional one-on-one interviews, group and panel interviews, and characteristics of the MMI format. In our own program, applicants complete three, hour-long interviews in small groups, each of which includes three applicants and two interviewers. Interviews are unstructured and encourage role play and discussion between applicants. The model demonstrates face validity but has not been assessed for evidence of predictive validity. The University of Michigan School of Medicine has collected preliminary validity evidence for an interview format that combines six, short, highly structured, scenario-focused interviews, but also includes two, 30-minute semistructured one-on-one interviews (Bibler Zaidi, Santen, Purkiss, Teener, & Gay, 2016).

Setting Standards

Setting standards for selected admissions variables (e.g., GPA, hours of clinical experience) is challenging. The first hurdle is determining whether or not a variable is quantitative or qualitative in nature. The GPA constitutes an objective and quantitative measure. Review of a personal statement represents a subjective and qualitative judgment, but will require development of a numeric scoring protocol (e.g., Likert-type ratings). The second hurdle is assigning reliable thresholds for both quantitative and qualitative variables. Programs prioritizing academic achievement may set a higher bar on the GPA. Conversely, some programs greatly value personal characteristics, setting lower academic bars. Justifying numeric cutoffs benefits from inspection of historical data (e.g., has GPA previously predicted performance), exploring the beliefs and values of faculty and staff, and comparison with national data. Admissions personnel should not assume they can develop unequivocal cutoffs. Standards must be routinely reviewed and adjusted.

Holistic Review

Structure and consistency are associated with the success of admissions processes. Whether it is the final stage of an admissions process where all the data are reviewed and rated by admissions personnel, during initial file review, or in-person interviews, a holistic rubric presents a useful tool to increase validity (Peeters, Schmude, & Stein miller, 2014; Urban Universities for Health, 2014). Holistic review combines multiple selection variables and is driven by core principles, as shown in Exhibit 31.3.

EXHIBIT 31.3 Core Principles of Holistic Admissions Process

1. Broad-based selection criteria linked to school or program vision, mission, and goals
2. Balanced consideration of applicant experience, attributes, and academic metrics
3. Assessment of applicant's potential to contribute to the school or program learning community and the profession
4. Respect for cognitive diversity and inclusion

CLEAR AND TRANSPARENT PROGRAM ADMISSIONS POLICIES

When developing or changing admissions policies, it is important that policies comply with local, state, and federal regulations; university policies; and accreditation requirements. We believe training a diverse student body has a direct and positive impact on the overall health of increasingly diverse communities. However, policies designed to recruit, train, and support underrepresented minorities must be compliant with university diversity policy and state law. Transparency is particularly important when establishing policy for student diversity. Race can be considered, but only when it is part of a broader mix of factors (Urban Universities for Health, 2014). However, in April 2014, the U.S. Supreme Court ruled that states have the right to amend their constitution to ban race-based affirmative action by referendum ("Fourteenth Amendment: Equal Protection," 2016). This ruling upheld state initiatives that banned affirmative action, including Washington, Michigan, Arizona, New Hampshire, California, and Florida. Applying race- or ethnic-based selection processes in these states can be difficult and has the potential to violate state initiatives. Working with university leadership to develop policies compliant with state regulations and having access to legal advice when developing these policies will help programs understand the limits set by state legislation.

It is important to create policies that standardize requirements and expectations for all applicants. Exceptions must be clearly stated. If the university requires special standardized exams for international students or additional documentation for military students, this must be clearly noted in any public communications. Policies and instructions for completing these additional requirements must be made clear to applicants. It is in a program's interest to have staff members who understand these requirements and can help applicants navigate required steps. International students can sometimes be admitted to a university, but visa status, state licensing requirements, and national exams may set limits for students who are not U.S. citizens.

The Family Educational Rights and Privacy Act (FERPA, 1974) protects the privacy of students in institutions receiving funding from the U.S. Department of Education (DOE). These rules do not apply to private institutions that do not receive DOE funding. FERPA dictates what and how much information can be disclosed with and without permission from students, how and when student records should be reviewed, what type of information can be disclosed to financial aid offices, what can be provided to entities conducting research, and more. It is important that admissions personnel are familiar with these rules and have access to institutional subject matter experts to ensure programs remain compliant.

Programs may receive requests from applicants with special circumstances. These requests can range from requests for advanced standing based on prior degree or experience, international students requesting acceptance of education credits earned in their home country, or persons looking to transfer credits from another training program. Although these requests are not common, programs must establish policies about each in alignment with program accreditation requirements and institutional rules. In the case of international credits, for example, institutions may require original transcripts, but also require course-by-course evaluated transcripts completed by an accredited translation agency in the United States. Students requesting advanced standing or transferring credits from one training program to another are likely subject to program rules and accreditation requirements.

The recommendations and references provided in this chapter are not intended to be exhaustive. Many admissions processes are program or institution specific and general recommendations may not be broadly relevant. For example, consider applicant notification policies. In some cases, programs seek to fill open positions as soon as a qualified applicant is recognized, whereas others programs process all applicants before making selection decisions. Programs commonly build a waitlist of applicants. However, these program-level policies can be constrained by institutional policies. Telephone notifications of acceptance are recommended. However, the response to rejected applicants and the type and level of feedback provided is impacted by program resources. Rejection messages are most commonly mailed or emailed to the applicant. Providing specific feedback is not common, but programs can provide generalized feedback statements for how the applicant might improve subsequent applications. Some programs encourage and others discourage reapplication. Programs that allow repeat applications are strongly urged to provide this opportunity to all reapplicants to avoid the appearance of inconsistency.

EVALUATION

Ongoing evaluation and adjustment to admissions processes are necessary to respond to changing applicant pools, changing program goals, and shifts in program leadership. Quality assurance (process monitoring) and quality control (testing against standards) constitute two arms of admissions program evaluation. They are needed to monitor and maintain quality, and as a requirement for program accreditation. Our summarized recommendations draw from standards published by the WHO and the Kellogg Foundation. Key variables include operational feasibility, efficiency, effectiveness, adequacy, equity, sustainability, and propriety in the administration and conduct of program activities.

Logic models provide a visual representation (Figure 31.2) of the elements of admissions programs' functioning. Programs have resources (e.g., faculty, staff) to conduct activities (e.g., applicant file review, interviews) and generate short-term outcomes (e.g., attracting and matriculating students) to establish long-term impacts (e.g., success of graduates). An experienced evaluator, integrated early into the admissions process, is essential. Resource-level metrics may include routine cost analyses to assess the cost per matriculant. Activities metrics address what is accomplished at each stage of the admissions process (e.g., file review). Judging the adequacy of resources and activities requires collection of short-term outcomes and long-term impacts. Examples of short-term metrics include applications received, files reviewed, applicants interviewed and selected, and the percentage of selected applicants who accept positions. Examples of long-term impacts include drop-out and graduation rates, licensure, and alignment of graduates' clinical practice with program mission.

CONCLUSIONS

Health sciences training programs share a common goal to graduate competent clinicians. We want our graduates to be clinically adept, professional, able to work in teams, able to lead or follow as needed, be kind and empathetic to patients, and contribute to their profession and practice. We support holistic admissions processes that focus on mission and recognize the importance of both short-term outcomes and long-term impacts. Holistic approaches are wide ranging. They embrace traditional demonstrations of academic potential, but equally important, appraise an applicant's personal character. Holistic processes seek the best fit between applicants and program missions, seeking students as engaged contributors, not simply vessels. The full range of

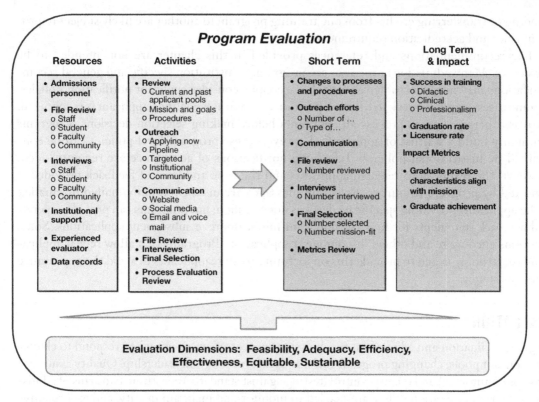

FIGURE 31.2 Summarized logic model for admissions evaluation.

holistic admissions data is extensive. Admissions personnel must be selective in determining what can be practically collected and reviewed, and carefully assess the validity of each data source and metric. Building a strong admissions program, or bolstering the effectiveness of an existing program, is difficult. Think in years, not months.

Before beginning training, before graduating to practice, and before establishing a career, we each encounter admissions. Admission to clinical training is rarely the first time an applicant will have encountered admissions processes. However, it may be the most significant as it involves entrance to a career. In good faith, admissions teams establish practices that comply with institutional and professional expectations, apply best evidence techniques, understand each technique's limitations, and continuously monitor and modify processes to maintain quality. This is not a simple goal. All those involved in admissions will make mistakes, some observable, some not. We honor our applicants, our students, our program, and health care practice by doing our best.

REFERENCES

Albanese, M. A., Snow, M. H., Skochelak, S. E., Huggett, K. N., & Farrell, P. M. (2003a). Assessing personal qualities in medical school admissions. *Academic Medicine*, 78(3), 313–321.

Albanese, M. A., Snow, M., Skochelak, S., Huggett, K., & Farrell, P. M. (2003b). Matriculating student perceptions of changes to the admissions interview process at the University of Wisconsin Medical School: A prospective, controlled comparison. *Wisconsin Medical Journal*, 102(2), 30–33.

Artino, A. R., Gilliland, W. R., Waechter, D. M., Cruess, D., Calloway, M., & Durning, S. J. (2012). Does self-reported clinical experience predict performance in medical school and internship? *Medical Education*, 46(2), 172–178.

Basco, W. T., Gilbert, G. E., Chessman, A. W., & Blue, A. V. (2000). The ability of a medical school admission process to predict clinical performance and patients' satisfaction. *Academic Medicine*, 75(7), 743–747.

Basco, W. T., Lancaster, C. J., Gilbert, G. E., Carey, M. E., & Blue, A. V. (2008). Medical school application interview score has limited predictive validity for performance on a fourth year clinical practice examination. *Advanced Health Science Education Theory and Practice, 13*(2), 151–162.

Bibler Zaidi, N. L., Santen, S. A., Purkiss, J. A., Teener, C. A., & Gay, S. E. (2016). A hybrid interview model for medical school interviews: Combining traditional and multisampling formats. *Academic Medicine, 91*(11), 1526–1529.

Brownell, K., Lockyer, J., Collin, T., & Lemay, J. F. (2007). Introduction of the multiple mini interview into the admissions process at the University of Calgary: Acceptability and feasibility. *Medical Teacher, 29*(4), 394–396.

Carr, S. E. (2009). Emotional intelligence in medical students: Does it correlate with selection measures? *Medical Education, 43*(11), 1069–1077.

Carrothers, R. M., Gregory, S. W., & Gallagher, T. J. (2000). Measuring emotional intelligence of medical school applicants. *Academic Medicine, 75*(5), 456–463.

Chamberlain, T. C., Catano, V. M., & Cunningham, D. P. (2005). Personality as a predictor of professional behavior in dental school: Comparisons with dental practitioners. *Journal of Dental Education, 69*(11), 1222–1237.

Chamorro-Premuzic, T., & Farnham, A. (2003). Personality predicts academic performance: Evidence from two longitudinal university samples. *Journal of Research in Personality, 37*, 319–338.

Chew, B. H., Zain, A. Md., & Hassan, F. (2015). The relationship between the social management of emotional intelligence and academic performance among medical students. *Psychological Health and Medicine, 20*(2), 198–204.

Chew, B. H., Zain, A. M., & Hassan, F. (2013). Emotional intelligence and academic performance in first and final year medical students: A cross-sectional study. *BioMed Central Medical Education, 13*, 44.

Conrad, M. (2006). Aptitude is not enough: How personality and behavior predict academic performance. *Journal of Research in Personality, 40*, 339–346.

DeZee, K. J., Magee, C. D., Rickards, G., Artino, A. R., Gilliland, W. R., Dong, T., . . . Durning, S. J. (2014). What aspects of letters of recommendation predict performance in medical school? Findings from one institution. *Academic Medicine, 89*(10), 1408–1415.

Didier, T., Kreiter, C. D., Buri, R., & Solow, C. (2006). Investigating the utility of a GPA institutional adjustment index. *Advanced Health Science Education Theory and Practice, 11*(2), 145–153.

Dipboye, R., Gouger, B., Hayes, T., & Parker, D. (2001). The validity of unstructured panel interviews: More than meets the eye? *Journal of Business and Psychology, 16*(1), 35–49.

Donnon, T., Oddone-Paolucci, E., & Violato, C. (2009). A predictive validity study of medical judgment vignettes to assess students' noncognitive attributes: A 3-year prospective longitudinal study. *Medical Teacher, 31*(4), e148–e155.

Donnon, T., & Paolucci, E. O. (2008). A generalizability study of the medical judgment vignettes interview to assess students' noncognitive attributes for medical school. *BioMed Central Medical Education, 8*, 58.

Dore, K. L., Kreuger, S., Ladhani, M., Rolfson, D., Kurtz, D., Kulasegaram, K., . . . Reiter, H. I. (2010). The reliability and acceptability of the multiple mini-interview as a selection instrument for postgraduate admissions. *Academic Medicine, 85*(Suppl. 10), S60–S63.

Edwards, D., Friedman, T., & Pearce, J. (2013). Same admissions tools, different outcomes: A critical perspective on predictive validity in three undergraduate medical schools. *BioMed Central Medical Education, 13*, 173.

El-Banna, M. M., Briggs, L. A., Leslie, M. S., Athey, E. K., Pericak, A., Falk, N. L., & Greene, J. (2015). Does prior RN clinical experience predict academic success in graduate nurse practitioner programs? *Journal of Nursing Education, 54*(5), 276–280.

Eva, K. W., & Macala, C. (2014). Multiple mini-interview test characteristics: 'Tis better to ask candidates to recall than to imagine. *Medical Education, 48*(6), 604–613.

Eva, K. W., Reiter, H. I., Rosenfeld, J., & Norman, G. R. (2004). The ability of the multiple mini-interview to predict preclerkship performance in medical school. *Academic Medicine, 79*(Suppl. 10), S40–S42.

Eva, K. W., Rosenfeld, J., Reiter, H. I., & Norman, G. R. (2004). An admissions OSCE: The multiple mini-interview. *Medical Education, 38*(3), 314–326.

Family Educational Rights and Privacy Act, 20 U.S.C. § 1232g; 34 CFR Part 99 (1974). Retrieved from http://www2.ed.gov/policy/gen/reg/ferpa/index.html

Ferguson, E., James, D., & Madeley, L. (2002). Factors associated with success in medical school: Systematic review of the literature. *British Medical Journal, 324*(7343), 952–957.

Ferguson, E., Sanders, A., O'Hehir, F., & James, D. (2000). Predictive validity of personal statements and the role of the five-factor model of personality in relation to medical training. *Occupational and Organizational Psychology, 73*(3), 321–344.

Friedman, R. B. (1983). Sounding board: Fantasy land. *New England Journal of Medicine, 308*(11), 651–653.

Gillespie, B. M., Chaboyer, W., & Wallis, M. (2009). The influence of personal characteristics on the resilience of operating room nurses: A predictor study. *International Journal of Nursing Studies, 46*(7), 968–976.

Gillespie, B. M., Chaboyer, W., Wallis, M., & Grimbeek, P. (2007). Resilience in the operating room: Developing and testing of a resilience model. *Journal of Advanced Nursing, 59*(4), 427–438.

Grice, K. O. (2014). Use of multiple mini-interviews for occupational therapy admissions. *Journal of Allied Health, 43*(1), 57–61.

Griffin, B., & Wilson, I. (2012). Associations between the big five personality factors and multiple mini-interviews. *Advances in Health Sciences Education: Theory and Practice, 17*(3), 377–388.

Hegmann, T., & Iverson, K. (2016). Does previous healthcare experience increase success in physician assistant training? *Journal of American Association of Physician Assistants, 29*(6), 54–56.

Higgins, R., Moser, S., Dereczyk, A., Canales, R., Stewart, G., Schierholtz, C., . . . Arbuckle, S. (2010). Admission variables as predictors of PANCE scores in physician assistant programs: A comparison study across universities. *Journal of Physician Assistant Education, 21*(1), 10–17.

Hojat, M., Erdmann, J. B., & Gonnella, J. S. (2013). Personality assessments and outcomes in medical education and the practice of medicine: AMEE Guide No. 79. *Medical Teacher, 35*(7), 1267–1301.

Husbands, A., & Dowell, J. (2013). Predictive validity of the Dundee multiple mini-interview. *Medical Education, 47*(7), 717–725.

Iddekinge, C., Sager, C., Burn field, J., & Hefner, T. (2006). The variability of criterion-related validity estimates among interviewers and interview panels. *International Journal of Selection and Assessment, 14*(3), 193–205.

Jerant, A., Fancher, T., Fenton, J. J., Fiscella, K., Sousa, F., Franks, P., & Henderson, M. (2015). How medical school applicant race, ethnicity, and socioeconomic status relate to multiple mini-interview-based admissions outcomes: Findings from one medical school. *Academic Medicine, 90*(12), 1667–1674.

Jones, P. E., Simpkins, S., & Hocking, J. A. (2014). Imperfect physician assistant and physical therapist admissions processes in the United States. *Journal of Education Evaluation and Health Professions, 11*, 11.

Kleshinski, J., Shriner, C., & Khuder, S. A. (2008). The use of professionalism scenarios in the medical school interview process: Faculty and interviewee perceptions. *Medical Education Online, 13*, 2.

Knorr, M., & Hissbach, J. (2014). Multiple mini-interviews: Same concept, different approaches. *Medical Education, 48*(12), 1157–1175.

Komarraju, M., Karau, S., Schmeck, R., & Avdic, A. (2011). The Big Five personality traits, learning styles, and academic achievement. *Personality and Individual Differences, 51*(4), 472–477.

Lemay, J. F., Lockyer, J. M., Collin, V. T., & Brownell, A. K. (2007). Assessment of non-cognitive traits through the admissions multiple mini-interview. *Medical Education, 41*(6), 573–579.

Levashina, J., Hartwell, C., Morgeson, F., & Campion, M. (2014). The structured employment interview: Narrative and quantitative review of the research literature. *Personnel Psychology, 67*, 243–293.

Lievens, F., Peeters, H., & Schollaert, E. (2008). Situational judgment tests: A review of recent research *Personnel Review, 37*(4), 426–427.

Lin, D. T., Kannappan, A., & Lau, J. N. (2013). The assessment of emotional intelligence among candidates interviewing for general surgery residency. *Journal of Surgical Education, 70*(4), 514–521.

Mason, R., & Schroeder, M. (2014). The predictive validity of teacher candidate letters of reference. *Journal of Education and Learning, 3*(3), 67–75.

McCann, C., Beddoe, E., McCormick, K., Huggard, P., Kedge, S., Adamson, C., & Huggard, J. (2013). Resilience in the health professions: A review of recent literature. *International Journal of Wellbeing, 3*(1), 60–80.

McManus, I. C., Dewberry, C., Nicholson, S., Dowell, J. S., Woolf, K., & Potts, H. W. (2013). Construct-level predictive validity of educational attainment and intellectual aptitude tests in medical student selection: Meta-regression of six UK longitudinal studies. *BioMed Central Medical Education, 11*, 243.

Milem, J. (2003). The educational benefits of diversity: Evidence from multiple sectors. In M. Chang, D. Witt, J. Jones, & K. Hakuta (Eds.), *Compelling interest: Examining the evidence on racial dynamics in higher education* (pp. 126–169). Stanford, CA: Stanford University Press.

Palmer, J. K., & Loveland, J. M. (2008). The influence of group discussion on performance judgments: Rating accuracy, contrast effects, and halo. *Journal of Psychology, 142*(2), 117–130.

Patterson, F., Knight, A., Dowell, J., Nicholson, S., Cousans, F., & Cleland, J. (2016). How effective are selection methods in medical education? A systematic review. *Medical Education, 50*(1), 36–60.

Patterson, F., Prescott-Clements, L., Zibarras, L., Edwards, H., Kerrin, M., & Cousans, F. (2016). Recruiting for values in healthcare: A preliminary review of the evidence. *Advanced Health Science Education Theory and Practice, 21*(4), 859–881.

Patterson, F., Rowett, E., Hale, R., Grant, M., Roberts, C., Cousans, F., & Martin, S. (2016). The predictive validity of a situational judgement test and multiple mini-interview for entry into postgraduate training in Australia. *BioMed Central Medical Education, 16*, 87.

Pau, A., Chen, Y. S., Lee, V. K., Sow, C. F., & De Alwis, R. (2016). What does the multiple mini interview have to offer over the panel interview? *Medical Education Online, 21*, 29874.

Pau, A., Jeevaratnam, K., Chen, Y. S., Fall, A. A., Khoo, C., & Nadarajah, V. D. (2013). The multiple mini-interview (MMI) for student selection in health professions training—A systematic review. *Medical Teacher, 35*(12), 1027–1041.

Peeters, M., Schmude, K., & Stein miller, C. (2014). Inter-rater reliability and false confidence in precision: Using standard error of measurement within PharmD admissions essay rubric development. *Currents in Pharmacy Teaching and Learning, 6*, 298–303.

Poole, P., Moriarty, H., Wearn, A., Wilkinson T. J., & Weller, J. (2009). Medical student selection in New Zealand: Looking to the future. *New Zealand Medical Journal, 122*, 88–100.

Prideaux, D., Roberts, C., Eva, K., Centeno, A., McCrorie, P., McManus, C., . . . Wilkinson, D. (2011). Assessment for selection for the health care professions and specialty training: Consensus statement and recommendations from the Ottawa 2010 Conference. *Medical Teacher, 33*(3), 215–223.

Razack, S., Faremo, S., Drolet, F., Snell, L., Wiseman, J., & Pickering, J. (2009). Multiple mini-interviews versus traditional interviews: Stakeholder acceptability comparison. *Medical Education, 43*(10), 993–1000.

Reiter, H. I., Eva, K. W., Rosenfeld, J., & Norman, G. R. (2007). Multiple mini-interviews predict clerkship and licensing examination performance. *Medical Education, 41*(4), 378–384.

Roberts, C., & Prideaux, D. (2010). Selection for medical schools: Re-imaging as an international discourse. *Medical Education, 44*(11), 1054–1056.

Rothbart, M., Ahead, S., & Evans, D. (2000). Temperament and personality: Origins and outcomes. *Journal of Personality and Social Psychology, 78*(1), 125–130.

Saguil, A., Dong, T., Gingerich, R. J., Swygert, K., LaRochelle, J. S., Artino, A. R., . . . Durning, S. J. (2015). Does the MCAT predict medical school and PGY-1 performance? *Military Medicine, 180*(Suppl. 4), 4–11.

Salvatori, P. (2001). Reliability and validity of admissions tools used to select students for the health professions. *Advanced Health Science Education Theory and Practice, 6*(2), 159–175.

Schripsema, N. R., van Trigt, A. M., Borleffs, J. C., & Cohen-Schotanus, J. (2014). Selection and study performance: Comparing three admission processes within one medical school. *Medical Education, 48*(12), 1201–1210.

Schuette, Attorney General of Michigan v. Coalition to Defend Affirmative Action, Integration and Immigration Rights and Fight for Equality By Any Means Necessary (BAMN) et al.2013/12–682.

Sebok, S. S., Luu, K., & Klinger, D. A. (2014). Psychometric properties of the multiple mini-interview used for medical admissions: Findings from generalizability and Rasch analyses. *Advanced Health Science Education Theory and Practice, 19*(1), 71–84.

Silver, B., & Hodgson, C. S. (1997). Evaluating GPAs and MCAT scores as predictors of NBME I and clerkship performances based on students' data from one undergraduate institution. *Academic Medicine, 72*(5), 394–396.

Sladek, R. M., Bond, M. J., Frost, L. K., & Prior, K. N. (2016). Predicting success in medical school: A longitudinal study of common Australian student selection tools. *BioMed Central Medical Education, 16*, 187.

Thomas, A., Young, M. E., Mazer, B. L., Lubarsky, S. E., & Razack, S. I. (2015). Candidates' and interviewers' perceptions of multiple-mini interviews for admission to an occupational therapy professional program. *Occupational Therapy Health Care, 29*(2), 186–200.

Tran, T., & Blackman, M. C. (2006). The dynamics and validity of the group selection interview. *Journal of Social Psychology, 146*(2), 183–201.

Urban Universities for Health. (2014). *Holistic admissions in the health professions findings from a national survey*. Washington, DC.

Utzman, R. R., Riddle, D. L., & Jewell, D. V. (2007a). Use of demographic and quantitative admissions data to predict academic difficulty among professional physical therapist students. *Physical Therapy*, *87*(9), 1164–1180.

Utzman, R. R., Riddle, D. L., & Jewell, D. V. (2007b). Use of demographic and quantitative admissions data to predict performance on the national physical therapy examination. *Physical Therapy*, *87*(9), 1181–1193.

Wilkinson, D., Zhang, J., Byrne, G. J., Luke, H., Ozolins, I. Z., Parker, M. H., & Peterson, R. F. (2008). Medical school selection criteria and the prediction of academic performance. *Medical Journal of Australia*, *188*(6), 349–354.

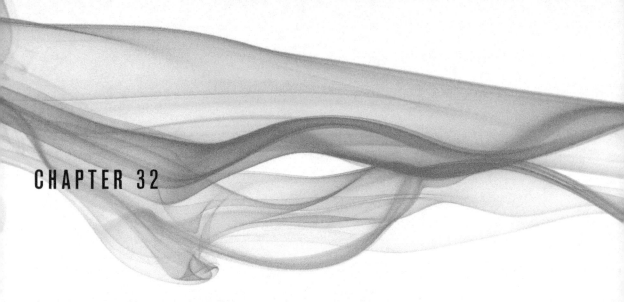

CHAPTER 32

Legal Matters for the Health Professions Educator

Gerald R. Weniger and John F. Knight

CHAPTER OBJECTIVES

- Review common legal issues in academia, including those related to the Family Educational Rights and Privacy Act (FERPA), Americans with Disabilities Act (ADA)
- Understand Title IX, academic freedom, academic dishonesty, and professionalism
- Describe best practices in management of litigation, public relations, and potential lawsuits

---

Academic freedom is but a facet of freedom in the larger society.

—*R. M. Pritchard*

OVERVIEW OF LAW IN HIGHER EDUCATION

Systems of Law

A great many aspects of the world are overwhelmed with laws and regulations, policies and procedures, risks, and insurance to provide protection against the liability associated with those risks. Those practicing in the health professions know this well. Those teaching in health professions programs in colleges and universities face the same reality, although some of the legal impositions may be different.

To successfully teach within an institution of higher education it is essential that instructors have not only a mastery of the subject matter, but also a firm understanding of the various laws within this complex system that regulates education—knowing not only what to teach and how to teach it, but also what schools and instructors must do and must refrain from doing in the course of such teaching. Academic programs involve a diverse population of students who may present with many challenges to instructors and administrators—challenges that the students themselves may need to overcome.

Overlaying all this is a framework of legal requirements and prohibitions that directly and significantly impact how you can, and should, educate and train students entering health professions. It can be daunting, especially given the many sources of requirements and prohibitions and the frequency with which they change. It is critical for anyone working in higher education to be familiar with a number of federal statutes and the manner in which those laws are implemented and interpreted. The most significant of these laws are discussed in this chapter. In addition, it is essential that health professionals new to the academic setting become familiar with applicable state laws and university policies specifically related to educational environments in general, and to students specifically. These are beyond the scope of this chapter given the sheer volume and potential variance among them. It is highly recommended that faculty members consult with the legal counsel of the university, if available, and request information or training specific to the state and institution. Furthermore, one would be wise to obtain copies or summaries of any risk management and/or insurance policies that cover the activities completed on behalf of the institution as a practitioner and educator.

Variations in Academic Settings

According to the U.S. Department of Education, there are approximately 4,726 degree-granting institutions in the United States (U.S. Department of Education, 2016). This includes both community colleges and 4-year institutions, and it includes both private and public schools. The fundamental difference between public and private institutions lies in how they are funded. This difference affects students because funding is directly tied to the cost of tuition. State governments help finance the operating costs of public institutions of higher education; therefore, tuition prices are generally lower at state schools because of this infusion of taxpayer money. Most public colleges and universities were established by state governments to give citizens the opportunity to receive an affordable college education. What seems like a cost of attendance is really a subsidized amount because funds raised from tuition do not need to cover all expenses of the institution. Conversely, private institutions do not receive state funding and therefore rely more heavily on tuition, donations, and private contributions to the school. This also means that tuition rates are generally much higher (The Pew Charitable Trusts, 2015).

There are other differences between public and private institutions—mostly the size of their enrollment and the number of degrees they offer. A comparison of characteristics of public and private institutions of higher education is shown in Table 32.1.

Variations in Governance

In the United States, a governing board is a group that oversees the affairs and activities of an organization, corporation, or institution. Most colleges and universities are directed and managed by a governing board. This includes both private and public institutions. Board members may be appointed by the state governor or the institution itself. Boards vary in size, power, membership, and especially in formal name. In fact, over time the terminology that is used to describe those who serve on governing boards, and those who lead them, has changed dramatically. In the nonprofit sector, it is common for a governing board to be called a *board of directors*. This has always been confusing, however, because it does not comprise individuals who call themselves *directors*, but rather individuals who are considered *members*. This is because when one hears the term director it often implies a position of leadership, rather than membership.

TABLE 32.1 Characteristics of Public Versus Private Institutions of Higher Education

Public Institutions	Private Institutions
• Larger enrollment (often > 10,000)	• Smaller enrollment (often <2,000)
• Larger class size, especially in general education courses	• Smaller class size
• Possibly reduced access to professors (due to class size)	• Possibly increased access to professors
• Wide range of majors	• Small range of majors, may put emphasis on specific fields (e.g., liberal arts)
• Often research intensive	• Research focus/subsidy varies
• Secular foundation	• May have religious affiliation
• May have principles of community that guide student, faculty conduct	• May have moral code that guides student, faculty conduct

Source: Adapted from Douglas (2006) and Peterson's Staff (2015).

Other terms that are used, especially in higher education settings, include *board of regents*, *board of governors*, or *board of trustees*. In most cases regents are the same as members, directors, governors, or trustees. There are some who believe the term *trustee* indicates more of a safekeeping role and is therefore a more appropriate term for nonprofit organizations as opposed to the for-profit sector. There are also some who believe that director is a more favorable term for the business sector because it conveys leadership rather than followership. Trustee more than any of the other terms tends to have a positive connotation that conveys attitudes of trust and altruism—traits associated with a higher purpose. In the business world though, trustee is a legal term. Therefore, it can be problematic for a board member to use the title of trustee because it implies that the member is accountable to state trust laws. Legally speaking, a trustee can be held liable for simple acts of negligence. To make things more confusing, there remain even more variations in what members of governing boards are called. Other examples include *board of overseers*, *board of curators*, *board of supervisors*, and *board of visitors*.

The head-of-the-board position is the second area where changing terminology over time has left things unclear and complicated. Several decades ago, the highest paid employee of an organization in the nonprofit sector was referred to as the *general secretary*. Later the title *executive secretary* also surfaced. Now it is common for this person to be called an *executive director*. This is a term that better conveys the leadership aspect of the position. In the for-profit sector, the titles *president* or *chief executive officer* (CEO) are more common, although many nonprofit leaders have also adopted these two terms. One could speculate that the shift from two previously favorable terms that both included the word *secretary*, to the terms director, CEO, or president could be the result of the executive moving away from a subservient role to more of a leadership role. This means that boards expect more leadership from the president or director rather than simply serving the will of the other members.

KEY LEGAL ISSUES FOR HEALTH PROFESSIONAL PROGRAMS

Academic Freedom

The term *academy* is sometimes used to refer to the entirety of faculty among colleges and universities. Academic freedom is a concept that many consider fundamental to the mission of the academy. It is unclear where the concept originated from but in the United States it was first well defined in 1940 by a statement of principles on academic freedom and tenure that was released by the American Association of University Professors and the Association of American Colleges and Universities (Brown & Kurland, 1990).

Academic freedom is the belief that faculty members should have the freedom to explore and inquire; therefore, it safeguards academic institutions as places where critical inquiry and academic debate can take place. It allows professors to teach or communicate ideas and philosophies that may be inconvenient or considered troublesome by external groups, including the government. In essence, a violation of academic freedom is an interference with the subject matter that is taught and/or discussed within academic institutions (Brown & Kurland, 1990). As former Supreme Court Justice William O. Douglas said, "The most important aspect of freedom of speech is freedom to learn. All education is a continuous dialogue—questions and answers that pursue every problem on the horizon. That is the essence of academic freedom, of all scientific inquiry" (Komlik, 2015).

Supporters of academic freedom believe that the academy should be allowed to control the flow of information. This places the responsibility to protect this right on academic institutions and the faculty themselves. Academic freedom and freedom of speech (which is guaranteed by the First Amendment to the Constitution) are very similar but not identical ideas. Supporters of academic freedom believe that faculty should have the freedom to teach ideas without being threatened with termination of employment. However, although university professors have the constitutional right to free speech, free-speech rights do not guarantee employment of a faculty member at a university. Academic freedom is itself not a legal concept. Academic freedom allows for faculty to express their expert opinions in teaching and scholarship, but it is not an unrestricted free-speech right (Brown & Kurland, 1990; Byrne, 1989; Komlik, 2015; Poch, 1993). Therefore, professors must still exercise their professional judgment.

Does academic freedom lie with the institution or with the individual? A 1978 landmark legal case (*Regents of the University of California vs. Bakke*, 1978) determined that the academic institution has the right to determine who may teach, who may be taught, and how information should be taught. Therefore, the authority to define and enforce academic freedom rests with each academic institution. It is also important to remember that faculty members have academic freedom in a professional capacity only, not as individuals. Academic freedom is not the right to be able to teach or discuss whatever one pleases, whenever one pleases. In public settings, professors and university administrators must indicate that what is being said is their own personal viewpoint and does not represent the opinions of the institutions that they are affiliated with. In addition, academic institutions may specifically limit academic freedom for religious beliefs of faculty as long as this is unequivocally stated in writing at the time of appointment.

Academic freedom is closely tied to the concept of tenure. Without job security, academic freedom is an ideal that is often not a reality for nontenured faculty. Therefore, tenure protects academic freedom by ensuring that professors can only be fired from an academic institution for reasons such as gross professional misconduct or the inability to perform his or her job duties. Academic freedom should be defended by the faculty of a university. Faculty may choose to establish committees or workgroups to dispute any attempt to undermine academic freedom. Professors should also endeavor to develop policies and a campus culture that supports and encourages academic freedom (Brown & Kurland, 1990).

Academic Dishonesty

Academic dishonesty is a comprehensive term that includes both cheating and plagiarism. At the root of all academic dishonesty is bearing false witness, otherwise known as *being deceitful, lying,* or *not telling the truth.* According to the *Oxford Living Dictionary plagiarism* means to take someone else's work or ideas and to passing those words off as one's own. Plagiarism is therefore a derivative of lying because one is not being truthful about who completed the work. Cheating on exams, quizzes, or assignments is also lying at its root, because one is lying about who truly knows (or does not know) the information.

Most educators would agree that academic dishonesty is a major problem among students. One study by Hamlin, Barczyk, Powell, and Frost (2013) revealed that "at some point during their academic careers, estimates are that 50–70% of all college students engage in cheating, plagiarism and other forms of dishonesty" (p. 35). Most educational institutions have specific policies on academic dishonesty and also have a committee that enforces the policies. The specifics on policy enforcement vary per institution. However, having an independent campus department or division (e.g., Student Judicial Affairs) is considered very important, otherwise faculty members find themselves as the enforcers. Faculty enforcement of academic honesty policies can lead to a conflict of interest, as students who were disciplined for academic dishonesty may take out their frustration and anger on the faculty member in the form of poor evaluations. This, in turn, is problematic because faculty course evaluations typically play a vital role in the tenure and promotion process.

Burnett, Enyeart Smith, and Wessel (2016, p. 63) performed a qualitative study using focus groups of undergraduate health science students. They found that students had justified cheating as a social norm because "everyone cheats everywhere" and "every school has cheaters." The respondents also self-reported a high degree of "pressure" to obtain acceptance into graduate programs and professional schools that also influenced their decision to cheat. The authors' concern was that cheating in an academic setting would likely transfer to dishonest behavior in their future health professions.

In a 2013 review article, Kusnoor and Falik examined cheating in medical school. There was a wide range of variability—the reported prevalence of cheating within medical schools was 0% to 58%. Nevertheless, their article broadly assessed many types of cheating, well beyond simply cheating on exams or plagiarism. The authors considered the use of unauthorized notes, the sharing of information about practical exams, and dishonesty about parts of a physical exam performed or not performed as cheating as well. The aggregate data from two medical schools had an overall response rate of 95%, and the authors found that almost 88% of participants cheated at least once during their undergraduate studies and 58% cheated at least once during medical school. It was postulated that two key factors may encourage dishonest behavior in this population: pressure to succeed and an inadequate understanding of what constitutes cheating (Kusnoor & Falik, 2013). Among nursing students, Krueger (2014) found that more than 50% reported having cheated on exams or during clinical experiences. Similarly, Hegmann (2008) found that 57% of physician assistant (PA) students self-reported cheating behaviors on patient encounter logs.

In conclusion, cheating and plagiarism are widespread within academia. A large percentage of students have normalized dishonesty. The belief that cheating "does not hurt anyone" is widespread and lends itself to the belief that cheating and plagiarism are acceptable (Kraus, 2002; Menon & Sharland, 2011). Students may not understand that they are hurting themselves by short-changing their own education and are potentially putting their future patients in harm's way. Educators are the gatekeepers of academic integrity, responsible for modeling ethical behavior to their students and for teaching the principles of ethical behavior as well.

Professionalism

What is a *profession*? Loosely, it is simply any occupation, and more specifically it is a vocation or occupation requiring advanced training, involving certain skills. Some may go slightly further and define a profession as an occupation that is formally qualified in some way. This formal qualification could be a specialized degree from an accredited institution, a passing score on a specialized exam, or the need to possess a state license and/or national certification to practice. Typically, some component of the required advanced education consists of training in ethics, moral codes, conduct, and behavior. So, what is professionalism? Loosely, professionalism is the practice of being a professional. More specific, professionalism encompasses the conduct, skills, civility, and wise discernment that are expected from any professional.

In an ideal sense, one can assume that all health professions aspire to maintain the highest standards of professionalism. More realistic, since professions are made up of people, a professional's individual level of success and failure will most certainly vary. It is often when patients are suffering or in their most vulnerable state that they are interacting with health professionals. Consider this: Patients are undressed and touched by the health professional, invasive procedures are performed, personal space is invaded, and matters of life and death are discussed. For these reasons, the general public expects a high level of professionalism from health professionals. Most health professions have some type of standard—a code of ethics or code of conduct—to which they ascribe as part of joining the profession. Typically, becoming a member and remaining a member of the profession demands strict adherence to these codes. In general, the profession is strengthened when the ethical standards of the profession are elevated and enforced.

Sometimes conflict arises when a profession's code of ethics clashes with a person's own personal code of ethics or behavior. In the health professions, common examples of some of these issues are end-of-life decisions, organ donation, stem cell use, assisted suicide, and abortion—just to name a few. These also tend to be the situations in which professionalism crosses into the realm of legal matters. Because health professionals encounter many complicated ethical situations with legal implications, a certain level of honesty and integrity must be expected of students in health professions programs. Admissions committees *must* take this into account by assessing professionalism in some way prior to admittance. A high level of integrity is also necessary because many health professionals will have access to dangerous substances in the form of medications and drugs. Therefore, health professions programs must develop and adhere to consistent policies regarding the admission of any applicant with a prior history of felony conviction, including illegal drug use.

What can often be difficult for a student to understand is the expectation that individual health professionals are accountable to their professional codes of ethics in both their public and private lives. The physician, nurse, PA, or pharmacist who is ethical in all parts of his or her daily practice but is arrested for driving under the influence (DUI) over the weekend is still subject to legal sanctions that will affect his or her practice. The nurse who violates the Health Insurance Portability and Accountability Act of 1996 (HIPAA) in the form of an inappropriate Facebook post on his or her personal account will still face the loss of professional privileges, the loss of employment, and potentially even litigation. It is imperative that students understand that choices and behavior in their personal lives can very much affect their professional careers.

These same sanctions apply to health professions students. Ethical or legal violations that occur during the academic program may violate university policies and result in dismissal from school, thus preventing graduation. Should a student successfully complete the health professions program despite an ethical or legal violation, the student may still face sanction from the state licensing board. Such sanction may prevent licensure or result in a restricted license.

Investigating Breaches of Professionalism

Health professionals have been inherently granted the right to self-govern the regulations and responsibilities of their individual professions. Actual enforcement of ethical standards and professional conduct is formally done within the legal system. Each state has laws that require health professionals to practice under a license that is granted by the state government. Requiring this license to practice is what allows the profession to maintain control and, in effect, self-govern because a license can be revoked when ethical standards are violated. State law varies, but most require health professionals to report any clinician who is exhibiting behavior that may interfere with his or her ability to practice to the appropriate licensing board. Because many health professions programs are prelicensure (e.g., medical, pharmacy, PA, social work, prelicensure nursing), students are not under the direct jurisdiction of state licensing boards. Therefore, health professions programs must have a committee or board that handles student violations of ethical or professional standards. Standard policies and procedures must be adopted to ensure due process and students' rights in the adjudication of any alleged violations.

Family Educational Rights and Privacy Act

FERPA, 20 U.S.C. § 1232g, may be one of the most frequently cited and yet least understood laws applicable to educational institutions. It establishes requirements regarding universities' maintenance of student educational records and limitations on the use and disclosure of those records. FERPA and its implementing regulations, 34 C.F.R. Part 99, apply to all private and public educational institutions that receive federal funds from the U.S. Department of Education or whose students receive federal funds and pay them to the institution (U.S. Department of Education, n.d.).

Student Rights Under FERPA

FERPA establishes several important rights for university students, the three most significant being: (a) the right to inspect their own records, (b) the right to request corrections to the records if they contain inaccurate information, and (c) restriction on the ability of others to access a student's records unless an exception applies. Of these three, regulation of the disclosure of students' education records causes the biggest day-to-day impact on the actions of educators and administrators (U.S. Department of Education, n.d.).

Information from educational records may be disclosed to any person or entity with specific consent of the student. Generally, FERPA prohibits the disclosure of personally identifiable information in a student's education record without the student's consent unless an exception to the law's general consent requirement applies. Personally identifiable information includes name, address, personal identifiers like Social Security number or date of birth, or any information that could be used alone or in combination to identify a student. FERPA also permits students to have access to, and correct inaccurate information in, their student record. *Education records* are records that are directly related to a student and maintained by an educational institution (U.S. Department of Education, n.d.).

Potential Sanctions for FERPA Violations

Violations of FERPA or its regulations may result in federal fines and/or a loss of federal funding to the school. In addition, individual employees may face legal or institutional penalties for FERPA violations, including temporary suspension, termination of employment, or possible prosecution under criminal codes. FERPA does not include a private cause of action; students may not bring a lawsuit to enforce the Act's provisions or to seek a remedy for violations of the Act. In *Gonzaga University v. Doe*, 536 U.S. 273 (2002), the U.S. Supreme Court ruled that Congress had not created a private right of action under FERPA.

Exceptions to FERPA Nondisclosure Rules

An educator or administrator is likely to encounter situations in which the disclosure of information from a student's education record without consent could be convenient and some in which such disclosure could be exceedingly necessary. Thus, there are multiple exceptions to FERPA's nondisclosure rule, discussed in the following sections. FERPA requires institution-specific policies regarding these exceptions. Therefore, it is incumbent upon educators to familiarize themselves with their institutions' policies and procedures.

General Directory Information   Directory information about a student may be disclosed without consent unless a student has informed the school that he or she does not wish for such information to be disclosed. Directory information is information contained in a student's education record that would not generally be considered harmful or an invasion of privacy if disclosed. For the most part, this information can be shared freely unless the student has specifically elected to have his or her directory information withheld. FERPA requires each institution to define its directory items, therefore one should refer to each individual institution's policy (U.S. Department of Education, n.d.).

Officials with Legitimate Educational Interests   Records may also be disclosed to "school officials with legitimate educational interests." The law does not, however, define who these school officials are or how to determine what constitutes a legitimate educational interest. Each university should have policies or written criteria for determining which persons and/or situations fit this exception. In essence, a legitimate educational interest is one that is necessary for a university employee to carry out his or her responsibilities in support of the institution's mission. This could be to evaluate a student's academic performance, provide academic or career advising, institute discipline for misconduct, or potentially for other reasons (U.S. Department of Education, n.d.).

Disclosure in Emergency Situations   FERPA permits disclosure without written consent in certain emergency situations if the information is necessary to protect the health and safety of the student or other individuals. Campus safety is a top priority for educational institutions and when a student's conduct or written or verbal communication raise concerns about his or her safety or the safety of others, disclosing records may be necessary to prevent harm from occurring. Safety concerns prompting disclosure may arise from a student's making statements about suicide, demonstrating unusual angry and/or erratic behavior, or other conduct that reasonably would cause someone to see the student as posing a risk of serious harm. It is important to note that FERPA does not prohibit anyone from disclosing his or her own personal observations of or describing interactions with a student. FERPA addresses the disclosure of information from education records—not behavior one has observed (U.S. Department of Education, n.d.).

OVERVIEW OF TITLE IX

Title IX of the Education Amendments of 1972 (Title IX) is a federal civil rights law that prohibits discrimination, including harassment and sexual violence, on the basis of gender in all of its educational programs and activities that receive federal financial assistance. This includes academics, employment, athletics, and other extracurricular activities at the institution. If only one of an educational institution's programs or activities receives federal funding, all of the programs within the institution must comply with Title IX and its implementing regulations. It protects any person from gender-based discrimination, regardless of his or her real or perceived gender, gender identity, or gender expression.

Examples of sex- or gender-based discrimination include allegations of different admission treatment to certain academic programs because of gender or gender identity, repeated comments of a sexual nature from one individual to or about another, a faculty member requesting or demanding sexual favors from a student while stating or implying that refusal may impact a grade or the student's standing in the academic program, determining assignment to clinical placements based on students' gender, or other similar circumstances. It also includes instances of sexual misconduct and sexual violence.

Title IX requires that a university, upon becoming aware of any incident of sexual harassment and misconduct, respond appropriately to protect and maintain the safety of the university community, including students, faculty, and staff. Schools must take immediate steps to address any gender discrimination, harassment, or violence to prevent it from affecting students further. If a school knows about or should reasonably know about gender-based discrimination, harassment, or violence that is creating a hostile environment, it must act to eliminate it, remedy the harm, and prevent it from recurring. This response requirement also applies to students who are completing internships or clinical placements in facilities off-campus or not directly affiliated with the school.

Every school must have a Title IX coordinator who manages gender discrimination complaints and an established procedure for handling those complaints. It is important that all members of a university community, especially employees of the university, know who the coordinator is and have a basic understanding of the complaint process and what resources may be available to victims, or know who can provide such information.

Faculty and staff members should consult with legal counsel and/or the Title IX coordinator to ensure they have an understanding of their reporting obligations in light of the law's requirement to take immediate action in response to instances of sexual harassment and sexual violence. These actions are the school's responsibility whether or not the individual who was harassed makes a complaint or otherwise asks the school to take action; reasonable steps to promptly respond are still required.

Some states have also passed their own statutes specifically aimed at reducing sexual violence on college campuses and each university is likely to have differences in policy and procedure, so faculty and staff ought to seek out information on the laws and rules unique to their campuses to ensure a proper response to reports of gender-based discrimination.

THE AMERICANS WITH DISABILITIES ACT

The ADA (US House of Representatives, 1990) and the Rehabilitation Act of 1973 were established to provide a clear comprehensive national mandate for the elimination of discrimination against individuals with disabilities. Section 504 is the section of the Rehabilitation Act of 1973 that specifically created civil rights for individuals with disabilities. Section 504 provides that no qualified individual with a disability should, only by reason of his or her disability, be excluded from the participation in, be denied the benefits of, or be subjected to discrimination under any program or activity receiving federal financial assistance (U.S. Department of Labor, n.d.-a).

Prohibition of Discrimination

The ADA, enacted in 1990, prohibits discrimination solely on the basis of disability in employment, public services, and accommodations. The person must be otherwise qualified for the program, service, or job. The ADA details administrative requirements, complaint procedures, and the consequences for noncompliance related to both services and employment. The ADA requires provision of reasonable effective accommodations for eligible students across educational activities and settings (Gordon & Keiser, 2000).

Definition of *Disability*

An individual with a disability is defined as a person who (a) has a physical or mental impairment that substantially limits one or more life activities, (b) has a record of such impairment, or (c) is regarded as having such impairment. Major life activities include but are not limited to walking, seeing, hearing, speaking, breathing, learning, working, caring for oneself, and performing manual tasks (U.S. Department of Labor, n.d.-b).

Types of Disabilities

The need for accommodations may arise in a variety of ways. Students with physical disabilities may need an accommodation in order to access certain buildings, classrooms, or lab spaces on campus. They may also need an accommodation in order to access facilities connected with a clinical placement or internship. Students with learning disabilities, psychiatric disabilities, or other nonphysical disabilities may likewise require some type of accommodation to fully participate in or have equal access to the benefits of higher education and the components thereof: academic courses and activities, training programs, examinations, and coursework (Orr & Hammig, 2009).

Reasonable Accommodations

Students with disabilities are entitled to access, support, and, when appropriate, reasonable accommodations. Reasonable and appropriate accommodations are determined based on a variety of factors, all of which should be considered in determining whether a student is disabled as defined by the ADA. These factors include the submitted documentation supporting a specific diagnosis, evaluation of a student's strengths and weaknesses, and specific course or classroom requirements. A reasonable accommodation is any modification or adjustment to academic program requirements, class assignments, and so forth that will enable the student to fully participate and have equal access to the educational benefits of his or her university and academic program (Gordon & Keiser, 2000). Accommodations can take many forms: preferential seating in a classroom; use of a notetaker or recording device in class; exams given in alternate format; extended time for test taking; exams individually proctored in a separate, quiet, and nondistracting room; substitute assignments offered in specific circumstances; use of assistive listening devices; and many others (Getzel, 2008). An accommodation is not reasonable if making the accommodation means making a substantial change in an essential nature of a program or an element of the curriculum. Accommodations are also not reasonable if they impose an undue financial or administrative burden or create a direct threat to the health or safety of others. Again, consultation with university legal counsel and an institution's office of disability services can help determine what is reasonable and whether accommodations are required at all.

Determination of Eligibility

In order to demonstrate eligibility for an accommodation a student will need to provide documentation of a recognized disability from a qualified professional. A qualified professional may be a physician, educational diagnostician, licensed psychologist, psychiatrist, or another individual qualified to make a determination of a disability. Having a medical condition alone is not enough to make a student eligible for an accommodation. To participate in specific academic programs such as the health sciences, a student must also still show that he or she is qualified.

Under the ADA, a "qualified individual with a disability is one who, with or without reasonable modification to rules, policies, or practices, the removal of architectural, communication, or transportation barriers, or the provisions of auxiliary aids and services, meets the essential eligibility requirements for the receipt of services or participation in programs or activities provided by a public entity" (ADA, PL101-336).

An institution should have established policies and procedures for an interactive process with students who request accommodations to determine whether they are (a) required, (b) reasonable, and (c) effective. It is the responsibility of individual instructors to provide accommodations determined to be reasonable. It is the student's responsibility to fulfill the academic requirements of the course. This interactive process applies to accommodations in traditional classroom settings, laboratory settings, and clinical placements or internships.

Students with disabilities have legal remedies available in the event of a university's noncompliance. Thus, individuals who are discriminated against may file a complaint with the relevant federal agency or sue in federal court. Where possible, enforcement agencies encourage informal mediation and voluntary compliance.

HEALTH INSURANCE PORTABILITY AND ACCOUNTABILITY ACT OF 1996

HIPAA regulates health care providers (covered entities [CEs]) that electronically maintain or transmit protected health information (PHI) in connection with a covered transaction. HIPAA requires each CE to maintain reasonable and appropriate administrative, technical, and physical safeguards for privacy and security. Entities or individuals who contract to perform services for a CE with access to PHI (business associates) are also required to comply with the HIPAA privacy and security standards. HIPAA does preempt state laws that conflict with its provisions, but state privacy laws that are more protective of individuals' health care information are not preempted.

HIPAA's Privacy Rule creates compliance, training, and information protection issues for universities. An in-depth review of HIPAA is beyond the scope of this chapter, and the majority of health professionals are likely already familiar with HIPAA and its requirements. Within the academic setting, the largest burden with regard to HIPAA is typically ensuring that students are also fully aware of those requirements, in particular before they report to clinical placement or internship sites.

Often universities enter into affiliation agreements, memoranda of understanding, or business associate agreements with medical and health service providers specifically to form relationships for the purpose of creating internships and clinical placements. These agreements also establish the obligations for the site and the school with respect to the training and academic training of students. Typically, these agreements address the sharing of student records for the purpose of evaluating students' performance and set forth the obligations of the school and individual students for compliance with HIPAA regarding the protection of patient privacy as well as awareness of and compliance with a facility's training, treatment, and record-keeping policies. Careful review of such agreements is essential. Individual students, staff, and faculty, as well as the university, may face civil and criminal penalties for violations of HIPAA's Privacy Rule. Regular consultation with your institution's legal counsel is recommended.

CONCLUSIONS

Health professions programs involve a diverse population of faculty, staff, and students who may present many legal challenges to an institution. In order to successfully teach within an institution of higher education, it is essential that health professions educators have not only a mastery of the subject matter, but also a firm understanding of the various laws within this complex system that regulates education. Common legal challenges include cheating and plagiarism, professionalism, academic dishonesty and academic freedom, diversity, inclusion, and equity. Educators also need to be familiar with laws that relate to FERPA, HIPAA, ADA, and Title IX. When in doubt, always seek guidance from your institution's legal counsel. Higher education attorneys provide effective counsel and can help individual faculty in the understanding of legal issues surrounding academia.

REFERENCES

Brown, R. S., & Kurland, J. E. (1990). Academic tenure and academic freedom. *Law and Contemporary Problems, 53*(3), 325–355.

Burnett, A. J., Enyeart Smith, T. M., & Wessel, M. T. (2016). Use of the social cognitive theory to frame university students' perceptions of cheating. *Journal of Academic Ethics, 14*(1), 49–69.

Byrne, J. P. (1989). Academic freedom: A "special concern of the First Amendment." *Yale Law Journal, 99*(2), 251–340.

Douglas, M. (2006). Public and private: What's the difference? Inside Higher Ed. Retrieved from https://www.insidehighered.com/views/2006/03/06/lombardi

Family Rights and Education Act, 20 U.S.C. § 1232g. (1974).

Getzel, E. E. (2008). Addressing the persistence and retention of students with disabilities in higher education: Incorporating key strategies and supports on campus. *Exceptionality, 16*(4), 207–219.

Gonzaga University v. Doe, 536 U.S. 273. (2002). Retrieved from https://supreme.justia.com/cases/federal/us/536/273/case.html

Gordon, M., & Keiser, S. (Eds.). (2000). *Accommodations in higher education under the Americans with Disabilities Act (ADA): A no-nonsense guide for clinicians, educators, administrators, and lawyers.* New York, NY: Guilford Press.

Hamlin, A., Barczyk, C., Powell, G., & Frost, J. (2013). A comparison of university efforts to contain academic dishonesty. *Journal of Legal, Ethical and Regulatory Issues, 16*(1), 35.

Hegmann, T. E. (2008). Cheating by physician assistant students on patient encounter logs. *Journal of Physician Assistant Education, 19*(2), 4–9.

Komlik, O. (2015). What is academic freedom? Economic Sociology and Political Economy. Retrieved from https://economicsociology.org/2015/03/04/what-is-academic-freedom

Kraus, J. (2002). Rethinking plagiarism: What our students are telling us when they cheat. *Issues in Writing, 13*(1), 80.

Krueger, L. (2014). Academic dishonesty among nursing students. *Journal of Nursing Education, 53*(2), 77–87.

Kusnoor, A. V., & Falik, R. (2013). Cheating in medical school: the unacknowledged ailment. *Southern Medical Journal, 106*(8), 479–83.

Menon, M. K., & Sharland, A. (2011). Narcissism, exploitative attitudes, and academic dishonesty: An exploratory investigation of reality versus myth. *Journal of Education for Business, 86*(1), 50–55.

Orr, A. C., & Hammig, S. B. (2009). Inclusive postsecondary strategies for teaching students with learning disabilities: A review of the literature. *Learning Disability Quarterly, 32*(3), 181–196.

Peterson's Staff. (2015). Public university vs. private college. Retrieved from https://www.petersons.com/college-search/public-university-vs-private.aspx

The Pew Charitable Trusts. (2015). Federal and state funding of higher education: A changing landscape. Retrieved from http://www.pewtrusts.org/en/research-and-analysis/issue-briefs/2015/06/federal-and-state-funding-of-higher-education

Plagiarism. (n.d.). In *Oxford Living Dictionaries* (online). Retrieved from https://en.oxforddictionaries.com/definition/plagiarism

Poch, R. K. (1993). *Academic freedom in American higher education: Rights, responsibilities, and limitations.* San Francisco, CA: Jossey-Bass.

Pritchard, R. M. (1998). Academic freedom and autonomy in the United Kingdom and Germany. *Minerva, 36*(2), 101–124.

Profession. (n.d.-a). In *Merriam-Webster's* online dictionary. Retrieved from http://www.yourdictionary.com/profession#websters

Profession (n.d.-b). In *Oxford Living Dictionaries* (online). Retrieved from https://en.oxforddictionaries.com/definition/profession

Regents of the University of California vs. Bakke, 438 U.S. 265. (1978). Retrieved from https://supreme
.justia.com/cases/federal/us/438/265

U.S. Department of Education (n.d.). Family Education Rights and Privacy Act (FERPA). Retrieved
from https://www2.ed.gov/policy/gen/guid/fpco/ferpa/index.html

U.S. Department of Education, National Center for Education Statistics. (2016). Digest of Education
Statistics, 2014 (NCES 2016–006). Retrieved from https://nces.ed.gov/fastfacts/display.asp?id=84

U.S. Department of Labor. (n.d.-a). Section 504, Rehabilitation Act of 1973. Retrieved from https://www
.dol.gov/oasam/regs/statutes/sec504.htm

U.S. Department of Labor. (n.d.-b). Americans With Disabilities Act. Retrieved from https://www.dol
.gov/general/topic/disability/ada

U.S. House of Representatives. (1990). *Americans With Disabilities Act, Pub. L. No. 101–336*. Retrieved from
http://library.clerk.house.gov/reference-files/PPL_101_336_AmericansWithDisabilities.pdf

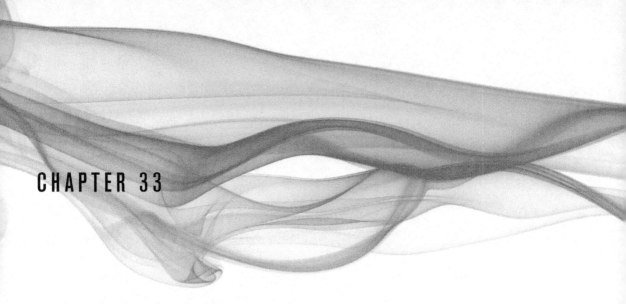

CHAPTER 33

Creating a Culture of Restorative Justice

Joao Salm, Gerald Kayingo, and Virginia McCoy Hass

CHAPTER OBJECTIVE

- Apply habits of the heart and mind to create a culture of restorative justice for students, faculty, and staff
- Review the core principles and best practices of restorative justice such as peacemaking circles

---

Justice is what we discover, you and I, when we walk together, listen together and even love one another in our curiosity about what justice is and where justice comes from.

—Socrates

Let us begin with a story. I was admitted to a hospital with an acute illness. The pain and the anxiety were pretty intense. Despite the rigid rules and regulations of the hospital and my fragile condition, I knew I had to engage my health care providers in my recovery process. This was about justice—a collective healing process for all of us—and we needed to be in it together, with a bond, in relation to one another. My efforts to engage these professionals were mostly effective. It was evident that their work had meaning for them, was part of a sense of accomplishment, which is its own reward. Their care followed values that reside in the human heart and mind, such as kindness and compassion.

But unfortunately, Dr. X did not follow suit. She seemed cold and distant, apparently tied closer to medical checklists than to me. She was an excellent professional, probably the best in the business, but our relationship, if there was one, lacked engagement, dialogue, and compassion. As the days went by, I felt neglected by Dr. X, despite her telling me I would be released only when she had "covered all the bases and done all her due diligence." I thought about calling the hospital administration and telling them I no longer wanted Dr. X's services. What bothered me most was that she appeared to lack those habits of the heart I knew she must have within her. As an "advocate for restorative justice" who needed health care, I was frustrated. Then I started to notice that the conflict between us could be worked on if I coaxed her to share her humanity as I did mine—through dialogue, storytelling, even an occasional joke—and I set my mind on bringing out the human in this excellent professional.

By the weekend, I had a plan. I would strengthen my relationship with her, and we would share our habits of the heart—compassion, care, and mutual respect—and justice would be constructed by both of us, a concept I had learned from the indigenous people of Canada. So, I started sharing my stories, my concerns, my thoughts on my situation. There was no dramatic response, but the first day she stayed longer than she usually did. On the second day, I told her I felt good when she came by and talked to me, shared some updates, and I then started asking her about her professional life. She hesitated, then shared a little, just enough to start warming up. I also engaged her in conversation with my visiting friends. Every now and then I cracked a joke and she would smile. When she came by on the third day, she said: "Last night I was thinking about you," and I felt she was transitioning to thinking of me in a relational way. From then on, my engagement with her strengthened, as did my emotional and physical state.

I was gratified to discover that even under such initially hostile circumstances, Dr. X and I could strengthen our relationship and construct a sense of healing and justice together. My physical care was directly related to my relational care, which made my healing experience rich for body and mind. This experience inspired me to share the concept of restorative justice with health care workers who are passionate about caring for others.

In this chapter we consider possibilities for creating a culture of restorative justice by empowering students, faculty, and staff not only for conflict resolution, but for living the principles and practices of restorative justice throughout all aspects of their lives. We observe how health care workers can strive to make their work meaningful through values and relationships, and that healing can be accomplished by creating interactions that foster compassion, interconnection, and collective decision making.

We examine the five main guiding principles of restorative justice—*humanizing values, strengthening relationships, sharing responsibility, addressing harm,* and *strengthening community*—and how putting these principles into action through dialogue, inclusion, and understanding can make a difference in the lives of the people we serve. Then we consider how creativity, innovation, and a sense of action can begin to transform the way we perceive and face our challenges during social interactions. We conclude by examining the idea that resisting the institutional mind-set can help us cultivate habits of the heart and mind to achieve a restorative and healing justice.

WHAT IS RESTORATIVE JUSTICE?

The concept of restorative justice has been highly debated. In a very broad sense, restorative justice is justice based on a set of principles and practices that allow us to humanize and be humanized—in other words, to act, to participate, to dialogue, to engage, and to make decisions with others, anywhere and at any time. Restorative justice invites us to heal collectively, in our curiosities about one another, without hostility, vengeance, or the infliction of pain on others. Restorative justice focuses on our human potential, the habits within our hearts and minds that can lead to great things (Doolin, 2007; Karp 2015). Thus, we can find restorative justice anywhere. To do so, we need to consciously bring out restorative habits from our hearts and minds in the face of challenges, especially in institutions that tend to break down relationships and collective responsibility, and that prevent the possibility of shared decision making. Restorative justice is less about the setting and more about holding, carrying, and living those principles and practices with a sense of interconnectedness. Still, context matters (Stout & Salm 2011); if we are to implement these value-relational-based justice practices collectively, we need the settings as well to be founded on a value-relational rationale (Ramos 1981). As Evans and Vaandering (2016) remind us:

It is now evident that addressing discipline and harmful behavior apart from the context of community interconnectedness, while maintaining a hierarchical power structure often found in schools, will be ineffective. (p. xii)

Next we consider a broad overview of the five principles of restorative justice.

PRINCIPLES OF RESTORATIVE JUSTICE

The philosophy of restorative justice is based on five core pillars: humanizing values, strengthening relationships, shared responsibility, addressing harm, and strengthening community (Figure 33.1).

Humanizing Values

Values and relationships are the first pillars of restorative justice. We all have values, whether inherent, cultivated by institutions, or even treated as universal human rights. Brincat and Wike define *values* as, "those goods that our theories, rules, and decisions work to bring about in the world" (2000, p. 141, cited in Elliott, 2011). Elliot also describes values as "virtues or positive qualities" and reminds us that there is a difference between "using values to judge others and using values to guide one's own actions" (Elliott, 2011, p. 106). Because we are human, we have some shared understanding of respect, honesty, truth, humility, sharing, empathy, courage, forgiveness, and love, and thus these values are the foundation of restorative justice (Braithwaite, 2000; Pranis, Stuart, & Wedge, 2003). Values go beyond labels or preconceived ideas shaped by our collective experiences in relationships. Here we refer to values in communities in which the ethics of responsibility and care go beyond a certain group, a physical space, or any ideology (Gilligan, 1982; Weber, 1944).

Human societies have taught us to think not according to a value-relational rationale, but rather according to human predictability and calculability (Ramos, 1981)—that is, according to

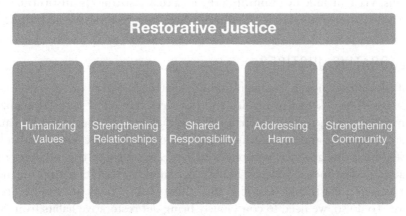

FIGURE 33.1 The five pillars of restorative justice.

laws and institutional rules and regulations, without an analysis of who we are as collective beings (as opposed to individuals without relationships). The goal of restorative justice is to change this paradigm. In restorative justice, the central proposition is that commission of a crime is a violation not only of norms and rules, but of people, values, and relationships (Zehr, 1990). For example, the indigenous people of Canada see themselves as part of a collective, not as autonomous independent agents in the world, community, and environment: "I am I plus my relationships." For them, if we do not think of our identity in relation to all others in a holistic way, the values of justice are no longer ethical, but moral codes that suit a certain reality regardless of the whole—a mechanical view of the world (Capra, 1982). We can extrapolate this premise to the general concept of harm, which in health care and health professions education may occur as malpractice, cheating, or other forms of misconduct.

Strengthening Relationships

In many formal institutions, including educational and health care systems, relationships are impersonal, and roles are structured around a hierarchy in which subordination is evident. In such settings, little time is possible for actualization and getting to know others (Elliott, 2011). In the U.S. system of health care, professionalization prevents meaningful relationships from flourishing. For example, nurses, physician, dentists, pharmacists, and social workers have traditionally been educated in silos. Yet, their practice requires them to work as a team. This situation must be challenged so that those working in health care see relationship strengthening as a priority. These relationships form the second pillar of restorative justice.

Within the health care arena, one of the barriers to strengthening relations lies in our conceptualization of "the patient." Too often health care professionals are divorced from the knowledge of and involvement in the communities of their "patients." Elliott (2011) notes that, lacking this knowledge and involvement, lawyers, social workers, therapists, police (and we add health care providers) may be accountable to institutional codes, norms, and procedures, but they lack responsiveness to needs of the people. As part of restorative justice, we can start by reconceptualizing the word *patient*, so that interactions are no longer transactional, but dialogical. As illustrated in my story, sometimes it felt that it was more important to follow the protocols and norms in the doctor's checklist than to engage with me, the patient. Following restorative justice principles, the two tasks should be complementary to each other.

A second barrier to strengthening relationships is the concept that human relationships are generally based on self-interest, distrust, and fear. This perspective lacks any emphasis on dialogue and story sharing, on how harm may have affected a person's life and relationships. We must thus reevaluate human relations within a new justice/healing system. Restorative justice in health care—we might call it *restorative health justice*—can provide us tools for reevaluating our social interactions.

As educators, we need to create an environment of trust and reduce fear among our students if we are to apply restorative justice principles in the classroom. For example, if students lack trust in fear of a punitive response, they may not provide constructive feedback about clinical preceptor experiences or report instances of cheating. We can use restorative justice principles to increase trust, reduce fear, and strengthen relationships.

Buber (1986) describes this relationship as "I–You," in which humans treat each other not as commodities but as other human beings who are part of their existence and who share mutual responsibilities. Accordingly, Pavlich quotes Umberto Eco's explanation of the relationship and the "I–You or the other in us":

This is not a sentimental vague propensity, but a basic condition. As we are told by the most secular of the social sciences, it is the other, his gaze, that defines us and determines us. Just as we couldn't live without eating or sleeping, we cannot understand who we are without the gaze and response of the other. Even those who kill, rape, rob, and violate do so in exceptional moments, and the rest of the time beg for love, respect praise from others. And even from those they humiliate, they seek recognition in the form of fear and submission. We might die or go insane if we lived in a community in which everyone had systematically decided never to look at us and behave as if we didn't exist. (Eco & Martini, 1997, p. 94, cited in Pavlich, 2002, p. 11)

This degree of reciprocal recognition of the other allows some people to seek justice within the context of the other. In other words, the "other" is connected to you and to me and cannot be viewed as entities separate from the whole. The premise of this collective thinking, of being part of a whole, may be to take responsibility for nature and the other. Using restorative justice principles and practices may enable us to make collective decisions to resolve conflicts without violence and the destruction of nature. To make this happen, we need to rethink our collective responsibility toward others and the environment. Without the ethics of care and responsibility in all institutions (including the health care system), there is no justice. Being responsible is to act, to take a position. For example, in the story at the beginning of the chapter, I, as a complex being, was as responsible for my healing process as anyone, including Dr. X.

Shared Responsibility

A story of a young man convicted of committing a crime illustrates the third pillar of restorative justice—shared responsibility. After his sentence was handed out, his community's leader requested of the judge that he be allowed to speak, "Your Excellency, we would like to take turns serving the sentence in prison." The judge was surprised by this request and said, "But you and the others have done nothing wrong. It was he who committed the hurtful behavior; he should be held accountable and therefore pay for it." The community leader replied, "Your Excellency, in our community we think that if one of us does something good, we all did something good, because we provided to that individual the conditions for a good life: education, food, care, health, and all the support a person needs. Now, if one of us performed a harmful act, it is because we failed as a community, and therefore we must all be responsible for that act."

Many speak of responsibility in restorative justice, but from an individualistic perspective: If one person harms another, then that person should be responsible and "pay for" the harmful act. Within this model of justice there is no shared responsibility or assigning collective in which human relations shape good or bad behavior (Boyes-Watson, 2000; Elliott, 2011; Pavlich, 2005; Ross, 1986). We must continue to highlight the need for collective or shared responsibility when it comes to dealing with issues in the justice or health care systems. The story illustrates the degree of ethical commitment on which some communities are still based today.

In restorative justice, collective or shared responsibility allows us to participate more completely and comprehensively in the construction of justice. A plan is laid out and the responsibilities are distributed collectively among the community, so that an action plan is implemented by the community in collaboration with the offender and the harmed, in order to reintegrate both into the community (Karp, 2015).

Addressing Harm

The fourth pillar of restorative justice is addressing harm. When we talk about the first principle of restorative justice, humanizing values, we refer to restorative justice as the possibility of justice that asks, "Who suffered harm by a certain behavior, and what relationships were broken?" In this section, we do not ask, "What norm or rule has been broken? But rather,

"How do we deal with the harm?" In restorative justice, we address the shame and trauma that resulted from some maltreatment, and then healing may begin to take place.

The shame (and guilt) aspect of restorative justice is closely linked to the idea of "avoidance behaviors, such as isolation detachment, withdrawal, cancellation of appointments, surrenders of responsibilities, emotional constriction and so on" (Wilson, Drozdek, & Turkovic, 2006, p. 138, cited in Elliott, 2011, p. 173). Dealing with shame in a stigmatizing way—by using labels or reinforcing stereotypes—makes the aftermath of the harm worse. However, dealing with shame in community can reintegrate the person into the company of those affected by the behavior.

Stigmatizing (or disintegrative shaming) is the effect of punishment whereby the offender feels cast aside and abandoned by the community (Braithwaite & Mugford, 1994, p. 332). The result is that the degree of inclusion and shared responsibility for the wrongdoing decreases. Reintegrative shaming speaks to the "idea that certain types of punishment can lead to a reduction of recidivism as long as they do not involve banishment and they induce healthy shame in the individual" (Pollock, 2014, p. 332). Even though studies have not found strong support for reintegrative shaming, they have found that, for example, "parental forgiveness and peer shaming had significant effects on reducing the likelihood of being involved in predatory offenses again" (Elliott, 2011, p. 163).

Trauma is the result of physical and/or psychological pain or injury caused by another. Historical or recurrent experiences of oppression and trauma can lead to long-term scars within communities, limiting the ability of people to learn, grow, and change at the individual or community level (Bopp & Bopp, 2011). This is one reason for making the community, not the individual, the main focus in restorative justice. Furthermore, restorative justice should reinforce the importance of strengthening the community.

Take the case of a student who is caught cheating on an exam by the staff proctor. In this case, the harmed individuals include the proctor, the fellow students, faculty, and the student who cheated—that is, the entire learning community. To address the harm, we ask, "What relationships are broken as a result of this cheating incident and what is the harm?" The incident results in disruption of trust between the student and faculty and staff, and among peers when faculty members conduct a general discussion of academic dishonesty with the class. A traditional punitive approach to academic dishonesty would involve review of university policies and disciplinary proceedings, possibly including dismissal. Using restorative justice principles, the community comes together with the offending student to discuss the breach of values, impact on relationships, and harms done to the learning community (staff, faculty, peers) and develops strategies for restoration, such as creating a process for greater understanding and self reflection of how the incident affected others. This process does not involve only faculty and the "cheating" student, it also involves rebuilding relationships and restoring trust with harmed staff and peers.

Strengthening Community

Strengthening community is the final pillar in restorative justice. In this context, *community* refers to human relationships and the bonds that reinforce them (Boyes-Watson, 2005). In situations in which we see ourselves as more than simply economic beings, we recognize our various dimensions in human relationships (Ramos, 1981). The community is no longer reduced to a group of people with common interests or goals, as occurs in the market society. Communities are composed of people who recognize their spiritual, political, social, physical, emotional, and economic dimensions, and their complex and diverse relationships (Salm & Leal, 2012). Elliott (2011) sums it up: "Community is a multi-dimensional concept that includes relational affective, political, creative and collective aspects. They are the micro-societies in which we feel some level of engagement outside of our homes" (p. 196).

Restorative justice operates on the assumption that the mindful and heartfelt habit of knowing the other in all of the other's diversity strengthens the community. Therefore, there is no space for exclusion, labels, and reductionism within community. As people cherish this complexity of community, we create what Block (2008) calls a "sense of belonging" (p. 1). We are in a community every time we find a space in which we belong, and that increases our sense of responsibility for others. Pavlich (2004) argues that community should not be a fixed entity in which there is a constant threat of totalitarianism. In restorative justice, community encompasses the idea of relationships, of heterogeneous and complex bonds, of embracing differences and coming together to dialogue about (in)justice. According to Pavlich (2004, cited in Zehr & Towes) an alternative to community should be centered on the idea of hospitality. Thus, people can take the principles and practices of restorative justice wherever they go. Restorative justice resides not in certain institutions or specific settings, but in the hearts and minds of each of us. We are all hosts when it comes to restorative justice.

PRACTICES OF RESTORATIVE JUSTICE

In this section, we discuss how the five core principles of restorative justice are operationalized. Practices vary according to each community's culture. The most cited forms of practices are family group conferencing, victim offender mediation, and peacemaking circles. Here we focus only on peacemaking circles, given its broad and inclusive scope of use.

Peacemaking Circles

Peacemaking circles have roots in indigenous Canadian culture. They provide a way to bring people together to engage in difficult dialogue, address conflict or differences, encourage collective responsibility, and strengthen relationships. Worldwide, peacemaking circles have been adopted for decision making, problem solving, conflict resolution, and community building in various settings such as families, neighborhoods, schools, workplaces, and criminal justice systems (Gray & Lauderdale, 2007; Pranis, 2005; Pranis et al., 2003).

Elements of Peacemaking Circles

Peacemaking circles borrow elements from indigenous traditions, especially the practice of using a "talking piece" (Table 33.1). The stage is set with participants arranged in a circle with nothing separating them. Dialogue is facilitated by the circle keeper, who proposes that the group establish values to guide the dialogue. Participants share their thoughts on those values with the group and decide whether or not they are in agreement. The circle keeper passes a talking piece, an object that is meaningful to the person facilitating the dialogue, from one person to the next, clockwise around the circle. Only the person who holds the talking piece can speak; the rest of the group actively listens. Those who have nothing to say may pass the talking piece on, but then must wait until the next round for their next turn to speak. Suggested topics for each round are listed in Table 33.1. Quite often people in the circle share their most intimate thoughts and reflections, and gain empathy without judgment from others. This openness is a consequence of trust within a circle. At times, the circle keeper may ask for clarification or suspend the dialogue for a break, so people have time to reflect on what has been said. Confidentiality and volunteerism should be respected, so that people feel safe that what is being shared will not be divulged (Karp, 2015; Pranis et al., 2003, 2005).

TABLE 33.1 Elements of Peacemaking Circles

Element	Strategy
Setting the stage	• Participants sit in a circle with nothing separating them • Facilitator (circle keeper) sets tone
Establishing trust	• Circle keeper facilitates dialogue using a talking piece • Group establishes values for discussion • Participation is voluntary • Confidentiality is maintained

Format	• Typically four rounds, though there can be as many as needed
	• First round (introductory):
	  • Circle keeper welcomes group, summarizes issue
	  • Participants introduce themselves, explain what they hope to achieve with the circle
	  • Circle keeper summarizes hopes expressed by the group
	• Second round (discuss the harm):
	  • Participants share their perceptions and feelings about the issue
	  • Facilitator summarizes themes, areas of agreement or disagreement
	• Third round (brainstorming):
	  • Participants share ideas about possible resolutions
	  • No debate about relative merits of proposed actions
	• Fourth round (reflection and reaction)
	  • Participants make final comments, share what the circle meant for them

Circles have extraordinary power to create a place of understanding, safety, and healing. Let us look at an example in which a peacemaking circle was used to address disruptive student behavior. A student who was always late with assignments and for class entered the classroom 50 minutes after class started. While the other students and I looked on in disbelief, he approached the front of the class, handed in his late assignment, and walked out. I felt not only hurt, but profoundly disrespected. My initial inclination was to take a punitive approach, knowing I had the power to expel him from the class. When I mentioned this episode to a colleague, her response was cutting: "But you don't believe in expulsion and inflicting pain on someone because they hurt you, that would be punishment, right?" This perspective led me to request a peacemaking circle in which I could constructively share my experience with the class; this was a teachable moment.

To begin, I asked students to form a circle with their chairs. I asked the students what human values might guide our interactions during the circle. We wrote them on a piece of paper, which we placed in the middle of the circle. I opened the session by reading a quote by Plato about justice. Then, using a talking piece, we shared each of our perspectives on how we felt we might have been disrespectful to one another all semester—not just one to one, but everyone toward the collective. Many expressed the need to apologize for arriving late or not doing their work, explaining that they were overwhelmed with family- or work-related problems, had little time to sleep, and sometimes lacked time to eat. During the first two rounds of passing the talking piece the student whom I felt insulted by had nothing to say. In fact, he seemed oblivious of any disrespectful behavior on his part.

As the talking piece went around the circle a few more times and other students shared, this particular student decided he had something to add: "I need to apologize for coming in late and not staying for our last class. Another professor asked me to meet at the same time as our class and I am about to flunk that class. But I felt the need to hand in my assignment so I would not lose participation points. I apologize, I did not mean to be disrespectful to you."

I acknowledged his contribution and then shared how I had felt. The opportunity helped me frame the interaction more clearly. I better understood that the student's actions were not malicious; his goal was to get through school and it influenced his behavior that day. Given this new perspective and understanding, I accepted his apology, and from that day forward, he was always on time and engaged in class.

Restorative justice practices thus provide meaningful ways to achieve dialogue on a particular subject. Integrating the principles and practices of restorative justice into everyday spaces can be highly beneficial. We have seen that peacemaking circles should be guided by principles and rituals. But how do we get there? We consider how we can establish the habit of living a restorative, meaningful, and just life in the following section.

Cultivating Habits of the Heart—Values, Relationships, Responsibility, and Dialogue

The sincerest and most authentic way to cultivate restorative justice is through education, by sharing what we know about the philosophy, principles, and practices of restorative justice. We need to examine critically the ethics of the marketplace and current institutions, and allow the ethics of care and responsibility for others and nature to flourish. It is fundamental that the state does its part in supporting community restorative justice initiatives (Ashworth, 2002). Restorative justice also invites us to challenge our perceptions of justice, that our perceptions may be influenced by institutions and the media (Evans & Vaandering, 2016; Karp, 2015). Furthermore, we cultivate the habits of contemplating and living restorative justice by getting to know people and by strengthening our relationships through seeking and pursuing justice together. When including others takes centrality in our lives, we bring down the walls that separate us by embracing our complexities and diversities.

More difficult than promoting our habits of the heart is revisioning and creating institutions that allow a culture of those habits to exist. We must ask, "If we are to create a culture of restorative justice, and the habits of living a life of value and relationships, do the orientations of our institutions need to be changed?" "Do our institutions need to function in a nonpunitive, caring, and relational way?" Thus there is value in health professions programs rethinking their curricula so that they are no longer based on a "banking system" of education in which teachers "deposit" skills in students as if they were banks (Freire, 1993, 1997, 1998). For Freire, education should instead be a provocative experience in which consciousness and autonomy are raised, and people become active participants, not passive subjects, in life. Such a new educational orientation would include many new ideas, including restorative justice.

CONCLUSIONS

We have considered the importance of restorative justice principles and briefly touched on one of its main practices, peacemaking circles. We have seen the importance of creating habits of the heart to heal and transform people, especially those who have experienced harm. This cultural change can occur through education and training in restorative justice principles and practices, and by rethinking the contexts in which these principles and practices play out.

We have seen that restorative justice requires institutions to have a value-relational rationale. It advocates critical thinking and the restoration of ethics concerning our responsibility toward others and nature. As illustrated in the story of Dr. X, involving others; cultivating a community of friends and family; and emphasizing values, relationships, and responsibility can enable all of us to experience physical, emotional, and social transformation, and can effect healing and health care in a collective and meaningful way.

REFERENCES

Ashworth, A. (2002). Responsibilities, rights and restorative justice. *British Journal of Criminology, 42*(3), 578–595.

Block, P. (2008). *Community: The structure of belonging.* San Francisco, CA: Berrett-Koehler.

Bopp, M., & Bopp, J. (2011). *Recreating the world: A practical guide to building sustainable communities* (3rd ed.). Calgary, Alberta, Canada: Four Worlds Press.

Boyes-Watson, C. (2000). Reflections on the purist and maximalist models of restorative justice. *Contemporary Justice Review, 3*(4), 441–450.

Boyes-Watson, C. (2005). Community is not a place but a relationship: Lessons for organizational development. *Public Organization Review, 5*(4), 359–374.

Braithwaite, J. (2000). Shame and criminal justice. *Canadian Journal of Criminology, 42*(3), 281–298.

Braithwaite, J., & Mugford, S. (1994). Conditions of successful reintegration ceremonies: Dealing with juvenile offenders. *British Journal of Criminology, 34*(2), 139–171.

Buber, M. (1986). *I and thou* (R. G. Smith, Trans.). New York, NY: Scribner Classics.

Capra, F. (1982). *The turning point.* New York, NY: Bantam Books.

Doolin, K. (2007). But what does it mean? Seeking definitional clarity in restorative justice. *Journal of Criminal Law, 71*(5), 427–440.

Elliott, E. (2011). *Security with care: Restorative justice and healthy societies.* Nova Scotia, Canada: Fernwood.

Evans, K., & Vaandering, D. (2016). *The little book of restorative justice in education: Fostering responsibility, healing and hope in schools.* New York, NY: Good Books.

Freire, P. (1993). *Pedagogy of the oppressed.* New York, NY: Continuum.

Freire, P. (1997). *Pedagogy of the heart.* New York, NY: Continuum.

Freire, Paulo. (1998). *Pedagogy of freedom: Ethics, democracy, and civic courage.* Lanham, MD: Rowman and Littlefield.

Gilligan, C. (1982). *In a difference voice: Psychological theory and women's development.* Cambridge, MA: Harvard University Press.

Gray, B. A., & Lauderdale, P. (2007). The great circle of justice: North American indigenous justice and contemporary restoration programs. *Contemporary Justice Review, 10*(2), 215–225.

Karp, D. (2015). *The little book of restorative justice for colleges and universities.* New York, NY: Skyhorse.

Pavlich, G. (2002). Towards an ethics of restorative justice. In L. Walgrave (Ed.), *Restorative justice and the law* (pp. 1–18). New York, NY: Routledge.

Pavlich, G. (2004). What are the dangers as well as the promises of community involvement? In B. Toews & H. Zehr (Eds.), *Critical issues in restorative justice.* Monsey, NY: Criminal Justice Press.

Pavlich, G. C. (2005). *Governing paradoxes of restorative justice.* London, UK: GlassHouse Press.

Pollock, J. M. (2014). Ethical dilemmas and decisions in criminal justice. Scarborough, ON, Canada. Nelson Education.

Pranis, K. (2005). *The little book of circle process: A new/old approach to peacemaking.* Intercourse, PA: Good Books.

Pranis, K., Stuart, B., & Wedge, M. (2003). *Peacemaking circles: From crime to community.* St. Paul, MN: Living Justice Press.

Ramos, A. G. (1981). *The new science of organizations: A reconceptualization of the wealth of nations.* Buffalo, NY: University of Toronto Press.

Ross, R. (1996). *Return to teaching: Exploring aboriginal justice.* Toronto, Canada: Penguin.

Salm, J., & Leal, J. (2012.) Restorative justice—Multidimensionality and its invited guest. *Revista Sequencia, 64*(33), 195–226.

Stout, M., & Salm, J. (2011). What restorative justice might learn from administrative theory. *Contemporary Justice Review, 14*(2), 203–225.

Weber, M. (1944). *Economy and society* (Vol. 1). New York, NY: Bedminster Press.

Zehr, H. (1990). *Changing lenses: A new focus for crime and justice.* Scottsdale, PA: Herald Press.

Zehr, H., & Toews, B. (2004). *Critical issues in restorative justice.* Monsey, NY: Criminal Justice Press.

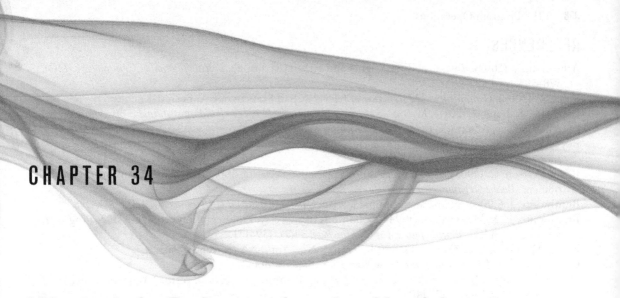

CHAPTER 34

Work–Life Balance for the Health Professions Educator

Patrick Auth and Michael Howley

CHAPTER OBJECTIVES

- Distinguish predictors and how to recognize them
- Discuss tools to measure burnout
- Implement strategies for achieving work–life balance and avoiding burnout

---

In dealing with those who are undergoing great suffering, if you feel "burnout" setting in, if you feel demoralized and exhausted, it is best, for the sake of everyone, to withdraw and restore yourself. The point is to have a long-term perspective.

—Dalai Lama

Job burnout is one of the most important threats to health professions faculty (e.g., physician assistant [PA], physical therapy, nursing, or occupational therapy). Health professions faculty are particularly prone to burnout because they not only educate a high volume of students, but often also care for patients in clinical settings. Burnout can result in decreased productivity, poor instructional quality, faculty turnover, and a variety of other consequences as described in Table 34.1). Each year, for example, about 20% of PA faculty leave their job because of reduced job satisfaction due to stressors (Forister & Blessing, 2007). A study of Canadian medical faculty found that "50% thought about leaving academic medicine every week" (Wallace, Lemaire, & Ghali, 2009, p. 1717). In nursing there is a 6.9% vacancy rate among faculty positions nationally (Maslach & Martin, 2014).

TABLE 34.1	Consequences of Burnout to the Individual, the Organization, and the Profession	

Individual	Organization	Profession
Excessive stress/anxiety	Decreased productivity	Negative attitude toward profession
Fatigue	Absenteeism	Lower tolerance for change
Vulnerability to illness	Increased errors at work	Increase risk for immoral or unethical behavior
Substance abuse	Poor quality of work	Negative publicity for dysfunctional behavior
Family deteriorations	Higher turnover rate	Legislative or regulatory censor

Source: Bianchi, Schonfeld, and Laurent (2015).

Faculty burnout can be an insidious problem. Health professions faculty are absorbed in a barrage of pressing issues such as responding to student or patient demands or trying to prepare that lecture at the last minute. Health professions faculty often lack insight into their internal states because they are trained to focus on their patients and students. Colleagues who are often astute diagnosticians may not see the early signs of burnout in themselves because they are immersed in the same day-to-day stresses and deadlines. Many of the interactions in meetings or casual hallway conversations do not activate a diagnostic mind-set. The purpose of this chapter is to help health professions faculty recognize burnout at the earliest stages so that they can intervene early.

The following exemplar is provided to enhance faculty members' ability to recognize and effectively manage burnout.

EXEMPLAR: BURNOUT IN A LONG-TERM EMPLOYEE

Jennifer is a 43-year-old clinical coordinator who has worked for a long-standing PA program for the past 7 years. She came to the PA program after a 10-year history of being a family practice PA and still works one afternoon a week in the clinic. For the past 3 to 4 years, her job has become increasingly stressful as she has experienced difficulties in obtaining clinical sites for her students. Six months ago, all of the OB/GYN sites withdrew their commitments. Increasingly, Jennifer is heard commenting on the stress in her job and her fatigue. Because she spends so much time traveling to site visits and trying to find additional OB/GYN sites, she is beginning to feel increasingly isolated from her students and faculty colleagues. She is becoming frustrated and wonders why she has been burdened with these difficult problems. She feels stuck and like she cannot get out. She has been heard yelling at staff and students—behavior that is out of character for her. In a brief discussion, Jennifer admitted to her colleague that she was frustrated but argued that it is important to find a good solution to these issues to maintain the quality of the students' education.

Does Jennifer have burnout? Although it may be obvious that Jennifer is beginning to struggle, can we say she is burned out?

DEFINING BURNOUT

Burnout is a syndrome of interrelated features, including emotional exhaustion, reduced personal accomplishment, and depersonalization, as illustrated in Figure 34.1 (Leiter, 1993; Maslach, Jackson, & Leiter, 1996). As a syndrome, diagnosing burnout can be difficult and these

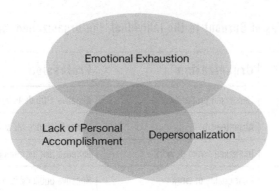

FIGURE 34.1 The key features of burnout.

symptoms may wax and wane over time. In considering the case over time, however, it is often possible to see a progression from exhaustion to reduced personal accomplishment, and then an end-stage depersonalization (Maslach et al., 1996). In order to diagnose job burnout, the symptoms should arise out of work activities and cannot be attributed to depression or other comorbid conditions.

The first factor, emotional exhaustion, is depletion or exhaustion of a person's mental and physical resources attributed to prolonged stress that results from striving toward some unrealized, work-related goal (Bianchi et al., 2015; Maslach et al., 1996). Jennifer is expending a lot of energy trying to achieve a goal that may not be attainable. The fact that Jennifer also has to deal with people (i.e., clinic relationships, students, patients) increases the energy expenditure and puts her at risk of burnout. The capriciousness of the OB/GYN sites suddenly withdrawing their commitments no doubt triggered an immense surge of catecholamines and other stress hormones, further depleting energy resources (Bianchi et al., 2015; Maslach et al., 1996). In the midst of these ongoing problems, Jennifer is not able to restore these psychological resources and becomes increasingly exhausted.

The second factor in burnout, lack of personal accomplishment, refers to a negative self-evaluation of one's own work (Bianchi et al., 2015; Kaschka, Korczak, & Broich, 2011; Leiter, 1993). Jennifer is getting nowhere with the clinic sites, so she is naturally not feeling a sense of personal accomplishment. At the same time, the emotional exhaustion prevents her from coping with these negative feelings (Leiter, 1993). Every day at work she faces her failure without any ability to compensate in a functional way, so she begins to miss work, becomes susceptible to illness, and starts to think about finding another job (Kaschka et al., 2011).

The third aspect of burnout, depersonalization, occurs when the individual develops negative attitudes toward the people that he or she serves, in the case of health professions educators this would be students, clinical preceptors, and institutional administration. Jennifer is overwhelmed and cannot cope in a functional way, and so may depersonalize the stressors as a protective mechanism. These attitudes can progress even to the point that the worker becomes callous and dehumanizing (Kaschka et al., 2011).

Given this discussion of job burnout, what do we make of the case of Jennifer and the OB/GYN sites? Although Jennifer is exhausted and lacks a personal sense of accomplishment, she has not begun to depersonalize. She still cares about her students. At the same time she seems to be on the road to burnout. How should her program director think about this "preburnout" situation? The organization does not want to lose a previously high-performing faculty member in the midst of the crisis. In the next section, we summarize the factors that cause job burnout before introducing the Job–Person Fit Model as an analytical tool to address Jennifer's early burnout symptoms.

WHAT CAUSES JOB BURNOUT?

Job burnout can result from various factors (Rupert, Miller, & Dorociak, 2015; Schaufeli, Leiter, & Maslach, 2009), including:

- **Lack of control:** Educators who have no control over their teaching schedule, the number of students they have in class, or the number of teaching credit hours will develop a sense of helplessness. In addition this could result from a lack of resources allotted to do the work.
- **Unclear job expectations:** If health professions educators are unclear about the job expectations or what their dean, associate dean, department chair, or program director expects from them, educators are likely feel uncomfortable in their jobs, which adds to stress.
- **Dysfunctional workplace dynamics:** Perhaps the work environment is hostile and faculty members feel undermined by colleagues or micromanaged by their department chair.
- **Poor job fit:** When the skills required to be a health professions educator do not fit with the interest and skills of the individual, there is poor job fit. As a result the job becomes increasingly stressful over time.
- **Extremes of activity:** When the job is monotonous or chaotic, coupled with limited time for recovery, fatigue and burnout will soon follow.

BURNOUT PREDICTORS AND HOW TO RECOGNIZE THEM

Burnout is a phenomenon in which the cumulative effects of a stressful work environment gradually overwhelm the defenses of the health professions educators, causing them to psychologically withdraw. To better understand the experience of health professions educators suffering from burnout, we examine the job cycle of burnout. Figure 34.2 illustrates a useful model for thinking about the cycle of burnout.

Do you remember your first day as a health professions educator? You were likely filled with lots of *enthusiasm*—it was a year of high hopes, high energy, and maybe, just maybe, some unrealistic expectations. This may also be a time when there is excessive identification with students and an inefficient expenditure of one's own energy.

If left unchecked this high level of enthusiasm can slowly move into *stagnation*—when one is still doing his or her job, but it is no longer thrilling (Maslach et al., 1996). Enough of the reality has come through to make one feel that it might be nice to have leisure time, a little time to spend with friends and family and/or at home. The emphasis now is on meeting one's own

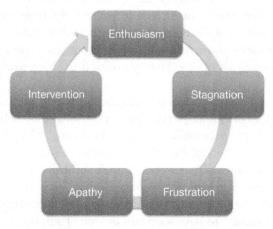

FIGURE 34.2 The cycle of burnout.

personal needs. At some point one migrates into *frustration* and calls into questions one's effectiveness in doing one's job. *Apathy* is typical and is a very natural defense mechanism against frustration. It occurs when a person is chronically frustrated on the job, yet needs the job to survive. Apathy is the attitude "a job is a job is a job." It can manifest in a variety of ways, such as (a) putting in the minimum required time (as against the overtime that is gladly taken during the enthusiasm stage), (b) avoiding challenges (even avoiding students whenever possible), and (c) seeking mainly to keep from endangering job security.

In addition, as clinicians transition into teaching there is a certain amount of role ambiguity that can occur. This role ambiguity has been found to correlate with emotional exhaustion, frustration, stagnation, and apathy (Warner, 2015). Individuals who are trying to gain competence as a teacher may feel that there is not enough time to accomplish all of the tasks required of a health professions educator. Moving from the clinical arena, where the faculty member was seen as a competent and respected clinician, to the educational environment, where he or she is now a novice, is a daunting task.

THE JOB–PERSON FIT MODEL

The Job–Person Fit Model explicitly integrates both individual and situational factors to better understand the antecedents or stressors that lead to burnout. In the Job–Person Fit Model, the greater the gap or mismatch between the individuals' internal resources and the demands of their job, the greater the likelihood of burnout. In the case of novice health professions educators, they are typically oriented to rational, evidence-based thinking and motivated to help others. The vagaries of an academic bureaucracy and the inevitable barriers that prevent helping others will create stresses for Jennifer or any health professions educator. Presumably, faculty members have been hired for their ability to cope with these challenges, but there are limits to these coping resources. The Job–Person Fit Model describes the dynamics between the stressors and coping resources, but health professions faculty are at risk of burnout because of these inherent mismatches (Maslach et al., 1996).

The Job–Person Fit Model organizes the potential mismatches between stressors and coping resources into six areas of work life that encompasses the central relationships with burnout: *workload, control, reward, community, fairness,* and *values* (Maslach et al., 1996). Burnout arises from a chronic mismatch in one or more of these areas.

Workload refers to an excessive volume of work that precludes a faculty member from recovering and is the most critical factor in creating exhaustion. Faculty members may also experience workload mismatch when their skill set or interests do not match the job. Helping other people, whether students or patients, is emotional work and can create overload when people must display emotions inconsistent with their feelings. Strategies to help faculty achieve a better workload job fit include adjusting the teaching schedule for an occasional free term or semester so faculty can focus on recovery, developing a shared workload for didactic and clinical faculty, and considering an off-site faculty position to share workload (Maslach et al., 1996).

Mismatches in the areas of *control* refers to situations in which individuals are responsible for outcomes but not resources or cannot pursue the work in what they believe is the most effective manner. Leaders may also experience a mismatch in control when they are overwhelmed by their levels of responsibility and feel that they do not have the necessary skills. This mismatch is reflected as one of responsibility exceeding one's authority. In addition, lack of control can be one of the most distressing aspects of burnout. Mismatches in control can bring on burnout by reducing personal accomplishments (Maslach et al., 1996). Strategies to avoid this mismatch include empowering faculty to have a certain degree of autonomy and decision-making responsibilities.

A mismatch in *rewards* refers to a lack of compensation and/or gratification for the demands of the job. Rewards may be financial, such as salary or benefits, or social, such as recognition and validation. Lack of social rewards or gratification is the more critical of the two. Workers who are not recognized and validated for their work are at high risk for a mismatch in rewards (Maslach et al., 1996). Lack of reward is closely associated with a lack of personal accomplishment. Faculty strategies to avoid a mismatch in rewards include developing an attitude that recognizes and celebrates accomplishments (submitting a manuscript, completing a curriculum revision, getting a student through a rough stretch), looking for ways to increase your professional competencies, and nourishing the creative side of faculty life.

A mismatch in *community* occurs when faculty members do not feel positively connected with others in the department or with students. Positive connection is derived from sharing praise, humor, respect, and comfort with colleagues (Maslach et al., 1996). On the other hand, chronic negative feelings of frustration and hostility create isolation and reduce social support (Maslach et al., 1996). Strategies to build a sense of community within a faculty include developing and implementing a new faculty development mentorship program, conducting off-campus retreats, and reminding colleagues to take an occasional break from technology and the community.

Another element in the Job–Person Fit Model is *lack of fairness*, which can exacerbate burnout by creating cynicism and emotional exhaustion (Maslach et al., 1996). Elements, such as unequal workload, compensation, or promotion and tenure practices, can all lead to unfairness in the workplace (Maslach et al., 1996). Strategies to ensure fairness in the health professions department include constructive and appropriate feedback from students, absence of mandatory and punitive instructor evaluations, and set boundaries with students.

A conflict between *values* also creates mismatch in the Job–Person Fit Model. This may manifest as perceived pressure to behave in an unethical manner or to do a job that contradicts one's values (Maslach et al., 1996). Values mismatch can also be between one's personal career goals and the goals of the institution, school, or department, college, or university. A common example is a mission statement that is not lived in day-to-day practice (Maslach et al., 1996). Strategies to help faculty members articulate their values include asking them: "What is it you value in our faculty position?" "What do you need in your faculty position to have a better work–life balance?" "What are your personal aspirations in your career?"

How does the Job–Person Fit Model apply to Jennifer's situation? How does this tool help us recognize burnout in ourselves or our colleagues? In this analysis, Jennifer is having mismatches in volume and rewards. In addition, she is beginning to have problems in community and fairness. Jennifer is stuck in a problem in which there is no apparent resolution. She has to do a lot of extra work to resolve this problem while also carrying her other work. This is leading to a mismatch in workload. The lack of results is creating a mismatch in rewards. These mismatches are then leading to mismatches in community and fairness. With these insights, Jennifer or one of her colleagues has a basis to analyze this complex situation and create a solution.

TOOL TO MEASURE BURNOUT

The primary tool used to measure burnout is the Maslach Burnout Inventory (MBI; Maslach & Jackson, 1981). In the case of health care professionals and educators, this tool is validated to assess emotional exhaustion, depersonalization, and reduced personal accomplishment (Bria, Spanu, Baban, & Dumitrascu, 2014; Cordes & Dougherty, 1993). The MBI include three sections—the Human Services Survey (MBI-HSS), the General Survey (MBI-GS), and the Educators Survey (MBI-ES). The MBI-ES evaluates the three dimensions of burnout in education, including teachers and administrators. The MBI-ES uses a 7-point scale to assess burnout, which ranges from "never" on the low end to "every day" on the high end. Health professions educators should be able to complete this assessment in 3 to 5 minutes per section.

Exemplar, Revisited

After thinking about the Job-Person Fit Model, one of Jennifer's senior faculty colleagues schedules time with Jennifer to discuss the situation. After allowing Jennifer to talk (i.e., vent) through the situation. Jennifer takes the MBI-ES, which suggests she is at risk for burnout. They discuss the alternatives and come up with the following approach. Jennifer generally likes her job and wishes she could get back to the balance she felt before the OB/GYN sites withdrew. To achieve this, the program director will give her assistance with finding new OB/GYN sites so Jennifer can restore her work balance. The program director will assign an administrative staffer to occasionally contact the previous sites in case new opportunities arise. In addition, the program director will feed her prospects for new OB/GYN sites so Jennifer does not have to generate her own leads. The program director will follow up with Jennifer periodically to assess how these interventions are working. Finally, Jennifer will schedule time off immediately for a restorative vacation.

CONCLUSIONS

We all continually experience tension between the stressors and demands of our jobs and our coping mechanisms. Health professions faculty are particularly at risk of job burnout because of a tendency to have a mismatch between their general approaches to a job (i.e., scientific and caring) and the demands of academic bureaucracy and business relationships. These mismatches between the person and the job can lead to decreased teaching effectiveness, student complaints, conflict, and turnover in health professions faculty. In this chapter, we have provided a framework by which health professions faculty can analyze these situations, restore a balance in the fit between health professions faculty members and their jobs, and prevent the devastating effects of burnout.

REFERENCES

Bianchi, R., Schonfeld, I. S., & Laurent, E. (2015). Is it time to consider the "burnout syndrome" A distinct illness? *Frontiers in Public Health, 3*, 158.

Bria, M., Spanu, F., Baban, A., & Dumitrascu, D. (2014). Maslach burnout inventory—General survey: Factorial validity and invariance among Romanian health professionals. *Burnout Research, 1*(3), 103–111.

Byrne, D. M., & Martin, B. N. (2014). A solution to the shortage of nursing faculty: Awareness and understanding of the leadership style of the nursing department head. *Nurse Educator, 39*(3), 107–112.

Cordes, C. L., & Dougherty, T. W. (1993). A review and integration of research on job burnout. *Academy of Management Review, 18*, 621–656.

Forister, J. G., & Blessing, B. (2007). Professional burnout: A study of physician assistant educators. *Physician Assistant Educator Journal, 18*(4), 10–15.

Kaschka, W. P., Korczak, D., & Broich, K. (2011). Burnout: A fashionable diagnosis. *Deutsches Ärzteblatt International, 108*(46), 781–787.

Leiter, M. P. (1993). Burnout as a developmental process: Consideration of models. In W. B. Schaufeli, C. Maslach, & T. Marek (Eds.), *Professional burnout: Recent developments in theory and research* (pp. 237–250). London, UK: Taylor & Francis.

Maslach, C., & Jackson, S. E. (1981). The measurement of experienced burnout. *Journal of Organizational Behavior, 2*(2), 99–113.

Maslach, C., Jackson, S. E., & Leiter, M. P. (1996). *Maslach burnout inventory* (3rd ed.). Palo Alto, CA: Consulting Psychologist Press.

Maslach, C., Schaufeli, W. B., & Leiter, M. P. (2001). Job burnout. *Annual Review of Psychology, 52*(1), 397–422.

Rupert, P. A., Miller, A. O., & Dorociak, K. E. (2015). Preventing burnout: What does the research tell us? *Professional Psychology: Research and Practice, 46*(3), 168–174.

Schaufeli, W. B., Leiter, M. P., & Maslach, C. (2009). Burnout: 35 years of research and practice. *Career Development International, 14*(3), 204–220.

Wallace, J. E., Lemaire, J. B., & Ghali, W. A. (2009). Physician wellness: A missing quality indicator. *Lancet, 374*(9702), 1714–1721.

Warner, M. (2015). From clinical practice to academia. *Journal of Physician Assistant Education, 26*(2), 109–110.

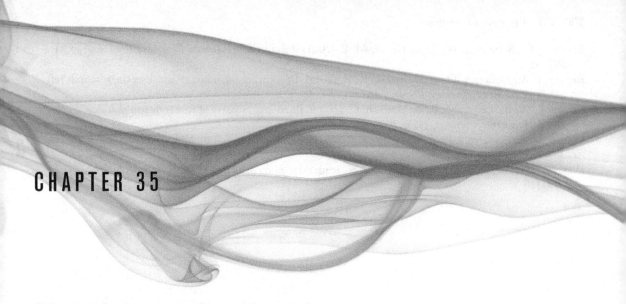

CHAPTER 35

Mindfulness for Health Professions Educators

Brenda Gustin

CHAPTER OBJECTIVE

- Discuss mindfulness practices and how educators can incorporate these practices into their routine to minimize stress, stay focused, and be productive

---

In the center of life's storms, I stand serene.

—*J. Donald Walters*

Physical and emotional stress is becoming an epidemic worldwide. Health professions educators are among the most affected as they experience stress both in clinical practice and in the classroom setting. Stress and burnout have a negative impact on compassion and resilience, which are some of the most important characteristics of health care providers and educators (Jazaieri et al., 2016; Smart et al., 2014). Mindfulness-based stress reduction techniques are safe and effective for reducing stress and burnout (Goyal et al., 2014), and are emerging as a strategy for reducing stress among clinicians (Praissman, 2008). Recent research provides strong evidence that practicing nonjudgmental, present-moment awareness (aka *mindfulness*) reduces stress, and increases concentration and productivity (Khoury, Sharma, Rush, & Fournier, 2015; Müller, Gerasimova, & Ritter, 2016). Mindfulness keeps our brains healthy, thereby supporting self-regulation and effective decision-making capabilities. These observations are backed by science. For instance, neuroscientists have shown that practicing mindfulness affects brain areas related to perception, body awareness, pain tolerance, emotion regulation, introspection, complex thinking, and sense of self (Fox et al., 2014). In this chapter, we discuss how to meditate, where to practice meditation, and how to integrate the benefits of meditation into daily life and be inspired by the benefits of mindfulness practices.

HOW TO MEDITATE

The practice of mindfulness through meditation opens access to deeper understanding of one's highest potential. Through conscious observance, mindfulness creates a state of being present and involved with the journey of life; and meditation is the key to mindfulness (Germer, 2004). The decision to inquire about meditation marks the beginning of a journey to discover the innate wellness within. Following is a guide of commonly used steps for beginning a meditation practice:

1. **Sit upright:** With your spine straight and both feet on the floor or sitting on the floor with legs crossed, align your ankles to the center of your body. Allow a gentle and deep breath into your belly. This deep breath expands the diaphragm and naturally lifts the torso up. Pull your shoulders gently up and back as you allow another gentle and deep breath. The upper back (thoracic spine) lengthens and opens the chest area. Oxygen and the cerebral spinal fluid will flow more easily helping your body to relax and allowing the parasympathetic system to be in charge. Place your hands gently upon your lap with palms upward if this feels good. If not, that is alright. If you feel tension in your hands, gently shake your wrists as if you are shaking water off them and flex your fingers a few times. This will activate your lymphatic system to assist in releasing stress and further open your circulatory systems. Adjust your chin parallel to the floor and gently support your back in the chair with a pillow at the lumbar space of your spine. If on the floor, place a small pillow or blanket under you to gently lift the base of your body. These adjustments support the four natural curves of an upright spine.

2. **Follow your breath:** Discover through observation where it flows. Consciously begin to enjoy its flow, not trying to control or regulate it.

3. **Feel your body breathe:** Place a hand on your belly and feel it rise and fall. If you do not feel this, breathe a little deeper until you do. You will then begin to feel some expansion in your ribs and then your chest cavity. You will notice a rhythm as these expand and contract. Notice its gentle flow into the nostrils and your throat. You may begin to feel the sinus cavity open and your arms, legs, and feet relax.

4. **Conscious observation:** Lift the interior gaze of your eyes up and outward to a 45° angle, as if you are basking in the rising sun. Allow your eyes to then gently relax and close. As you consider your body, you may become aware of body tension. A new dimension of conscious relationship to your body, bridging your mind–body connection through your breath, has begun. Breath, also known as *spirit*, derived from the Latin word, *spiritus*, provides insight and inspiration for you to move freely and with ease. It loosens constrictions from within the body to free mind-sets that may lead to inflexibility and stress. Tension is an important aspect of life. Stress occurs when tension becomes so tight that it may break.

5. **Breath as inspiration:** Using your breath as inspiration, inhale into the relaxed areas of your body by focusing your attention there and then exhale the feeling of relaxation into areas of body tension and stress. This brings oxygen and flow into the circulatory systems. Adjust your body position when needed to allow this flow. This is a form of *pranayama* (life force control). At first, creating this relaxed state may take 5 minutes. If this fills the time allotted to begin your meditation practice, that is fine. You have done well. You will feel a little better, and you will have established an inner connection and relationship with yourself. Serotonin will be secreted as you celebrate this first step and your body will

respond more quickly to this practice the next time as you begin to create new imprints through the neuroplasticity of your brain.

6. **Developing your practice:** Staying here longer now, or the next time, will move you to deeper and higher states of consciousness. Additional tools and techniques will help you adjust to changes in your meditation experience. Gently close your eyes and lift them gently upward. Inhale with a short and long breath through your nostrils as you tense your entire body gently then moderately. Hold the breath and then exhale with a short and long breath through your mouth and nostrils. This brings circulation to all body parts while releasing excess tension. With your next inhalation, feel this gentle lift of your eyes and as you exhale, feel how letting go of the breath is naturally followed by the letting go of pressure. This ebb and flow with the breath tunes you more deeply into the center of the body, closer to the path of least resistance. This pathway is where the life force flows. Access to this central axis begins to magnetize *prana* (life force, chi, etc.) through your conscious participation with the breath. Organs, glands, and systems will operate efficiently as you are not overtaxing them by bringing in new experiences for their processing. Instead, while awake, you are witnessing the body shift into the parasympathetic system and allowing it to process what has already been gathered. Allowing this state of rest, even if only for 5 or 10 minutes, reduces stress, lowers the heart rate, and regulates beneficial hormones throughout the endocrine system.

7. **Mind chatter:** After the body is relaxed, often even before body relaxation, the mind will wander. Sustaining a relationship with your body takes practice as you notice the rhythms of your breath and its circulation, and you are practicing how to relieve tension, stress, and blocks. Your body may think it is time for sleep; however, since you are sitting upright, thoughts can be quite strong. Thoughts have been stirring, interrupting your focus on the breath and as the body begins to drift into sleep, you are reminded by your thoughts that there are many other tasks or people that need your attention. Some people avoid meditation because this resultant activity occurs every time they try to meditate. This is the time to use your thoughts to learn and grow rather than become frustrated. Many people think they have failed meditation at this point. They cannot stop their thoughts and are looking for a blank slate and Zen-like feeling of bliss. Instead, they are thinking about their grocery list, an argument, their stomach is rumbling for food, something they forgot to do pops in, or a deadline approaching soon shouts out "you don't have time for this." So, they give up and give in. Rather than give up, give in to a deeper practice.

8. **Deepening your practice by "dialing in":** In the same way that a radio must be dialed to eliminate static, the breath, affirmations, mantras, or visualizations are tools and techniques to keep you focused and aligned to the state of consciousness (station) you desire. Your practice and observance of thoughts will enable you to know yourself more deeply. To know thyself is the beginning of wisdom. This saying, attributed to Socrates, is equally true today. You will learn, discern, and differentiate your thoughts from those of others. You will find thoughts you have picked up along your way and realize are no longer aligned with who you are now. Rather than try to understand and figure them out, you will find health and wellness is a process of letting go and tuning into that which is currently beneficial. You will begin to know and remember that if something is meant for you, it will bubble up and come around again. When it does, you can choose again. This process in meditation is the transition point in life when you get to choose what is best and appropriate for you right now. All else can be set aside or let go of entirely. These choices are levels and stages that evolve over time as you get to know yourself better. Through this conscious awareness, you will see and feel the lightness and joy that is your true state of being. You will see that which is yours and let go of all else with ease. There will be no need to collect and hold tightly to things and ways of doing life that cause dysfunction.

9. **Amaze yourself with wonder:** Think of your mind as the sky filled with clouds. The clouds are your thoughts. You can focus on the clouds (thoughts) individually and try to figure them out, or you can allow them to just be there. Like clouds, they will drift on by, come and go; some more than others. Feel your body breathing and begin to choose thoughts that are beneficial to you and let the rest float right on by. Clouds of thought will cycle around again. You can even write down ones you wish to keep and then continue to observe your thoughts moving by. As you direct your mind to focus on beneficial thoughts, you can focus on one. Noticing this, you may find this thought leading you to a state of mind and connection to your next best step. If not, just let it go and return to observing. You will begin to expand naturally into broader viewpoints. Each time you discover your mind drifting deeper and further away from the essence of a thought into details and questions such as how, when, and where, gently bring yourself back from this wandering to follow your breath and allow wonder to present itself again. Being kind to yourself is very important. This is a process and mastery comes from practicing the process. Kindness with yourself brings patience into your ability to *be* in ease and flow with your current circumstances.

10. **Align thoughts through affirmations and mantras:** *Pranayama*, a Sanskrit word, describes the control of life force: *prana* (life force) and *yama* (control). Through repetition and sound vibration, affirmations and mantras help control the life force by aligning the mind and body with beneficial feelings and states of consciousness (Yogananda, 2003a). Affirmations such as "I am calm, I am poised"; "I breathe in, I breath out"; "I am conscious, I am free"; and "I love myself, I love my life" bring forth feelings into the body and align with the vibratory and creative field of your cells. Mantras have been developed and recited for centuries. There are many for you to consider. *Hong Sau* is a Sanskrit mantra that means *I am* (*Hong*) he (*Sau*). Brought to the United States in the 1920s by Paramhansa Yogananda who said "this technique is 'the greatest contribution of India's spiritual science to the world,' and that one-hour of Hong Sau practice equals twenty-four hours of sitting in silence" (Cornell, 2013, p. 154).

In meditation, both systems are enhanced to optimally operate when the mind and body are relaxed and focused. The energy channel on the left side of the body (*ida*) moves upward with the inhalation, whereas the energy channel on the right side (*pingala*) moves downward with the exhalation. These "astral" currents waft with *prana* (life force) throughout the endocrine glands. As you focus deeper in meditation, body systems slow and conscious sensitivity to the subtle life force energy channels enhances the stillness within.

By raising focus to the midpoint between the eyes and bringing your inhalation to this point, negative energy within the body travels upward for integration with the function of the pituitary gland, the master gland of the endocrine system. Upon exhalation, release of the breath activates the pineal gland to release water throughout the body. In a simplified view of the endocrine system, oxygen affects bloodflow, the pituitary gland commands the endocrine system, and the pineal gland commands balance of the water to assist these movements. Conscious connection with the breath calms the adrenals and the sympathetic nervous system to support and enrich the parasympathetic nervous system (Chopra, 2007; Frawley, 1999).

11. **The oxytocin breath:** Allow a deep breath as before and as you exhale, relax, and open your mouth slightly. As you do so, bring forth a pleasurable thought and audibly say the word, "Hahhhhhh" with your exhalation. This sound, thought, and feeling of pleasure will notify the hypothalamus within the brain that you are safe. The fight, flight, and freeze mechanisms of the sympathetic nervous system that uses adrenaline and cortisol for survival will relax. The vagus nerve will vibrate and oxytocin will be secreted for the body

to function through the parasympathetic nervous system. Continued practice of the oxytocin breath will enhance secretion of hormones to support homeostasis within the endocrine system. Meditation, when combined with diaphragmatic and oxytocin breathing, stimulates the parasympathetic system to provide the balance of chemicals necessary to sustain health and vitality in life (Vago, 2012).

A sample guided visualization exercise that can be used to begin a meditation practice is found in Exhibit 35.1. It may be useful to have another person read it out loud or record it yourself for use. Exhibit 35.2 provides additional meditation resources.

EXHIBIT 35.1 Sample Guided Visualization Exercise

---

1. Relaxation: Relax completely, both physically and mentally.
2. Interiorization: Interiorize your attention and concentrate your focus upward at a 45° angle as if you are basking in the sun.
3. Expansion: Focus your concentrated attention on an aspect of your own deeper self; light, sound, peace, calmness, love, joy, wisdom, and power or an aspect of nature you enjoy. This will help you mindfully expand your consciousness beyond the current surroundings.
4. Now, allow yourself the naturally occurring wonder to:
   - Enjoy this aspect of self.
   - Enjoy this feeling.
   - Enjoy letting go of conditions.
5. As soon as your mind beings to wander,
   - Repeat the previous steps.
   - Repeat them again and again; a gain will occur.
   - Repetition will slowly train your mind and body.
   - It becomes much easier, even amid chaos.

When complete with your practice, write down the quality, feeling, or natural setting that came to you in your meditation. Writing this down will activate the kinesthetic memory in your cellular makeup and assist you in recalling this state of calmness and ease so that you can observe chaos, relax yourself, and look inward to follow the directions received from your inner strength to calmly speak and act from there. Practice is all it takes.

Tune in to your inner qualities: your inner strength.
Although life is ever-changing,
consistency lives deeper within . . . You!
Accept the changing exterior.
Expand your interior awareness.
Allow your breath to integrate the two.

EXHIBIT 35.2 Resources for Multiple Ways to Meditate

Free meditation programs:

- Ananda Center: http://anandasacramento.org/learn-to-meditate
- Chopra Meditation Center: www.chopracentermeditation.com
- Expanding Light Center: www.expandinglight.org/meditation
- Heal Your Body: Spoken Guided Meditation for Pain & Sickness: www.youtube.com/watch?v=_jD3VxSGM-k

(continued)

EXHIBIT 35.2 Resources for Multiple Ways to Meditate (*continued*)

- How to Meditate: www.youtube.com/watch?v=DyAOQj6FFEg
- How to Meditate Organization: www.how-to-meditate.org
- Learn to Meditate: A Free Mini Course: http://us8.campaign-archive1.com/?u=761f2a7978a0ff2f16853987a&id=bf81ea53b8
- Meditainment (for pain management): www.meditainment.com/pain-management
- Meditation: A simple, fast way to meditate: www.mayoclinic.org/tests-procedures/meditation/in-depth/meditation/art-20045858
- Meditation for Christians: www.thechristianmeditator.com/christian-meditation-techniques
- Mindbodygreen: www.mindbodygreen.com/0-16452/6-simple-meditation-techniques-for-real-people.html
- Vedanta Center: www.vedantasacto.org

Meditation apps for smartphones:

- Buddhify
- Calm
- Headspace
- Insight Timer
- OMG! I Can Meditate
- Omvana
- Smiling Mind
- Stop, Breathe & Think
- Take a Break
- The Mindfulness App

WHERE TO PRACTICE

The best practice of creating a quiet space for meditation practice can be one of the biggest excuses for a person to not begin. Individuals should not allow this to be a barrier to mindfulness practice. Meditation can be successfully practiced in virtually any environment, right in the middle of your living space, in your office, or on the train as you commute. Practicing within challenging situations can build a strong meditation practice. Everyday living is filled with distractions, and meditation provides new ways to live within distractions while remaining calm, responsive, and focused. You will and can find 5 to 10 minutes to sit and consciously breathe.

Once an individual has begun to practice, choosing a place that is comfortable and quiet can deepen the practice. In addition, it is important to be as consistent as possible in practicing meditation in the same location. This consistency supports a kinesthetic connection to the meditation practice that the body will begin to recognize. Lighting a candle and putting on soft music or earphones to deflect outside interference can support focus in the early stages of meditation practice. However, the music may eventually become a distractor. Quiet is best. Darkness or soft lighting can be beneficial if it does not provoke sleep. Sitting in nature with soft sunlight is also beneficial with proper protection of skin and hair. Meditation can be practiced at any time of day and establishing a consistent time of day for meditation promotes development of a regular practice.

INTEGRATING BENEFITS OF MEDITATION THROUGHOUT THE DAY

There are many ways health professions educators can integrate the benefits of meditation throughout each day. The following suggestions provide a guide:

1. **Stop, look, and listen:** Use transit points as a place to stop, look, and listen to your breath, your body and observe your thoughts. Transit points can be when you enter a classroom or a hallway, before a meeting or phone call, before responding to a complicated email, or before exiting or after entering your vehicle. This type of integrative practice heightens conscious awareness of physiologic stress cues or negative thoughts, allowing an intentional response. Even though outside circumstances play a large role in life, mindfulness permits a broader view and orients one toward solutions. Workplace, family, and friends will benefit as the individual creates and presents the very best of him- or herself.

2. **Meditating on a solution:** This can occur with ease. Draw a circle on a piece of paper and write a description of the challenge presenting itself to you on the line of the circle. Sit quietly and ask yourself for a few solutions and write them in the center of the circle. Just allow the free flow of ideas without editing. You will find this open space in time you created will bring solutions quickly and with ease.

3. **On the spot:** Noticing when you and/or others are operating in a state of fight, flight, or freeze is an opportunity to create calmness within yourself so that you respond rather than react. All you need do is notice the heightened level of energy and breathe deeply within. As you exhale, imagine you are exhaling the excess emotion surrounding the situation. In doing this, you are grounding yourself so you are not becoming swept up in the emotional context of the situation. Rather than being in the storm, become the eye of the storm, calm and centered.

4. **Check your EKG: E**xpress **k**indness and **g**ratitude whenever possible. The more you practice your regular meditation, these practices and more will become the normal way for you to respond to any situation, even emergencies.

WHY PRACTICE MEDITATION?

The body naturally accesses the adrenal system for increased energy and stamina during emergent situations when survival is at stake. The inability to process and differentiate emergencies from everyday occurrences creates exhaustion from constantly operating in "emergency mode" (Dobkin, 2008; Kabat-Zinn, 1990). Conscious awareness of this exhaustion can help people learn that reaction to stress has stopped the natural rhythm within and stimulated the sympathetic nervous system to increase adrenal output. Shallow breathing, holding the breath, and inconsistent use of diaphragmatic breathing become habit, which bypasses the intrinsic homeostatic mechanism to restore balance between the sympathetic and parasympathetic systems. Meditation and mindfulness training have been demonstrated to restore this balance and provide the following benefits.

1. **Reduce stress:** Studies show that meditation relaxes muscles and declutters the mind. The result is total mind and body rejuvenation, and increased resilience to stress and the pressures of everyday life (Aherne et al., 2016; Galante, Galante, Bekkers, & Gallacher, 2014; Goyal et al., 2014; Grossman, Niemann, Schmidt, & Walach, 2004; Irving, Dobkin, & Park, 2009; Khoury et al., 2015; Reibel, Greeson, Brainard, & Rosenzweig, 2001).

2. **Improve sleep patterns:** A regular meditation practice improves sleep patterns, particularly enhancing refreshing, rejuvenating, deeper sleep (Dentico et al., 2016; Nagendra, Maruthai, & Kutty, 2012).

3. **Increase creativity and cognitive flexibility:** Meditation is shown to amplify the ability to tap into ideas and create new ones; it also helps unlock new ideas with greater ease (Lebuda, Zabelina, & Karwowski, 2016; Müller et al., 2016).

4. **Sharpen focus and working memory:** Meditation sharpens focus resulting in improved goal orientation and efficiency. In addition, mindfulness training is shown to reduce functional impairment in working memory associated with high-stress environments such as

academia (Chan & Woollacott, 2007; Chiesa, Calati, & Serretti, 2011; Jha, Stanley, Kiyonaga, Wong, & Gelfand, 2010).

5. **Improve emotional regulation and increase compassion:** Meditation and mindfulness training with a specific focus in cultivating compassion (CCT) is demonstrated to improve all three domains of compassion—compassion for others, receiving compassion from others, and self-compassion (Jazaieri et al., 2013, 2014).

6. **A healthier mind and body:** Multiple studies have confirmed that meditation and mindfulness training have a powerful impact on every aspect of health, from lowering blood pressure to strengthening the immune system (Carlson, Speca, Faris, & Patel, 2007; Davidson et al., 2003; Jevning, Wallace, & Beidebach, 1992; Khoury et al., 2013).

CONCLUSIONS

The ability to see the overall picture in the scheme of things comes with time and experience. Practiced attunement to the inner self is the easiest way to observe and become familiar with thoughts, actions, behaviors, and emotions. Being an observer of oneself provides distancing from the personal to the impersonal. This practice expands the viewpoint beyond self-centeredness to see the center of self in all people and all things. This begins the disintegration of feeling separate from others and enhances a deeper connection based on unification, commonality, and the infinite number of possibilities available. Freedom, joy, and fulfillment are attained when possibilities become the normal vantage point from which to view life and its many opportunities from changing circumstances. These meditation techniques, practices, and the science behind them can be used to maintain balance in the face of the day-to-day challenges of health professions education.

In calmness, I touch my inner strength.

—J. Donald Walters

REFERENCES

Aherne, D., Farrant, K., Hickey, L., Hickey, E., McGrath, L., & McGrath, D. (2016). Mindfulness-based stress reduction for medical students: Optimising student satisfaction and engagement. *BMC Medical Education*, 16(1), 209.

Carlson, L. E., Speca, M., Faris, P., & Patel, K. D. (2007). One year pre-post intervention follow-up of psychological, immune, endocrine and blood pressure outcomes of mindfulness-based stress reduction (MBSR) in breast and prostate cancer outpatients. *Brain, Behavior, and Immunity*, 21, 1038–1049.

Chan, D., & Woollacott, M. (2007). Effects of level of meditation experience on attentional focus: Is the efficiency of executive or orientation networks improved?" *Journal of Alternative and Complementary Medicine*, 13(6), 651–658.

Chiesa, A., Calati, R., & Serretti, A. (2011). Does mindfulness training improve cognitive abilities? A systematic review of neuropsychological findings. *Clinical Psychology Review*, 31(3), 449–464.

Chopra, D. (2007). *Perfect health—Revised and updated: The complete mind body guide*. New York, NY: Three Rivers Press.

Cornell, J. B. (2013). *AUM, The melody of love; The spirit behind all creation*. Nevada City, CA: Crystal Clarity.

Davidson, R. J., Kabat-Zinn, J., Schumacher, J., Rosenkranz, M., Muller, D., Santorelli, S. F., . . . Sheridan, J. F. (2003). Alterations in brain and immune function produced by mindfulness meditation. *Psychosomatic Medicine*, 65(4), 564–570.

Dentico, D., Ferrarelli, F., Riedner, B. A., Smith, R., Zennig, C., Lutz, A., . . . Davidson, R. J. (2016). Short meditation trainings enhance non-REM sleep low-frequency oscillations. *PLOS ONE*, 11(2), e0148961. doi:10.1371/journal.pone.0148961

Dobkin, P. L. (2008). Mindfulness-based stress reduction: What processes are at work? *Complementary Therapies in Clinical Practice*, 14(1), 8–16.

Fox, K. C., Nijeboer, S., Dixon, M. L., Floman, J. L., Ellamil, M., Rumak, S. P., . . . Christoff, K. (2014). Is meditation associated with altered brain structure? A systematic review and meta-analysis of morphometric neuroimaging in meditation practitioners. *Neuroscience and Biobehavioral Reviews, 43*, 48–73.

Frawley, D. (1999). *Yoga and Ayurveda: Self-healing and self-realization.* Twin Lakes, WI: Lotus Press.

Galante, J., Galante, I., Bekkers, M., & Gallacher, J. (2014). Effect of kindness-based meditation on health and well-being: A systematic review and meta-analysis. *Journal of Consulting and Clinical Psychology, 82*(6), 1101–1114.

Germer, C. (2004). What is mindfulness? *Insight Journal, 22,* 24–29.

Goyal, M., Singh, S., Sibinga, E. M. S., Gould, N. F., Rowland-Seymour, A., Sharma, R., . . . Haythornthwaite, J. A. (2014). Meditation programs for psychological stress and well-being: A systematic review and meta-analysis. *JAMA Internal Medicine, 174*(3), 357–368.

Grossman, P., Niemann, L., Schmidt, S., & Walach, H. (2004). Mindfulness-based stress reduction and health benefits: A meta-analysis. *Journal of Psychosomatic Research, 57*(1), 35–43.

Irving, J. A., Dobkin, P. L., & Park, J. (2009). Cultivating mindfulness in health care professionals: A review of empirical studies of mindfulness-based stress reduction (MBSR). *Complementary Therapies in Clinical Practice, 15*(2), 61–66.

Jazaieri, H., Jinpa, G. T., McGonigal, K., Rosenberg, E. L., Finkelstein, J., Simon-Thomas, E., . . . Goldin, P. R. (2013). Enhancing compassion: A randomized controlled trial of a compassion cultivation training program. *Journal of Happiness Studies, 14*(4), 1113–1126.

Jazaieri, H., Lee, I. A., McGonigal, K., Jinpa, T., Doty, J. R., Gross, J. J., & Goldin, P. R. (2016). A wandering mind is a less caring mind: Daily experience sampling during compassion meditation training. *Journal of Positive Psychology, 11*(1), 37–50.

Jazaieri, H., McGonigal, K., Jinpa, T., Doty, J. R., Gross, J. J., & Goldin, P. R. (2014). A randomized controlled trial of compassion cultivation training: Effects on mindfulness, affect, and emotion regulation. *Motivation and Emotion, 38,* 23–35.

Jevning, R., Wallace, R. K., & Beidebach, M. (1992). The physiology of meditation: A review. A wakeful hypometabolic integrated response. *Neuroscience and Biobehavioral Reviews, 16,* 415–424.

Jha, A. P., Stanley, E. A., Kiyonaga, A., Wong, L., & Gelfand, L. (2010). Examining the protective effects of mindfulness training on working memory capacity and affective experience. *Emotion, 10*(1), 54.

Kabat-Zinn, J. (1990). *Full catastrophe living: Using the wisdom of your body and mind to face stress, pain and illness.* New York, NY: Delacorte.

Khoury, B., Lecomte, T., Fortin, G., Masse, M., Therien, P., Bouchard, V., . . . Hofmann, S. G. (2013). Mindfulness-based therapy: A comprehensive meta-analysis *Clinical Psychology Review, 33*(6), 763–771.

Khoury, B., Sharma, M. J., Rush, S. E., & Fournier, C. (2015). Mindfulness-based stress reduction for healthy individuals: A meta-analysis. *Journal of Psychosomatic Research, 78*(6), 519–528.

Lebuda, I., Zabelina, D. L., & Karwowski, M. (2016). Mind full of ideas: A meta-analysis of the mindfulness–creativity link. *Personality and Individual Differences, 93,* 22–26.

Müller, B. C. N., Gerasimova, A., & Ritter, S. M. (2016). Concentrative meditation influences creativity by increasing cognitive flexibility. *Psychology of Aesthetics, Creativity, and the Arts, 10*(3), 278–286.

Nagendra, R. P., Maruthai, N., & Kutty, B. M. (2012). Meditation and its regulatory role on sleep. *Frontiers in Neurology,* doi:10.3389/fneur.2012.00054

Praissman, S. (2008). Mindfulness-based stress reduction: A literature review and clinician's guide. *Journal of the American Academy of Nurse Practitioners, 20*(4), 212–216.

Reibel, D. K., Greeson, J. M., Brainard, G. C., & Rosenzweig, S. (2001). Mindfulness-based stress reduction and health-related quality of life in a heterogeneous patient population. *General Hospital Psychiatry, 23*(4), 183–192.

Smart, D., English, A., James, J., Wilson, M., Daratha, K. B., Childers, B., & Magera, C. (2014). Compassion fatigue and satisfaction: A cross-sectional survey among U.S. healthcare workers. *Nursing and Health Sciences, 16*(1), 3–10.

Vago, D. R. (2012). Self-awareness, self-regulation, and self-transcendence (S-ART): A framework for understanding the neurobiological mechanisms of mindfulness. *Frontiers in Human Neuroscience, 6,* 296.

Yogananda, P. (2003a). *Autobiography of a Yogi.* Nevada City, CA: Crystal Clarity Publishers.

Yogananda, P. (2003b). *Metaphysical meditations.* Los Angeles, CA: Self-Realization Fellowship.

PART VIII
Current Trends and Future Directions in Health Professions Education

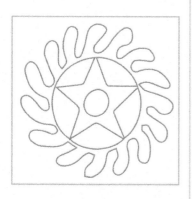

SESA WO SUBAN
"Change or transform your character."

Symbol of life transformation

This symbol combines two separate adinkra symbols, the "morning star," which can mean a new start to the day, placed inside the wheel, representing rotation or independent movement.

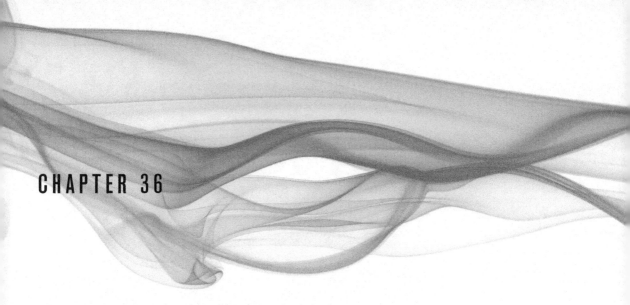

CHAPTER 36

Postgraduate Fellowships and Residency Programs

Vasco Deon Kidd, Dennis Tankersley, and Virginia McCoy Hass

CHAPTER OBJECTIVES

- Describe fellowships and residencies for physician assistants (PAs) and nurse practitioners (NPs), including pros and cons
- Discuss how to start a postgraduate residency program

Better than a thousand days of diligent study is one day with a great teacher.

—Japanese proverb

Enrolling in a formal postgraduate education program is one of several ways physician assistants (PAs) and nurse practitioners (NPs) may gain advanced knowledge and skill. Formal postgraduate training programs provide a structured education similar to that of a physician residency program. Although these postgraduate training programs are often referred to as either *residencies* or *fellowships*, residencies and fellowships are not necessarily synonymous.

In physician graduate medical education (GME), a residency is a mandatory training program that prepares medical graduates for board certification and independent practice of medicine in a specialty, whereas a fellowship provides elective subspecialty training following a residency and board certification (Accreditation Council for Graduate Medical Education [ACGME], 2013). Thus, postgraduate training for PAs and NPs is most accurately described as a fellowship in elective postgraduate specialty training sought by board-certified PAs or NPs. Still, no official governing body oversees the usage of these terms, and PA and NP postgraduate training programs frequently use the term that best fits the customs of the hospital or university system in which they are housed.

THE GROWTH OF PHYSICIAN ASSISTANT POSTGRADUATE RESIDENCIES AND FELLOWSHIPS

PA postgraduate education began in 1971; in the late 1980s and early 1990s, it experienced an uptick in program development that was driven by several factors. The first was the downsizing of physician residency programs (Verhoven, 1998). Furthermore, decreases in GME funding and restrictions on the number of resident duty hours allowed have contributed to the demand for PAs within teaching hospitals (Moote, Krsek, Kleinpell, & Todd, 2011). Students' attraction to postgraduate education most likely occurs during clinical rotations in which they are exposed to the various specialties. Tertiary referral hospitals provide excellent opportunities for students to work and learn from experts. The reputation of an institution and its faculty remains the primary selling point for students considering a residency or fellowship program (Verhoven, 1998).

Over the past decade, PA postgraduate training has intensified due to both surging demand for specialty PAs and the relative scarcity of primary care openings (Morgan, Himmerick, Leach, Dieter, & Everett, 2016; Morgan & Hooker, 2010). Recent research has shown that the overwhelming majority (82%) of PA job postings in 2014 were for positions in specialties ($n = 28,047$), whereas only 18% of PA job postings were for primary care positions ($n = 6,091$; Morgan et al., 2016). An increased demand for specialty health care coverage, a growing realization of the economic benefits of utilizing PAs to augment the delivery of specialty medical care, and a growing acceptance of team-based care have continued to fuel the demand for formal postgraduate PA educational programs. As a result, programs that mirror either the internship or physician academic model can be found in nearly all medical specialties (American Academy of Physician Assistants [AAPA], 2005), including (but not limited to) orthopedics, emergency medicine, general surgery, urology, critical care, dermatology, pediatrics, neurology, oncology/hematology, and psychiatry.

The majority of these programs are in some way associated with or housed in institutions that also have physician GME. Program length varies by specialty from 6 months to 24 months; the vast majority of programs offer a certificate of completion (Polansky, Garver, & Hilton, 2012; Wiemiller, Somers, & Adams, 2008). A small number of postgraduate programs offer a terminal degree such as a master's option or doctor of science (DSc) in PA studies (Wiemiller et al., 2008). Unlike physician residencies, PA and NP postgraduate training programs are not eligible for Medicare direct GME payments.

As part of the growth of PA residencies and fellowships, a formal organization, the Association of Postgraduate PA Programs (APPAP), was founded in 1988. The APPAP provides general guidelines for member programs in the areas of curricular delivery, sponsorship, faculty, administrative personnel, resident evaluation, and program governance. The APPAP does not have regulatory or policy-making authority, and not all PA postgraduate training programs are affiliated with APPAP (2017).

THE GROWTH OF NURSE PRACTITIONER POSTGRADUATE RESIDENCIES AND FELLOWSHIPS

The first NP postgraduate residency program started in 2007 at the Community Health Center, Inc. (CHCI) of Middletown, Connecticut (Flinter, 2012). Although no systematic review of NP residency programs has been done, there is evidence that their numbers are growing (Brown, Poppe, Kaminetzky, Wipf, & Woods, 2015; Flinter, 2012; Goudreau et al., 2011). In January

2012, the University of California, San Francisco (UCSF) and University of California, Los Angeles (UCLA) launched the NP residency partnership, which offers four 1-year residencies to certified NPs and is modeled after the CHCI residency. NP postgraduate residency and fellowship programs have not grown at the rate of those for PAs perhaps because NPs have two options for formal postgraduate education (i.e., research-focused and practice-focused) (American Association of Colleges of Nursing [AACN], 2010).

ACCREDITATION OF POSTGRADUATE RESIDENCIES AND FELLOWSHIPS

Accreditation of PA Postgraduate Residencies and Fellowships

The Accreditation Review Commission on Education for the Physician Assistant (ARC-PA) is the only accrediting body in PA education. The ARC-PA accredits entry-level PA programs, and, until 2014, it also accredited postgraduate residency and fellowship programs (ARC-PA, 2017). During the years in which accreditation was offered in postgraduate residency and fellowship programs, the ARC-PA granted accreditation to eight clinical postgraduate programs in the United States (Exhibit 36.1).

In 2013, the Society of Emergency Medicine Physician Assistants (SEMPA) convened the SEMPA Postgraduate Training Committee to provide existing program guidance in the development of educational curriculum and to support the development of new programs. This committee, composed of representatives from several postgraduate program across the country, published the *Emergency Medicine Physician Assistant Postgraduate Training Program Standards* in 2015. SEMPA is the only PA specialty organization to have provided this level of guidance to its specialty, and it has sought collaboration with both APPAP and ARC-PA in the development of a new process that recognizes the educational quality of postgraduate PA programs (SEMPA, 2015).

Accreditation of NP Postgraduate Residencies and Fellowships

Currently, there is no central organization or standardized curriculum for NP residency programs. The majority of NP postgraduate residencies and fellowships are offered through community health centers, federally qualified health centers, and other health care organizations.

EXHIBIT 36.1 ARC-PA Accredited Postgraduate PA Residency and Fellowship Programs

Arrowhead Postgraduate PA Orthopedics Residency
Duke University Medical Center Postgraduate PA Surgical Residency
Johns Hopkins Hospital Department of Surgery Postgraduate PA Surgical Residency
Mayo Clinic Postgraduate PA ENT Residency
Mayo Clinic Postgraduate PA Hospital Internal Medicine Residency
MD Anderson Cancer Center Postgraduate PA Program in Oncology
Naval Medical Center (Portsmouth) Postgraduate PA Program in Orthopedics
University of Iowa Postgraduate PA Emergency Medicine Residency

Source: ARC-PA (2017).

Although most of these are in primary care, some are in subspecialties such as hepatology (Bond, 2014; Brown et al., 2015).

PROS AND CONS OF POSTGRADUATE RESIDENCY AND FELLOWSHIP TRAINING

Physician Assistant Residency and Fellowship Programs

Since the inception of PA postgraduate training, little consensus has been reached over the value of these programs as they relate to on-the-job training. Research is limited on specific attitudes, experiences, capabilities, and expectations of residents or fellows who have completed postgraduate PA training programs. A recent study found high levels of satisfaction among graduates who completed a postgraduate training program; in fact, such graduates felt they were more marketable, required less onboarding time, and experienced increased confidence in their chosen specialty (Anick, Carlson, & Knott, 2003). Moreover, nearly 90% felt that postgraduate programs provided them the skill sets they needed to become leaders within their organization or specialty (Anick et al., 2003). Asprey and Helms (1999) surveyed 16 PA residency program directors (PDs) about the efficacy of their programs and found that the majority of PDs felt that residency-trained PAs were better prepared to practice their specialty than PAs with equivalent durations of on-the-job training in the same specialty area. Anecdotally, employers' recognition of residency programs is growing, especially in large integrated health systems and physician groups, which preferentially recruit graduates from these training programs. Further research is needed to validate this trend and the value added by residency training.

Among the potential drawbacks to PA postgraduate training programs is an increase in student debt resulting from the accumulation of additional interest owed and reduced income while enrolled. Although no programs currently require tuition, participants of postgraduate training programs are routinely paid at a level that is far below an entry-level salary. In addition, PA residents or fellows typically do not work a standard workweek and are often uncompensated for overtime. In addition, there is no evidence that residency training increases compensation in the long term (Dehn, 2007). These uncertainties could result in reduced interest in PA postgraduate training programs over time.

Nurse Practitioner Residency Programs

Current research focuses on strategies and potential barriers to starting an NP residency program (Brown et al., 2015). Little is known about the long-term cost–benefit implications of these programs on the health care system and the NPs who join them. Further research is needed to elucidate both the short- and long-term pros and cons of NP residencies.

WILL PA POSTGRADUATE TRAINING BE REQUIRED FOR FUTURE PRACTICE?

Peter Drucker is widely quoted as saying, "Trying to predict the future is like trying to drive down a country road at night with no lights while looking out the back window" (cited in Schweyer, Newman, & De Vries, 2009, p. 53). In a similar vein, it is too early to predict the impact of postgraduate training on the PA profession. However, for several reasons, it is unlikely that postgraduate PA residency training will be a requirement for clinical practice in the near future. First, it is estimated that fewer than 2% of PA graduates apply for postgraduate training programs (Polansky et al., 2012). Second, the value of extending PA training beyond the generalist model is questionable in light of the trend toward accelerated medical school curricula (Green, Welty, Thomas, & Curry, 2016; Raymond, Kerschner, Hueston, & Maurana, 2015). Third, rising PA salaries—especially in places such as California, Connecticut, Minnesota, Arizona, and Alaska, where the median salary is $105,000—may hamper efforts to recruit students for postgraduate training programs (Japsen, 2016). Finally, millennials approach medical education differently than other generations. Many PA postgraduate surgical training programs require 60 to 80 hours per week when factoring night, day, and weekend call shifts. Research has shown that millennials prefer life balance over working 80 hours a week, and they typically are not interested in sacrificing quality of life even for the prospect of higher salaries (Western Michigan University School of Medicine, 2013). Even the physician residency-training model, which has been in existence for more than 100 years, is being restructured to accommodate the expectations of millennial residents (Toohey, Wray, Wiechmann, Lin, & Boysen-Osborn, 2016). PA postgraduate residency may want to consider ways of restructuring its traditional postgraduate training programs to a modified version that incorporates greater life balance and newer technology (such as hybrid educational design; Toohey et al., 2016). In addition, incorporating quality improvement and leadership development opportunities into postgraduate training could better prepare millennials for an evolving health care system.

DEVELOPING A POSTGRADUATE RESIDENCY OR FELLOWSHIP PROGRAM

A crucial step in initiating a postgraduate training program is to determine whether the sponsoring institution, medical group, or health center can provide the financial, administrative, and didactic support, and the appropriate mix of clinical experiences for prospective trainees. Equally important is whether the culture of the practice site is supportive of PA or NP postgraduate residency training, because the clinical staff is responsible for the day-to-day delivery of care.

Approval Process

In some settings, particularly large health care organization or physician groups, the medical executive committee (MEC) has the final authority to endorse program approval. Also, PA or NP postgraduate trainees may require credentialing for practice. Getting the endorsements of the MEC and staff can be challenging; a recommended strategy for selling the idea of postgraduate residency training is to demonstrate how trainees can reduce physician residents' workloads, increase access, and improve care without substantial cost to the health system. It is also important to demonstrate to key stakeholders that the residency program will not infringe on funding and educational resources allocated for traditional Medicare ACGME-funded programs (i.e., physician residencies).

Program Funding

The next task is to secure start-up funding for the program. It is important to develop a business plan and budget that details the costs associated with resident or fellow stipends and benefits, administrative support, instructional faculty, recruitment, conferences, textbooks, supplies, and credentialing. Although no data on the average costs of developing PA or NP postgraduate training programs are available, a few financial considerations must be taken into account. For example, the hidden costs of trainee onboarding can affect the bottom line. The average U.S. company spends $12,000 per employee on training ("Bersin by Deloitte," 2015). This cost is potentially offset by PAs or NPs billing for services.

Program Leadership

It is vital to have an experienced PD, preferably a lead or chief PA or NP who has experience in program evaluation, curricular development, staff supervision, and health systems policies. The PD should remain current in the discipline and be able to oversee all aspects of postgraduate training. Administrative support will vary depending on the needs of the program. The program should also have a collaborating physician who represents the program at the MEC committee, subcommittee meetings, and internal review panels. The chairman works with the PD to develop the educational curriculum and measureable learning objectives to assess trainee competence.

Didactic Curriculum

The didactic component should encompass comprehensive learning experiences, including weekly lectures, seminars, grand rounds, simulation in procedure or surgical skills lab, journal club, radiology review, and research or quality-improvement opportunities. Specific objectives for each learning experience should be based on the competencies of each profession. Competencies for the PA profession include six general areas: medical knowledge, interpersonal and communication skills, patient care, professionalism, practice-based learning and improvement, and systems-based practice (AAPA/Accreditation Review Commission on Education for the Physician Assistant/Physician Assistant Education Association/National Commission on Certification of Physician Assistants, 2012). Core competencies for the NP profession include scientific foundation, leadership, quality improvement, practice inquiry, technology and information literacy, health policy and delivery systems, ethics, and independent practice (National Organization of Nurse Practitioner Faculties [NONPF], 2012).

The curriculum of postgraduate residency programs may be formatted as block rotations or longitudinal training. Before the didactic phase is implemented, clear expectations must be set regarding how postgraduate trainees will be supervised and interact with physician residents and clinical staff. Although physician residents may supervise medical residents, it is not appropriate for resident physicians to supervise postgraduate PA and NP trainees and they should not act as chart cosigners. Graduate PA and NP trainees must be supervised by a clinician who is certified and licensed in his or her respective field. The postgraduate program must adopt and follow health system and medical staff bylaws and policies.

Trainee Evaluation

Evaluations of postgraduate trainees should occur periodically throughout their training. Residents or fellows should receive continued timely feedback regarding their progress and potential areas needing improvement. We recommend evaluations based on the competencies specific to each profession, as described earlier. In each of the relevant competency domains, learning outcomes should be tied to program goals and objectives. It is important to have obtainable targets for resident performance using formal and informal assessments. Attending physicians, PAs, and/or NPs who serve as instructional faculty should be involved in assessing and mentoring postgraduate trainees.

Class Size

A final concern is class size. There is no standard formula or rubric for how many enrollees to accept. The maximum should be based on the resources (clinical space, human resources, funding, and so forth) available to the program. And in general, a minimum class size of two participants is preferred in order to create a "cohort." Current literature suggests that peer interaction and evaluation are important for professional development among medical residents (Dupras & Edson, 2011).

RECOMMENDATIONS FOR FUTURE RESEARCH

As previously noted, current research focusing on PA postgraduate residencies is limited. And we have just reached a decade of NP postgraduate residency programs. More research is needed to analyze the cost–benefit of these programs. Areas of exploration include employer and trainee satisfaction, best practices in curriculum development, educational quality and effectiveness, health care quality and safety outcomes, cost savings, and perceptions of other health care providers such as physicians regarding PA and NP residency programs.

CONCLUSIONS

Since its inception, PA postgraduate residency training has been met with optimism and criticism. Attitudes toward NP residency programs are similarly mixed. But one thing is clear: Formal postgraduate residencies for PAs and NPs have caught the eye of the professions, researchers, employers, and hospital administrators. Still, more research is needed to evaluate the effectiveness of these programs. Moreover, the question of whether residency or fellowship training is superior to on-the-job training can only be answered by research. Given the growing demand for both NPs and specialty PAs, we expect the development of postgraduate training programs to continue.

REFERENCES

Accreditation Council for Graduate Medical Education. (2013). Glossary of terms. Retrieved from http://www.acgme.org/Portals/0/PDFs/ab_ACGMEglossary.pdf?ver=2015-11-06-115749-460

Accreditation Review Commission on Education for the Physician Assistant. (2017). Accreditation History of Postgraduate Programs. Retrieved from http://www.arc-pa.org/accreditation/postgraduate-programs/accreditation-process/

American Academy of Physician Assistants. (2005). Maintaining professional flexibility. The case against accreditation of post graduate physician assistant programs. *Journal of the American Academy of Physician Assistants, 18*(8), 14–16.

American Academy of Physician Assistants Accreditation Review Commission on Education for the Physician Assistant/Physician Assistant Education Association/National Commission on Certification of Physician Assistants. (2012). Competencies for the physician assistant profession. Retrieved from http://www.nccpa.net/uploads/docs/pacompetencies.pdf

American Association of Colleges of Nursing. (2010). Retrieved from http://www.aacn.nche.edu/publications/position/DNPpositionstatement.pdf

Anick, M., Carlson, J., & Knott, P. (2003). Postgraduate PA residency training. *Advance NP/PAs, 11*(1), 50.

Association of Postgraduate PA Programs. (2017). A resource for postgraduate education for physician assistants. Retrieved from http://appap.org

Asprey, D., & Helms, L. (1999). A description of physician assistant postgraduate residency training: The director's perspective. *Perspective on Physician Assistant Education, 10*(3), 124–131.

Bersin by Deloitte. (2015). U.S. spending on recruitment rises, driven by increased competition for critical talent. Retrieved from http://www.bersin.com/News/Content.aspx?id=18439

Bond, J. (2014). 30 great nurse practitioner residency programs. Retrieved from http://www.bestmasterofscienceinnursing.com/great-nurse-practitioner-residency-programs

Brown, K., Poppe, A., Kaminetzky, C., Wipf, J., & Woods, N. F. (2015). Recommendations for nurse practitioner residency programs. *Nurse Educator, 40*(3), 148–151.

Dehn, R. (2007). PA-C. Is PA residency training worth it? *Clinical Advisor, 10*(2). Retrieved from http://www.clinicaladvisor.com/commentary/pa-is-pa-residency-training-worth-it/article/116919/

Dupras, D. M., & Edson, R. S. (2011). A survey of resident opinions on peer evaluation in a large internal medicine residency program. *Journal of Graduate Medical Education*, *3*(2), 138–143. doi:10.4300/JGME-D-10-00099.1

Flinter, M. (2012). From new nurse practitioner to primary care provider: Bridging the transition through FQHC-based residency training. *Online Journal of Issues in Nursing*, *17*(1). Retrieved from http://www.nursingworld.org/MainMenuCategories/ANAMarketplace/ANAPeriodicals/OJIN/TableofContents/Vol-17-2012/No1-Jan-2012/Articles-Previous-Topics/From-New-Nurse-Practitioner-to-Primary-Care-Provider.html

Goudreau, K. A., Ortman, M. I., Moore, J. D., Aldredge, L., Helland, M. K., Fernandes, L. A., & Gibson, S. (2011). A nurse practitioner residency pilot program: A journey of learning. *Journal of Nursing Administration*, *41*(9), 382–387.

Green, M. M., Welty, L., Thomas, J. X., & Curry, R. H. (2016). Academic performance of students in an accelerated baccalaureate/MD program: Implications for alternative physician education pathways. *Academic Medicine*, *91*(2), 256–261.

Japsen, B. (2016, January). Physician assistant pay reaches $100K annually. *Forbes*.

Moote, M., Krsek, C., Kleinpell, R., & Todd, B. (2011). Physician assistant and nurse practitioner utilization in academic medical centers. *American Journal of Medical Quality*, *26*(6), 452–460.

Morgan, P., Himmerick, K. A., Leach, B., Dieter, P., & Everett, C. (2016). Scarcity of primary care positions may divert physician assistants into specialty practice. *Medical Care Research and Review*, *74*(1), 109–122.

Morgan, P. A., & Hooker, R. S. (2010). Choice of specialties among physician assistants in the United States. *Health Affairs*, *29*(5), 887–892.

National Organization of Nurse Practitioner Faculties. (2012). Nurse practitioner core competencies. Retrieved from http://c.ymcdn.com/sites/www.nonpf.org/resource/resmgr/competencies/npcorecompetenciesfinal2012.pdf

Polansky, M., Garver, G. J. H., & Hilton, G. (2012). Postgraduate clinical education of physician assistants. *Journal of Physician Assistant Education*, *23*(1), 39–45.

Raymond, J. R., Sr., Kerschner, J. E., Hueston, W. J., & Maurana, C. A. (2015). The merits and challenges of three-year medical school curricula: Time for an evidence-based discussion. *Academic Medicine*, *90*(10), 1318–1323.

Schweyer, A., Newman, E., & De Vries, P. (2009). *Talent management technologies: A buyer's guide to new, innovative solutions*. AuthorHouse.

Society of Emergency Medicine Physician Assistants. (2015). Emergency medicine physician assistant postgraduate training program standards. Retrieved from https://www.sempa.org/uploadedFiles/SEMPA/PostGraduate_Programs/EMPA%20Postgraduate%20Training%20Standards%20PDF%20File%20for%20Website.pdf

Toohey, S. L., Wray, A., Wiechmann, W., Lin, M., & Boysen-Osborn, M. (2016). Ten tips for engaging the millennial learner and moving an emergency medicine residency curriculum into the 21st century. *Western Journal of Emergency Medicine*, *17*(3), 337.

Verhoven, A. (1998). Interest in and opinions on postgraduate emergency medicine physician assistant residency training programs: A national survey. *Perspective on Physician Assistant Education*, *9*(2), 64–70.

Western Michigan University School of Medicine. (2013). How are millennial students (and faculty) different from previous generations? Retrieved from http://www.med.wmich.edu/how-are-millennial-students-and-faculty-different-previous-generations

Wiemiller, M. J., Somers, K. K., & Adams, M. B. (2008). Postgraduate physician assistant training programs in the United States: Emerging trends and opportunities. *Journal of Physician Assistant Education*, *19*(4), 58–63.

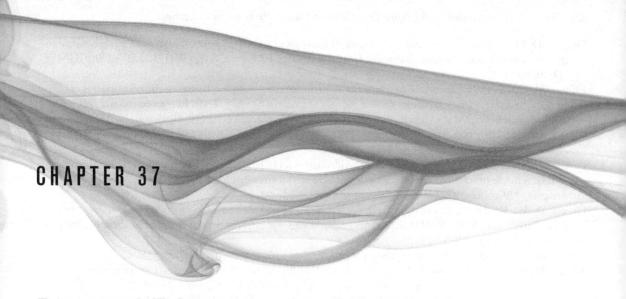

CHAPTER 37

Doctoral Education for Physician Assistants: Demand, Design, and Drawbacks

Lucy W. Kibe and James F. Cawley

CHAPTER OBJECTIVE

- Compare and contrast influences shaping the debate about doctoral degrees for physician assistants

---

It is the mark of an educated mind to be able to entertain a thought without accepting it.

—Aristotle

DOCTORAL EDUCATION FOR PHYSICIAN ASSISTANTS

Clinical doctorate degrees have become the terminal expected credential for a number of health professions. In the past decade, a lot has been written about the doctor of nursing practice (DNP; Carollo & Mason, 2017), but little is still known about doctoral education for physician assistants (PAs). This chapter focuses on doctoral education for PAs, which has surfaced in the past decade as part of the phenomena in U.S. higher education known as *degree creep*, in which a variety of health care professions have created doctoral-level degrees as the completion of professional training. This trend is obvious in pharmacy, physical therapy, advance practice nursing, and assorted others. PAs are the only clinical practitioners with prescribing authority who do not have a profession-specific doctorate option. Within the field of PA education, there are two

---

EXHIBIT 37.1 Relevant Definitions

- **Doctor:** Derived from Latin, equivalent to *doc (ēre)*, meaning to teach.
- **Doctorate** (aka *doctor's degree*): The highest award a student can earn for graduate study. Warrants the title *doctor*. This term is used in any field of study.
- **Professional doctorate** (aka *doctor's degree–professional practice, practice doctorate, or applied doctorate*): This is a doctoral degree conferred on "completion of a program providing the knowledge and skills for the recognition, credential, or license required for professional practice"and may be an entry level for the profession or obtained after the professional degree (National Center for Education Statistics, 2015). Either way, the total preprofessional and professional length of study is at least 6 years. Some examples of professional doctoral degrees: DC or DCM, DDS, DMD, DNP, DO, DPM, JD, and MD.
- **Postprofessional doctorate:** Not a specific degree designation. Refers to a doctoral degree earned after obtaining a professional credential. For example, a PA can obtain a postprofessional DHSc*, EdD, DrPH, PhD.
- **Clinical doctorate:** Refers to a professional doctorate, which includes clinical study, most commonly entry level, for example, MD, DO, DDS, DVM.
- **Postprofessional clinical doctorate:** Refers to a professional doctorate, which includes advanced clinical study (e.g., clinical specialization) obtained after obtaining a professional credential (e.g., DNP and DPT models that are not entry level, DSc-PA).
- **Doctor's degree-research/scholarship:** A doctoral degree that requires successful completion of empirical study of original work or execution of an original project, demonstrating substantial artistic or scholarly achievement (e.g., PhD).

DC or DCM, doctor of chiropractic; DDS, doctor of dental surgery; DHS or DHSC, doctor of health science; DMD, doctor of medicine in dentistry; DNP, doctor of nursing practice; DO, doctor of osteopathic medicine; DrPH, doctor of public health; DPM, doctor of podiatric medicine; DPT, doctor of physical therapy; DSc-PA, doctor of science physicians assistant; DVM, doctor of veterinary medicine; EdD, doctor of education; JD, doctor of jurisprudence; MD, doctor of medicine; OD, doctor of optometry; Pharm D, doctor of pharmacy; PhD, doctor of philosophy.

*In this chapter, *DHS* and *DHSc* refer to the same degree.

Source: National Center for Education Statistics (2015).

potential categories of doctoral education: an entry-level doctoral degree that would accompany professional education and a postprofessional doctorate in which some form of doctoral degree is obtained after professional education (Exhibit 37.1). This chapter examines both categories of PA doctoral degrees and discusses their emergence, advantages, and challenges. It also provides a summary of some of the things to consider for those interested in pursuing doctoral education (Exhibit 37.2).

CLINICAL DOCTORATE–BACKGROUND

Over the past several decades, there has been a steady growth in postprofessional clinical doctorate (PPD) degrees using transitional models from bachelor's or master's to doctoral degrees. These trends have more recently moved on to exclusively entry-level models for practice in their professions. For example, PharmD, DPT, and DNP first introduced transitional bachelor's-to-doctorate or master's-to-doctorate paths. By 2005, the American Association of Colleges of Pharmacy (AACP) phased out the transitional PharmD, and the entry-level PharmD became the only professional pharmacy degree (Accreditation Council for Pharmacy Education [ACPE], 2011). In 2000, the American Physical Therapy Association House of Delegates (APTA-HOD) announced that by 2020, "physical therapy will be provided by physical therapists who are doctors of physical therapy, recognized by consumers and other health care professionals as the practitioners" (APTA, 2015). Similarly, the American Association of Colleges of Nursing (AACN, 2015) voted to move the level of preparation of advanced nursing practice to the doctorate level by 2015 (DNP fact sheet; AACN, 2016). However, the transitions by these disciplines were not without controversy (Chase & Pruitt, 2006; Huggins & Choy, 2016; Pierce & Peyton, 1999; Plack & Wong, 2002). These evolutions took years, sometimes decades of debate before a consensus was reached (Pierce & Peyton, 1999). Others have criticized these doctorates, arguing

---

EXHIBIT 37.2 Things to Consider for PAs Interested in Pursuing Doctoral Education

---

1. Start With Self-Reflection
   a. What is your motivation for pursuing a doctoral degree?
   b. What are your interests in the areas of clinical practice, teaching, and research?
   c. What are your career goals: Leadership? Academia? Advanced and/or specialized clinical practice? Research?
   d. Will the cost, time, and effort pay off in a way that is meaningful to you? (cost-benefit analysis)
   e. Are you ready to handle the pressure of being a student at this time?
   f. Do you have the support of family, friends, peers, and your employer?
2. Do Your Homework: Questions to Ask When Exploring Doctoral Programs
   a. Is the institution accredited? (www.ed.gov/accreditation?src=rn)
   b. What program of study is offered (i.e., what is the culminating degree—PhD or professional doctorate)?
   c. What are the program goals and curriculum focus?
   d. Is there more than one track (e.g., clinical, education, leadership, global health)?
   e. What is the requirement and rigor of the scholarly product (e.g., dissertation vs. doctoral project)? Can you incorporate it at your place of employment?
   f. What mechanism is in place for student advising and support for scholarly project or research?
   g. Are the faculty actively involved in scholarly activities?
   h. How many faculty members are PAs? What are the credentials, research skills, and PA professional involvement of the PA faculty?
   i. Mode of education—distance (online), residential (on site), or blended?
   j. Is there a practicum/internship required? If yes, what is the focus?
   k. Do you have to find your own internship/practicum/fellowship (if required)?
   l. What is the length of study? Is there a cap on the number of years for completion?
   m. What is the weekly time commitment? Can you still work full time/part time? Do you need to take time from work?
   n. Do you have to maintain your PA licensure and certification while enrolled?
   o. Are students from other professions enrolled in the same classes? Are there interprofessional learning activities?
   p. Is there a system for peer networking?
   q. What type of financial aid/tuition assistance is available from the university? Will your employer offer tuition benefits?

PAs, physician assistants.

that one does not need a doctoral degree to be proficient in one's practice, and termed this movement *degree creep* (Coplan, Richardson, & Stoehr, 2009; Cornell, 2008; Royeen & Lavin, 2007). Similar arguments have been expressed in the PA community (Bushardt, 2014; Coplan & Meyer, 2011). Nevertheless, other health professions are continuing these debates and are at different levels of transition, including social work (Anastas, 2012), laboratory sciences (Doig, 2005), occupational therapy (Brown, Crabtree, Mu, & Wells, 2015), and athletic training, among others (Seegmiller, Nasypany, Kahanov, Seegmiller, & Baker, 2015). The PA profession is the only similar profession that has not moved to a profession-specific doctorate to date.

DOCTORAL DEGREES IN MEDICINE

The discipline of the PA profession is medicine, a domain that PAs share with physicians. Now accepted as an entry-level clinical doctorate, the MD was not originally offered as a doctoral degree, or even a master's degree, but as a bachelor of medicine (MB). The MB was first awarded in 1768 in the United States by the University of Pennsylvania as the terminal degree for the practice of medicine. At time, the title "doctor" was reserved only for those qualified to teach at the highest level of academia in any field of study (Bouchard, 2009; Royeen & Lavin, 2007).

These academic elites were awarded a PhD degree, which remains a terminal academic degree requiring empirical research with the focus on acquisition of new knowledge. Toward the end of the 18th century, the transition from the MB to the MD degree came about as part of medical education reforms. To obtain an MD, MB practitioners were required to have 7 years of medical practice, submit a dissertation, and successfully pass an examination. It was not until 1811 that all medical schools transitioned to the MD degree as an entry-level clinical doctorate (Royeen & Lavin, 2007). Later, other professions, such as DDS and DPM, followed suit (Bouchard, 2009). Accordingly, in the future the PA profession is likely to follow a similar path to an entry-level clinical doctorate.

THE PA PROFESSION'S POSITION

In 2009, the PA professional organizations, specifically the American Academy of Physician Assistants (AAPA) and Physician Assistant Education Association (PAEA) under pressure by their members, embarked on a project to investigate the clinical doctorate for PAs. The product was a 2-day summit in March 2009 to "develop recommendations to the profession on whether the clinical doctorate is appropriate as an entry-level degree, as a postgraduate degree, or not at all" (PAEA, 2009, p. 22). The summit recommendations endorsed the master's degree as the entry level and terminal degree for the profession (PAEA, 2009). This endorsement is not binding on PA education programs and places no restrictions on institutions by the Accreditation Review Commission on Education for PA (ARC-PA).

Here, we remind the reader that PA certification, independent of academic standing, indicates that a PA is fully qualified to practice medicine as a PA. In addition, the PA profession promotes the pursuit of lifelong learning with the doctoral degree being one avenue of achieving professional fulfillment (PAEA, 2009). This is in accord with the Institute of Medicine's call to enhance and diversify training for health care professionals (Greiner & Knebel, 2003).

ENTRY-LEVEL PA DOCTORATE

Some would say that the emergence of an entry-level doctoral degree for PAs is inevitable. Support for this view is based upon the rigor of current PA professional training, the high-performance expectations and responsibilities of PA graduates, and the fact that the PA profession is now the only major health profession that does not award the doctoral degree for professional education. The majority of studies on the perceptions of the clinical PA doctorate have focused on the entry-level option. The overall findings of these studies show that while practicing PAs and PA faculty did not support the entry-level PA doctorate, physicians and PAs students were more amenable (Menenez et al., 2015; Muma, 2011, 2012; Swanchak, 2011). Development of an entry-level doctorate for PA education would likely follow the patterns observed in the fields of pharmacy, physical therapy, and advanced practice nursing. It could be predicted that, once a sponsoring institution made such an educational offering available, others will follow so as to compete for the most qualified students.

CURRENT MODELS OF PA DOCTORAL EDUCATION

Swanchak (2010) proposed the application of the modified Maslow's hierarchy of needs for motivation in the workplace as a framework for studying the motivations for the PA clinical doctorate (Benson & Dundis, 2003). Theoretically, motivated PAs desire to reach the pinnacle of self-actualization by attaining full professional development. Without sufficient PA programs offering postprofessional degrees (clinical or otherwise), PAs interested in a doctoral degree have to obtain them in other specific or general health disciplines. Unfortunately, data on the current trends, demand, and opportunities for PAs with doctorates are not available, and the only data on the number of doctorally prepared PAs are limited to PA faculty surveyed by PAEA. In 2015, excluding medical directors, 27% of all PA faculty and 44% of PA program directors reported having a doctorate (PAEA Research Director, personal communication, April 1, 2017). The most common doctoral degrees among nonphysician PA faculty were: PhD, DHSc, and EdD (PAEA, 2015).

Multiple models of PPD for PAs have been developed and continue to be developed (Table 37.1). In 2007, the first four PAs with a PPD designed for PAs graduated from Baylor University through a partnership with the U.S. Army emergency medicine residency program (Salyer & Knott, 2008). This new DSc-PA degree intensified the doctorate discussion in the PA community, which had started a decade earlier (Bouchard, 2009; Cawley, 2008; Coplan & Meyer, 2011; Jones, 2009; Rahr, 2009). It was not until 2016 that a second PPD designed for PAs, the doctor of medical science (DMS), was established at Lincoln Memorial University, Tennessee (2016). Similar PPD programs for PAs are underway, for example, Lynchburg College offers such a program (Lynchburg College, 2016). These programs are not entry-level doctorate PA programs, but rather PPD degrees for board-certified PAs offering training in advanced medical practice. This is in keeping with the 2009 PAEA summit report, which opposed a clinical doctorate as the entry-level doctorate for PAs but supported *nonprofession-specific postgraduate or clinical doctorates*. Although these programs are designed to accept PAs only, they are not PA-specific per se because the resulting degree is not a "doctor of PA."

In 2014, Wake Forest University introduced a dual-degree option by pairing a master's degree in PA education with a PhD focused on basic science (Wake Forest University, 2016). This model

TABLE 37.1 Attributes of the Most Common Postprofessional Degrees Pursued by PAs

Degree Name	Characteristics
Research doctorate (PhD is the most common; others, such as DrPH, DSc, may have similar characteristics)	Usually 4 to 6 years May or may not require a prior master's degree Classmates will have different master's degrees (PA, NP, PT, OT, MPH, and so on) Academic study in a specific field Requires substantial original research dissertation Traditionally requires residence but can be done online Graduate/research assistantship common, in exchange for research/teaching
Professional doctorate (general health practice, e.g., DHSc)	Usually 3 to 4 years Usually requires a prior master's degree Academic study integrates disciplines, such as public health, education, leadership, and business Usually requires a less substantial dissertation or graduate project Usually distance education or blended
Professional doctorate (clinical focus—developed for PAs, DMS, DSc-PA, DO); as of 2016, there are only three programs	1.5 to 2 years Academic study in medical topics Requires master's degree in PA education Requires active PA certification and licensure Residency is required
Professional doctorate (other focus, e.g., EdD, JD, DMSc-education track)	Attributes vary by focus area

DHSc, doctor of health science; DMS or DMSc, doctor of medical science; DO, doctor of osteopathic medicine; DrPH, doctor of public health; DSc, doctor of science; DSc-PA, doctor of science in PA; EdD, doctor of education; JD, doctor of jurisprudence; MPH, master of public health; NP, nurse practitioner; OT, occupational therapist; PA, physician assistant; PT, physical therapist.

is neither an entry-level PA doctorate nor a PPD. Students earn the two degrees sequentially, with the PhD earned first. This model will graduate PA practitioners who are both clinicians and basic scientists, analogous to the MD–PhD Model.

Perhaps the most popular postprofessional doctorate training for credentialed PAs is the DHSc. Although several universities offer the DHSc degree, as of this writing the most popular programs among PAs are at Nova University in Florida and A.T. Still University in Arizona. DHSc programs are designed to enhance overall health care practice, leadership skills, and applied scholarship. They do not typically focus on substantially expanding the student's clinical or research knowledge and skills.

Finally, another model of doctoral education aimed at practicing PAs is the so-called "bridge" program. Some have suggested the further development of such programs for both PAs and NPs (Danielsen, 2008). One such program has been developed at Lake Erie College of Osteopathic Medicine and offers PAs with at least 3 years in practice to enter an accelerated medical education program to obtain a DO (Lake Erie College of Osteopathic Medicine, 2016). A handful of individuals began this program in 2011. A 2012 survey of the perceptions of PAs toward a PPD designed as a PA-to-physician bridge program showed that PAs overwhelmingly supported this model and agreed that this would be beneficial to the health care community and would be supported by physicians. They also agreed that PA and physician organizations should support such programs (Muma, 2012). The position taken by the AAPA and PAEA in the 2009 doctoral summit was that further study needs to be undertaken to assess the value of these programs. Others who are skeptical of "bridge" programs note that such programs pose a dilemma for the profession's organizations. Bridge programs are essentially a plan for PAs to leave the PA profession, making it difficult for either the AAPA or PAEA to have any kind of official position and/or endorse the notion. How can those whose role is to promote the PA profession support programs in which PAs in practice would exit the profession (Cawley, 2009)?

Benefits of Postprofessional Doctorate Degrees for PAs (Clinical and Nonclinical)

There are several potential benefits of PPD degrees for PAs:

1. **Increased clinical competence and self-confidence:** Professional doctorate programs designed to provide advanced clinical knowledge and training increase provider competence and self-confidence. This is especially true for programs that offer additional training in a given specialty (Seegmiller et al., 2015).
2. **Leadership skills:** Several professional doctorate programs focus on or incorporate leadership training. Data on whether this translates to clinical leadership opportunities are lacking. Doctoral programs that include leadership training are likely to expand PA leadership roles in academia, local, national, and global health care arenas.
3. **Expanded roles:** Most professional doctorate programs in health care take a generalist approach on health care (e.g., DHSc, DrPH), preparing students for a wide range of opportunities. Others, such as the EdD, prepare students for academia and PhD degrees prepare students for research.
4. **Scholarship:** Although varying in scope and rigor, most doctoral-level degrees involve a type of scholarly inquiry or project. This enhances the PAs abilities to be an independent thinker and catalyst for advances in health care. It is important to note that certain research funding is only awarded to those with doctoral degrees.
5. **A foundation for the future:** Just as the PA profession has evolved to an entry-level master's degree, the progression to an entry-level doctorate is on the horizon. Having a ready

workforce of doctorally prepared PA faculty and clinical mentors prior to this transition will avoid the crises other similar professions have experienced (Anastas, 2012).

6. **Professional parity:** The PA profession is the last in its cluster of similar professions (pharmacy, physical therapy, nursing, and so forth) to embrace entry-level or PPD degrees. Whether it should or should not, the title "doctor" accords rank. To maintain its recognition, the PA profession will not want to be the only clinician at the table without the "doctor" title.

7. **Reimbursement:** It is not clear whether a postprofessional degree for PAs would influence reimbursement for clinical services. Reimbursement for clinical services is compensated based on clinical skills, not academic credentials. However, postprofessional degrees may lead to increased PA practice autonomy in the practice setting (Seegmiller et al., 2015), which may in turn influence reimbursement.

8. **Compensation:** Although it is not clear whether for similar jobs, compensation would be higher for PAs with doctorates compared to those without; this may happen by increasing leadership opportunities for the former. In 2015, PA faculty with doctorates reported 6% higher salaries compared with those with master's degrees. However, it is unclear whether physician faculty were included in this group (PAEA, 2015). Other professions have reported increased salary with advanced degrees (Seegmiller et al., 2015).

9. **Interprofessional collaboration:** Most professional doctorate programs usually enroll students from diverse disciplines. This promotes interprofessional collaboration in training.

CHALLENGES FOR POSTPROFESSIONAL DOCTORATE DEGREES FOR PAs (CLINICAL AND NONCLINICAL)

Conversely, PPD degrees also pose potential challenges:

1. **Uncertainty of added benefit:** It is unclear whether postprofessional doctoral education for PAs has any benefits for patient outcomes, health policy, research, or PA training (Bushardt, 2014; Bushardt, Booze, Hewett, Hildebrandt, & Thomas, 2012; Cawley & Ritsema, 2013; Orcutt, Hildebrand, & Jones, 2006).

2. **Lack of uniformity:** Even with the same degree conferred, institutions have diverse designs and curricula, and different program requirements. An online search for *DHSc degree* found the DHSc degree varied from 33 to 72 course credits. Some required a practicum or internship, whereas some did not; some required a traditional dissertation, whereas others required no independent scholarly work.

3. **Workforce shortages:** Increasing PA training time and/or reducing work hours to meet the demands of the educational pursuit could lead to workforce shortages. However, most postprofessional doctorates (especially nonclinical) can be completed without changing employment status. And, in programs with a clinical fellowship, the PA continues to provide clinical care as a fellow.

4. **Financial burden:** PA education is already expensive. In 2015, the average cost was $43 thousand for public and $78 thousand for private institutions (PAEA, 2016). There are very few educational grants or fellowships available for postprofessional education; therefore, students commonly take loans or pay out of pocket (Anastas, 2012; Royeen & Lavin, 2007). Depending on the delivery of the training, students may incur additional costs if they have to relocate. Moreover, they may experience loss of income if they cannot continue with employment while enrolled.

5. **"Degree creep":** As indicated, *degree creep* refers to mandating that a higher degree now be attained to perform the same job that formerly required a lower degree. Other professions have reported feeling the pressure to transition to entry-level doctorate degrees as their standard (Cornell, 2008).

6. **Lack of qualified faculty:** Doctoral students in some professional doctoral programs have reported lack of satisfaction in their faculty's skills to teach and advise them (Anastas, 2012). Building a faculty base may be a necessary first step.

7. **Lack of research support:** Although most professional doctorate programs do not require extensive dissertations, most require a form of scholarly work independently performed by students. Students have reported dissatisfaction with their training and support to become scholar practitioners (Seegmiller et al., 2015).

8. **Risk for widening the diversity gap:** Some have argued that minorities, women, and students with larger financial responsibilities may not be able to spend additional money on higher academic degrees, thereby increasing the already significant disparity among health care providers (Randolph & Siler, 2007).

Title Dilemma: Doctor PA?

As defined in Exhibit 37.1, the doctoral degree warrants the use of the title "doctor," independent of area of specialization. In 2006, the American Medical Association (AMA) attempted to restrict the title "doctor" to physicians, dentists, and podiatrists, thus blocking the title from being used by other health care professionals regardless of academic achievement. The AMA claimed that the broad use of the title would confuse patients, compromise patient safety, and erode physician–patient trust. After an overwhelming response from individuals, health care organizations, and universities, the AMA House of Delegates rejected the resolution (Chism, 2016). The current AMA position is that it "(1) will advocate that professionals in a clinical healthcare setting clearly and accurately identify to patients their qualifications and degree(s) attained and develop model state legislation for implementation; and (2) supports state legislation that would make it a felony to misrepresent oneself as a physician (MD/DO)" (AMA, 2009). When the title "doctor" is used in a clinical setting, it should be followed by a role clarification. PAs with doctoral degrees should also be aware of their specific state legislation on the use of the title "doctor" in clinical settings.

CONCLUSIONS

As technology advances and health care becomes more complex, the PA profession will continue to feel the need for clinical and academic advancement. It is likely that with growth of doctoral degrees in the health professions, the PA profession will sooner or later adopt the entry-level doctorate as well as see the emergence of additional models of postprofessional doctoral degrees. It is possible that some current PA postgraduate residency programs will eventually link with educational institutions to offer doctoral degrees along the lines of the Army–Baylor DSc PA in emergency medicine program. The PA profession also sees the advances made by the nursing profession in terms of attaining independent practice authority, a circumstance aided by the establishment of the DNP degree for entry-level nurse practitioner education. For PAs, the nascent movement toward full-practice authority currently under consideration by the AAPA (n.d.) may be strengthened by the attainment of doctoral degrees by more practicing PAs.

Given the likely desire for parity among PAs toward other similarly trained health care professionals, the absence of any impediments on the part of the accreditation organization, the nonbinding nature of PAEA educational accords passed in 2008, and the opportunism of institutions within American higher education, the establishment of an entry-level doctorate for PAs seems only a matter of time. For postprofessional doctoral programs, the movement is well underway with a number of creative and innovative programs already established or under development. Educational advancement, regardless of model or credential, is not the antithesis of a sound clinical practice. It is the natural evolution of a health profession.

REFERENCES

Accreditation Council for Pharmacy Education. (2011). Accreditation standards and guidelines for the professional program in pharmacy leading to the doctor of pharmacy degree. Retrieved from https://www.acpe-accredit.org/pdf/FinalS2007Guidelines2.0.pdf

American Academy of Physician Assistants. (n.d.). Full practice authority and responsibility. Retrieved from http://news-center.aapa.org/wp-content/uploads/sites/2/2016/12/FAQ-Final_12_15.pdf

American Association of Colleges of Nursing. (2015). The doctor of nursing practice: Current issues and clarifying recommendations. Retrieved from http://www.aacn.nche.edu/aacn-publications/white-papers/DNP-Implementation-TF-Report-8-15.pdf

American Association of Colleges of Nursing. (2016). DNP fact sheet. Retrieved from http://www.aacn.nche.edu/media-relations/fact-sheets/dnp

American Medical Association. (2009). Protection of the titles "doctor," "resident" and "residency" H-275.925. Retrieved from https://policysearch.ama-assn.org/policyfinder/detail/H-275.925?uri=%2FAMADoc%2FHOD.xml-0-1903.xml

American Physical Therapy Association. (2015). *Vision 2020*. Retrieved from http://www.apta.org/Vision2020/

Anastas, J. W. (2012). *Doctoral education in social work*. New York, NY: Oxford University Press.

Benson, S. G., & Dundis, S. P. (2003). Understanding and motivating health care employees: Integrating Maslow's hierarchy of needs, training and technology. *Journal of Nursing Management, 11*(5), 315–320.

Bouchard, G. (2009). Doctoral education: Degrees of separation. *Journal of Physician Assistant Education, 20*(2), 29–32.

Brown, T., Crabtree, J. L., Mu, K., & Wells, J. (2015). The next paradigm shift in occupational therapy education: The move to the entry-level clinical doctorate. *American Journal of Occupational Therapy: Official Publication of the American Occupational Therapy Association, 69*(Suppl. 2), 6912360020p1-6912360020p6.

Bushardt, R. L. (2014). Growing pains. *Journal of the American Academy of Physician Assistants, 27*(5), 8–10.

Bushardt, R. L., Booze, L. E., Hewett, M. L., Hildebrandt, C., & Thomas, S. E. (2012). Physician assistant program characteristics and faculty credentials on physician assistant national certifying exam pass rates. *Journal of Physician Assistant Education, 23*(1), 19–23.

Carollo, S., & Mason, A. (2017). Doctor of nursing practice curricula redesign: Challenge, change and collaboration. *Journal for Nurse Practitioners, 13*(4), e177–e183.

Cawley, J. F. (2008). Doctoral degrees for PAs: What happens next? *Journal of the American Academy of Physician Assistants, 21*(3), 13.

Cawley, J. F. (2009). Bridge to nowhere. *Advance for Physicians Assistants, 17*(5–6), 16.

Cawley, J., & Ritsema, T. (2013). Where are the PA researchers? *Journal of the American Academy of Physician Assistants, 26*(5), 22.

Chase, S. K., & Pruitt, R. H. (2006). The practice doctorate: Innovation or disruption? *Journal of Nursing Education, 45*(5), 155.

Chism, L. (2016). *The doctor of nursing practice* (3rd ed.). Burlington, MA: Jones & Bartlett Learning.

Coplan, B., & Meyer, J. E. (2011). Physician assistants—One less doctor(ate) in the house. *Journal of the American Medical Association, 305*(24), 2571–2572.

Coplan, B., Richardson, L., & Stoehr, J. D. (2009). Physician assistant program medical directors' opinions of an entry-level physician assistant clinical doctorate degree. *Journal of Physician Assistant Education, 20*(2), 8–13.

Cornell, S. (2008). Degree creep: Are entry-level doctoral degrees and more postgraduate doctoral degrees in PA profession's future. *Advance for Physician Assistants, 19*, 47–50.

Danielsen, R. (2008). Fast-tracking PAs and NPs into medical school. *Clinician Review, 18*, 1–12.

Doig, K. (2005). The case for the clinical doctorate in laboratory science. *Clinical Laboratory Science, 18*(3), 132.

Greiner, A. C., & Knebel, E. (2003). *Health professions education: A bridge to quality*. Washington, DC: National Academies Press.

Huggins, C. E., & Choy, M. (2016). Raising the standard: Requiring a bachelor's degree for PharmD programs. *American Journal of Pharmaceutical Education, 80*(4), 72–73.

Jones, P. E. (2009). The dead-end clinical doctorate idea. *Journal of Physician Assistant Education, 20*(2), 4–5.

Lake Erie College of Osteopathic Medicine. (2016). Accelerated physician assistant pathway. Retrieved from https://lecom.edu/academics/the-college-of-medicine/accelerated-physician-assistant-pathway

Lincoln Memorial University. (2016). Doctor of medical science program. Retrieved from https://www
.lmunet.edu/academics/schools/debusk-college-of-osteopathic-medicine/dms

Lynchburg College. (2016). Doctor of medical science. Retrieved from http://www.lynchburg.edu/
graduate/physician-assistant-medicine/physician-assistant-doctoral-option

Menezes, P., Senkomago, V., & Coniglio, D. (2015). Physician assistant students' attitudes towards a
clinical doctoral degree. *Journal of Physician Assistant Education, 26*(1), 3–9.

Muma, R. D., Phipps, B., & Vredenburg, S. (2012). The perceptions of U.S. physician assistants regarding
physician assistant-to-physician bridge programs. *Journal of Physician Assistant Education, 23*(3), 7–11.

Muma, R. D., Smith, B. S., Anderson, N., Richardson, M., Selzer, E., & White, R. (2011). Perceptions of
U.S. physicians regarding the entry-level doctoral degree in physician assistant education: A comparative study with physician assistants and PA faculty. *Journal of Allied Health, 40*(1), 25–30.

National Center for Education Statistics. (2015). *Digest of education statistics.* Washington, DC: Author.
Retrieved from http://nces.ed.gov/programs/digest/d15/tables/dt15_324.10.asp?current=yes

Orcutt, V. L., Hildebrand, A., & Jones, P. E. (2006). The doctoral pipeline in physician assistant education. *Journal of Physician Assistant Education, 17*(1), 6–9.

Physician Assistant Education Association. (2009). *PA clinical doctorate summit final report and summary.*
Washington, DC: Author.

Physician Assistant Education Association. (2015). *Physician assistant education association, physician assistant program faculty and directors survey report, 2015.* Washington, DC: Author.

Physician Assistant Education Association. (2017). *Physician assistant education association, by the numbers:
Program report 31.* Washington, DC: Author.

Pierce, D., & Peyton, C. (1999). A historical cross-disciplinary perspective on the professional doctorate
in occupational therapy. *American Journal of Occupational Therapy: Official Publication of the American
Occupational Therapy Association, 53*(1), 64.

Plack, M. M., & Wong. C. K (2002). The evolution of the doctorate of physical therapy: Moving beyond
the controversy. *Journal of Physical Therapy Education, 16*(1), 48.

Rahr, R. R. (2009). The physician assistant clinical doctorate: Professional suicide in the making? *Journal
of Physician Assistant Education, 20*(2), 6–7.

Randolph, D. S., & Siler, W. L. (2007). A clinical look at clinical doctorates. *Audiology Today, 19*(1), 22.

Royeen, C., & Lavin, M. A. (2007). A contextual and logical analysis of the clinical doctorate for health
practitioners: Dilemma, delusion, or de facto? *Journal of Allied Health, 36*(2), 101–106.

Salyer, S. W., & Knott, P. (2008). A clinical doctorate in emergency medicine for physician assistants:
Postgraduate education. *Journal of Physician Assistant Education, 19*(3), 53–56.

Seegmiller, J. G., Nasypany, A., Kahanov, L., Seegmiller, J. A., & Baker, R. (2015). Trends in doctoral
education among healthcare professions: An integrative research review. *Athletic Training Education
Journal, 10*(1), 47–56.

Swanchak, L. E. (2010). *The perceptions of changing the entry-level degree for physician assistants to a clinical
doctorate among physician assistant students.* Available from ProQuest Dissertations and Theses Global:
The Sciences and Engineering Collection.

Wake Forest University. (2016). MMS-PhD dual degree. Retrieved from http://www.wakehealth.edu/
School/Physician-Assistant-Program/MMS-PhD-Dual-Degree.htm

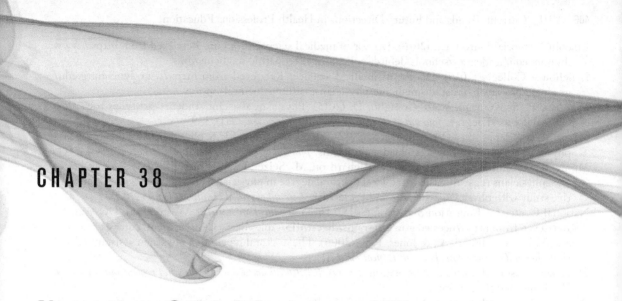

CHAPTER 38

Nurturing Social Accountability and Community Engagement

Nadia Cobb, Amy Clithero, Fortunato Cristobal, Julian Fisher,
Sarah Larkins, Lyn Middleton, André-Jacques Neusy, Robyn Preston,
Simone J. Ross, Roger Strasser, and Torres Woolley

CHAPTER OBJECTIVE

- Develop methods to nurture social accountability and community engagement to develop people-centered health professionals

---

Recall the face of the poorest and weakest man you have seen, and ask yourself if this step you contemplate is going to be any use to him.

—Mahatma Gandhi

The need to address the social determinants of health and to promote health equity has become a top priority for various health care organizations (High-Level Commission on Health Employment and Economic Growth, 2016). Part of the solution lies in developing a workforce that understands and has the will to address these issues. Health professionals and health organizations must be socially accountable to the communities they serve. Thus, they need to be people centered and willing to engage in community services (WHO, 2016). Preparing a health workforce that provides holistic or integrated, people-centered care in communities where people live and work demands that educators critically appraise and adjust their educational vision and health care practices.

The Training for Health Equity Network (THEnet; Larkins et al., 2013; Palsdottir, Neusy, & Reed, 2008; Ross et al., 2014) is a leading example of how institutions can create socially accountable health workforce education. THEnet's framework focuses on integrated people-centered services, community health needs and population health. There is an increased emphasis on teaching health promotion, disease prevention, and primary care. Around the world, THEnet partner institutions implement this mandate in locally responsive ways. In this chapter, we discuss four case studies as exemplars of how health education schools have transformed their education practices to nurture people-centered health professionals, social accountability, community engagement, and care for the underserved.

EXEMPLAR A: JAMES COOK UNIVERSITY COLLEGE OF MEDICINE AND DENTISTRY, TOWNSVILLE, AUSTRALIA

Northern Australia has a widely dispersed population over a vast geographical area, with no settlement of over 200,000. There is a geographical and vocational maldistribution of health professionals and historically, it has been challenging to attract and retain health professionals to this region. With a high proportion of Aboriginal peoples and Torres Strait Islanders in Northern Australia, there are significant local health care needs (Clucas et al., 2008; Hoy, Norman, Hayhurst, & Pugsley, 1997).

In 2000, after a long campaign, James Cook University College of Medicine and Dentistry (JCUCMD) was established as the first medical school in the north of Australia and only the second outside of a state capital city. JCUCMD has a clear mission to produce health professionals to serve the priority health needs of the unique northern population, with skills, knowledge, and competencies in rural, remote, tropical, and indigenous health. Staffing profile, curriculum, research priorities, and community and health sector partnerships encompass these priorities. The college also delivers innovative postgraduate training pathways, particularly in rural general practice and rural generalist streams, and partners with health systems to address the needs of the health workforce and medically underserved populations (James Cook University College of Medicine and Dentistry, 2017).

The values of "social justice, innovation, and excellence" are espoused throughout the 6-year undergraduate degree. Years 1 to 3 are delivered in Townsville, and years 4 to 6 delivered in a distributed service learning education model in either Townsville, Cairns, Mackay, or Darwin. The Australian Standard Geographical Classification (ASGC) is based on road distance from a locality to the closest service centre in each of the five classes of population size. Townsville, Mackay, Darwin, and Cairns are classified as outer regional areas (Australian Institute of Health and Welfare [AIHW], 2004).

Community-Focused Admissions and Integrated Curriculum

The student selection process favors rural and remote applicants, Australian Aboriginal and Torres Strait Islander peoples. Communities are involved in the selection interview and students facilitate educational outreach programs to rural high schools.

The integrated curriculum includes a primary care focus and early exposure to rural practice. All JCUCMD students undertake at least 20 weeks of placement in a small rural town across the course: 4 weeks in year 2; 6 weeks in year 4; and 10 weeks in year 6.

Regional health services, both public and private, have been supportive since the college's establishment. In 2016, there were 1,009 students across the 6-year undergraduate degree, with class size ranging from 171 in year 1 to 167 in year 6. These numbers illustrate the influence of the health systems support as well as the impact of JCUCMD's student support services on student retention. Notably, the JCUCMD has now graduated 20 Australian Aboriginal and/or Torres Strait Islander doctors.

Community Engagement/Partnerships

Student placements are an important way that students interact with rural communities through both junior placements and year-6 service learning rural internships. The idea that students are attached to "a community" rather than a doctor was an early innovation of the school. As part of their 4-week rural placement in second year, students are encouraged to undertake community activities such as visiting a local high school to talk with year 10 and 12 students about health careers and participating in recreational activities. An interesting requirement for assessment was that students had to describe their interactions with a community person who had assisted them during their placement. Reflecting on their involvement in the social side of community life, such as speaking to service clubs, is part of a learning portfolio for JCUCMD students undertaking rural placements.

Outcomes and Success

The college's comprehensive graduate tracking system demonstrates successful outcomes. Eighty-two percent of graduates (2006–2012) grew up outside of major cities, with 5% having remote or very remote backgrounds, 20% are from inner regional areas, and 57% from outer regional areas. Approximately 65% of JCUCMD medical graduates undertake their intern year in a nonmetropolitan area (Sen Gupta, Woolley, Murray, Hays, & Mccloskey, 2014). Furthermore, over the first 9 working years following graduation, graduates whose hometown was rural or remote were shown to practice predominantly in rural and remote towns, areas that have traditionally been designated as medically underserved (Ray, Woolley, & Sen Gupta, 2015). This is strong evidence that the admissions and educational practices at the JCU medical school are successful in meeting the school's mission to produce doctors for rural and northern Australia.

EXEMPLAR B: UNIVERSITY OF NEW MEXICO SCHOOL OF MEDICINE, ALBUQUERQUE, NEW MEXICO

New Mexico is a geographically large state with some of the poorest health outcomes that are driven by social determinants, including healthy-food access, living conditions, education achievement, and economic poverty (Kaiser Family Foundation, 2017). Compared to the United States, New Mexico is a majority-minority state, with 46.4% Hispanic/Latin Americans (compared to 16.9% on average in other states) and 8.8% American Indian/Alaska Native (compared to 0.8% in other states) comprising more than half of the population in 2015 (Kaiser Family Foundation, 2017; New Mexico Indicator-Based Information System [NM-IBIS], 2016). Close to one third of the population live in nonmetropolitan areas. New Mexico ranks sixth among the U.S. states for uninsured persons and has the second highest percentage of women and children living in poverty in the United States (Kaiser Family Foundation, 2017; National Women's Law Center, 2016).

The University of New Mexico School of Medicine (UNMSOM) is the only allopathic medical school in New Mexico and is responsible for training physicians who are likely to remain in New Mexico to practice. Established in 1961, improving population health has always been a guiding mandate of the medical school. A strong focus on community medicine, health disparity reduction, and education on the social determinants of health demonstrates a commitment to the state and the conditions and needs of its population. The UNMSOM actively engages New Mexico community members in designing and implementing education and service programs to recognize and utilize their rich culture and community assets and strengths. UNMSOM is not only responsible for serving community needs as the state's only medical school, it is responsive to community needs as identified by the community and, most important, is accountable, as demonstrated by its actions. This accountability is best demonstrated by operationalization through admissions and innovative pipeline programs, community partnerships and community immersion, and the medical school curriculum (University of New Mexico School of Medicine, n.d.).

Admissions and Pipelines

Conventional Admission to the MD Program

A holistic admission process is one that considers experience and cognitive attributes as much as or more than admission test scores. At the UNMSOM, admitted students are nearly exclusively state residents or from states that have no medical school. In accordance with social accountability mandates, including students who represent the communities served and a focus on primary care, special consideration in the admission process is given to (UNMSOM, 2004):

• Underrepresented minorities (URMs)
• Students from rural areas
• Students from disadvantaged backgrounds
• Individuals with a record of work, service, or volunteerism with disadvantaged populations
• Individuals committed to work in underserved areas
• Individuals committed to primary care

This emphasis reflects the diversity of the state in both racial composition and socioeconomic characteristics. A little under half (48% in 2016) of the student body come from backgrounds that are underrepresented in medicine (University of New Mexico School of Medicine, 2015).

Innovative Admission to the MD Program Through the BA/MD Program

Beginning with the matriculating class of 2010, the UNMSOM class size increased with the addition of students from the UNM bachelor of arts (BA)/MD program. This "new" pool of applicants was comprised of students from a separately admitted, state-funded educational track whereby high school students from the state are selected during their senior year to complete 4 years of undergraduate education, leading to a BA degree with guaranteed admission to the medical school upon successful completion of the BA degree. The majority of students selected for the BA/MD program are from rural areas and, quite often, disadvantaged backgrounds. Applicants must be New Mexico residents, with the exception of Navajos and students from other reservations, and have a strong desire to remain and practice in New Mexico. Since 2010, students have been recruited from virtually every rural school in the state, many of which have limited educational resources. These graduates are impressive in their achievements despite attending schools in low-income areas. This unconventional pathway is a strategy to enhance the diversity of the UNMSOM student body and to achieve the state's rural workforce goals.

Pipeline Programs Invest in the Next Generation of Clinicians

Research on characteristics of clinicians practicing in remote areas consistently finds that a rural and underserved background is a strong predictor of the type of clinician who will serve these type of areas (Laven & Wilkinson, 2003; Rabinowitz, Diamond, Veloski, & Gayle, 2000). UNM has statewide pipeline programs that extend from middle school to high school to college support initiatives that actively reach out to rural residents, students from diverse cultural and ethnic backgrounds, and first-generation college attendees. These strategies increase access to health care by encouraging and then assisting youth in considering and successfully pursuing a health professions career.

Community Partnerships and Community Immersion

Communities themselves know what their needs are and these are often in conflict with what a school of medicine thinks they are. Through strong collaborative processes, the UNMSOM has joined with communities to find community-driven solutions to major health problems affecting New Mexicans that are rooted in community wisdom and experience. Community members are active stakeholders throughout the state, empowering them to address their own needs and to improve their health status. Health extension agents, who live and work full time in communities throughout New Mexico, link community-identified priorities, including community-based education, health professional recruitment, and technical assistance such as grant writing, with academic resources. The UNMSOM and partner states created the Health Extension Toolkit (www.healthextensiontoolkit.org) to assist these workers and others in implementing a similar community engagement program (Agency for Healthcare Research and Quality, 2013).

Early clinical exposure off the university campus is a cornerstone of the UNMSOM curriculum. Starting in their first 2 weeks of education, students begin community-immersion experiences by visiting local community centers and organizations that address community needs such as food banks and homeless shelters. By the second half of their first year, students are actively training in both inpatient and outpatient settings, including Native American urban population and reservation sites. Rural farming and ranching communities are also part of the educational and care activities. These off-site experiences occur in more than 155 New Mexico communities and are offered throughout the 4-year curriculum, comprising at least half of the clinical experience.

An example of patient care and service to a disadvantaged community is the Pajarito Mesa initiative. Beginning as a student project, Pajarito Mesa is now a sustainable program. Pajarito Mesa is an unincorporated "colonia" 30 miles west of Albuquerque, New Mexico's most populous city. This community consists of undocumented immigrants without access to health insurance as well as persons choosing to "live off the grid." Until recently, this community was without water or electricity and their roads are still often unpassable. A UNM medical student coordinated volunteer faculty and student outreach services, partnered with a private health care organization (Blue Cross) to use their health services van and the local food bank to provide ongoing outreach services such as assisting with the paperwork required to be seen by a regular primary care provider.

Outcomes and Success

A combination of a holistic approach to admissions, an emphasis on public health education, and early community immersion experiences that emphasize rural communities and primary care can lead to successful recruitment and retention of practitioners after they complete their education. As of 2016, graduates from the combined BA/MD program are still in the early stages of residency programs and thus information on practice location is not yet available. Using 2015 graduate data, about one third of graduates from the traditional MD track are licensed in New Mexico. Approximately 65.7% of all physicians who completed both medical school and residency at UNM have New Mexico medical licenses. This percentage has steadily increased over the past 10 years, such that UNM-trained physicians practice in 30 of New Mexico's 33 counties (UNSOM, 2016).

EXEMPLAR C: ATENEO DE ZAMBOANGA UNIVERSITY SCHOOL OF MEDICINE, ZAMBOANGA CITY, PHILIPPINES

Comprising over 700 inhabited Islands, the Philippines is the fourth highest disaster-prone country in the world with 13 of the 17 WHO-recognized neglected tropical diseases endemic to the country, a high incidence of communicable diseases, and a growing prevalence of noncommunicable diseases (Global Health Observatory, 2015). Forty-one percent of the population lives on less than $2/day. The inequities in the southern Philippines, particularly Mindanao, are significant. Compared to Manila, child mortality is four to five times higher, and neonatal mortality accounts for 50% of all deaths of children younger than age 5. Currently, the Philippines is one of nine countries with the fastest growing rate of HIV, with a 587% increase in cases over the past 5 years (Global Health Observatory, 2015). In 1994, more than 68% of medical graduates from the Philippines worked overseas. In Zamboanga, there were no physicians in 80% of the 100 municipalities, most of which were rural with limited human and physical resources for health care, largely as a result of the continued civil unrest between government forces and rebel groups (Cristobal & Worley, 2012).

In response to this dire situation, Ateneo de Zamboanga University School of Medicine (ADZU-SOM) was founded in 1993, as a voluntary not-for-profit community effort to train physicians in community-based, people-centered care to increase access to care for the most underserved and isolated communities in Western Mindanao (Cristobal & Worley, 2012). In 2012, the school had three paid employees, with all the teaching and precepting done by volunteer providers within the local health services. Innovative educational strategies include developing strong medical skills oriented to the social determinants of health, community participation, and intersectoral collaboration in curriculum development and delivery.

Curriculum/Community Immersion

Community and problem-based learning are central tenets of ADZU-SOM. During the first year, students live, learn, and work in communities off and on for a period of 2 months. In the first segment, students work with the local community members in assessing health needs that the community has to develop comprehensive intersectional plans to address identified needs. In the second segment, students design research projects aligned with the community's plan, remaining longitudinally involved in the implementation of the research until graduation, when the research is completed. Over the course of the program, students spend increasing amounts of time in the communities devoting close to 50% of the total clinical training period in communities and 50% in hospital rotations in medicine; pediatrics; surgery; obstetrics and gynecology; ear, nose, and throat; laboratory; and radiology (Cristobal & Kreutz, 2001).

Outcomes and Success

Graduates pass the national board certification at close to 100%. Based on the ranking of graduates in the national board certifying examination, Ateneo de Zamboanga University School of Medicine (ADU-SOM) is ranked number one among small medical schools, and ranked 10th out of the 38 medical schools in the Philippines. Ninety-seven percent of ADZU-SOM graduates stay in the Philippines, of these, 48% serve in the most remote and rural areas and 65% are employed by the government (Cristobal & Worley, 2012). By comparison, in 2011 the national average for physician graduates staying in the Philippines was 32% (Cristobal & Worley, 2012). Graduates represent diverse ethnicities and religious backgrounds and 50% are female.

Student and community projects have contributed to improved community health and public health outcomes, such as increased potable water access through the building of pit latrines in 80% of the region; development of home vegetable gardens to address nutritional deficiencies and generate income; and a 90% decrease in infant mortality in Zamboanga between 1994 and 2008, in comparison to a 50% nationally (Cristobal & Worley, 2012). Although causality is difficult to attribute fully to any one intervention, ADZU-SOM's broad and deep community engagement is highly credited for these achievements.

EXEMPLAR D: NORTHERN ONTARIO SCHOOL OF MEDICINE, ONTARIO, CANADA

In Canada, Northern Ontario province is geographically vast (more than 800,000 sq. km) with a volatile resource-based economy, including forestry and mining and socioeconomic characteristics that differ from the southern part of the province of Ontario. Forty percent of the population of Northern Ontario lives in rural and remote areas where there are diverse communities and cultural groups, most notably Indigenous and Francophone peoples (Bains et al., 2004). The health status of people in the region is worse than in the province as a whole, and there is a chronic shortage of doctors and other health professionals (Pong & Pitblado, 2005).

In this context, the Northern Ontario School of Medicine (NOSM) in Canada opened in 2005 with a social accountability mandate focused on improving the health of the people and communities of Northern Ontario (Strasser et al., 2009). Uniquely developed through a community consultative process, the holistic cohesive curriculum for the NOSM undergraduate program is grounded in the Northern Ontario health context, organized around five themes and relies heavily on electronic communications and interdependent community partnerships to support distributed community engaged learning (DCEL; Strasser et al., 2009). The five themes—northern and rural health, professional medical practice, social and population health, foundations of medicine, and clinical and communication skills—are integrated into every teaching module, clerkship, and assessment throughout the training (www .nosm.ca/ume).

Student Body and Integrated Curriculum

Northern Ontario students make up 92% of NOSM's learners, with substantial inclusion of Indigenous (7%) and Francophone (22%) students (Strasser et al., 2009). In the classroom and in clinical settings, students learn in the context of providing health care in Northern Ontario. NOSM's Indigenous Elders are vital at all levels of school structure, student learning, faculty development, and connection to the communities served. The weekly presence of the Elders and their work promote persistence and success in the Indigenous students, as the Elders provide balance between school and home, as well as a heightened understanding and appreciation of the deep ancestral heritage that many of the learners have. The Elders' roles have been attributed to empowering the Indigenous learners to recognize that studying is better achieved through oral methods, as storytelling is a strong part of their culture (Northern Ontario School of Medicine [NOSM], 2011).

Community Partnerships

Through community engagement, community members are active participants and stakeholders in various aspects of the school, including participating in the admissions process, serving as standardized patients, ensuring that learners feel "at home" in their community, and encouraging an understanding and knowledge of the social determinants of health at the local level. There is a strong emphasis on interprofessional education and integrated clinical learning, which takes place in more than 90 communities and many different health service settings, so that students have personal experience of the diversity of the region's communities and cultures (Strasser, 2016; Strasser et al., 2009).

Outcomes and Successes

There is evidence that NOSM is successful in graduating doctors who have the skills and the commitment to practice in rural/remote communities and that NOSM is having a largely positive socioeconomic impact on Northern Ontario. Sixty-two percent of NOSM graduates have chosen family practice (predominantly rural) training (Strasser et al., 2013). Ninety-four percent of the doctors who completed undergraduate and postgraduate education with NOSM are practicing in Northern Ontario (Hogenbirk et al., 2016). The socioeconomic impact of NOSM includes new economic activity such as salaries and benefits, spending on travel, supplies and services, stipends paid to clinical teachers, spending by learners, and research expenditures. This economic activity totals $67 to $82 million per year, which is more than double the school's budget. Additional benefits include enhanced retention and recruitment of personnel for the universities and hospitals/health services, and a sense of empowerment among community participants that is attributable to their work with NOSM (Hogenbirk et al., 2015).

CONCLUSIONS

There is a critical need for a health care workforce that provides holistic, or integrated people-centered care and that is socially accountable to the communities it serves. Educators hold the key to preparing this type of health workforce. Evidence from existing programs demonstrates that curriculum design positively influences graduates' disposition to work in areas of unmet need. There is a need to transform health professions curricula to expand opportunities for community engagement and increase social justice awareness. When integrated in an institutional mission and properly implemented in its health care workforce, social accountability has great potential to improve community health outcomes, advance health equity, and provide cost-effective integrated services to people where they live, learn, and work.

REFERENCES

Agency for Healthcare Research and Quality. (2013). Health Extension Toolkit. Tools for implementing the health extension model. Retrieved from http://healthextensiontoolkit.org

Australian Institute of Health and Welfare. (2004). *Rural, regional and remote health: A guide to remoteness classifications* (Rural health series no. 4. Cat. no. PHE 53). Canberra, Australia: Author.

Bains, N., Dall, K., Hay, C., Pacey, M., Sarkella, J., & Ward, M. (2004). *Population health profile: North East LHIN*. Toronto, Canada: Government of Ontario Publications.

Clucas, D. B., Carville, K. S., Connors, C., Currie, B. J., Carapetis, J. R., & Andrews, R. M. (2008). Disease burden and health-care clinic attendances for young children in remote Aboriginal communities of northern Australia. *Bulletin of the World Health Organization, 86*(4), 275–281.

Cristobal, F., & Worley, P. (2012). Can medical education in poor rural areas be cost-effective and sustainable: The case of the Ateneo de Zamboanga University School of Medicine. *Rural and Remote Health, 12*, 1835.

High-Level Commission on Health Employment and Economic Growth. (2016). Working for health and growth: Investing in the health workforce. Retrieved from http://apps.who.int/iris/bitstream/10665/250047/1/9789241511308-eng.pdf?ua=1

Hogenbirk, J. C., Robinson, J. R., Hill, M. E., Minore, B., Adams, K., Strasser, R. P., & Lipinski, J. (2015). The economic contribution of the Northern Ontario School of Medicine to communities participating in distributed medical education. *Canadian Journal of Rural Medicine, 20*(1)25–32.

Hogenbirk, J. C., Timony, P., French, M. G., Strasser, R., Pong, R. W., Cervin, C., & Graves, L. (2016). Milestones on the social accountability journey: Family medicine practice locations of Northern Ontario School of Medicine graduates. *Canadian Family Physician, 62*, e138–e145.

Hoy, W. E., Norman, R. J., Hayhurst, B. G., & Pugsley, D. J. (1997). A health profile of adults in a Northern Territory Aboriginal community, with an emphasis on preventable morbidities. *Australian and New Zealand Journal of Public Health, 21*(2), 121–126.

James Cook University College of Medicine and Dentistry. (2017). College philosophy. Retrieved from https://www.jcu.edu.au/college-of-medicine-and-dentistry/about-us/our-teaching-philosophy

Kaiser Family Foundation. (2013). Health insurance coverage of the total population. Retrieved from http://kff.org/other/state-indicator/total-population

Kaiser Family Foundation. (2017). State health facts. New Mexico: Health status. Retrieved from http://kff.org/state-category/health-status/?state=NM

Larkins, S., Preston, R., Matte, M., Lindemann, I. C., Samson, R., Tandinco, F. D., . . . Neusy, A.-J. (2013). Measuring social accountability in health professional education: Development and international pilot testing of an evaluation framework. *Medical Teacher, 35*(1), 32–35.

Laven, G., & Wilkinson, D. (2003). Rural doctors and rural backgrounds: How strong is the evidence? A systematic review. *Australian Journal of Rural Health, 11*(6), 277–284.

National Women's Law Center. (2016). Women and poverty, state by state. Retrieved from https://nwlc.org/resources/women-and-poverty-state-state

New Mexico Indicator-Based Information System. (2016). Health indicator report of New Mexico population demographic—Race/ethnicity. Retrieved from https://ibis.health.state.nm.us/indicator/view/NMPopDemoRacEth.NM.html

Northern Ontario School of Medicine. (2011). Elders handbook, how the medical school engages and works with Aboriginal elders. Retrieved from https://www.nosm.ca/uploadedFiles/Communities/Aboriginal_Affairs_Unit/Publications/Elders_Handbook_-_for_web.pdf

Palsdottir, B., Neusy, A., & Reed, G. (2008). Building the evidence base: Networking innovative socially accountable medical education programs. *Education for Health, 8,* 177.

Pong, R. W., & Pitblado, J. R. (2005). *Geographic distribution of physicians in Canada: Beyond how many and where.* Ottawa, Canada: Canadian Institute for Health Information.

Rabinowitz, H. K., Diamond, J. J., Veloski, J. J., & Gayle, J. A. (2000). The impact of multiple predictors on generalist physicians' care of underserved populations. *American Journal of Public Health, 90*(8), 1225.

Ray, R., Woolley, T., & Sen Gupta, T. (2015). James Cook University's rurally orientated medical school selection process: Quality graduates and positive workforce outcomes. *Rural and Remote Health, 15,* 1–11.

Ross, S. J., Preston, R., Lindemann, I. C., Matte, M. C., Samson, R., Tandinco, F. D., . . . Neusy, A.-J. (2014). The training for health equity network evaluation framework: A pilot study at five health professional schools. *Education for Health: Change in Learning and Practice, 27*(2), 116–126.

Sen Gupta, T., Woolley, T., Murray, R., Hays, R., & Mccloskey, T. (2014). Positive impacts on rural and regional workforce from the first seven cohorts of James Cook University medical graduates. *Rural Remote Health, 14,* 2657.

Strasser, R. (2016) Delivering on social accountability: Canada's Northern Ontario School of Medicine. *The Asia-Pacific Scholar, 1*(1), 1–6.

Strasser, R., Hogenbirk, J. C., Minore, B., Marsh, D. C., Berry, S., McCready, W. G., & Graves, L. (2013). Transforming health professional education through social accountability: Canada's Northern Ontario School of Medicine. *Medical Teacher, 35,* 490–496.

Strasser, R., Lanphear, J., McCready, W., Topps, M., Hunt, D., & Matte, M. (2009). Canada's new medical school: The Northern Ontario School of Medicine—social accountability through distributed community engaged learning. *Academic Medicine, 84,* 1459–1464.

University of New Mexico School of Medicine. (n.d.). About undergraduate medical education. Retrieved from http://som.unm.edu/education/md/ume

University of New Mexico School of Medicine. (2004). Admissions policy statement. Retrieved from http://som.unm.edu/leadership/policies/pdf/admissions-statement.pdf

University of New Mexico School of Medicine. (2015). UNM Health Sciences Center School of Medicine. Medical students (M.D. candidates). Student enrollment for academic year fall 2015. Year, gender and ethnicity. Retrieved from http://hsc.unm.edu/assets/doc/databook/2015-16/medical-students-enrollment-year-gender-and-ethnicity.pdf

University of New Mexico School of Medicine. (2016). Location report 2016. Retrieved from http://som.unm.edu/leadership/reports/locationreport/locationreport2016.pdf

World Health Organization. Global strategy on human resources for health: Workforce 2030. Retrieved from http://www.who.int/hrh/resources/pub_globstrathrh-2030/en

World Health Organization. (2016, April 15). Framework on integrated, people-centred health services: Report by the secretariat. Retrieved from http://apps.who.int/gb/ebwha/pdf_files/WHA69/A69_39-en.pdf?ua=1&ua=1

World Health Organization. The global strategy and action plan on aging and health, 2016–2020. Retrieved from http://who.int/ageing/global-strategy/en

World Health Organization. (2016). Global health sector strategies for HIV, viral hepatitis, STIs, 2016–2021. Retrieved from http://www.who.int/hiv/strategy2016-2021/en

World Health Organization. (2017). Health Observatory country views. Philippines statistics summary (2002-present). Retrieved from http://apps.who.int/gho/data/node.country.country-PHL?lang=en

World Health Organization. Global health sector strategy on viral hepatitis, 2016–2021. Retrieved from http://www.who.int/hepatitis/strategy2016-2021/ghss-hep/en

Index

AACN. *See* American Association of Colleges of Nursing

AACP. *See* American Association of Colleges of Pharmacy

AAC&U. *See* Association of American Colleges and Universities

AAHHE. *See* American Association of Hispanics in Higher Education Multidisciplinary Faculty Fellows Program

AAMC. *See* Association of American Medical Colleges

AAP. *See* American Academy of Pediatrics

AAPA. *See* American Academy of Physician Assistants

ABIM. *See* American Board of Internal Medicine

academia
building feedback into work environment, 320
direct reports, 319
exemplars, 321–322
managing down, 320
managing up, 319
navigating, 264–265
scholarship and, 264–265
setting expectations and understanding roles, 318–319
tools to facilitate group interactions, 321
transitioning to, 317–318

academic dishonesty, 348–349

academic freedom, 347–348

academic health professions
diversity as driver for excellence in, 223–224
equity as driver for excellence in, 223–224
evolution of diversity in, 224

academic leadership, 285–295

academic portfolios, 263–264

academic resources, 209–210

academy, 347

ACAPT. *See* American Council of Academic Physical Therapy

accreditation
of NP postgraduate residencies and fellowships, 391–392
of PA postgraduate residencies and fellowships, 391

Accreditation Council for Graduate Medical Education (ACGME), 25, 168, 211

Accreditation Review Commission on Education for the Physician Assistant (ARC-PA), 26, 391, 400

accreditation standards, 17
curriculum mapping and, 43

ACGME. *See* Accreditation Council for Graduate Medical Education

ADA. *See* Americans with Disabilities Act

ADDIE Model of curriculum design, 15

admissions best practices, 327–339
application review, 331–335
clear and transparent program admissions policies, 337–338

admissions best practices (*cont.*)
  communication, 329–330
  evaluation, 338
  interviews, 335–337
  outreach, 328–329
admissions policies, 337–338
advertising, minority faculty and, 238–239
ADZU-SOM. *See* Ateneo de Zamboanga
  University School of Medicine
AllofE, 126
AltSchool, 97
AMA. *See* American Medical Association
American Academy of Pediatrics (AAP), 200
American Academy of Physician Assistants
  (AAPA), 26, 179, 238, 291, 400
American Association of Colleges of Nursing
  (AACN), 238, 398
American Association of Colleges of Pharmacy
  (AACP), 200, 242, 398
American Association of Hispanics in Higher
  Education (AAHHE) Multidisciplinary
  Faculty Fellows Program, 241
American Association of University Professors,
  348
American Board of Internal Medicine (ABIM),
  200
American Council of Academic Physical Therapy
  (ACAPT), 242
American Medical Association (AMA), 404
  House of Delegates, 404
American Nurses Association (ANA), 179, 200
  *Code of Ethics for Nurses with Interpretive
    Statements*, 200
  Nursing: A Social Policy Statement, 200
American Physical Therapy Association House
  of Delegates (APTA-HOD), 398
Americans with Disabilities Act (ADA), 353–355
  determination of eligibility, 354–355
  disabilities, types of, 354
  disability, defined, 354
  prohibition of discrimination, 353
  reasonable accommodations, 354
ANA. *See* American Nurses Association
analytical tools, 98–100
  Facebook Insights, 98–99
  Google analytics, 98
  social media management dashboard, 99–100
  Twitter Analytics, 99
Annie E. Casey Foundation Leaders in Equitable
  Evaluation and Diversity (LEEAD)
  Program, 241
APAMSA. *See* Asian Pacific American Medical
  Student Association
apathy, 373

APPAP. *See* Association of Postgraduate PA
  Programs
application review, in admissions, 331–335
  academic record, 331–332
  clinical experience, 332
  cognitive evidence, 331–332
  demographics, 333
  noncognitive evidence, 333–335
  personal statements and reference letters,
    334–335
  personality variables, 333
appreciation, 297–298
APTA-HOD. *See* American Physical Therapy
  Association House of Delegates
ARC-PA. *See* Accreditation Review Commission
  on Education for the Physician Assistant
arts, learner-centered pedagogy and, 9–10
ASGC. *See* Australian Standard Geographical
  Classification
Asian Pacific American Medical Student
  Association (APAMSA), 253
assessment
  clinical training sites, 126–127
  leadership, 293
  of learning, 189–195
  peer, 71
  problem-based learning (PBL), 63
  professionalism, 202–203
  summative, 298
assessment methodologies, global examples of,
  195–196
  Canada, 195–196
  Myanmar, 196
  Netherlands, 196
  South Africa, 195
assessment software, 92
Association of American Colleges and
  Universities (AAC&U), 248, 348
Association of American Medical Colleges
  (AAMC), 32, 129, 179, 238, 266, 293
Association of Postgraduate PA Programs
  (APPAP), 390
asynchronous distance education, 106, 110–111
A.T. Still University, Arizona, 402
Ateneo de Zamboanga University School of
  Medicine (ADZU-SOM), 412–413
  community immersion, 412
  curriculum, 412
  outcomes and success, 412–413
Australian Standard Geographical Classification
  (ASGC), 408
authentic leadership, 287–288
*Authentic Leadership: Rediscovering the Secrets to
  Creating Lasting Value* (George), 287

backward design, TBL, 73–75
backward reasoning, 59
Banks, James, 224–225, 252
barriers
   to giving feedback, 298–299
   to inclusion, 250
Bass, B. M., 287
Bay Path University Physician Assistant
      Program, 190
Baylor Medical College, 68
BBS. *See* Bulletin Board System
Becoming a Culturally Diverse Learning
      Community seminars, 229
behavior, unprofessional, 203
bias, unconscious, 229, 240, 253
big data, 96–97
   challenges to integration, 102–103
   defined, 95
   health professions education programs,
      95–96
Blackboard, 97, 107
blended courses, 108–110
blended education, 106. *See also* hybrid
      education
blogging, 6–7
Bloom's taxonomy, 17, 19–20
BMJ Publishing Group, 282
board of curators, 347
board of directors, 346
board of governors, 347
board of overseers, 347
board of regents, 347
board of supervisors, 347
board of trustees, 347
board of visitors, 347
Bolman, Lee G., 288
book clubs, 229–231
brand loyalty, 305
branding
   program, 102
   self-branding, 179
breaches of professionalism, 350–351
Brief Structured Clinical Observation (BSCO),
      142
BSCO. *See* Brief Structured Clinical
      Observation
Bulletin Board System (BBS), 98
burnout
   causes of, 372
   consequences of, 370
   cycle of, 372
   defining, 370–371
   Job–Person Fit Model, 373–374
   key features of, 371

   in long-term employees, 370
   predictors, recognizing, 372–373
   tool to measure, 374–375
Burns, J. M., 287

Canada, 195–196
Canadian Physician Competency Framework
      (CanMEDS), 188
career development, nature of, 183
career development curriculum, 177–183
   career development, nature of, 183
   checklist for the transition from health care
      student to licensed clinician, 182
   cover letters, writing, 180
   curriculum vitae development, 180
   effective feedback, 178
   importance of self-branding to future
      professionals, 179
   interview preparation and follow-up, 181
   job-search strategies, 180–181
   negotiation concerning job offers, 181–182
career development programs (CDP), 294
career discovery, 179
Carnegie Foundation for the Advancement of
      Teaching, 14
Carr, Phyllis, 306–307
case-based learning (CBL), 226–228
case-log analysis, 101
CATS. *See* Communication and Teamwork Skills
      assessment
CBL. *See* case-based learning
CDC. *See* Centers for Disease Control and
      Prevention
CDP. *See* career development programs
ceiling microphones, 112
Center for Creative Leadership, 294
Centers for Disease Control and Prevention
      (CDC), 96
character
   defined, 290
   development, leadership and, 291–293
   faculty leadership and, 288–291
   strengths, 291
   student leadership and, 288–291
character-based leadership, 291–293
charismatic leadership, 288
Charon, Rita, 293
CHCI. *See* Community Health Center, Inc.
checklist for transition from health care student
      to licensed clinician, 182
CHIRP. *See* Collaborative Healthcare
      Interdisciplinary Relationship Planning
      scale

classroom
  face-to-face, 89–94
  online, 89–94
  redefining time in, 81
  technology in, 87–94
clerkships, 151. *See also* international clinical
  education
clickers, 91–92
clinical doctorate, 398–399
clinical IPE curricula, 50–52
  conducting a needs assessment and selecting an
    ideal IPE site, 50–51
  description and timeline, 52
  developing and implementing effective teaching
    strategies, 51–52
  evaluation of clinical activity, 52
  learning objectives and competencies, 51
  participants, 52
  purpose, 51
clinical learning, 162–163
clinical micro-skills, 141
clinical simulation, 131–136
  common challenges and practical suggestions,
    134–136
  disaster preparedness, 132
  examples of simulation incorporated into
    curriculum, 132–133
  history-taking and physical exam skills, 133
  interprofessional simulation exercise,
    implementation of, 133–134
  interprofessional simulation scenario, 134
  learning procedures, 132
  learning to respond to emergency situations,
    132
  OB/GYN education, 133
  OSCE and remediation, 133
  surgical preparation, 132
clinical site factors, in ICE, 157–160
  faculty ambassador, 157–158
  initial evaluation, 158–159
  ongoing evaluation, 159–160
  site identification, 158
clinical sites assessment form, 124–125
clinical teaching, 139–143
  preparing the environment, 140
  preparing the faculty/preceptor/field instructor,
    141–143
  preparing the learner, 140–141
clinical training sites
  acquisition, 122–123
  assessments, 126–127
  recruiting and maintaining, 121–130
  retaining preceptors, 127–130
  scheduling, 123–126

clinical work, scholarship, 265–266
CLT. *See* cognitive learning theory
coaching, 298
  feedback, 298
cognitive information processing, 72
cognitive learning theory (CLT), 72
cognitivism, 72
coherence, as element of professional writing,
  276–277
Collaborative Healthcare Interdisciplinary
  Relationship Planning (CHIRP) scale, 52
collaborative testing, 190
commitment
  faculty leadership and, 288–291
  student leadership and, 288–291
communication, holistic admissions and,
  329–330
Communication and Teamwork Skills (CATS)
  assessment, 53
community, 374
  defined, 364
  restorative justice and, 364–365
  strengthening, 364–365
community engagement, 407–414
  models, 231–233
Community Health Center, Inc. (CHCI), 390
competence, defined, 26–27
competence in medicine, defined, 187
competencies, 26–29
  clinical IPE curricula and, 51
  developing, 27–29
  entrustable professional activities, 32–33
  faculty leadership and, 288–291
  student leadership and, 288–291
complex sentence, 276. *See also* sentence
compound sentence, 276. *See also* sentence
compound–complex sentence, 276. *See also*
  sentence
Conger, Jay A., 288
Conscious Competence Learning Model, 188
content integration, 225
contingency theory, 286–287
control, defined, 373
Corporation for National and Community
  Service, 172
cost in time, 42
course management tools, 92
courses
  blended, 108–110
  online, 107–108
  web-facilitated, 107
cover letters, writing, 180
Crossing the Quality Chasm (Institute of Medicine),
  247

cultural competency, 252
cultural humility, 240
curriculum, 13
    clinical simulation and, 132–133
    competency-based, 26
    didactic, 394
    and distance education, 113–114
    elements of, 14
    evolving, 42
    hidden, 202
    integrated, 14
    lecture-based, 65
    models of, 14–15
    planning and preparing for service learning in, 168–169
    traditional, 26
curriculum design, 13–23
    elements of curricula, 14
    instructional objectives, forming, 18–22
    models of curricula, 14–15
    process, 15–18
    syllabi, 22–23
curriculum design process, 15–18
    accreditation standards, 17
    analysis, 16–17
    design, 17
    development, 17–18
    evaluation, 18
    goals and outcomes, 16
    implementation, 18
    logistical considerations, 17
    needs assessment, 16
    target audience, 16
curriculum map matrix, 38–40
curriculum mapping, 35–44
    assures compliance with accreditation standards, 43
    benefits of, 42–44
    challenges of, 41–42
    cost in time, 42
    demonstrates relevance, 43
    evolving curriculum, 42
    faculty buy-in, 41–42
    getting started with, 36–41
    helps to bridge the gaps and dissolve the overlaps, 43
    promotes collaboration, 42
    promotes program self-study, 44
    purpose of, 36
    supports in data reporting, 43–44
    visualizes alignment, 43
curriculum vitae, 270–271
curriculum vitae development, 180
cycle of burnout, 372

Daily Briefing, 293
data analytics, defined, 98
data reporting, 43–44
DataStar, 254
Deal, Terrence E., 288
death, 10
debate
    implementing as a learner-centered strategy, 8–9
    learner-centered pedagogy and, 7–9
    role in learner-centered health professions education, 7–9
degree creep, 397, 399, 403
Dell Children's Medical Center, Austin, Texas, 141, 146
DES. *See* Diversity Engagement Survey
desk microphones, 112
"Developing Leadership Character" (Gandz, Crossan, Seijts, Stephenson, and Mazutis), 289
Diamond, Dan, 293
didactic (top-down) curricula, 50
didactic (bottom-up) curriculum, 48–50, 394
    assembling an education team, 48
    basics, 48
    continuation and follow-through, 49
    day of the event, 49–50
    postevent wrap-up and debriefing, 50
    preparing for first team meeting, 48
    preparing for the next event, 49
    sample agenda, 48–49
    situation, 48
didactic IPE curricula, 47–50
    bottom-up approach, 48–50
    summary of, 50
    top-down approach, 50
"digital natives," 6
direct reports, 319
disabilities
    defined, 354
    types of, 354
disaster preparedness, 132
discrimination, gender-based, 353
distance education
    asynchronous, 106, 110–111
    blended courses, 108–110
    classroom setup, 112
    common problems and solutions in, 115
    curriculum and, 113–114
    defined, 106
    history of, 105–106
    online courses, 107–108
    pedagogical approaches for, 114
    practical teaching tips and best practices, 114–116

distance education (*cont.*)
  synchronous, 106, 110–111
  technology and, 106–107, 111–113
diversity
  benefits of, 248–249
  communities of support, creating, 253–254
  defined, 248
  as driver for excellence, 223–224
  equity pedagogy and, 252–253
  microaggressions, 253
  multicultural education strategies and,
    252–253
  organizational transparency, creating, 254
  promoting education and scholarship in
    cultural competency, 252
  stereotype threat, 253
  strategies to excellence in, 250–254
  unconscious bias, 253
  underrepresented faculty and, 251–252
  underrepresented students and, 251
diversity burden, 238
Diversity Engagement Survey (DES), 254
diversity tax, 238
diversity versus inclusion, 248
doctor, defined, 398
doctoral degrees in medicine, 399–400
doctoral education for physician assistants,
    397–404
  challenges for postprofessional doctorate
    degrees for PAs, 403–404
  clinical doctorate, 398–399
  definitions, 398
  doctoral degrees in medicine, 399–400
  entry-level PA doctorate, 400
  models of, 400–403
  PA profession's position, 400
  title dilemma: doctor PA, 404
doctorate, defined, 398
DOE. *See* U.S. Department of Education
Douglas, William O., 348
drawing activity, 9
Dunham-Taylor, Janne, 306
Dust Bowl, 230
Dweck, Carol, 303
dying, 10

EdPACT. *See* Education in Patient-Aligned Care
    Teams
education
  blended, 106
  cultural competency and, 252
  equity, 223. *See also* equity
  hybrid, 106

interprofessional, 45–53
  online, 106
  scholarship, 266–267
  traditional, 106
  web-assisted, 106
Education in Patient-Aligned Care Teams
    (EdPACT), 140, 143–144
education records, 351
"Educational Outcomes and Leadership to Meet
    the Needs of Modern Health Care" (Spencer
    and Jordon), 285
educational technology. *See* technology
effective feedback, 178
  characteristics of, 178
electronic medical record (EMR), 126
eMedley, 126
*Emergency Medicine Physician Assistant Postgraduate
    Training Program Standards*, 391
employees, burnout and, 370
empowerment
  faculty leadership and, 288–291
  student leadership and, 288–291
EMR. *See* electronic medical record
engagement, defined, 98
enthusiasm, defined, 372
entrustable professional activities (EPA), 32–33,
    194
entry-level PA doctorate, 400
EPA. *See* entrustable professional activities
equity
  defined, 223
  as driver for excellence, 223–224
  education, 223
  health, 224
equity pedagogy, 223–233, 225
  book clubs, 229–231
  community engagement models, 231–233
  diversity and, 252–253
  diversity as driver for excellence in health
    professions, 223–224
  equity as driver for excellence in health
    professions, 223–224
  inclusion and, 252–253
  integrated case-based learning, 226–228
  multicultural education in health professions,
    224–226
  Teamwork for Professionalism, Ethics, and
    Cultural Enrichment (Team PEACE)
    Culture in Health Series, 228–229
ethical considerations, in international clinical
    education, 152–153
ethical leadership, 287–288
evaluation, 298
E*Value, 101, 126

exemplary leadership, 288–291
Experience and Education (Dewey), 15
external minority leadership programs, 242

Facebook, 98–99, 181, 200
Facebook Insights, 98–99
  advantages, 99
  disadvantages, 99
FaceTime, 307
face-to-face classroom, 89–94
faculty, 141–143
  assessment, 142
  clinical micro-skills, 141
  evaluation, 142
  faculty development, 142–143
  feedback for clinical performance, 141
  interprofessional clinical teaching skills, 142
  team-based learning, 75
  underrepresented, 251–252
faculty buy-ins, 41–42
faculty development, 142–143
  IPE curricula and, 47
  need for, 202
  professionalism and, 202
faculty leadership
  character and, 288–291
  commitment and, 288–291
  competencies and, 288–291
  empowerment and, 288–291
Family Educational Rights and Privacy Act
    (FERPA), 103, 337, 351–352
  disclosure in emergency situations, 352
  exceptions to FERPA nondisclosure rules, 352
  general directory information, 352
  officials with legitimate educational interests,
    352
  sanctions for violations, 351
  student rights under, 351
Fanlight Productions, 229
feedback, 297–303
  barriers to giving, 298–299
  coaching, 298
  defined, 297
  essential qualities of giving effective, 299–301
  giving, 297–298
  models of giving effective, 301–302
  problem-based learning (PBL), 63–64
  qualities of effective, 300
  receiving, 302–303
  work environment and, 320
feedback sandwich, 301
fellowship programs. *See* postgraduate residencies
    and fellowships

FERPA. *See* Family Educational Rights and
    Privacy Act
Fiedler, Fred, 286–287
field instructors, in clinical teaching, 141–143
  assessment, 142
  clinical micro-skills, 141
  evaluation, 142
  faculty development, 142–143
  feedback for clinical performance, 141
  interprofessional clinical teaching skills, 142
file review, 331
Flexner, Abraham, 14
Flexner Report, 14, 26
"The Flipped Approach to a Learner-Centered
    Class" (Honeycutt and Garrett), 83
flipped classroom, 79–85
  benefits and concerns of lecturing versus, 80
  building space in teaching day, 81
  closing, 84
  fight the urge to flip everything, 81
  in-class activities, 84
  prior-to-class activities, 84
  purpose, 84
  redefining time in the classroom, 81
  refrain from jamming it all in, 81
  skills needed to be successful to, 82–83
  small steps, 81
  starting, 82–84
  steps to creating a flipped classroom experience,
    83
  thoughts to consider before you flip, 81
  unprepared students, 83
Friendster site, 98
funding for service learning, 173

Gallery Walk, 70–71
Gardner, John W., 286
gender-based discrimination, 353
GenSilent, 229
George, Bill, 287
giving feedback, 297–298
  barriers to, 298–299
goals, 16
  defined, 18
Gold Rush migrations, 230
Gonzaga University v. Doe, 351
Google, 96, 98
Google analytics, 98
  advantages, 98
  disadvantages, 98
Google Docs, 113
governance, 346–347
grading in TBL courses, 71

Graduate Record Examination (GRE), 332
  General Test, 332
grammatical correctness, as element of
    professional writing, 277
Gray Paper (assignment), 7
Gray Paper blog, 7
GRE. *See* Graduate Record Examination
Great Migration, 230
Greenleaf, Robert, 287
Gregory, Krista, 146
group interviews, 335

harm, restorative justice and, 363–364
Harvard Business School, 227
Health and Care Professions Council, 289
health educational management tools, 101
health equity, 224. *See also* equity
Health Insurance Portability and Accountability
    Act (HIPAA), 103, 350, 355
health professions curriculum, professionalism in,
    201
health professions education
  attrition of minority faculty in, 238
  big data, 95–96
  content integration, 225, 226
  empowering school culture and social
    structure, 226
  equity pedagogy, 225, 226
  health educational management tools, 101
  integration opportunities for, 100–102
  interdisciplinary team, building, 100
  international clinical education as part of,
    151–153
  knowledge construction, 225, 226
  multicultural approaches to teaching, 226
  online learning management platform
    analytics, 100–101
  personalized modules, 101–102
  prejudice reduction, 225–226
  social media, 95–96
  team-based learning (TBL) and, 67–68
health professions mentoring. *See* mentoring
Healthy People 2020, 173
hidden curriculum, 202
higher education
  characteristics of public versus private
    institutions of, 347
  law in, 345–347
high-fidelity simulation, 131
history
  of distance education, 105–106
  of mentoring, 306–307
  of service learning, 167

holistic admissions, 327–328
Hong Sau (Sanskrit mantra), 380
Hootsuite, 99
horizontal integration, 14
Hurwitz, Craig, 146
hybrid education, 106. *See also* blended education

IBM. *See* International Business Machines
ICE. *See* international clinical education
identity trigger, 303
Ifill, Gwen, 308
Implicit Association Test (Project Implicit), 141
in-class activities, 84
in-class readiness assurance process, 70
inclusion
  barriers to, 250
  communities of support, creating, 253–254
  defined, 248
  diversity versus, 248
  equity pedagogy and, 252–253
  making central to organization's mission, 251
  measuring, 254
  microaggressions, 253
  multicultural education strategies and,
    252–253
  organizational transparency, creating, 254
  promoting education and scholarship in
    cultural competency, 252
  stereotype threat, 253
  strategies to excellence in, 250–254
  unconscious bias, 253
  underrepresented faculty and, 251–252
  underrepresented students and, 251
inclusive excellence, 248
Indeed, 180
individual readiness assurance test (iRAT), 70
information management, as element of
    professional writing, 276–277
Instagram, 181
Institute of Medicine, 25
instructional objectives, forming, 18–22
  action, 21
  assessment and reflection, 19–21
  audience and time, 21
  Bloom's taxonomy, 19–20
  confounding factors, 21
  description, 21
  evaluation and refinement, 22
  formulation of components, 21
  learning audience, 19
  overall goals, 19
  testing objectives, 21–22
integrated case-based learning, 226–228

integrated curriculum, 14
integration
    defined, 89
    horizontal, 14
    spiral, 14
    vertical, 14
Integrative Case-Based Learning, 134
interdisciplinary team, building, 100
International Business Machines, 224
international clinical education (ICE), 151–164
    affiliation, 155–156
    challenges and risks of, 153
    clinical site factors, 157–160
    coordination, 157
    curriculum, 156
    ethical considerations, 152–153
    evaluation, 156–157, 163–164
    goals and benefits of, 154
    learner factors, 160–163
    learning objectives for, 156–157
    logistical tasks for learner preparation, 161
    main stakeholders in, 153–163
    mission, 154
    as part of health professions education,
        151–153
    policies, 155
    postreturn debriefing, 163–164
    program factors, 153–154
    program policies, 155
    asks for initial site evaluation, 159
International Journal of Market Research, 96
international rotations, 151. *See also* international
    clinical education
interpreters, 30
interprofessional clinical teaching, 139–149, 143
    skills, 142
Interprofessional Collaborative Competencies
    Attainment Survey (ICCAS), 142, 145
interprofessional collaborative practice, core
    competencies for, 46
interprofessional education, 45–53, 139–149
    clinical teaching, 139–143
    exemplars, 143–148
    interprofessional simulation exercise—
        University of North Carolina, Wilmington,
        144–145
    Pono Clinic, University of Hawaii, 146–148
    Schwartz Rounds, 145–146
    Veterans Affairs Center and EdPACT, 140,
        143–144
interprofessional simulation exercise, 133–134,
    145–146
    debrief, 145
    evaluation and feedback, 145

impact, 145
    learners, 144
    prebrief process, 145
    simulation design, 144–145
interprofessional simulation scenario, 134
interventional research, 282
interview(s), 335–337
    group, 335
    holistic review, 336
    hybrid approaches, 336
    multiple mini-interviews, 335–336
    one-on-one, 335
    panel, 335
    preparation and follow-up, 181
    setting standards, 336
IPE curricula
    clinical, 50–52
    didactic, 47–50
    early steps in development of, 47
    faculty development, role of, 47
    tools for evaluating students, 52–53
    types of, 46–47
iRAT. *See* individual readiness assurance test

James Cook University College of Medicine and
    Dentistry (JCUCMD), 408–409
    community engagement/partnerships, 409
    community-focused admissions and integrated
        curriculum, 408–409
    outcomes and success, 409
JCUCMD. *See* James Cook University College of
    Medicine and Dentistry
job burnout. *See* burnout
job offers, 181–182
Job–Person Fit Model, 373–374
job-search strategies, 180–181
Jones, Barbara, 146
Journal of Economics Education, 79

Kail, Eric, 291
Kanungo, Rabindra N., 288
Keirsey Personality Testing, 321
Kellogg Foundation, 338
knowledge abstraction, 63
knowledge construction, 225
Kouzes, James, 288

lack of fairness, 374
Laney, Doug, 96
language standards for professionals, 277–280
Latina Researchers Network, 241

Latino Medical Student Association (LMSA), 253
law
in higher education, 345–347
systems of, 345–346
variations in academic settings, 346
variations in governance, 346–347
Lawlor, Richard, 146
leadership
academic, 285–295
assessment, 293
authentic, 287–288
character development and, 291–293
character-based, 291–293
charismatic, 288
contingency theory and situational, 286–287
ethical, 287–288
faculty, 288–291
five practices of exemplary, 288–291
four frames for, 288
servant, 287
situational, 286–287
student, 285–295
theoretical basis of, 286–293
transactional, 287–288
transformational, 287–288
on trial, 290
women and, 293–294
*The Leadership Challenge: How to Make
Extraordinary Things Happen in Organizations*
(Kouzes and Posner), 288
Leadership Education in Neurodevelopmental
and Related Disabilities (LEND) programs,
146
learner, in clinical teaching, 140–141
attitude, 140–141
culture, 140–141
knowledge, 140
skills, 140
learner assessment and remediation, 207–217.
See also remediation
academic factors, addressing, 210
academic resources, 209–210
admissions and, 210
determining success, 215–217
faculty framework and evaluator role, 212–214
feedback, 217
identification and diagnosis, 210–211
importance of, 209
learning prescription, 211–212
learning to learn, 208–209
preventive measures, 209–210
progression policies, 209–210
remediation strategies, 214–215, 216
starting from the ground up, 217

learner assessment strategies, 187–196
in Canada, 195–196
diverse exemplars of, 195–196
in Myanmar, 196
in Netherlands, 196
in South Africa, 195
learner factors, in ICE, 160–163
clinical learning, 162–163
predeparture training, 161–162
selection, 160–161
learner-centered health professions education
debate, 7–9
learner-centered pedagogy, 3–10
domains of, 5–6
focus in, 5
implementing an arts and medicine
curriculum, 9
role of debate in, 7–9
social media and, 6–10
social media and blogging as tools in, 6–7
student-centered pedagogy versus teacher-
centered pedagogy, 4–5
teacher-centered versus, 4
technology and, 6–10
use of the arts as a driver for, 9–10
learning
assessment of, 189–195
case-based, 226–228
integrated case-based, 226–228
principles of, 188–189
problem-based, 57–65
scholarship and, 266–267
service, 167–174
team-based, 67–76
learning, principles of, 188–189
learning audience, 19
learning management software (LMS),
106
learning prescription, 211–212
learning theories and outcomes, 71–73
learning to learn, 208–209
lecture-based curriculum, 65
lecture-capture tools, 92
lecturing, flipped classroom versus, 80
LEEAD. *See* Annie E. Casey Foundation Leaders
in Equitable Evaluation and Diversity
Program
legal issues, for health professions educator,
345–356
academic dishonesty, 348–349
academic freedom, 347–348
Americans with Disabilities Act, 353–355
Family Educational Rights and Privacy Act,
351–352

HIPAA, 355
  law in higher education, 345–347
  professionalism, 349–351
  Title IX of the Education Amendments of 1972,
    352–353
lesbian, gay, bisexual, transgender, and queer
    (LGBTQ) community, 229
Licklider, J. C. R., 97
Likert scale questionnaire, 142
Lincoln Memorial University, Tennessee, 401
LinkedIn, 179, 180
logistical considerations, in curriculum design,
    17
long-term memory, 73
low-fidelity simulation, 131

managers, 30
marketing campaigns, 102
Maslach Burnout Inventory, 374
Maslow's hierarchy of needs, 400
massive open online courses (MOOCs), 106–107
MassPat program, 182
Master Interview Rating Scale, 27
McMaster University, 58
McMaster University Physician Assistant
    Education Program, 195
McMaster–Ottawa Scale, 53
MCQ. See multiple-choice questions
Mead, Margaret, 4
MedEdPORTAL, 266–267
MedHub, 126
Medical College Admission Test (MCAT), 332
medical tourism, 152
medicine, doctoral degrees in, 399–400
meditation
  benefits of, 382–383
  quiet space for practicing, 382
  reasons for, 383–384
  resources for multiple ways to, 381–382
  sample guided visualization exercise, 381
  steps for beginning, 378–381
memoranda of understanding (MOU), 170
memory
  long-term, 73
  short-term, 73
  working, 73
mentee(s), 312
  commonalities of, 308
  role of, 308
mentor(s), 312
  characteristics, 307–308
  commonalities of, 308
  finding, 307

mentoring, 305–310
  definition and characteristics, 312–313
  finding a mentor, 307
  history of, 306–307
  of minority faculty, 243–244
  nature of, 305–306
  situations, 308–309
  successful, 312–313
  types of, 307
mentoring pair, 312, 314
mentoring program, 312–315
  design of, 314–315
  mentoring pair, 314
  right matching, 313
  successful mentoring, 312–313
mentoring relationship, 312
  elements of, 313
Michaelsen, Larry, 67–68
microaggressions, 253
  racial, 253
milestones, 29–32
  developing, 31–32
  entrustable professional activities, 32–33
  Miller's pyramid of clinical competence, 29–30
  RIME (recorder, interpreter, manager, and
    expert) Model, 30–31
Miller Analogies Test (MAT), 332
Miller's prism, 189, 194
Miller's pyramid of clinical assessment, 29
Miller's pyramid of clinical competence, 29–30
mindfulness, 377–384
  meditation practice, quiet space for, 382
  through meditation, 378–382
mindfulness-based stress reduction techniques,
    377
minority faculty, 237–244
  attrition of, 238
  competitive hiring packages and promotion
    opportunities, 241
  cutting edge advertising and outreach, 238–239
  diverse and well-trained search committees,
    240
  external minority leadership programs, 242
  institutional strategies supporting culture of
    diversity and inclusion, 239
  leadership workshops, 242
  mentoring and sponsorship, 243–244
  scholarship, 242
  strategies for recruitment and retention,
    238–241
  strategies for succeeding in academic
    environment, 241–242
  strong mission statements and inclusive campus
    climate, 239–240

models of giving effective feedback, 301–302
   feedback sandwich, 301
   Pendleton Model, 301–302
   reflective feedback conversation model, 301–302
Monster.com, 180
Moodle, 107
multicultural education
   applied dimensions of, 228, 230, 231, 233
   content integration, 225, 226
   diversity and, 252–253
   empowering school culture and social
      structure, 226
   equity pedagogy, 225, 226
   five dimensions of, 225–226
   in health professions, 224–226
   inclusion and, 252–253
   knowledge construction, 225, 226
   prejudice reduction, 225–226
Multimedia Educational Resource for Learning
   and Online Teaching, 267
multiple mini-interviews, 335–336
multiple-choice questions (MCQ), 70
Myanmar, 196
Myers–Briggs Type Indicator, 179

Narrative Practice seminars, 229
National Academy of Sciences, 268
National Center for Education Statistics, 238
National Center for Faculty Development and
   Diversity (NCFDD), 241
National Center for Interprofessional Practice
   and Education (NEXUS), 48, 142–143
National Commission on Certification of
   Physician Assistants (NCCPA), 26, 37
National Institute for Health and Care
   Excellence, United Kingdom, 285
National League for Nursing (NLN), 225–226
National Organization of Nurse Practitioner
   Faculties (NONPF), 26, 242
NCCPA. *See* National Commission on
   Certification of Physician Assistants
NCFDD. *See* National Center for Faculty
   Development and Diversity
needs assessment, 16
   clinical IPE curricula and, 50–51
negotiation concerning job offers, 181–182
Netflix, 97
Netherlands, 196
New England Journal of Medicine, 14
NEXUS. *See* National Center for
   Interprofessional Practice and Education
Nivet, Marc, 224, 250
NLN. *See* National League for Nursing

NONPF. *See* National Organization of Nurse
   Practitioner Faculties
Northern Ontario School of Medicine (NOSM),
   Canada, 413–414
   community partnerships, 413–414
   outcomes and successes, 414
   student body and integrated curriculum, 413
NOSM. *See* Northern Ontario School of
   Medicine, Canada
Nova University, 402
nurse practitioner residency programs, 392
Nursing: A Social Policy Statement, 200

OB/GYN education, 133
objective structured clinical examination (OSCE),
   63, 194
objectives
   achievable and realistic, 22
   measurable, 22
   specific, 21
   time-bound, 22
observable practice activities (OPA), 194
one-on-one interviews, 335
online classroom, 89–94
online collaboration tools, 92
online courses, 107–108
online discussions, 92–93
online education, 106
online electronic portfolios, 272–273
online learning management platform analytics,
   100–101
online videoconferencing, 93
online writing tools, 93
OPA. *See* observable practice activities (OPA)
organizational transparency, 254
OSCE. *See* objective structured clinical
   examination
outcomes, 16
outreach
   holistic admissions and, 328–329
   minority faculty and, 238–239
Oxford Living Dictionary, 348
oxytocin breath, 380–381

PACKRAT. *See* Physician Assistant Clinical
   Knowledge Rating and Assessment Tool
PAEA. *See* Physician Assistant Education
   Association
PANCE. *See* Physician Assistant National
   Certifying Exam
panel interviews, 335
peacemaking circles, 365–367

pedagogy
  learner-centered, 3–10
  student-centered, 4–5
  teacher-centered, 4–5
peer assessment, 71
Pendleton Model, 301–302
personal statements, 334–335
personality variables, 333
personalized modules, 101–102
Physician Assistant Clinical Knowledge Rating
    and Assessment Tool (PACKRAT), 101
Physician Assistant Education Association
    (PAEA), 26, 123, 127, 242, 400
Physician Assistant National Certifying Exam
    (PANCE), 127
physician assistant residency and fellowship
    programs, 390, 392
physician assistants (PA)
  benefits of postprofessional doctorate degrees
    for, 402–403
  challenges for postprofessional doctorate
    degrees for, 403–404
  doctoral education for, 397–404
  entry-level doctorate, 400
  models of doctoral education, 400–403
  profession's position, 400
Pierce, Chester, 253
plagiarism, 348–349
P-MEX. *See* Professionalism Mini-Evaluation
    Exercise
Pono Clinic, University of Hawaii, 146–148
portfolio(s)
  as method for service learning assessment, 173
  scholarship. *See* scholarship portfolio
Posner, Barry, 288
postgraduate residencies and fellowships,
    389–395
  accreditation of, 391–392
  approval process, 393
  class size, 394–395
  didactic curriculum, 394
  nurse practitioner (NP), 390–391
  nurse practitioner residency programs, 392
  PA postgraduate training and, 392–393
  physician assistant (PA), 390, 392
  postgraduate residency or fellowship program,
    developing, 393–395
  program funding, 393
  program leadership, 394
  pros and cons of training, 392
  recommendations for future research, 395
  trainee evaluation, 394
postprofessional clinical doctorate, defined, 398
postprofessional doctorate, defined, 398

postreturn debriefing, 163–164
prana, 379, 380
pranayama, 378, 380
*Preceptor Orientation Handbook: Tips, Tools, and
    Guidance for Physician Assistant Preceptors*,
    123
preceptors, in clinical teaching, 141–143
  assessment, 142
  clinical micro-skills, 141
  evaluation, 142
  faculty development, 142–143
  feedback for clinical performance, 141
  interprofessional clinical teaching skills, 142
predeparture training, 161–162
prejudice reduction, 225
presentation software, 89–91
Prideaux, David, 13
prior-to-class activities, 84
problem-based learning (PBL), 57–65
  advantages of, 58–59
  assessment, 63
  basic principles of, 60–65
  case-based learning (CBL) and, 59
  climate setting, 62
  closing the case, 63
  contrasting with similar pedagogies, 59
  disadvantages of, 58–59
  feedback, 63–64
  format of, 58
  goals, 62
  history of, 58
  integrating into a lecture-based curriculum,
    65
  learning issues, 62–63
  management of the process, 64–65
  patient encounter, 62
  team-based learning and, 59
profession, defined, 349–350
professional doctorate, defined, 398
professional socialization, 200. *See also*
    professionalism
professional writing
  coherence, 276–277
  elements of, 276–280
  grammatical correctness, 277
  information management, 276–277
  language standards for professionals, 277–280
  sentence development, 276–277
  unity of message, 276
professionalism, 199–203, 349–351. *See also*
    professional socialization;
    professionalization
  ABIM definition of, 200
  assessment, 202–203

professionalism (*cont.*)
  breaches of, 350–351
  defined, 350
  defining, 200
  factors influencing student, 200–201
  faculty development, need for, 202
  in health professions curriculum, 201
  remediation and consequences for
    unprofessional behavior, 203
Professionalism Mini-Evaluation Exercise
    (P-MEX), 202–203
professionalization, 200. *See also* professionalism
professionals, language standards for, 277–280
program branding
  social media spotlighting, 102
  tailored marketing campaigns, 102
  use of social media for, 102
program factors, in ICE, 153–157
  affiliation, 155–156
  coordination, 157
  curriculum, 156
  learning and evaluation, 156–157
  mission, 154
  policies, 155
program self-study, 44
progression policies, 209–210
Protagoras of Abdera, 7

qualitative research, 282
quantitative research, 282

racial microaggressions, 253
randomized controlled trials, 282
RAT. *See* readiness assurance tests
reach, defined, 98
readiness assurance tests (RAT), 68
Readiness for Interprofessional Learning Scale
    (RIPLS), 52
reasonable accommodations, 354
reference letters, 334–335
reflection, 172
reflective feedback conversation, 301–302
Regents of the University of California vs. Bakke, 348
Rehabilitation Act of 1973, 353
relationship trigger, 303
relationships
  restorative justice and, 362–363, 367
  strengthening, 362–363
remediation, 207–217. *See also* learner assessment
    and remediation
  academic factors, addressing, 210
  academic resources, 209–210

admissions and, 210
determining success, 215–217
faculty framework and evaluator role, 212–214
feedback, 217
identification and diagnosis, 210–211
importance of, 209
learning prescription, 211–212
preventive measures, 209–210
progression policies, 209–210
setting a framework for, 212–214
starting from the ground up, 217
strategies for, 214–215, 216
structured approach to remedial assessment,
    211
using team approach to, 211
research
  interventional, 282
  involving human subjects, 268
  qualitative, 282
  quantitative, 282
  scholarship, 268–269
  study, 282
residency program. *See* postgraduate residencies
    and fellowships
resource and file sharing, 93
responsibility, shared, 363
restorative health justice, 362. *See also* restorative
    justice
restorative justice, 359–367. *See also* restorative
    health justice
  addressing harm, 363–364
  community, strengthening, 364–365
  concept of, 360–361
  dialogue and, 367
  five pillars of, 361
  peacemaking circles, 365–367
  practices of, 365–367
  principles of, 361–365
  relationships, strengthening, 362–363, 367
  responsibility and, 367
  shared responsibility, 363
  values, humanizing, 361–362, 367
retaining preceptors, and clinical training sites,
    127–130
rewards, 374
RIME (recorder, interpreter, manager, and
    expert) Model, 30–31
RIPLS. *See* Readiness for Interprofessional
    Learning Scale
Robert Wood Johnson Foundation, 231
Robert Wood Johnson Foundation Harold Amos
    Medical Faculty Development Program, 241
Ross, Howard, 248
Rotterdam University, 196

scheduling, clinical training sites, 123–126
scholarship, 263–273
  academic and the scholarship portfolio, 264
  of application and engagement, 266
  clinical work, 265–266
  contributions of health professions educators to,
      282–283
  cultural competency and, 252
  defining, 263–265, 275
  of discovery, 266
  education and teaching, 266–267
  four legs of, 265–269
  for health professions educators, 280–283
  of integration, 266
  of learning, 266–267
  minority faculty and, 242
  navigating academia, 264–265
  objectives, 265
  portfolio, 269–273
  research, 268–269
  service, 267–268
Scholarship Assessed (Glassick, Huber, Maeroff, and
    Boyer), 281
scholarship portfolio, 269–273
  components, 270–272
  curriculum vitae, 270–271
  professional goal statement, 270
  scholarship philosophy statement, 272
  teaching philosophy statement, 271–272
school(s)
  culture, 226
  health professions, 239
  health sciences, 3
Schools of Isolated and Distance Education
    (SIDE), 105. *See also* Western Australia
    Correspondence School
Schwartz Rounds, 141, 145–146
screencasting, 93–94
sculpture reflection activity, 10
self-assessment, 71
self-branding, 179
self-paced, defined, 106
SEMPA Postgraduate Training Committee,
    391
sensory register, 72
sentence
  complex, 276
  compound, 276
  compound–complex, 276
  simple, 276
sentence development, as element of professional
    writing, 276–277
sentence diagramming, 277
servant leadership, 287

service, scholarship, 267–268
service learning, 167–174, 268
  activities, types of, 170–171
  advocacy, 171
  benefits of, 168
  building relationships, 169–170
  definition and pedagogy of, 168
  developing assessments, 172–173
  direct, 170
  funding for, 173
  history of, 167
  indirect, 170–171
  planning, in the curriculum, 168–169
  preparing, in the curriculum, 169
  research, 171
  staff development, 171–172
service learning activities, 170–171
  advocacy, 171
  direct, 170
  indirect, 170–171
  research, 171
shared responsibility, restorative justice and,
    363
Shoemaker, Harry, 58
short-term memory, 73
SIDE. *See* Schools of Isolated and Distance
    Education
simple sentence, 276. *See also* sentence
simulation, 131–136
  benefits of, 131–132
  common challenges and practical suggestions,
      134–136
  disaster preparedness, 132
  examples of simulation incorporated into
      curriculum, 132–133
  high-fidelity, 131
  history-taking and physical exam skills, 133
  interprofessional simulation exercise,
      implementation of, 133–134
  interprofessional simulation scenario, 134
  learning procedures, 132
  learning to respond to emergency situations,
      132
  low-fidelity, 131
  OB/GYN education, 133
  OSCE and remediation, 133
  surgical preparation, 132
  virtual reality, 135
site acquisition, 122–123
situational leadership, 286–287
SkillScan Career Drivers, 179
Skype, 307
SMART objectives, 21–22
smartphones, 91–92

SNMA. *See* Student National Medical Association
social accountability, 407–414
Social Determinants of Health seminars, 229
social media
    challenges to integration, 102–103
    defined, 97
    health professions education programs, 95–96
    learner-centered pedagogy and, 6–10
    spotlighting, 102
    tailored marketing campaigns, 102
    use for program branding, 102
social media analytics, 97–100
    analytical tools, 98–100
    Facebook Insights, 98–99
    Google analytics, 98
    social media management dashboard, 99–100
    Twitter Analytics, 99
social media management dashboard, 99–100
    advantages, 100
    disadvantages, 100
social networks, 97
social structure, 226
Society of Emergency Medicine Physician Assistants (SEMPA), 391
Socrates, 379
software
    assessment, 92
    presentation, 89–91
Souba, F., 307
South Africa, 195
Southwest Airlines, 96
span of control, 319
spiral integration, 14
sponsorship, of minority faculty, 243–244
staff development, 171–172
stagnation, 372
stakeholders in ICE, 153–163
    clinical site factors, 157–160
    curriculum, learning and evaluation, coordination, 156–157
    learner factors, 160–163
    mission, policies, affiliation, 154–156
    program factors, 153–154
stereotype threat, 253
StrengthsFinder 2.0, 179
Strong, Colin, 96
Strong Interest Inventory, 179
student(s)
    effective feedback, giving and receiving, 178
    sample of standard form for preceptor evaluation of, 128–129
    team-based learning (TBL), 75–76
    tools for evaluating, 52–53

underrepresented, 251
unprepared, 83
student leadership, 285–295
    character and, 288–291
    commitment and, 288–291
    competencies and, 288–291
    empowerment and, 288–291
Student National Medical Association (SNMA), 253
student professionalism, 200–201. *See also* professionalism
student-centered pedagogy, 4–5
    versus teacher-centered pedagogy, 4–5
summative assessment, 298
Summer Medical and Dental Education Program (SMDEP) program, 231
syllabi, 22–23
    classroom etiquette, 23
    course specifics, 22
    evaluation and assessment, 23
    instructor specifics, 22
    plan, 22–23
    policies, 23
    required and recommended resources, 22
synchronous distance education, 106, 110–111

tailored marketing campaigns, 102
target audience, 16
TBL. *See* team-based learning
TBL Collaborative, 75
teacher-centered pedagogy, 4–5
    focus in, 4
    versus learner-centered pedagogy, 4
    student-centered pedagogy versus, 4–5
teaching
    scholarship, 266–267
    strategies, 51–52
team-based learning (TBL), 67–76
    application activities, 70–71
    creating a quality TBL session using backward design, 73–75
    creating teams, 68–69
    grading in TBL courses, 71
    health professions education, application in, 67–68
    in-class readiness assurance process, 70
    learning theories and outcomes, 71–73
    long-term memory and, 73
    minilecture, 70
    origin of, 67–68
    preparing faculty for, 75
    preparing students for, 75–76
    process of, 68–71

self- and peer assessments, 71
short-term memory and, 73
student preparation for class, 69
working memory and, 73
Teamwork for Professionalism, Ethics, and
    Cultural Enrichment (Team PEACE)
    Culture in Health Series, 228–229
technology
    active learning and, 88
    benefits of using, 88
    and distance education, 111–113
    in education, 106–107
    in face-to-face classroom, 89–94
    learner-centered pedagogy and, 6–10
    in online classroom, 89–94
    used in health professions education, 90–91
technology in classroom, 87–94
    assessment software, 92
    clickers and smartphones, 91–92
    course management tools, 92
    lecture-capture tools, 92
    online collaboration tools, 92
    online discussions, 92–93
    online videoconferencing, 93
    online writing tools, 93
    presentation software, 89–91
    resource and file sharing, 93
    screencasting, 93–94
    technology integration, 89
    using, 87–89
technology integration, 89
technology-enhanced learning strategies, 88–89
telelearning, 106
A Theory of Leadership Effectiveness (Fiedler), 286
time, cost in, 42
Title IX of the Education Amendments of 1972
    (Title IX), 352–353
To Err Is Human, 25
tourism, medical, 152
traditional education, 106
Training for Health Equity Network (THEnet),
    408
transactional leadership, 287–288
transformational leadership, 287–288
transitioning to academia, 317–318
The Triangular Model, 314
truth trigger, 303
tweet, defined, 99
Twitter, 98, 99, 181
Twitter Analytics, 99
    advantages, 99
    disadvantages, 99
Twitter handle, 99
Typhon Group, 126

UCLA. See University of California, Los Angeles
UCSF. See University of California, San Francisco
unconscious bias, 240, 253
Unconscious Bias seminars, 229
underrepresented faculty
    diversity and, 251–252
    inclusion and, 251–252
underrepresented minority (URM) faculty, 238
underrepresented students
    diversity and, 251
    inclusion and, 251
Unequal Treatment: Confronting Racial and Ethnic
    Disparities in Healthcare (Institute of
    Medicine), 247
unity of message, as element of professional
    writing, 276
University of British Columbia Department of
    Oceanic and Atmospheric Sciences, 190
University of California, Davis, 134
University of California, Los Angeles (UCLA),
    391
University of California, San Francisco (UCSF),
    140, 143–144, 391
University of Cambridge, 96
University of Community Health, Magway,
    Myanmar, 196
University of Hawaii, 141
University of London, 105
University of Massachusetts Medical School, 254
University of Michigan School of Medicine, 336
University of New Mexico School of Medicine
    (UNMSOM), 409–411
    admissions and pipelines, 410–411
    community partnerships and community
        immersion, 411
    outcomes and success, 411
University of North Carolina, Wilmington,
    144–145
University of Oklahoma, 68
University of Otago, 100
University of Otago Technology-Enhanced
    Analytics (UO-TEA), 100–101
University of Pennsylvania, 399
University of San Francisco, 282
University of Washington, 231
UNMSOM. See University of New Mexico
    School of Medicine
unprofessional behavior
    consequences for, 203
    remediation for, 203
UO-TEA. See University of Otago Technology-
    Enhanced Analytics
URM. See underrepresented minority faculty
U.S. Army Signal Corps, 58

U.S. Census Bureau, 247
U.S. Department of Defense, 15
U.S. Department of Education (DOE), 337, 346, 351
U.S. Department of State, 155
U.S. Supreme Court, 337, 351

values
 defined, 361
 humanizing, 361–362
 restorative justice and, 361–362, 367
variations
 in academic settings, 346
 in governance, 346–347
VBO. *See* Virtue-Based Orientation Model
Ventilla, Max, 97
vertical integration, 14
Veterans Affairs Center, 143–144
Veterans Affairs Education in Patient-Aligned Care Teams (EdPACT) program, 140, 143–144
videoconferencing, 93, 106
virtual reality simulation, 135
Virtue-Based Orientation (VBO) Model, 292
visual thinking activity, 9
volume, defined, 96
Vroom–Yetton Model of Leadership, 287

Wake Forest University, 401
Wal-Mart, 96

Walter Sisulu Medical School, 195
The Warmth of Other Suns (Wilkerson), 230
Web 2.0, 97
web-assisted education, 106
web-facilitated courses, 107
Wee Keng Neo, 64
Western Australia Correspondence School, 105. *See also* Schools of Isolated and Distance Education (SIDE)
WHO. *See* World Health Organization
Wilkerson, Isabel, 230
women and leadership, 293–294
work environment, feedback and, 320
working memory, 73
work–life balance, 369–375
 job burnout, 369–373
 Job–Person Fit Model, 373–374
 tool to measure burnout, 374–375
workload, 373
World Health Organization (WHO), 45, 327, 338
Worlds Apart: A Four-Part Series on Cross-Cultural Health Care, 229
writing tools, online, 93
written exams, 173

yama, 380
YouTube, 181

Zion, Libby, 25
Zuckerberg, Mark, 98

Made in the USA
Monee, IL
10 May 2024

58296957R10256